The Health Benefits of SMOKING CESSATION

a report of the Surgeon General

1990

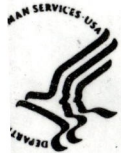

U.S. DEPARTMENT OF HEALTH AND HUMAN SERVICES
Public Health Service
Centers for Disease Control
Center for Chronic Disease Prevention and Health Promotion
Office on Smoking and Health
Rockville, Maryland 20857

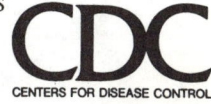

THE SECRETARY OF HEALTH AND HUMAN SERVICES
WASHINGTON, D.C. 20201

SEP 13 1990

The Honorable Thomas S. Foley
Speaker of the House of
   Representatives
Washington, D.C. 20515

Dear Mr. Speaker:

It is my pleasure to transmit to the Congress the 1990 Surgeon General's Report on the health consequences of smoking as mandated by Section 8(a) of the Public Health Cigarette Smoking Act of 1969 (Pub. L. 91-222). The report was prepared by the Centers for Disease Control's Office on Smoking and Health.

This report, entitled <u>The Health Benefits of Smoking Cessation</u>, examines how an individual's risk of smoking-related diseases declines after quitting smoking. The evidence is overwhelming that smoking cessation has major and immediate health benefits for men and women of all ages. Smoking cessation increases overall life expectancy and reduces the risk of lung cancer, other cancers, heart attack, stroke, and chronic lung disease such as emphysema. The health benefits of smoking cessation far exceed any risks from the average 5-pound weight gain or any adverse psychological effects that may follow quitting.

Cigarette smoking is the most important preventable cause of death in our society. It is responsible for approximately 390,000 deaths each year in the United States, or more than one of every six deaths. We must do all we can to prevent young people from taking up this deadly addiction, and we must help smokers quit. Given the enormous benefits of smoking cessation, and the fact that good smoking cessation programs can achieve abstinence rates of 20 to 40 percent at one-year followup, these programs are likely to be extremely cost-effective compared with other preventive or curative services. Therefore, I would encourage health insurers to provide payment for smoking cessation treatments that are shown to be effective. At a minimum, the treatment of nicotine addiction should be considered as favorably by third-party payors as treatment of alcoholism and illicit drug addiction.

This report should help convince all smokers of the compelling need to quit smoking.

Sincerely,

Louis W. Sullivan
Louis W. Sullivan, M.D.
Secretary

Enclosure

THE SECRETARY OF HEALTH AND HUMAN SERVICES
WASHINGTON, D.C. 20201

SEP 13 1990

The Honorable Dan Quayle
President of the Senate
Washington, D.C. 20515

Dear Mr. President:

It is my pleasure to transmit to the Congress the 1990 Surgeon General's Report on the health consequences of smoking as mandated by Section 8(a) of the Public Health Cigarette Smoking Act of 1969 (Pub. L. 91-222). The report was prepared by the Centers for Disease Control's Office on Smoking and Health.

This report, entitled The Health Benefits of Smoking Cessation, examines how an individual's risk of smoking-related diseases declines after quitting smoking. The evidence is overwhelming that smoking cessation has major and immediate health benefits for men and women of all ages. Smoking cessation increases overall life expectancy and reduces the risk of lung cancer, other cancers, heart attack, stroke, and chronic lung disease such as emphysema. The health benefits of smoking cessation far exceed any risks from the average 5-pound weight gain or any adverse psychological effects that may follow quitting.

Cigarette smoking is the most important preventable cause of death in our society. It is responsible for approximately 390,000 deaths each year in the United States, or more than one of every six deaths. We must do all we can to prevent young people from taking up this deadly addiction, and we must help smokers quit. Given the enormous benefits of smoking cessation, and the fact that good smoking cessation programs can achieve abstinence rates of 20 to 40 percent at one-year followup, these programs are likely to be extremely cost-effective compared with other preventive or curative services. Therefore, I would encourage health insurers to provide payment for smoking cessation treatments that are shown to be effective. At a minimum, the treatment of nicotine addiction should be considered as favorably by third-party payors as treatment of alcoholism and illicit drug addiction.

This report should help convince all smokers of the compelling need to quit smoking.

Sincerely,

Louis W. Sullivan, M.D.
Secretary

Enclosure

FOREWORD

More than 38 million Americans have quit smoking cigarettes, and nearly half of all living adults who ever smoked have quit. Unfortunately, some 50 million Americans continue to smoke cigarettes, despite the many health education programs and anti-smoking campaigns that have been conducted during the past quarter century, despite the declining social acceptability of smoking, and despite the consequences of smoking to their health.

Twenty previous reports of the Surgeon General have reviewed the health effects of smoking. Scientific data are now available on the consequences of smoking cessation for most smoking-related diseases. Previous reports have considered some of these data, but this Report is the first to provide a comprehensive and unified review of this topic.

The major conclusions of this volume are:

1. **Smoking cessation has major and immediate health benefits for men and women of all ages. Benefits apply to persons with and without smoking-related disease.**
2. **Former smokers live longer than continuing smokers. For example, persons who quit smoking before age 50 have one-half the risk of dying in the next 15 years compared with continuing smokers.**
3. **Smoking cessation decreases the risk of lung cancer, other cancers, heart attack, stroke, and chronic lung disease.**
4. **Women who stop smoking before pregnancy or during the first 3 to 4 months of pregnancy reduce their risk of having a low birthweight baby to that of women who never smoked.**
5. **The health benefits of smoking cessation far exceed any risks from the average 5-pound (2.3-kg) weight gain or any adverse psychological effects that may follow quitting.**

With the long-standing evidence that smoking is extremely harmful to health and the mounting evidence that smoking cessation confers major health benefits, we remain faced with the task of developing effective strategies to curtail the use of tobacco. Two broad categories of intervention are available: prevention of smoking initiation among youth and smoking cessation. Resources for tobacco control are limited, and policymakers must decide how best to allocate those resources to smoking prevention and cessation.

The goal of public health is to intervene as early as possible to prevent disease, disability, and premature death. From that standpoint, prevention of smoking initiation should be a major priority. More than 3,000 teenagers become regular smokers *each day* in the United States. Because of the strength of nicotine addiction, some have argued that public health efforts should focus on smoking prevention rather than smoking cessation. However, this need not be an "either-or" situation.

Public health practitioners have categorized interventions into primary, secondary, and tertiary prevention. Primary prevention generally refers to the elimination of risk factors for disease in asymptomatic persons. Secondary prevention is defined as the early detection and treatment of disease, and is practiced using tools such as Pap smears and blood pressure screening. Tertiary prevention consists of measures to reduce impairment, disability, and suffering in people with existing disease.

Smoking cessation falls under the category of primary prevention as does the prevention of smoking initiation. Smoking cessation meets the definition of primary prevention by reducing the risk of morbidity and premature mortality in asymptomatic people. In addition, parents who quit smoking reduce or eliminate the risk of passive-smoking-related disease among their children and reduce the probability that their children will become smokers. Thus, there should be no debate about the need for smoking prevention versus cessation—both are important.

Public awareness of the health effects of smoking has increased substantially through the years. Nevertheless, important gaps in public knowledge still exist. Some smokers may have failed to quit because of a lack of appreciation of the health hazards of smoking and the benefits of quitting. In the 1987 National Health Interview Survey of Cancer Epidemiology and Control, respondents were asked whether smoking increases the risk of various diseases (lung cancer, cancer of the mouth and throat, heart disease, emphysema, and chronic bronchitis) and whether smoking cessation reduces the risk. Thirty to forty percent of smokers either did not believe that smoking increases these risks or did not believe that cessation reduces these risks. These proportions correspond to 15 to 20 million smokers in the United States. Clearly, our efforts to educate the public on the health hazards of smoking and the benefits of quitting are not yet complete.

As we continue and intensify our efforts to inform the public of these findings, we must make available smoking cessation programs and services to those who need them. Although 90 percent of former smokers quit without using smoking cessation programs, counseling, or nicotine gum, smokers who do need this assistance should have it available. We endorse the view expressed in the Preface to the 1988 Surgeon General's Report that treatment of nicotine addiction should be considered at least as favorably by third-party payors as treatment of alcoholism and illicit drug addiction. Good smoking cessation treatments can achieve abstinence rates of 20 to 40 percent at 1-year followup. Those success rates, combined with the enormous health benefits of smoking cessation, would likely make payment for some smoking cessation treatments cost-beneficial. For example, research by the Centers for Disease Control suggests that a smoking cessation program offered to all pregnant smokers could save $5 for every dollar spent by preventing low birthweight-associated neonatal intensive care and long-term care.

This Report should galvanize the health community to stress repeatedly at every opportunity the value of smoking cessation to the 50 million Americans who continue to smoke.

James O. Mason, M.D., Dr.P.H.
Assistant Secretary for Health
Public Health Service

William L. Roper, M.D.
Director
Centers for Disease Control

PREFACE

This Report of the Surgeon General is the 21st Report of the U.S. Public Health Service on the health consequences of smoking and the first issued during my tenure as Surgeon General. Whereas previous reports have focused on the health effects of smoking, this Report is devoted to the benefits of smoking cessation.

The public health impact of smoking is enormous. As documented in the 1989 Surgeon General's Report, an estimated 390,000 Americans die each year from diseases caused by smoking. This toll includes 115,000 deaths from heart disease; 106,000 from lung cancer; 31,600 from other cancers; 57,000 from chronic obstructive pulmonary disease; 27,500 from stroke; and 52,900 from other conditions related to smoking. More than one of every six deaths in the United States are caused by smoking. For more than a decade the Public Health Service has identified cigarette smoking as the most important preventable cause of death in our society.

It is clear, then, that the elimination of smoking would yield substantial benefits for public health. What are the benefits, however, for the individual smoker who quits? A large body of evidence has accumulated to address that question and derives from cohort and case–control studies, cross-sectional surveys, and clinical trials. In studies of the health effects of smoking cessation, persons classified as former smokers may include some current smokers; this misclassification is likely to cause an underestimation of the health benefits of quitting. Taken together, the evidence clearly indicates that smoking cessation has major and immediate health benefits for men and women of all ages.

Overall Benefits of Smoking Cessation

People who quit smoking live longer than those who continue to smoke. To what extent is a smoker's risk of premature death reduced after quitting smoking? The answer depends on several factors, including the number of years of smoking, the number of cigarettes smoked per day, and the presence or absence of disease at the time of quitting. Data from the American Cancer Society's Cancer Prevention Study II (CPS-II) were analyzed in this Report to estimate the risk of premature death in ex-smokers versus current smokers. These data show, for example, that persons who quit smoking before age 50 have one-half the risk of dying in the next 15 years compared with continuing smokers.

Smoking cessation increases life expectancy because it reduces the risk of dying from specific smoking-related diseases. One such disease is lung cancer, the most common cause of cancer death in both men and women. The risk of dying from lung cancer is

22 times higher among male smokers and 12 times higher among female smokers compared with people who have never smoked. The risk of lung cancer declines steadily in people who quit smoking; after 10 years of abstinence, the risk of lung cancer is about 30 to 50 percent of the risk for continuing smokers. Smoking cessation also reduces the risk of cancers of the larynx, oral cavity, esophagus, pancreas, and urinary bladder.

Coronary heart disease (CHD) is the leading cause of death in the United States. Smokers have about twice the risk of dying from CHD compared with lifetime nonsmokers. This excess risk is reduced by about half among ex-smokers after only 1 year of smoking abstinence and declines gradually thereafter. After 15 years of abstinence the risk of CHD is similar to that of persons who have never smoked.

Compared with lifetime nonsmokers, smokers have about twice the risk of dying from stroke, the third leading cause of death in the United States. After quitting smoking, the risk of stroke returns to the level of people who have never smoked; in some studies this reduction in risk has occurred within 5 years, but in others as long as 15 years of abstinence were required.

Cigarette smoking is the major cause of chronic obstructive pulmonary disease (COPD), the fifth leading cause of death in the United States. Smoking increases the risk of COPD by accelerating the age-related decline in lung function. With sustained abstinence from smoking, the rate of decline in lung function among former smokers returns to that of never smokers, thus reducing the risk of developing COPD.

Influenza and pneumonia represent the sixth leading cause of death in the United States. Cigarette smoking increases the risk of respiratory infections such as influenza, pneumonia, and bronchitis, and smoking cessation reduces the risk.

Cigarette smoking is a major cause of peripheral artery occlusive disease. This condition causes substantial mortality and morbidity; complications may include intermittent claudication, tissue ischemia and gangrene, and ultimately, loss of limb. Smoking cessation substantially reduces the risk of peripheral artery occlusive disease compared with continued smoking.

The mortality rate from abdominal aortic aneurysm is two to five times higher in current smokers than in never smokers. Former smokers have half the excess risk of dying from this condition relative to current smokers.

About 20 million Americans currently have, or have had, an ulcer of the stomach or duodenum. Smokers have an increased risk of developing gastric or duodenal ulcers, and this increased risk is reduced by quitting smoking.

Benefits at All Ages

According to a 1989 Gallup survey, the proportion of smokers who say they would like to give up smoking is lower for smokers aged 50 and older (57 percent) than for smokers aged 18–29 (68 percent) and 30–49 (67 percent). Older smokers may be less motivated to quit smoking because the highly motivated may have quit already at younger ages, leaving a relatively "hard-core" group of older smokers. But many long-term smokers may lack motivation to quit for other reasons. Some may believe they are no longer at risk of smoking-related diseases because they have already survived smoking for many years. Others may believe that any damage that may have been caused by smoking is irreversible after decades of smoking. For similar reasons, many physicians may be less likely to counsel their older patients to quit.

CPS-II data were used to estimate the effects of quitting smoking at various ages on the cumulative risk of death during a fixed interval after cessation. The results show that the benefits of cessation extend to quitting at older ages. For example, a healthy man aged 60–64 who smokes 1 pack of cigarettes or more per day reduces his risk of dying during the next 15 years by 10 percent if he quits smoking.

These findings support the recommendations of the Surgeon General's 1988 Workshop on Health Promotion and Aging for the development and dissemination of smoking cessation messages and interventions to older persons. I am pleased that a coalition of organizations and agencies is now working toward implementation of those recommendations, including the Centers for Disease Control; the National Cancer Institute; the National Heart, Lung, and Blood Institute; the Administration on Aging; the Department of Veterans Affairs; the Office of Disease Prevention and Health Promotion; the American Association of Retired Persons; and the Fox Chase Cancer Center. The major message of this campaign will be that it is never too late to quit smoking.

Two facts point to the urgent need for a strong smoking cessation campaign targeting older Americans: (1) 7 million smokers are aged 60 or older; and (2) smoking is a major risk factor for 6 of the 14 leading causes of death among those aged 60 and older, and is a complicating factor for 3 others.

Benefits for Smokers with Existing Disease

Many smokers who have already developed smoking-related disease or symptoms may be less motivated to quit because of a belief that the damage is already done. For the same reason, physicians may be less motivated to advise these patients to quit. However, the evidence reviewed in this Report shows that smoking cessation yields important health benefits to those who already suffer from smoking-related illness.

Among persons with diagnosed CHD, smoking cessation markedly reduces the risk of recurrent heart attack and cardiovascular death. In many studies, this reduction in risk has been 50 percent or more. Smoking cessation is the most important intervention in the management of peripheral artery occlusive disease; for patients with this condition, quitting smoking improves exercise tolerance, reduces the risk of amputation after peripheral artery surgery, and increases overall survival. Patients with gastric and duodenal ulcers who stop smoking improve their clinical course relative to smokers who continue to smoke. Although the benefits of smoking cessation among stroke patients have not been studied, it is reasonable to assume that quitting smoking reduces the risk of recurrent stroke just as it reduces the risk of recurrence of other cardiovascular events.

Even smokers who have already developed cancer may benefit from smoking cessation. A few studies have shown that persons who stopped smoking after diagnosis of cancer had a reduced risk of acquiring a second primary cancer compared with persons who continued to smoke. Although relevant data are sparse, longer survival might be expected among smokers with cancer or other serious illnesses if they stop smoking. Smoking cessation reduces the risk of respiratory infections such as pneumonia, which are often the immediate causes of death in patients with an underlying chronic disease.

The important role of health care providers in counseling patients to quit smoking is well recognized. Health care providers should give smoking cessation advice and assistance to all patients who smoke, including those with existing illness.

Benefits for the Fetus

Maternal smoking is associated with several complications of pregnancy including abruptio placentae, placenta previa, bleeding during pregnancy, premature and prolonged rupture of the membranes, and preterm delivery. Maternal smoking retards fetal growth, causes an average reduction in birthweight of 200 g, and doubles the risk of having a low birthweight baby. Studies have shown a 25- to 50-percent higher rate of fetal and infant deaths among women who smoke during pregnancy compared with those who do not.

Women who stop smoking before becoming pregnant have infants of the same birthweight as those born to women who have never smoked. The same benefit accrues to women who quit smoking in the first 3 to 4 months of pregnancy and who remain abstinent throughout the remainder of pregnancy. Women who quit smoking at later stages of pregnancy, up to the 30th week of gestation, have infants with higher birthweight than do women who smoke throughout pregnancy.

Smoking is probably the most important modifiable cause of poor pregnancy outcome among women in the United States. Recent estimates suggest that the elimination of smoking during pregnancy could prevent about 5 percent of perinatal deaths, about 20 percent of low birthweight births, and about 8 percent of preterm deliveries in the United States. In groups with a high prevalence of smoking (e.g., women who have not completed high school), the elimination of smoking during pregnancy could prevent about 10 percent of perinatal deaths, about 35 percent of low birthweight births, and about 15 percent of preterm deliveries.

The prevalence of smoking during pregnancy has declined over time but remains unacceptably high. Approximately 30 percent of U.S. women who are cigarette smokers quit after recognition of pregnancy, and others quit later in pregnancy. However, about 25 percent of pregnant women in the United States smoke throughout pregnancy. A shocking statistic is that half of pregnant women who have not completed high school smoke throughout pregnancy. Many women who do not quit smoking during pregnancy reduce their daily cigarette consumption; however, reduced consumption without quitting may have little or no benefit for birthweight. Of the women who quit smoking during pregnancy, 70 percent resume smoking within 1 year of delivery.

Initiatives have been launched in the public and private sectors to reduce smoking during pregnancy. These programs should be expanded, and less educated pregnant women should be a special target of these efforts. Strategies need to be developed to address the problem of relapse after delivery.

Benefits for Infants and Children

As a pediatrician, I am particularly concerned about the effects of parental smoking on infants and children. Evidence reviewed in the 1986 Surgeon General's Report, *The Health Consequences of Involuntary Smoking*, indicates that the children of parents who smoke, compared with the children of nonsmoking parents, have an increased frequency of respiratory infections such as pneumonia and bronchitis. Many studies have found a dose–response relationship between respiratory illness in children and their level of tobacco smoke exposure.

Several studies have shown that children exposed to tobacco smoke in the home are more likely to develop acute otitis media and persistent middle ear effusions. Middle ear disease imposes a substantial burden on the health care system. Otitis media is the most frequent diagnosis made by physicians who care for children. The myringotomy-and-tube procedure, used to treat otitis media in more than 1 million American children each year, is the most common minor surgical operation performed under general anesthesia.

The impact of smoking cessation during or after pregnancy on these associations has not been studied. However, the dose–response relationship between parental smoking and frequency of childhood respiratory infections suggests that smoking cessation during pregnancy and abstinence after delivery would eliminate most or all of the excess risk by eliminating most or all of the exposure.

If parents are unwilling to quit smoking for their own sake, I would urge them to quit for the sake of their children. Passive-smoking-induced infections in infants and young children can cause serious and even fatal illness. Moreover, children whose parents smoke are much more likely to become smokers themselves.

Smoking Cessation and Weight Gain

The fear of postcessation weight gain may discourage many smokers from trying to quit. The fear or occurrence of weight gain may precipitate relapse among many of those who already have quit. In the 1986 Adult Use of Tobacco Survey, current smokers who had tried to quit were asked to judge the importance of several possible reasons for their return to smoking. Twenty-seven percent reported that "actual weight gain" was a "very important" or "somewhat important" reason why they resumed smoking; 22 percent said that "the possibility of gaining weight" was an important reason for their relapse. Forty-seven percent of current smokers and 48 percent of former smokers agreed with the statement that "smoking helps control weight."

Fifteen studies involving a total of 20,000 persons were reviewed in this Report to determine the likelihood of gaining weight and the average weight gain after quitting. Although four-fifths of smokers who quit gained weight after cessation, the average weight gain was only 5 pounds (2.3 kg). The average weight gain among subjects who continued to smoke was 1 pound. Thus, smoking cessation produces a 4-pound greater weight gain than that associated with continued smoking. This weight gain poses a minimal health risk. Moreover, evidence suggests that this small weight gain is accompanied by favorable changes in lipid profiles and in body fat distribution.

Smoking cessation programs and messages should emphasize that weight gain after quitting is small on average.

Not only is the average postcessation weight gain small, but the risk of large weight gain after quitting is extremely low. Less than 4 percent of those who quit smoking gain more than 20 pounds. Nevertheless, special advice and assistance should be available to the rare person who does gain considerable weight after quitting. For these individuals, the health benefits of cessation still occur, and weight control programs rather than smoking relapse should be implemented.

Increases in food intake and decreases in resting energy expenditure are largely responsible for postcessation weight gain. Thus, dietary advice and exercise should be helpful in preventing or reducing postcessation weight gain. Unfortunately, minor weight control modifications to smoking cessation programs do not generally yield beneficial effects in terms of reducing weight gain or increasing cessation rates. A few studies have investigated pharmacologic approaches to postcessation weight control; preliminary results are encouraging but more research is needed. High priority should be given to the development and evaluation of effective weight control programs that can be targeted in a cost-effective manner to those at greatest need of assistance.

Psychological and Behavioral Consequences of Smoking Cessation

Nicotine withdrawal symptoms include anxiety, irritability, frustration, anger, difficulty concentrating, increased appetite, and urges to smoke. With the possible exception of urges to smoke and increased appetite, these effects soon disappear. Nicotine withdrawal peaks in the first 1 to 2 days following cessation and subsides rapidly during the following weeks. With long-term abstinence, former smokers are likely to enjoy favorable psychological changes such as enhanced self-esteem and increased sense of self-control.

Although most nicotine withdrawal symptoms are short-lived, they often exert a strong influence on smokers' ability to quit and maintain abstinence. Nicotine withdrawal may discourage many smokers from trying to quit and may precipitate relapse among those who have recently quit. In the 1986 Adult Use of Tobacco Survey, 39 percent of current smokers reported that irritability was a "very important" or "somewhat important" reason why they resumed smoking after a previous quit attempt.

Smokers and ex-smokers should be counseled that adverse psychological effects of smoking subside rapidly over time. Smoking cessation materials and programs, nicotine replacement, exercise, stress management, and dietary counseling can help smokers cope with these symptoms until they abate, after which favorable psychological changes are likely to occur.

Support for a Causal Association Between Smoking and Disease

Tens of thousands of studies have documented the associations between cigarette smoking and a large number of serious diseases. It is safe to say that smoking represents the most extensively documented cause of disease ever investigated in the history of biomedical research.

Previous Surgeon General's reports, in particular the landmark 1964 Report of the Surgeon General's Advisory Committee on Smoking and Health and the 1982 Surgeon General's Report on smoking and cancer, examined these associations with respect to the epidemiologic criteria for causality. These criteria include the consistency, strength, specificity, coherence, and temporal relationship of the association. Based on these criteria, previous reports have recognized a causal association between smoking and cancers of the lung, larynx, esophagus, and oral cavity; heart disease; stroke; peripheral artery occlusive disease; chronic obstructive pulmonary disease; and intrauterine growth retardation. This Surgeon General's Report is the first to conclude that the evidence is now sufficient to identify cigarette smoking as a cause of cancer of the urinary bladder; the 1982 Report concluded that cigarette smoking is a contributing factor in the development of bladder cancer.

The causal nature of most of these associations was well established long before publication of this Report. Nevertheless, it is worth noting that the findings of this Report add even more weight to the evidence that these associations are causal. The criterion of coherence requires that descriptive epidemiologic findings on disease occurrence correlate with measures of exposure to the suspected agent. Coherence would predict that the increased risk of disease associated with an exposure would diminish or disappear after cessation of exposure. As this Report shows in great detail, the risks of most smoking-related diseases decrease after cessation and with increasing duration of abstinence.

Evidence on the risk of disease after smoking cessation is especially important for the understanding of smoking-and-disease associations of unclear causality. For example, cigarette smoking is associated with cancer of the uterine cervix, but this association is potentially confounded by unidentified factors (in particular by a sexually transmitted etiologic agent). The evidence reviewed in this Report indicates that former smokers experience a lower risk of cervical cancer than current smokers, even after adjusting for the social correlates of smoking and risk of sexually acquired infections. This diminution of risk after smoking cessation supports the hypothesis that smoking is a contributing cause of cervical cancer.

Conclusion

The Comprehensive Smoking Education Act of 1984 (Public Law 98–474) requires the rotation of four health warnings on cigarette packages and advertisements. One of those warnings reads, "SURGEON GENERAL'S WARNING: Quitting Smoking Now Greatly Reduces Serious Risks to Your Health." The evidence reviewed in this Report confirms and expands that advice.

The health benefits of quitting smoking are immediate and substantial. They far exceed any risks from the average 5-pound weight gain or any adverse psychological effects that may follow quitting. The benefits extend to men and women, to the young and the old, to those who are sick and to those who are well. Smoking cessation represents the single most important step that smokers can take to enhance the length and quality of their lives.

Public opinion polls tell us that most smokers want to quit. This Report provides smokers with new and more powerful motivation to give up this self-destructive behavior.

                        Antonia C. Novello, M.D., M.P.H.
                        Surgeon General

ACKNOWLEDGMENTS

This Report was prepared by the Department of Health and Human Services under the general editorship of the Office on Smoking and Health, Ronald M. Davis, M.D., Director. The Managing Editor was Susan A. Hawk, Ed.M., M.S.

The scientific editors of the Report were:

Jonathan M. Samet, M.D. (Senior Scientific Editor), Professor of Medicine and Chief, Pulmonary Division, Department of Medicine and the New Mexico Tumor Registry, Cancer Center, University of New Mexico, Albuquerque, New Mexico

Ronald M. Davis, M.D., Director, Office on Smoking and Health, Center for Chronic Disease Prevention and Health Promotion (CCDPHP), Centers for Disease Control (CDC), Rockville, Maryland

Neil E. Grunberg, Ph.D., Professor, Department of Medical Psychology, Uniformed Services University of the Health Sciences, Bethesda, Maryland

Judith K. Ockene, Ph.D., Professor of Medicine, and Director, Division of Preventive and Behavioral Medicine, Department of Medicine, University of Massachusetts Medical School, Worcester, Massachusetts

Diana B. Petitti, M.D., M.P.H., Associate Professor, Department of Family and Community Medicine, University of California at San Francisco, School of Medicine, San Francisco, California

Walter C. Willett, M.D., Dr.P.H., Professor of Epidemiology and Nutrition, Harvard School of Public Health, and The Channing Laboratory, Department of Medicine, Harvard Medical School and Brigham and Women's Hospital, Boston, Massachusetts

The following individuals prepared draft chapters or portions of the Report:

Robert Anda, M.D., Epidemiologist, Office of Surveillance and Analysis, CCDPHP, CDC, Atlanta, Georgia

John Baron, M.D., Associate Professor of Medicine, Department of Medicine, Dartmouth Medical School, Hanover, New Hampshire

Tim Byers, M.D., M.P.H., Chief, Epidemiology Branch, Division of Nutrition, CCDPHP, CDC, Atlanta, Georgia

Arden G. Christen, D.D.S., M.S.D., M.A., Chairman, Professor, Department of Preventive and Community Dentistry, Indiana University School of Dentistry, Indianapolis, Indiana

Graham Colditz, Dr.P.H., Assistant Professor of Medicine, Harvard School of Public Health, and the Channing Laboratory, Department of Medicine, Harvard Medical School and Brigham and Women's Hospital, Boston, Massachusetts

Carlo C. DiClemente, Ph.D., Associate Professor, Department of Psychology, University of Houston, Houston, Texas

Douglas W. Dockery, Sc.D., Associate Professor, Department of Environmental Health, Environmental Epidemiology Program, Harvard School of Public Health, Boston, Massachusetts

Gary A. Giovino, Ph.D., Acting Chief, Epidemiology Branch, Office on Smoking and Health, CCDPHP, CDC, Rockville, Maryland

Deborah Grady, M.D., Assistant Professor, Departments of Epidemiology and Medicine, University of California at San Francisco, School of Medicine, San Francisco, California

Neil E. Grunberg, Ph.D., Professor, Department of Medical Psychology, Uniformed Services University of the Health Sciences, Bethesda, Maryland

John R. Hughes, M.D., Associate Professor, Human Behavioral Pharmacology Laboratory, Departments of Psychiatry, Psychology, and Family Practice, University of Vermont, Burlington, Vermont

Robert W. Jeffery, Ph.D., Professor, Division of Epidemiology, School of Public Health, University of Minnesota, Minneapolis, Minnesota

LTC James W. Kikendall, M.D., Assistant Chief, Gastroenterology Section, Walter Reed Army Medical Center, Washington, D.C.

Robert Klesges, Ph.D., Associate Professor, Department of Psychology, Memphis State University, Memphis, Tennessee

Lynn Kozlowski, Ph.D., Head, Behavioral Tobacco Research, Socio-behavioral Research Department, Addiction Research Foundation, Toronto, Ontario, Canada

Stephen Marcus, Ph.D., Epidemiologist, Office on Smoking and Health, CCDPHP, CDC, Rockville, Maryland

James L. McDonald, Jr., Ph.D., Assistant Chairman, Professor, Department of Preventive and Community Dentistry, Indiana University School of Dentistry, Indianapolis, Indiana

Sherry L. Mills, M.D., M.P.H., Medical Officer, Office on Smoking and Health, CCDPHP, CDC, Rockville, Maryland

Judith K. Ockene, Ph.D., Professor of Medicine, and Director, Division of Preventive and Behavioral Medicine, Department of Medicine, University of Massachusetts Medical School, Worcester, Massachusetts

Carole Tracy Orleans, Ph.D., Director, Smoking Cessation Services, Fox Chase Cancer Center, Cheltenham, Pennsylvania

Diana B. Petitti, M.D., M.P.H., Associate Professor, Department of Family and Community Medicine, University of California at San Francisco, School of Medicine, San Francisco, California

John P. Pierce, Ph.D., Associate Professor, Director, Population Studies and Cancer Prevention, Tobacco Control Project, University of California, San Diego Cancer Center, San Diego, California

Paul R. Pomrehn, Ph.D., M.S., Associate Professor, Department of Preventive Medicine and Environmental Health, University of Iowa College of Medicine, Iowa City, Iowa

James O. Prochaska, Ph.D., Professor, Director, Cancer Prevention Research Unit, Department of Psychology, University of Rhode Island, Kingston, Rhode Island

Barbara Rimer, Dr.P.H., Director, Behavioral Research, Fox Chase Cancer Center, Philadelphia, Pennsylvania

Mary Ann Salmon, Ph.D., Research Specialist, School of Social Work, C.A.R.E.S., University of North Carolina, Chapel Hill, North Carolina

Jonathan M. Samet, M.D. (Senior Scientific Editor), Professor of Medicine and Chief, Pulmonary Division, Department of Medicine and the New Mexico Tumor Registry, Cancer Center, University of New Mexico, Albuquerque, New Mexico

David Savitz, Ph.D., Associate Professor, Department of Epidemiology, School of Public Health, University of North Carolina, Chapel Hill, North Carolina

Charles B. Sherman, M.D., Director, Pulmonary Division, Miriam Hospital, Providence, Rhode Island

Meir Stampfer, M.D., Dr.P.H., Associate Professor of Epidemiology, Harvard School of Public Health, and The Channing Laboratory, Department of Medicine, Harvard Medical School and Brigham and Women's Hospital, Boston, Massachusetts

Wayne F. Velicer, Ph.D., Professor, Co-Director, Cancer Prevention Research Unit, Department of Psychology, University of Rhode Island, Kingston, Rhode Island

Thomas Vogt, Ph.D., Principle Investigator, Center for Health Research, Portland, Oregon

Scott T. Weiss, M.D., Associate Professor, Harvard School of Public Health, and The Channing Laboratory, Department of Medicine, Harvard Medical School and Brigham and Women's Hospital, Boston, Massachusetts

Anna H. Wu-Williams, Ph.D., Associate Professor, Department of Preventive Medicine, University of Southern California, Los Angeles, California

The editors acknowledge with gratitude the following distinguished scientists, physicians, and others who lent their support in the development of this Report by coordinating manuscript preparation, contributing critical reviews, or assisting in other ways. In particular, the editors express appreciation to the American Cancer Society for making available data from its Cancer Prevention Study II.

David B. Abrams, Ph.D., Director, Division of Behavioral Medicine, The Miriam Hospital, Associate Professor, Psychiatry and Human Behavior, Brown University Program in Medicine, Providence, Rhode Island

Duane Alexander, M.D., Director, National Institute of Child Health and Human Development, National Institutes of Health, Bethesda, Maryland

David Bates, M.D., FRCP, FRCPC, FACP, FRSC, Professor Emeritus of Medicine, Department of Health Care, University of British Columbia, Vancouver, British Columbia

James S. Benson, Acting Commissioner, Food and Drug Administration, Rockville, Maryland

Trudy S. Berkowitz, Ph.D., Associate Professor, Department of Obstetrics, Gynecology, and Reproductive Science, Mount Sinai School of Medicine, New York, New York

Ruth Bonita, M.P.H., Ph.D., Masonic Senior Research Fellow, Geriatric Unit, University of Auckland, Auckland 9, New Zealand

Lester Breslow, M.D., M.P.H., Professor of Public Health and Director, Health Services Research, Division of Cancer Control, Jonsson Comprehensive Cancer Center, University of California, Los Angeles, Los Angeles, California

Samuel Broder, M.D., Director, National Cancer Institute, National Institutes of Health, Bethesda, Maryland

David Burns, M.D., Associate Professor, Pulmonary Division, Division of Pulmonary Medicine and Critical Care, University of California at San Diego Medical Center, San Diego, California

Benjamin Burrows, M.D., Director, Division of Respiratory Sciences, University of Arizona Health Sciences Center, University of Arizona School of Medicine, Tucson, Arizona

Jane Cauley, Dr.P.H., Assistant Professor of Epidemiology, Department of Epidemiology, University of Pittsburgh, Pittsburgh, Pennsylvania

Gregory N. Connolly, D.M.D., M.P.H., Director, Office on Nonsmoking and Health, Massachusetts Department of Public Health, Boston, Massachusetts

Thomas M. Cooper, D.D.S., Professor, University of Kentucky Medical Center, College of Dentistry, Lexington, Kentucky

Stephen Corbin, D.D.S., M.P.H., Policy Analyst, Disease Prevention, Center for Preventive Services (CPS), CDC, Bethesda, Maryland

K. Michael Cummings, Ph.D., M.P.H., Cancer Control and Epidemiology, Roswell Park Cancer Institute, Buffalo, New York

Joseph W. Cullen, Ph.D., Director, AMC Cancer Research Center, Denver, Colorado

Sir Richard Doll, ICRF Cancer Studies Unit, Oxford, United Kingdom

Virginia Ernster, Ph.D., Professor of Epidemiology, Department of Epidemiology and International Health, University of California, San Francisco, San Francisco, California

Jonathan E. Fielding, M.D., M.P.H., Vice President and Health Director, Johnson and Johnson Health Management, Inc., Santa Monica, California

Gary D. Friedman, M.D., M.S., Division of Research, Kaiser Permanente Medical Care Program, Northern California Region, Oakland, California

William Foege, M.D., Executive Director, The Carter Center of Emory University, Atlanta, Georgia

Lawrence J. Furman, D.D.S., M.P.H., Chief, Dental Disease Prevention Activity, CPS, CDC, Atlanta, Georgia

Lawrence Garfinkel, Vice President for Epidemiology and Statistics, Director of Cancer Prevention, American Cancer Society, Inc., New York, New York

Barbara A. Gilchrest, M.D., Professor and Chairman, Department of Dermatology, Boston University Medical Center, Boston, Massachusetts

Frederick K. Goodwin, M.D., Administrator, Alcohol, Drug Abuse, and Mental Health Administration, Rockville, Maryland

Robert O. Greer, Jr., D.D.S., Sc.D., Professor and Chairman, Division of Oral Pathology and Oncology, Department of Diagnostic and Biological Sciences, School of Dentistry, University of Colorado Health Sciences Center, Boulder, Colorado

Ellen Gritz, Ph.D., Director, Division of Cancer Control, Jonsson Comprehensive Cancer Center, University of California, Los Angeles, Los Angeles, California

Nancy J. Haley, Ph.D., Associate Chief, Division of Nutrition and Endocrinology, American Health Foundation, Valhalla, New York

Sharon M. Hall, Ph.D., Professor of Medical Psychology, Department of Psychiatry, University of California, San Francisco, San Francisco Veterans Administration Medical Center, San Francisco, California

Robert Harmon, M.D., Administrator, Health Resources and Services Administration, Rockville, Maryland

Jeffrey E. Harris, M.D., Ph.D., Associate Professor, Department of Economics, Massachusetts Institute of Technology, Cambridge, Massachusetts, Clinical Associate, Medical Services, Massachusetts General Hospital, Boston, Massachusetts

Norman O. Harris, D.D.S., M.S., University of Texas Health Science Center, San Antonio, Texas

Jack Henningfield, Ph.D., Chief, Clinical Pharmacology Branch, National Institute on Drug Abuse Addiction Research Center, National Institutes of Health, Baltimore, Maryland

Robert A. Hiatt, M.D., Ph.D., Senior Epidemiologist, Division of Research, Kaiser Permanente Medical Care Program, Oakland California

Millicent Higgins, M.D., Associate Director, Epidemiology and Biometry Program, Division of Epidemiology and Clinical Applications, National Heart, Lung, and Blood Institute, National Institutes of Health, Bethesda, Maryland

Carol Hogue, Ph.D., M.P.H., Director, Division of Reproductive Health, CCDPHP, CDC, Atlanta, Georgia

John Holbrook, M.D., Professor of Internal Medicine, Department of Internal Medicine, University of Utah School of Medicine, Salt Lake City, Utah

Richard Hunt, M.D., Division of Gastroenterology, McMaster University Medical Center, Hamilton, Ontario, Canada

Dwight Janerich, D.D.S., M.P.H., Professor of Epidemiology, Department of Epidemiology and Public Health, Yale University School of Medicine, New Haven, Connecticut

William Kannel, M.D., Professor of Medicine, Department of Preventive Medicine, Boston University School of Medicine, Boston, Massachusetts

LTC James W. Kikendall, M.D., Assistant Chief, Gastroenterology Section, Walter Reed Army Medical Center, Washington, D.C.

Dushanka V. Kleinman, D.D.S., M.Sc.D., Section Chief, National Institute on Dental Research, National Institutes of Health, Bethesda, Maryland

C. Everett Koop, M.D., Sc.D., U.S. Surgeon General, 1981–89, Bethesda, Maryland

Jeffrey P. Koplan, M.D., M.P.H., Director, CCDPHP, CDC, Atlanta, Georgia

Lewis H. Kuller, M.D., Dr.P.H., Professor and Chairperson, Department of Epidemiology, University of Pittsburgh Graduate School of Public Health, Pittsburgh, Pennsylvania

Charles L. LeMaistre, M.D., President, The University of Texas M.D. Anderson Cancer Center, Houston, Texas

Claude Lenfant, M.D., Director, National Heart, Lung, and Blood Institute, National Institutes of Health, Bethesda, Maryland

Richard J. Levine, M.D., M.S., M.P.H., Chief Epidemiologist, Chemical Industry Institute of Toxicology, Research Triangle Park, North Carolina

Edward Lichtenstein, Ph.D., Research Scientist, Oregon Research Institute, Eugene, Oregon

Jay H. Lubin, Ph.D., National Cancer Institute, National Institutes of Health, Rockville, Maryland

Alfred C. Marcus, Ph.D., Director, Community Research and Applications, AMC Cancer Research Center, Denver, Colorado

Denis M. McCarthy, M.D., M.Sc., Chief, Division of Gastroenterology, University of New Mexico, Department of Medicine, Veterans Administration Medical Center, Albuquerque, New Mexico

J. Michael McGinnis, M.D., Deputy Assistant Secretary for Health, Disease Prevention and Health Promotion, Department of Health Human Services, Washington, D.C.

Sonja M. McKinlay, Ph.D., M.Sc., M.A., B.A., ASA, APHA, AER, SCt, Biometrics Society, Institute of Mathematical Statistics, International Menopause Society, American Association for the Advancement of Science, President, New England Research Institute, Inc., Watertown, Massachusetts

Robert E. Mecklenberg, D.D.S., M.P.H., Potomac, Maryland

L. Joseph Melton, III, M.D., Head, Section of Clinical Epidemiology, Department of Health Sciences Research, Mayo Clinic and Foundation, Rochester, Minnesota

Anthony Miller, B.A., M.B.B., M.R.C.P., M.F.C.M., F.R.C.P.C., Professor, Department of Preventive Medicine and Biostatistics, University of Toronto, Toronto, Ontario, Canada

Gregory Morosco, Ph.D., M.P.H., Chief, Health Education Branch and Coordinator, Smoking Education Program, National Heart, Lung, and Blood Institute, National Institutes of Health, Bethesda, Maryland

Richard L. Naeye, M.D., Professor and Chairman, Department of Pathology, Pennsylvania State University School of Medicine, Hershey, Pennsylvania

Thomas A. Pearson, M.D., M.P.H., Ph.D., Director, Mary Imogene Bassett Research Institute, Cooperstown, New York, Professor of Public Health in Medicine, Columbia University, New York, New York

Terry Pechacek, Ph.D., Acting Chief, Smoking, Tobacco, and Cancer Branch, National Cancer Institute, National Institutes of Health, Bethesda, Maryland

Michael G. Perri, Ph.D., Professor and Deputy Chairman, Psychology Department, Fairleigh Dickinson University, Teaneck, New Jersey

Richard Peto, FRS, ICRF Cancer Studies Unit, Oxford, United Kingdom

John M. Pinney, Executive Director, Institute for the Study of Smoking Behavior and Policy, John F. Kennedy School of Government, Harvard University, Cambridge, Massachusetts

William F. Raub, Ph.D., Acting Director, National Institutes of Health, Bethesda, Maryland

Patrick L. Remington, M.D., Bureau of Community Health Prevention, Wisconsin Division of Health, Madison, Wisconsin

Everett R. Rhoades, M.D., Director, Indian Health Service, Rockville, Maryland

Julius Richmond, M.D., John D. MacArthur Professor of Health Policy, Emeritus, Division of Health Policy, Research, and Education, Harvard University, Boston, Massachusetts

William A. Robinson, M.D., M.P.H., Director, Office of Minority Health, Department of Health and Human Services, Washington, D.C.

William L. Roper, M.D., M.P.H., Director, CDC, Atlanta, Georgia

Richard B. Rothenberg, M.D., Assistant Director for Science, CCDPHP, CDC, Atlanta, Georgia

Thomas C. Schelling, Ph.D., Director, Institute for the Study of Smoking Behavior and Policy, Lucius N. Littauer Professor of Political Economy, Harvard University, Cambridge, Massachusetts

Marc B. Schenker, M.D., M.P.H., Associate Professor and Division Chief, Occupational and Environmental Medicine, University of California, Davis, Davis, California

David Schottenfeld, M.D., Professor and Chairman, Department of Epidemiology, University of Michigan School of Public Health, Ann Arbor, Michigan

Kathleen L. Schroeder, D.D.S., M.Sc., Assistant Professor, Section of Oral Biology, The Ohio State University College of Dentistry, Columbus, Ohio

Mary J. Sexton, Ph.D., M.P.H., Professor, Department of Epidemiology and Preventive Medicine, University of Maryland School of Medicine, Baltimore, Maryland

Saul Shiffman, Ph.D., Associate Professor, Department of Psychology, University of Pittsburgh, Pittsburgh, Pennsylvania

Donald Shopland, Smoking, Tobacco, and Cancer Branch, National Cancer Institute, National Institutes of Health, Bethesda, Maryland

Amnon Sonnenberg, M.D., Associate Professor, Gastroenterology Section, Medical College of Wisconsin, Veterans Administration Medical Center, Milwaukee, Wisconsin

Frank E. Speizer, M.D., Professor of Medicine, Harvard Medical School, Professor of Environmental Epidemiology, Harvard School of Public Health, Co-Director, The Channing Laboratory, Department of Medicine, Brigham and Women's Hospital, Boston, Massachusetts

Jesse Steinfeld, M.D., San Diego, California

Steven D. Stellman, Ph.D., Assistant Commissioner, New York City Department of Health, New York, New York

Ira B. Tager, M.D., M.P.H., Associate Professor of Medicine and Epidemiology and Biostatistics, University of California, San Francisco, Veterans Administration Medical Center, San Francisco, San Francisco, California

Kenneth Warner, Ph.D., Senior Fellow, Institute of Gerontology, University of Michigan, Ann Arbor, Michigan

Jonathan S. Weiss, M.D., Assistant Professor of Dermatology, Section of Dermatology, Emory Clinic, Atlanta, Georgia

Noel S. Weiss, M.D., Dr.P.H., Professor and Chairman, Department of Epidemiology, University of Washington, Seattle, Washington

Gail R. Wilensky, Ph.D., Administrator, Health Care Financing Administration, Washington, DC

Deborah Winn, Ph.D., Deputy Director, Division of Health Interview Statistics, National Center for Health Statistics, CDC, Hyattsville, Maryland

Philip A. Wolf, M.D., Professor of Neurology, Department of Neurology, Boston University School of Medicine, Boston, Massachusetts

Ernst L. Wynder, M.D., President, American Health Foundation, New York, New York

The editors also acknowledge the contributions of the following staff members and others who assisted in the preparation of this Report:

Carmen Aguirre, Secretary, Office on Smoking and Health, CCDPHP, CDC, Rockville, Maryland
Andrea Anderson, Student Intern, Office on Smoking and Health, CCDPHP, CDC, Rockville, Maryland
Margaret Anglin, Secretary, Office on Smoking and Health, CCDPHP, CDC, Rockville, Maryland
Cathy Arney, Graphic Artist, The Circle, Inc., McLean, Virginia
John Artis, Courier, The Circle, Inc., McLean, Virginia
Michele Asrael, Conference Coordinator, The Circle, Inc., McLean, Virginia
John L. Bagrosky, Associate Director for Program Operations, Office on Smoking and Health, CCDPHP, CDC, Rockville, Maryland
Sonia Balakirsky, Secretary, Office on Smoking and Health, CCDPHP, CDC, Rockville, Maryland
Barbara Barnes, Administrative Assistant, The Circle, Inc., McLean, Virginia
Carol A. Bean, Ph.D., Acting Managing Editor, Artemis Technologies, Inc., Springfield, Virginia
Marissa A. Bernstein, Editor, The Circle, Inc., McLean, Virginia
Em' Ria Briscoe, Conference Coordinator, The Circle, Inc., McLean, Virginia
Karen Broder, Public Information Specialist, Office on Smoking and Health, CCDPHP, CDC, Rockville, Maryland
Barbara M. Brown, Editorial Assistant, Office on Smoking and Health, Rockville, Maryland
Catherine E. Burckhardt, Public Information Specialist, Office on Smoking and Health, CCDPHP, CDC, Rockville, Maryland
Lee Chapell, Courier, The Circle, Inc., McLean, Virginia
Won Choi, Research Assistant, Office on Smoking and Health, CCDPHP, CDC, Rockville, Maryland
Trish Davidson, Student Intern, Office on Smoking and Health, CCDPHP, CDC, Rockville, Maryland
Susan E. Day, Secretary, Office on Smoking and Health, CCDPHP, CDC, Rockville, Maryland
Karen M. Deasy, Associate Director for Policy, Office on Smoking and Health, CCDPHP, CDC, Rockville, Maryland
June Dow, Public Health Service Congressional Reports Coordinator, Office of Health Planning and Evaluation, Office of the Assistant Secretary for Health, Washington, D.C.
Joanna Ebling, Word Processing Specialist, The Circle, Inc., McLean, Virginia
Pam Edwards, System Administrator, MSA, Inc., Rockville, Maryland
Rita Elliott, Technical Editor, New Mexico Tumor Registry, University of New Mexico, Albuquerque, New Mexico
Seth Emont, Ph.D., Epidemic Intelligence Service Officer, Office on Smoking and Health, CCDPHP, CDC, Rockville, Maryland

Sharon K. Faupel, Staff Assistant, Office on Smoking and Health, CCDPHP, CDC, Rockville, Maryland

Leanna Fernando, Administrative Assistant, New Mexico Tumor Registry, University of New Mexico, Albuquerque, New Mexico

David Fry, Editor, The Circle, Inc., McLean, Virginia

Lynn Funkhauser, Word Processing Specialist, The Circle, Inc., McLean, Virginia

Amy Garson, Student Intern, Office on Smoking and Health, CCDPHP, CDC, Rockville, Maryland

Mary Graber, Secretary, University of California at San Francisco, School of Medicine, Department of Family and Community Medicine, San Francisco, California

Gwen Harvey, Program Analyst, CCDPHP, CDC, Atlanta, Georgia

Patricia Healy, Technical Information Specialist, Office on Smoking and Health, CCDPHP, CDC, Rockville, Maryland

Phyllis E. Hechtman, Editorial Assistant, The Circle, Inc., McLean, Virginia

Timothy K. Hensley, Technical Publications Writer-Editor, Office on Smoking and Health, CCDPHP, CDC, Rockville, Maryland

Julian Hudson, Courier, The Circle, Inc., McLean, Virginia

Beth Jacobsen, Student Intern, Office on Smoking and Health, CCDPHP, CDC, Rockville, Maryland

Renee Kolbe, Program Specialist, Office on Smoking and Health, CCDPHP, CDC, Rockville, Maryland

Matt Kreuter, Public Information Specialist, Office on Smoking and Health, CCDPHP, CDC, Rockville, Maryland

Peggy Lytton, Editor, The Circle, Inc., McLean, Virginia

Diana Lord, Research Psychologist, Department of Medical Psychology, Uniformed Services University of the Health Sciences, Bethesda, Maryland

Daniel F. McLaughlin, Editor, The Circle, Inc., McLean, Virginia

Jackie L. Meador, Desktop Publishing/Word Processing Specialist, The Circle, Inc., McLean, Virginia

Elaine Medoff-McGovern, Medical Secretary, Division of Preventive and Behavioral Medicine, Department of Medicine, University of Massachusetts Medical School, Worcester, Massachusetts

Nancy A. Miltenberger, M.A., Production Editor, The Circle, Inc., McLean, Virginia

Rebecca Mosher, Staff Assistant, New Mexico Tumor Registry, University of New Mexico, Albuquerque, New Mexico

Millie R. Naquin, Research Assistant, Office on Smoking and Health, CCDPHP, CDC, Rockville, Maryland

Thomas E. Novotny, M.D., Chief, Program Services Activity, Office on Smoking and Health, CCDPHP, CDC, Rockville, Maryland

Cathie M. O'Donnell, Project Director, The Circle, Inc., McLean, Virginia

Christine Pappas, Editorial Research Assistant, The Channing Laboratory, Harvard School of Public Health, Boston, Massachusetts

Stacey M. Parcover, Secretary, Office on Smoking and Health, CCDPHP, CDC, Rockville, Maryland

Lida Peterson, Computer Systems Manager, The Circle, Inc., McLean, Virginia

Renate J. Phillips, Graphic Artist, Desktop Publishing Designer, The Circle, Inc., McLean, Virginia

Margaret E. Pickerel, Public Information and Publications Specialist, Office on Smoking and Health, CCDPHP, CDC, Rockville, Maryland

Elizabeth Precup, Student Intern, Office on Smoking and Health, CCDPHP, CDC, Rockville, Maryland

Cary R. Prince, Editor, The Circle, Inc., McLean, Virginia

Dick Ray, Director of Computer Services, The Circle, Inc., McLean, Virginia

Nancy J. Rhodes, Editor, The Circle, Inc., McLean, Virginia

Rose Mary Romano, Chief, Public Information Branch, Office on Smoking and Health, CCDPHP, CDC, Rockville, Maryland

Lisa Phelps, Computer Systems Analyst, The Circle, Inc., McLean, Virginia

Sel Semler, Secretary, Office on Smoking and Health, CCDPHP, CDC, Rockville, Maryland

James Sliwa, Student Intern, Office on Smoking and Health, CCDPHP, CDC, Rockville, Maryland

Mattie Smith, Secretary, CCDPHP, CDC, Rockville, Maryland

Linda R. Spiegelman, Administrative Officer, Office on Smoking and Health, CCDPHP, CDC, Rockville, Maryland

Traion C. Stallings, Project Secretary, The Circle, Inc., McLean, Virginia

Sophia Stewart, Student Intern, Office on Smoking and Health, CCDPHP, CDC, Rockville, Maryland

Daniel R. Tisch, Director of Publications, The Circle, Inc., McLean, Virginia

Anne Trontell, M.D., Epidemic Intelligence Service Officer, Office on Smoking and Health, CCDPHP, CDC, Rockville, Maryland

Karen Tyler, Conference Coordinator, The Circle, Inc., McLean, Virginia

Godfrey R. Vaz, M.D., Student Intern, Office on Smoking and Health, CCDPHP, CDC, Rockville, Maryland

Susan Von Braunsberg, Information Specialist, The Circle, Inc., McLean, Virginia

Elyse Watson, Administrative Assistant, New Mexico Tumor Registry, University of New Mexico, Albuquerque, New Mexico

Michael F. White, Associate Director for Program Development, CCDPHP, CDC, Rockville, Maryland

Charles Wiggins, M.S.P.H., Epidemiologist, New Mexico Tumor Registry, University of New Mexico, Albuquerque, New Mexico

Louise G. Wiseman, Technical Information Specialist, Office on Smoking and Health, CCDPHP, CDC, Rockville, Maryland

Rebecca B. Wolf, Program Analyst, Office of Program Planning and Evaluation, CDC, Atlanta, Georgia

S. Tanner Wray, Technical Information Specialist, Office on Smoking and Health, CCDPHP, CDC, Rockville, Maryland

TABLE OF CONTENTS

Foreword i

Preface v

Acknowledgments xiii

List of Tables xxv

List of Figures xxxi

1. Introduction, Overview, and Conclusions 1
2. Assessing Smoking Cessation and Its Health Consequences 17
3. Smoking Cessation and Overall Mortality and Morbidity 71
4. Smoking Cessation and Respiratory Cancers 103
5. Smoking Cessation and Nonrespiratory Cancers 143
6. Smoking Cessation and Cardiovascular Disease 187
7. Smoking Cessation and Nonmalignant Respiratory Diseases 275
8. Smoking Cessation and Reproduction 367
9. Smoking, Smoking Cessation, and Other Nonmalignant Diseases 425
10. Smoking Cessation and Body Weight Change 469
11. Psychological and Behavioral Consequences and Correlates of Smoking Cessation 517

Volume Appendix. National Trends in Smoking Cessation 579

Glossary 617

Index 619

LIST OF TABLES

Chapter 2

Table 1. Measures of false reports of not smoking from studies using nicotine and cotinine as a marker 38

Table 2. Measures of false reports from studies using CO as a marker 41

Table 3. Examples of potential methodologic problems in investigating the health consequences of smoking cessation 47

Chapter 3

Table 1. Summary of longitudinal studies of overall mortality ratios relative to never smokers among male current and former smokers according to duration of abstinence (when reported) 76

Table 2. Overall mortality ratios among current and former smokers, relative to never smokers, by sex and duration of abstinence at date of enrollment, ACS CPS-II 78

Table 3. Estimated probability of dying in the next 16.5-year interval for quitting at various ages compared with never smoking and continuing to smoke, by amount smoked and sex 83

Table 4. Summary of overall mortality ratios in intervention studies in which smoking cessation was a component 84

Table 5. Summary of studies of medical care utilization among smokers and former smokers 88

Table 6. Relation of smoking cessation to various measures of general health status 90

Table 7. Age- and sex-specific mortality rates among never smokers, continuing smokers, and former smokers by amount smoked and duration of abstinence at time of enrollment for subjects in ACS CPS-II study who did not have a history of cancer, heart disease, or stroke and were not sick at enrollment 95

Table 8. Estimated probability of dying in the next 16.5-year interval (95% CI) for quitting at various ages compared with never smoking and continuing to smoke, by amount smoked and sex 97

Chapter 4

Table 1. Histologic changes (%) in bronchial epithelium by smoking status ... 109

Table 2. Relative risks of lung cancer among never, former, and current smokers in selected epidemiologic studies ... 111

Table 3. Lung cancer mortality ratios among never, current, and former smokers by number of years since stopped smoking (relative to never smokers), prospective studies ... 112

Table 4. Relative risks of lung cancer among former smokers, by number of years since stopped smoking, and current smokers, from selected case–control studies ... 115

Table 5. Relative risks of lung cancer among never, current, and former smokers, by number of years since stopping smoking and histologic type ... 119

Table 6. Relative risks of lung cancer among never, former, and current smokers by types of tobacco products smoked ... 120

Table 7. Standard mortality ratios of lung cancer among former smokers in ACS CPS-II (relative to never smokers) by years of smoking abstinence, daily cigarette consumption at time of cessation, and history of chronic disease ... 130

Table 8. Histologic changes in laryngeal epithelium by smoking status ... 132

Table 9. Relative risks of laryngeal cancer by smoking status ... 133

Chapter 5

Table 1. Studies of oral cancer and smoking cessation ... 148

Table 2. Studies of esophageal cancer that have examined the effect of smoking cessation ... 153

Table 3. Studies of cancer of the pancreas and smoking cessation ... 156

Table 4. Studies of bladder cancer and smoking cessation ... 160

Table 5. Bladder cancer risk according to smoking dose, duration of smoking, and smoking status ... 165

Table 6. Studies of cervical cancer and smoking cessation ... 167

Table 7. Studies of breast cancer and smoking cessation ... 170

Table 8. Studies of cancer at selected sites that have examined the effect of smoking cessation ... 173

Chapter 6

Table 1. Case–control studies of CHD risk among former smokers 201

Table 2. Cohort studies of CHD risk among former smokers 206

Table 3. Estimated probability of dying from ischemic heart disease in the next 16.5-year interval (95% CI) for quitting at various ages compared with never smoking and continuing to smoke, by amount smoked and sex 216

Table 4. Intervention trials of smoking cessation and CHD risk 225

Table 5. Studies of the effect of smoking cessation on persons with diagnosed CHD 231

Table 6. Studies of smoking cessation and risk of death due to aortic aneurysm 242

Table 7. Case–control studies of smoking cessation and risk of stroke 247

Table 8. Prospective cohort studies of smoking cessation and risk of stroke 253

Chapter 7

Table 1. Percentages of subjects in cross-sectional studies with respiratory symptoms, by cigarette smoking status and gender 289

Table 2. Percentages of subjects in cross-sectional surveys with respiratory symptoms by smoking and occupational exposure status 297

Table 3. Change (%) in presence of respiratory symptoms, longitudinal studies, by cigarette smoking status 300

Table 4. Percentage of subjects with respiratory symptoms by smoking status, 1961 and 1971, in a cohort of middle-aged, rural Finns 305

Table 5. Age-standardized mortality ratios for influenza and pneumonia for current and former smokers compared with never smokers 309

Table 6. Association between cigarette smoking status and FEV_1 levels in selected cross-sectional studies of adult populations 311

Table 7. Spirometric studies of participants in smoking cessation programs 320

Table 8. Studies of closing volume (CV/VC%), closing capacity (CC/TLC%), and slope of alveolar plateau (SBN_2/L) among participants in smoking cessation programs 324

Table 9. Population-based longitudinal studies of annual decline in pulmonary function 330

Table 10. Decline of FEV_1 (mL/yr) in subjects in the Copenhagen City Heart Study 337

Table 11. Mortality attributable to COPD, United States, 1986 342

Table 12. Prospective studies of COPD mortality in relation to cigarette smoking status 343

Table 13. Standardized mortality ratios for COPD among current and former smokers broken down by years of abstinence 346

Chapter 8

Table 1. Possible mechanisms for effect of smoking on pregnancy and pregnancy outcome 372

Table 2. Summary of studies of fertility among smokers and former smokers 375

Table 3. Summary of studies of perinatal and neonatal mortality in smokers and nonsmokers during pregnancy 377

Table 4. Estimated relative risk of fetal plus infant mortality for maternal smoking in several birthweight groups, adjusting for maternal marital status, education, age, and parity 378

Table 5. Summary of studies of perinatal mortality in smokers throughout pregnancy, smokers who quit in the early months of pregnancy, and nonsmokers during pregnancy 379

Table 6. Summary of studies of mean birthweight, by smoking status 382

Table 7. Summary of nonexperimental studies of smoking cessation after conception, mean increase (+) or decrease (–) in birthweight (g) according to timing of cessation 384

Table 8. Summary of nonexperimental studies of relative risk of low birthweight for smoking cessation after conception 385

Table 9. Summary of birthweight outcome in randomized trials of smoking cessation in pregnancy 388

Table 10. Smoking and smoking cessation during pregnancy, summary of results of two surveys of national probability samples 391

Table 11. Patterns of smoking cessation during pregnancy among selected populations 394

Table 12. Summary of studies that estimated relative risk of various pregnancy outcomes for smoking based on a "synthesis" of the literature, and attributable risk percent based on several estimates of the prevalence of smoking during pregnancy 395

Table 13. Summary of studies reporting relationship of cigarette smoking and age at natural menopause 397

Table 14. Summary of studies of age of natural menopause among former smokers 399

Table 15. Sexual performance among male former smokers 404

Table 16. Sperm quality among smokers and nonsmokers 406

Table 17. Estimated relative risk of azoospermia or oligospermia among smokers versus nonsmokers or never smokers 408

Table 18. Sperm quality among former smokers 409

Chapter 9

Table 1. Percentage of healed duodenal ulcers among smoking and nonsmoking patients 434

Table 2. Results of statistical analysis of pooled data from Table 1 437

Table 3. Recurrences of duodenal ulcer in smokers and nonsmokers in clinical trials 438

Table 4. Recurrences of gastric ulcer in smokers and nonsmokers in clinical trials 442

Table 5. Summary of studies of smoking and bone mass 445

Table 6. Summary of case–control studies of smoking and fractures 450

Table 7. Summary of cohort studies of smoking and fractures 454

Chapter 10

Table 1. Summary of prospective studies on smoking and body weight 474

Table 2. Details of prospective studies in which change in weight relative to continuing smokers was reported 477

Table 3. Mortality ratios for all ages combined in relation to the death rate of those 90–109% of average weight 493

Table 4. Mortality ratios for all ages combined according to smoking status in relation to those 90–109% of average age 494

Chapter 11

Table 1. Diagnostic categorization and criteria for nicotine withdrawal—Nicotine-induced organic mental disorder 522

Table 2. Prospective studies of quitting-related changes in mood, anxiety, stress reactivity, perceived stress, self-image, and psychological well-being 536

Table 3. Summary of data from 1985 NHIS, behaviors of never, former, and current smokers aged 20 and older 548

Table 4. Summary of data from 1987 NHIS, behaviors of never, former, and current smokers aged 18 and older 549

Table 5. Summary of data from 1987 BRFSS, behaviors of former smokers and current smokers aged 18 and older 550

Table 6. Summary of data from 1987 BRFSS, behaviors of former smokers aged 18 and older by duration of abstinence 552

Table 7. Percent distribution of persons aged 18 and older by tobacco product and use status, according to gender and cigarette smoking status, United States, 1987 557

Table 8. Physician visits and medical tests within the past year among AARP members aged 50 and older, by smoking status 563

Volume Appendix

Table 1. Quit ratio in selected States, by age group and gender—BRFSS, 1988 586

Table 2. Cigarette smoking continuum by year, percentage of ever cigarette smokers, by NHISs, United States, 1978–87, adults aged 20 and older 589

Table 3. Trends in quit ratio (%) (percentage of ever cigarette smokers who are former cigarette smokers), by age and by education, NHISs, United States, 1965–87, adults aged 20 and older 592

Table 4. Effect of adjusting for use of other tobacco products on quit ratio (percentage of ever cigarette smokers who are former cigarette smokers), 1987, NHIS, United States 594

Table 5. Selected measures of quitting activity (%), NHISs, United States, adults aged 20 and older 600

Table 6. Percentage of those intending to smoke in 5 years, by gender, AUTSs, United States, 1964–86, current smokers aged 21 and older 609

Table 7. Percentage who report having ever received advice to quit from a doctor, by smoking status and gender, United States, 1964–87, adults aged 21 and older 610

LIST OF FIGURES

Chapter 2

Figure 1. Cyclical model of the stages of change 23

Figure 2. Hypothetical examples of disease incidence rates for current, former, and never smokers, by age 55

Chapter 3

Figure 1. Compared with never smokers, relative risk of mortality in current and former smokers aged 50–54, 60–64, and 70–74 at enrollment, by amount smoked and duration of abstinence 81

Figure 2. Estimated probability of dying in the next 16.5-yr interval for quitting at ages 55–59 compared with never smoking and continuing to smoke, by sex 98

Chapter 4

Figure 1. Risk of lung cancer by number of cigarettes smoked per day before quitting, number of years of abstinence, sex, and histologic types ... 121

Figure 2. Relative risk of lung cancer among ex-smokers compared with continuing smokers as a function of time since stopped smoking, estimated from logistic regression model, pattern adjusted for smoking duration compared with pattern unadjusted for duration 123

Figure 3. Incidence of bronchial carcinoma among continuing cigarette smokers in relation to age and duration of smoking and among never smokers in relation to age, double logarithmic scale 127

Chapter 6

Figure 1. Hypothetical effects of smoking cessation on risk of CHD if mechanisms are predominantly rapidly reversible 198

Figure 2. Estimated relative risk of MI after quitting smoking among men under age 55, adjusted for age 204

Figure 3. Mortality ratios due to coronary artery diseases; rates for men who have stopped smoking are compared with those for men who never smoked and those for men still smoking in 1952 214

Figure 4. Mortality ratios for all cardiovascular diseases and CHD, by daily cigarette consumption, US Veterans Study, 1954–69 219

Figure 5. Mortality ratio for current and former cigarette smokers by years of smoking cessation, US Veterans Study, 1954–69 220

Figure 6. Effect of smoking cessation on survival among men with documented coronary atherosclerosis; pooled survival among quitters (N=1,490) and continuers (N=2,675) 238

Figure 7. Mortality ratios for stroke for current smokers and ex-smokers compared with never smokers, by daily cigarette consumption, US Veterans Study, 1954–69 252

Figure 8. Survival free of stroke in cigarette smokers, never smokers, and former smokers, aged 60, using Cox proportional hazard regression model, among men and women 259

Chapter 7

Figure 1. Nonproportional Venn Diagram of the interrelationship among chronic bronchitis, emphysema, asthma, and airways obstruction 280

Figure 2. Theoretical curves depicting varying rates of decline of FEV_1 281

Figure 3. Hypothesized mechanisms by which airway hyperresponsiveness may be associated with developing or established COPD without necessarily being a preexisting risk factor 284

Figure 4. Symptom ratio (number of observed symptoms to number of possible symptoms) in nonmodifiers, modifiers, and quitters at each test period; symptoms are cough, sputum production, wheezing, and shortness of breath 287

Figure 5. Prevalence of cough and phlegm by smoking group 293

Figure 6. Prevalence of dyspnea by smoking group 295

Figure 7. Sex-specific mean height-adjusted FEV_1 residuals versus pack-years for current and ex-smokers, and distributions of number of subjects by pack-years 317

Figure 8. Mean values FVC and FEV_1, expressed as a percentage of predicted values, in 15 quitters and 42 smokers during 30 months after 2 smoking cessation clinics 322

Figure 9. Mean values for the ratio of CV/VC, of CC/TLC, and slope for phase III of the single breath N_2 test (N_2/L), expressed as a percentage of predicted values in 15 quitters and 42 smokers during 30 months after 2 smoking cessation clinics 326

Figure 10. Percent-predicted diffusing capacity (%pDL) by pack-years of smoking, current smokers and former smokers, in a study of adults in Tucson, AZ 329

Figure 11. Mean ΔFEV_1 values in never smokers, consistent ex-smokers, subjects who quit smoking during followup, and consistent smokers in several age groups 334

Figure 12. Effects of quitting smoking during followup among men aged 50–69 336

Chapter 8

Figure 1. Perinatal, neonatal, and fetal mortality rates by birthweight in singleton white males, 1980 380

Chapter 11

Figure 1. Performance on a meter (i.e., visual) vigilance task. Performance on the continuous clock task, a visual vigilance task 527

Figure 2. Self-reported withdrawal discomfort among abstinent smokers 531

Figure 3. Drinking relative to smoking status for men, 1983 NHIS 558

Figure 4. Drinking relative to smoking status for women, 1983 NHIS 559

Appendix

Figure 1. Trends in the quit ratio, United States, 1965–87, by gender 590

Figure 2. Trends in the quit ratio, United States, 1965–87, by race 591

Figure 3. Flow chart of quitting history, attempts lasting longer than 1 year, NHEFS 597

Figure 4. Estimated duration of abstinence on first 1-year or longer quit attempt, product–limit method, N=3,363 598

Figure 5. Percentage of ever smokers who never tried to quit, by education, United States, 1974–87 601

Figure 6. Percentage of persons smoking at 12 months prior to the survey interview who quit for at least 1 day during those 12 months, United States, 1978–80, 1987, by education 602

Figure 7. Percentage of ever smokers who had been abstinent for less than 1 year, United States, 1966–87, by education 603

Figure 8. Percentage of ever smokers who had been abstinent for 1–4 years, United States, 1966–87, by education 604

Figure 9. Percentage of ever smokers who had been abstinent for 5 years or more, United States, 1966–87, by education 605

CHAPTER 1
INTRODUCTION, OVERVIEW, AND CONCLUSIONS

CONTENTS

Introduction 5

Major Conclusions 8

Development of the Report 8

Chapter Conclusions 9
    Chapter 2: Assessing Smoking Cessation and Its Health Consequences 9
    Chapter 3: Smoking Cessation and Overall Mortality and Morbidity 9
    Chapter 4: Smoking Cessation and Respiratory Cancers 10
    Chapter 5: Smoking Cessation and Nonrespiratory Cancers 10
    Chapter 6: Smoking Cessation and Cardiovascular Disease 10
    Chapter 7: Smoking Cessation and Nonmalignant Respiratory Diseases 11
    Chapter 8: Smoking Cessation and Reproduction 11
    Chapter 9: Smoking, Smoking Cessation, and Other Nonmalignant Diseases .. 12
    Chapter 10: Smoking Cessation and Body Weight Change 12
    Chapter 11: Psychological and Behavioral Consequences and Correlates of
        Smoking Cessation 13
    Volume Appendix: National Trends in Smoking Cessation 13

References 15

INTRODUCTION

The 1964 Report of the Surgeon General's Advisory Committee on Smoking and Health (US PHS 1964) concluded that cigarette smoking is a cause of lung cancer and laryngeal cancer in men, a probable cause of lung cancer in women, and the most important cause of chronic bronchitis. Other diseases, including emphysema and cardiovascular disease, also were found to be associated with cigarette smoking, although the evidence available at that time was not viewed as sufficient to establish the associations as causal. Even in 1964, however, the evidence for adverse health consequences of cigarette smoking was sufficient for the Committee to conclude that "cigarette smoking is a health hazard of sufficient importance in the United States to warrant appropriate remedial action" (US PHS 1964, p. 33).

Subsequent reports of the Surgeon General on smoking and health expanded and strengthened the conclusions of the 1964 Report on active smoking and documented the benefits of smoking cessation. (See US DHHS 1989 for review.) For some diseases, such as cardiovascular disease, newer evidence warranted a determination that associations with cigarette smoking were causal. Further associations of cigarette smoking with disease were identified, and involuntary (passive) smoking was found to be a cause of disease in nonsmokers (US DHHS 1986). Although cigarette smoking has been investigated intensively since the 1950s, new associations of smoking with adverse effects continue to be identified. For example, in a recent study smoking was associated with cataracts (West et al. 1989).

Evidence substantiates cigarette smoking as a cause of disease in smokers and, through involuntary smoking, in never smokers as well. This evidence has motivated the implementation of diverse and far-reaching programs for smoking prevention and cessation. The proportion of U.S. adults who smoke decreased substantially since the 1964 Report. In 1965, 29.6 percent of persons who had ever smoked had quit; by 1987, this percentage had increased to 44.8, representing more than 38 million adults. As the numbers of formerly smoking adults increased in the United States and other countries (US DHHS 1989), epidemiologic and clinical studies provided increasingly extensive information on the health benefits of smoking cessation. Thus, the 1964 Report noted that former smokers had lower overall mortality rates and lower lung cancer risk than current smokers, but the cited evidence was limited. Scientific data are now available on the consequences of cessation for most smoking-related diseases. Major benefits have been shown for overall mortality and for many specific diseases. Although past reports have considered much of the evidence, these data have not received a comprehensive and unified review. This Report systematically reviews the findings on the health benefits and consequences of cessation.

This Report includes a Foreword by the Assistant Secretary for Health and the Director of the Centers for Disease Control, a Preface by the Surgeon General of the U.S. Public Health Service, and the following chapters:

Chapter 1. Introduction, Overview, and Conclusions

Chapter 2. Assessing Smoking Cessation and Its Health Consequences

Chapter 3. Smoking Cessation and Overall Mortality and Morbidity

Chapter 4. Smoking Cessation and Respiratory Cancers

Chapter 5. Smoking Cessation and Nonrespiratory Cancers

Chapter 6. Smoking Cessation and Cardiovascular Disease

Chapter 7. Smoking Cessation and Nonmalignant Respiratory Diseases

Chapter 8. Smoking Cessation and Reproduction

Chapter 9. Smoking, Smoking Cessation, and Other Nonmalignant Diseases

Chapter 10. Smoking Cessation and Body Weight Change

Chapter 11. Psychological and Behavioral Consequences and Correlates of Smoking Cessation

Volume Appendix. National Trends in Smoking Cessation

A key to acronyms and terms used throughout the Report is found at the end of the volume.

Other publications of the Public Health Service have reviewed determinants of smoking cessation and abstinence (US DHEW 1979; US DHHS 1980, 1988) and methods of smoking cessation and relapse prevention (Schwartz 1987; US DHHS 1988); hence, these topics are not covered in this Report.

Beginning with the 1964 Report, the evidence on active smoking and disease has been reviewed for causality to evaluate the associations of smoking with disease. The explicit criteria used in this evaluation include the consistency, strength, specificity, temporal relationship, and coherence of the association (US PHS 1964; US DHHS 1989). These criteria have provided a consistent and effective framework for examining the epidemiologic, clinical, and experimental data on active smoking. Although the criteria cannot be applied in the same fashion to associations of smoking cessation with changes in disease occurrence, the criteria of consistency, an appropriate temporal relationship, and coherence must be maintained with evidence on smoking cessation and health.

Thus, this Report examines data for consistency among investigations of the associations of cessation with disease occurrence and other outcomes, and considers the biologic plausibility of the known or presumed associations in the context of the mechanisms by which cigarette smoking is known or thought to cause disease. The appropriate time sequence of cessation with its effect is evident; cessation must always precede its presumed effect. In an observational study, this sequence may be reversed by the tendency of persons with initial symptoms of a cigarette-related disease or with frank disease to reduce cigarette consumption or to stop smoking (Chapter 2). The findings of longitudinal studies among former smokers document high mortality rates among short-term former smokers, which is consistent with reversal of the causal sequence of cessation followed by reduced disease occurrence; that is, disease has caused a change in exposure (Rogot and Murray 1980).

Cigarette smoke in its gaseous and particulate phases contains thousands of agents, many of which can damage tissues and cause disease (US DHEW 1979; US DHHS 1986, 1989). The pathogenetic mechanisms by which cigarette smoking causes disease are diverse, ranging from longer term processes, such as carcinogenesis, to shorter term processes, such as interference with tissue oxygenation by carbon monoxide. Thus, the biologic context in which the evidence on cessation is considered must be disease-specific; a unified biologic framework for evaluating the evidence on cessation cannot be offered.

For example, cigarette smoking causes emphysema, an irreversible destruction of the gas-exchanging structure of the lung, and permanent or only partially reversible damage to the airways of the lung. Little improvement of lung function after cessation would be anticipated for a long-term smoker with disabling chronic obstructive pulmonary disease (COPD) and extensive irreversible damage to the lung. However, cessation would benefit a smoker who has less extensive damage by slowing the rate of lung function decline and thereby reducing the likelihood of clinically significant impairment. By contrast with COPD, smoking cessation following myocardial infarction has both relatively immediate and longer term benefits. The immediately decreased risk of death in those who stop smoking in comparison with those who continue to smoke may reflect a decrease of blood coagulability, improved tissue oxygenation, and less predisposition to cardiac arrhythmias after cessation.

The findings of studies on the health consequences of smoking cessation also provide evidence relevant to determining the causality of associations of active smoking with disease. A decline in disease incidence after cessation needs to be considered as a positive indication of such a causal association. However, the pattern of changing risk after cessation must be interpreted in the context of the mechanism of disease causation by active smoking.

In interpreting individual studies on the consequences of smoking cessation, difficult methodologic and conceptual issues must be considered. Chapter 2 addresses these issues in depth. Because smoking cessation is a dynamic process, often involving multiple relapses to active smoking, accurate characterization of the former smoker is difficult and best accomplished by longitudinal observation. Misclassification of cigarette smoking status may lead to biased estimates of the consequences of smoking cessation. In observational studies and trials some subjects may report that they are former smokers, even though they continue to smoke; the resulting misclassification tends to result in underestimation of the benefits of cessation. Unraveling the consequences of smoking cessation from the effects of other factors determining the occurrence of disease poses a substantial analytical challenge. In reviewing individual reports on the consequences of smoking cessation, the approaches to these potential methodologic issues were assessed (Chapter 2).

MAJOR CONCLUSIONS

More than 38 million Americans have quit smoking, and almost half of all living adults in the United States who ever smoked have quit (Volume Appendix). Nevertheless, more than 50 million Americans continue to smoke. This Report reviews in detail the health consequences of smoking cessation for those who have quit and for those who will quit in the future. The following major volume conclusions summarize the health consequences of smoking cessation for those who quit smoking in comparison with those who continue to smoke:

1. **Smoking cessation has major and immediate health benefits for men and women of all ages. Benefits apply to persons with and without smoking-related disease.**

2. **Former smokers live longer than continuing smokers. For example, persons who quit smoking before age 50 have one-half the risk of dying in the next 15 years compared with continuing smokers.**

3. **Smoking cessation decreases the risk of lung cancer, other cancers, heart attack, stroke, and chronic lung disease.**

4. **Women who stop smoking before pregnancy or during the first 3 to 4 months of pregnancy reduce their risk of having a low birthweight baby to that of women who never smoked.**

5. **The health benefits of smoking cessation far exceed any risks from the average 5-pound (2.3-kg) weight gain or any adverse psychological effects that may follow quitting.**

DEVELOPMENT OF THE REPORT

This Report was developed by the Office on Smoking and Health (OSH), Center for Chronic Disease Prevention and Health Promotion, Centers for Disease Control, Public Health Service of the U.S. Department of Health and Human Services, as part of the Department's responsibility under Public Law 91–222 to report new and current information on smoking and health to the U.S. Congress.

The scientific content of this Report was produced through the efforts of more than 120 scientists in the fields of medicine, psychology, the biologic and social sciences, and public health. Manuscripts for the Report, constituting drafts of chapters or sections of chapters, were prepared by 26 scientists selected for their expertise in specific content areas. An editorial team, including the Director of OSH, a medical psychologist with the Uniformed Services University of the Health Sciences, and four non-Federal experts, edited and consolidated the individual manuscripts into chapters. These draft chapters were subjected to an intensive outside peer review, with each chapter reviewed by an average of five individuals knowledgeable about the chapter's subject matter. Incorporating the reviewers' comments, the editors revised the chapters and assembled a draft of the complete Report. The draft Report was then submitted to 25 distinguished scientists for their review and comment on the entirety of its contents. Simultaneously, the draft Report was submitted to 10 institutes and agencies within the U.S. Public Health Service for review. Comments from the senior scientific reviewers and the agencies were then used to prepare the final draft of the Report, which was then reviewed by the Office of the Assistant Secretary for Health and the Secretary, Department of Health and Human Services.

CHAPTER CONCLUSIONS

Chapter 2: Assessing Smoking Cessation and Its Health Consequences

1. Most former smokers have cycled several times through the process of smoking cessation and relapse before attaining long-term abstinence. Any static measure of smoking status is thus a simplification of a dynamic process.

2. In studies of the health effects of smoking cessation, persons classified as former smokers may include some current smokers. Consequently, the health benefits of smoking cessation are likely to be underestimated.

3. In contexts other than intervention trials, self-reported smoking status at the time of measurement and concurrent biochemical assessment are highly concordant. This high concordance supports self-report as a valid measure of smoking status in observational studies of the health effects of smoking cessation.

Chapter 3: Smoking Cessation and Overall Mortality and Morbidity

1. Former smokers live longer than continuing smokers, and the benefits of quitting extend to those who quit at older ages. For example, persons who quit smoking before age 50 have one-half the risk of dying in the next 15 years compared with continuing smokers.

2. Smoking cessation at all ages reduces the risk of premature death.

3. Among former smokers, the decline in risk of death compared with continuing smokers begins shortly after quitting and continues for at least 10 to 15 years. After 10 to 15 years of abstinence, risk of all-cause mortality returns nearly to that of persons who never smoked.

4. Former smokers have better health status than current smokers as measured in a variety of ways, including days of illness, number of health complaints, and self-reported health status.

Chapter 4: Smoking Cessation and Respiratory Cancers

1. Smoking cessation reduces the risk of lung cancer compared with continued smoking. For example, after 10 years of abstinence, the risk of lung cancer is about 30 to 50 percent of the risk in continuing smokers; with further abstinence, the risk continues to decline.

2. The reduced risk of lung cancer among former smokers is observed in males and females, in smokers of filter and nonfilter cigarettes, and for all histologic types of lung cancer.

3. Smoking cessation lowers the risk of laryngeal cancer compared with continued smoking.

4. Smoking cessation reduces the severity and extent of premalignant histologic changes in the epithelium of the larynx and lung.

Chapter 5: Smoking Cessation and Nonrespiratory Cancers

1. Smoking cessation halves the risks for cancers of the oral cavity and esophagus, compared with continued smoking, as soon as 5 years after cessation, with further reduction over a longer period of abstinence.

2. Smoking cessation reduces the risk of pancreatic cancer, compared with continued smoking, although this reduction in risk may only be measurable after 10 years of abstinence.

3. Smoking is a cause of bladder cancer; cessation reduces risk by about 50 percent after only a few years, in comparison with continued smoking.

4. The risk of cervical cancer is substantially lower among former smokers in comparison with continuing smokers, even in the first few years after cessation. This finding supports the hypothesis that cigarette smoking is a contributing cause of cervical cancer.

5. Neither smoking nor smoking cessation are associated with the risk of cancer of the breast.

Chapter 6: Smoking Cessation and Cardiovascular Disease

1. Compared with continued smoking, smoking cessation substantially reduces risk of coronary heart disease (CHD) among men and women of all ages.

2. The excess risk of CHD caused by smoking is reduced by about half after 1 year of smoking abstinence and then declines gradually. After 15 years of abstinence, the risk of CHD is similar to that of persons who have never smoked.

3. Among persons with diagnosed CHD, smoking cessation markedly reduces the risk of recurrent infarction and cardiovascular death. In many studies, this reduction in risk of recurrence or premature death has been 50 percent or more.

4. Smoking cessation substantially reduces the risk of peripheral artery occlusive disease compared with continued smoking.

5. Among patients with peripheral artery disease, smoking cessation improves exercise tolerance, reduces the risk of amputation after peripheral artery surgery, and increases overall survival.

6. Smoking cessation reduces the risk of both ischemic stroke and subarachnoid hemorrhage compared with continued smoking. After smoking cessation, the risk of stroke returns to the level of never smokers; in some studies this has occurred within 5 years, but in others as long as 15 years of abstinence were required.

Chapter 7: Smoking Cessation and Nonmalignant Respiratory Diseases

1. Smoking cessation reduces rates of respiratory symptoms such as cough, sputum production, and wheezing, and respiratory infections such as bronchitis and pneumonia, compared with continued smoking.

2. For persons without overt chronic obstructive pulmonary disease (COPD), smoking cessation improves pulmonary function about 5 percent within a few months after cessation.

3. Cigarette smoking accelerates the age-related decline in lung function that occurs among never smokers. With sustained abstinence from smoking, the rate of decline in pulmonary function among former smokers returns to that of never smokers.

4. With sustained abstinence, the COPD mortality rates among former smokers decline in comparison with continuing smokers.

Chapter 8: Smoking Cessation and Reproduction

1. Women who stop smoking before becoming pregnant have infants of the same birthweight as those born to never smokers.

2. Pregnant smokers who stop smoking at any time up to the 30th week of gestation have infants with higher birthweight than do women who smoke throughout pregnancy. Quitting in the first 3 to 4 months of pregnancy and abstaining

throughout the remainder of pregnancy protect the fetus from the adverse effects of smoking on birthweight.

3. Evidence from two intervention trials suggests that reducing daily cigarette consumption without quitting has little or no benefit for birthweight.

4. Recent estimates of the prevalence of smoking during pregnancy, combined with an estimate of the relative risk of low birthweight outcome in smokers, suggest that 17 to 26 percent of low birthweight births could be prevented by eliminating smoking during pregnancy; in groups with a high prevalence of smoking (e.g., women with less than a high school education), 29 to 42 percent of low birthweight births might be prevented by elimination of cigarette smoking during pregnancy.

5. Approximately 30 percent of women who are cigarette smokers quit after recognition of pregnancy, with greater proportions quitting among married women and especially among women with higher levels of educational attainment.

6. Smoking causes women to have natural menopause 1 to 2 years early. Former smokers have an age at natural menopause similar to that of never smokers.

Chapter 9: Smoking, Smoking Cessation, and Other Nonmalignant Diseases

1. Smokers have an increased risk of development of both duodenal and gastric ulcer, and this increased risk is reduced by smoking cessation.

2. Ulcer disease is more severe among smokers than among nonsmokers. Smokers are less likely to experience healing of duodenal ulcers and are more likely to have recurrences of both duodenal and gastric ulcers within specified timeframes. Most ulcer medications fail to alter these tendencies.

3. Smokers with gastric or duodenal ulcers who stop smoking improve their clinical course relative to smokers who continue to smoke.

4. The evidence that smoking increases the risk of osteoporotic fractures or decreases bone mass is inconclusive, with many conflicting findings. Data on smoking cessation are extremely limited at present.

5. There is evidence that smoking is associated with prominent facial skin wrinkling in whites, particularly in the periorbital ("crow's foot") and perioral areas of the face. The effect of cessation on skin wrinkling is unstudied.

Chapter 10: Smoking Cessation and Body Weight Change

1. Average weight gain after smoking cessation is only about 5 pounds (2.3 kg). This weight gain poses a minimal health risk.

2. Approximately 80 percent of smokers who quit gain weight after cessation, but only about 3.5 percent of those who quit smoking gain more than 20 pounds.

3. Increases in food intake and decreases in resting energy expenditure are largely responsible for postcessation weight gain.

Chapter 11: Psychological and Behavioral Consequences and Correlates of Smoking Cessation

1. Short-term consequences of smoking cessation include anxiety, irritability, frustration, anger, difficulty concentrating, increased appetite, and urges to smoke. With the possible exception of urges to smoke and increased appetite, these effects soon disappear.

2. Smokers who abstain from smoking show short-term impairment of performance on a variety of simple attention tasks, which improves with nicotine administration. Memory, learning, and the performance of more complex tasks have not been clearly shown to be impaired. Whether the self-reported improvement in attention tasks upon nicotine administration is due entirely to relief of withdrawal effects or is also due in part to enhancement of performance above the norm is unclear.

3. In comparison with current smokers, former smokers have a greater perceived ability to achieve and maintain smoking abstinence (self-efficacy) and a greater perceived control over personal circumstances (locus of control).

4. Former smokers, compared with current smokers, practice more health-promoting and disease-preventing behaviors.

Volume Appendix: National Trends in Smoking Cessation

1. By 1987, more than 38 million Americans had quit smoking cigarettes, nearly half of all living adults who ever smoked.

2. The percentage of ever cigarette smokers who are former cigarette smokers (quit ratio) has increased from 29.6 percent in 1965 to 44.8 percent in 1987 at an average rate of 0.68 percentage points per year. The quit ratio has increased among men and women, among blacks and whites, and among all age and education subgroups. Between 1966 and 1987, the rate of increase in the quit ratio among college graduates was twice the rate among high school dropouts.

3. About one-third of all former cigarette smokers who have maintained abstinence for at least 1 year may eventually relapse. As the duration of abstinence increases, relapse becomes less likely.

4. Quitting activity, as measured by the proportion of people smoking at 12 months before a survey who quit for at least 1 day during those 12 months, has increased slightly over time. Between 1978 and 1987, this proportion increased from 27.8 to 31.6 percent.

5. Female smokers were more likely than male smokers to have quit smoking cigarettes for at least 1 day during the previous year; however, there were no gender differences in the proportion abstinent for 1 to 4 years. Men were more likely than women to have been abstinent for 5 years or more. These findings do not take into account the use of tobacco products other than cigarettes.

6. Black smokers were more likely than white smokers to have quit for at least 1 day during the previous year. Blacks, however, were less likely than whites to have been abstinent for 1 year or more.

7. Younger smokers (aged 20 to 44) were more likely than older smokers to have quit for at least 1 day during the previous year.

8. Smokers with less education tend to be less likely to have quit for at least 1 day during the previous year compared with those having more education. In addition, those with lower levels of education are less likely to have been abstinent for 1 year or more.

9. In 1964, about three-fourths of all current smokers predicted that they would "definitely" or "probably" be smoking in 5 years. In 1986, fewer than half of all current smokers felt the same way. Moreover, while more than 20 percent of current smokers in 1964 predicted that they would "definitely" be smoking in 5 years, only about 7 percent of current smokers in 1986 so predicted.

10. Current smokers in 1987 were more than three times as likely as current smokers in 1964 to report having received advice from a doctor to stop smoking.

References

ROGOT, E., MURRAY, J.L. Smoking and causes of death among U.S. veterans: 16 years of observation. *Public Health Reports* 95(3):213–222, May–June 1980.

SCHWARTZ, J.L. *Review and Evaluation of Smoking Cessation Methods: United States and Canada, 1978–1985.* U.S. Department of Health and Human Services, Public Health Service, National Institutes of Health, NIH Publication No. 87-2940, April 1987.

U.S. DEPARTMENT OF HEALTH AND HUMAN SERVICES. *The Health Consequences of Smoking for Women. A Report of the Surgeon General.* U.S. Department of Health and Human Services, Public Health Service, Office of the Assistant Secretary for Health, Office on Smoking and Health, 1980.

U.S. DEPARTMENT OF HEALTH AND HUMAN SERVICES. *The Health Consequences of Involuntary Smoking. A Report of the Surgeon General.* U.S. Department of Health and Human Services, Public Health Service, Centers for Disease Control. DHHS Publication No. (CDC) 87-8398, 1986.

U.S. DEPARTMENT OF HEALTH AND HUMAN SERVICES. *The Health Consequences of Smoking: Nicotine Addiction. A Report of the Surgeon General, 1988.* U.S. Department of Health and Human Services, Public Health Service, Centers for Disease Control, Center for Health Promotion and Education, Office on Smoking and Health. DHHS Publication No. (CDC) 88-8406, 1988.

U.S. DEPARTMENT OF HEALTH AND HUMAN SERVICES. *Reducing the Health Consequences of Smoking: 25 Years of Progress. A Report of the Surgeon General.* U.S. Department of Health and Human Services, Public Health Service, Centers for Disease Control, Center for Chronic Disease Prevention and Health Promotion, Office on Smoking and Health. DHHS Publication No. (CDC) 89-8411, 1989.

U.S. DEPARTMENT OF HEALTH, EDUCATION, AND WELFARE. *Smoking and Health. A Report of the Surgeon General.* U.S. Department of Health, Education, and Welfare, Public Health Service, Office of the Assistant Secretary for Health, Office on Smoking and Health. DHEW Publication No. (PHS) 79-50066, 1979.

U.S. PUBLIC HEALTH SERVICE. *Smoking and Health. Report of the Advisory Committee to the Surgeon General of the Public Health Service.* U.S. Department of Health, Education, and Welfare, Public Health Service, Center for Disease Control. PHS Publication No. 1103, 1964.

WEST, S., MUÑOZ, B., EMMETT, E.A., TAYLOR, H.R. Cigarette smoking and risk of nuclear cataracts. *Archives of Opthalmology* 107(8):1166–1169, August 1989.

CHAPTER 2
ASSESSING SMOKING CESSATION AND ITS HEALTH CONSEQUENCES

CONTENTS

Introduction	21
Part I. Assessing the Dynamic Process of Smoking Cessation	22
The Process of Smoking Behavior Change	22
Behavioral Measures	25
Self-Report: Questionnaires and Interviews	25
Temporal and Frequency Issues	27
Improving Self-Report Measures	28
Alternative Behavioral Measures	29
Surrogate Assessments	30
Nonbehavioral Measures	31
Physiologic Measures	32
Biochemical Markers	33
Terminology	33
Carbon Monoxide	34
Thiocyanate	35
Cotinine	36
Bogus Pipeline	37
Contextual Issues Affecting Biochemical Assessment	37
Part II. Assessing the Consequences of Smoking Cessation	46
Study Designs Used To Assess the Consequences of Cessation	46
Overview of Study Design	46
Ecologic Studies	47
Cross-Sectional Studies	47
Cohort Studies	48
Case–Control Studies	49
Intervention Trials	50
Methodologic Issues	51
Introduction	51
Statistical Considerations	52
Bias	52
Analytic Issues in Observation Studies	55
Summary	57
Conclusions	58
References	59

INTRODUCTION

Smoking cessation is a dynamic process that begins with a decision to stop smoking and ends with abstinence from cigarettes maintained over a long period of time. Typically, initiation of regular cigarette smoking occurs at a young age, usually during the teenage years (US DHHS 1989); cessation may be contemplated and initiated at any age. The spectrum of factors motivating cessation is diverse; some smokers quit before being adversely affected by cigarette smoking whereas others quit as a result of developing smoking-related disease. Most attempts to quit are temporarily successful, and most smokers attempting to quit return several times to regular smoking before achieving long-term abstinence.

For the purpose of health research, smoking status (i.e., never, former, or current smoker) can be evaluated by using an interview or questionnaire to query subjects about their smoking behavior. However, self-reports may not fully characterize the process of cessation in individual smokers, particularly if information is collected retrospectively or cross-sectionally. Moreover, persons who are smoking may falsely report themselves as former or never smokers. Biochemical markers, such as cotinine and thiocyanate (SCN^-) levels in body fluids, provide complementary measures of tobacco product use.

However, reliance solely on biochemical markers of smoking also may lead to some misclassification. For example, intake of some foods can result in high SCN^- levels unrelated to smoking behavior. Individuals who accurately report being quitters may fail to participate in the validation process and therefore may be misclassified as continuing smokers if nonparticipants in biochemical testing are assumed to be smoking. Because proper classification of smoking behavior is critical for conducting research on the health consequences of smoking cessation and for evaluating the results of such research, it is important to consider how smoking status is assessed.

The health consequences of smoking cessation have been studied using conventional approaches of epidemiologic and clinical research: ecologic study, cross-sectional study or survey, case–control study, cohort study, and intervention trial. Each design has well-described advantages for studying causes of disease and preventive factors among human populations (Kleinbaum, Kupper, Morgenstern 1982). In addition, each design type is subject to the three types of bias potentially affecting any epidemiologic study: selection bias, information bias, and confounding bias (Rothman 1986) (Chapter 2, Part II). Misclassification resulting from information bias is of particular concern in studies of smoking cessation; misclassification is addressed in detail in this Chapter.

These conventional research designs have been used successfully to characterize the adverse effects of active cigarette smoking and to amass the scientific information on smoking cessation reviewed in this Report. For example, the evidence on smoking cessation and mortality derives from cohort studies (Chapter 3); evidence on cancer comes largely from case–control and cohort studies (Chapters 4 and 5); and information on respiratory morbidity and mortality is based primarily on cross-sectional and cohort studies (Chapter 7).

This Chapter establishes a methodologic framework for interpreting the evidence on smoking cessation obtained from observation studies and intervention trials. Part I describes the process of smoking cessation and the methods used to assess smoking behavior. Part II reviews research methods used to study smoking cessation as well as the potential limitations of data obtained from observational studies and intervention trials including biases that may affect the results.

PART I. ASSESSING THE DYNAMIC PROCESS OF SMOKING CESSATION

This Section describes the dynamic nature of smoking behavior, the various measures of smoking status applied in observational and intervention studies, and the effect of these measures on classification of smoking status.

The Process of Smoking Behavior Change

Smoking behavior in U.S. populations has been changing, and three-fourths of all smokers have attempted to quit (Volume Appendix). The proportion of adult former smokers in the population is now about the same as the proportion of current smokers. These population changes have provided opportunity to describe the consequences and, thereby, the benefits of cessation.

Progressing from smoking to former smoking is a complex, dynamic process and not a one-time event. Retrospective, cross-sectional, and longitudinal studies of how people quit smoking on their own have demonstrated that smokers move through a series of stages in their cessation efforts (DiClemente and Prochaska 1982; Lichtenstein and Brown 1980; Prochaska and DiClemente 1983; Prochaska et al. 1985; Rosen and Shipley 1983). These stages have been labeled motivation and commitment, initial change, and maintenance by Brownell and coworkers (1986); contemplating change, decidingt change, short-term change, and long-term change by Horn (1976); motivation and commitment, cessation and possible relapse, and maintenance by Marlatt and Gordon (1985); precontemplation, contemplation, action, and maintenance and/or relapse by Prochaska and DiClemente (1983); and initial decision, initial control, and maintenance by Rosen and Shipley (1983).

The stage model of Prochaska and DiClemente (1983; Prochaska et al., in press) has generated the most research and is described in more detail below (Figure 1). Precontemplation is a period in which smokers are not thinking about quitting smoking, or at least not about quitting within the next 6 months. The basis for the 6-month timeframe is the assumption that 6 months into the future is as far as most people plan a specific behavior change. Contemplation is the period in which smokers seriously consider quitting smoking within the next 6 months. Action is the period that begins when actual cessation occurs and continues for 6 months after stopping smoking. Maintenance is defined as the period beginning 6 months after cessation occurrence. In all of the proposed stage models, differentiation is made between short-term (generally up to 6 months) and long-term (generally 6 months and longer) change or between initial cessation and maintenance of cessation. Maintenance continues until relapse to regular smoking, or until a return to regular smoking is of minimal or no concern and "termination" of the behavior occurs for the confirmed ex-smoker.

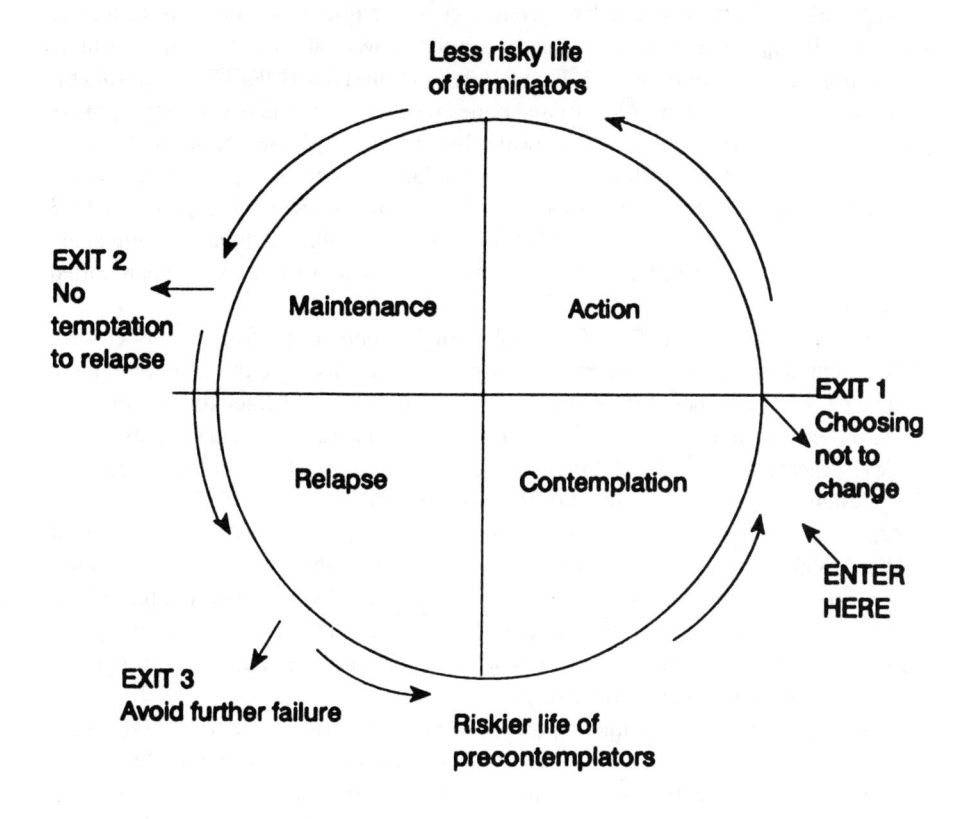

FIGURE 1.—Cyclical model of the stages of change
SOURCE: Prochaska et al. (in press).

On any single cessation attempt (action stage), the majority of smokers relapse and return to regular smoking. A National Heart, Lung, and Blood Institute consensus conference defined relapse as at least one puff per day for 7 days and recommended that this definition be applied uniformly (Shumaker and Grunberg 1986); however, this definition is not used in all studies. Any return to smoking that is less than the criterion for relapse is considered a "lapse" or a "slip," which may or may not cause a return to regular smoking (Brownell et al. 1986; Marlatt, Curry, Gordon, 1988).

Although 75 to 80 percent of relapse occurs at 6 months and before (Hunt, Barnett, Branch 1971; Hunt and Bespalec 1973; Hughes et al. 1981; Garvey, Heinold, Rosner 1989), individuals who maintain abstinence for 6 months continue to relapse by 12 months and beyond. For example, in a review of 10 studies in which minimal or no intervention occurred (i.e., self-change studies), relapse rates at 12 months for smokers who had previously maintained abstinence for at least 6 months ranged from 7 to 35 percent (Cohen et al. 1989). Data from the National Health and Nutrition Examination

Survey I (NHANES-I) Epidemiologic Followup Study demonstrate that even after 1 year of prolonged abstinence, relapse continues to occur in about one-third of former smokers. Relapse continues to occur at a much lower rate after 2 years (Volume Appendix). In the Multiple Risk Factor Intervention Trial (MRFIT), a multifactor intensive intervention study, Ockene and colleagues (1982) found that among smokers who had stopped with the aid of intensive intervention, relapse continued to occur throughout the 6 years of followup. However, relapse was at a much higher rate in the first year than in years two through six. Kirscht and colleagues (1987) reported that 9.5 percent of adults who had been abstinent for 24 to 119 months reported smoking again in a followup survey. Even after 120 months, 2.3 percent of former smokers reported smoking again.

Research would be simplified if the probability of remaining a former smoker were 100 percent after a prolonged period of abstinence. If this were the case, then there would be no concern about future misclassification of these confirmed former smokers. However, the continuous nature of the relapse process and the curves that represent this process indicate that the probability of maintained cessation will never be 100 percent. The available data (Garvey, Heinold, Rosner 1989; Ockene et al. 1982; Cohen et al. 1989; Volume Appendix) suggest that for most research purposes, 24 months of continuous abstinence can be used as a practical criterion for categorizing individuals as confirmed former smokers. However, use of this timeframe is often not feasible or applicable in many research studies, and as a general guideline for interpreting outcomes—the longer the duration of continuous abstinence, the greater the probability that individuals will remain former smokers.

Cessation is a cyclical, not linear, process; smokers can enter or leave the process at any point (Prochaska and DiClemente 1983; Prochaska et al., in press) (Figure 1). Research on self-change approaches to smoking cessation suggests that the average smoker cycles three to four times through the stages before attaining long-term continuous abstinence and becoming a confirmed former smoker (Prochaska and DiClemente 1984, 1986; Marlatt, Curry, Gordon 1988; Schachter 1982). In a review of self-change studies, Cohen and colleagues (1989) found that only 4.3 percent of the participants in the reviewed studies shifted immediately from current smokers to former smokers without experiencing any lapses or relapses. Most smokers who relapse return to a point where they think about stopping again, that is, the contemplation stage. A smaller proportion lose their motivation to change and regress back to the precontemplation stage (Prochaska and DiClemente 1984).

In summary, because of the dynamic nature of change in smoking behavior, any categorization of smoking status at a single point in time becomes a simplification. A group of former smokers will include individuals who have stopped recently or who have been abstinent for varying lengths of time; some will maintain abstinence, and some will relapse. Knowledge of the dynamics of smoking cessation and its usual time course can help investigators minimize misclassification by choosing the most appropriate methods for assessing smoking behavior and the appropriate sampling procedures (e.g., number of measurements made and time between repeated measures of smoking status).

Behavioral Measures

Self-Report: Questionnaires and Interviews

For health research purposes, smoking status is usually assessed by using self-administered questionnaires or interviews. However, other behavioral methods, surrogate assessments, and nonbehavioral methods such as biochemical assessments are also used as sources of smoking data. These other sources will be reviewed in subsequent sections. (See also reviews by Pechacek, Fox et al. 1984 and Marsh et al. 1988.)

Questionnaires and interviews may include information concerning smoking at the time of the assessment or concerning a complete or partial retrospective lifetime history. Assessment can be made once or serially over time, thus providing more valid data regarding cessation and possible relapse. Information gathered from an interview or questionnaire about smoking categorizes respondents as never, current, or former smokers. Two standard items used in the National Health Interview Survey (Volume Appendix) to classify smoking status are "Have you smoked at least 100 cigarettes in your entire life?" and "Do you smoke cigarettes now?" Someone responding "yes" to the first question and "no" to the second would be classified as a former smoker. Such a broad definition for former smokers combines persons who experimented with smoking enough to have smoked 100 cigarettes with individuals who may have smoked during their entire adult life and quit in the week prior to being interviewed.

The commonly used item, "Have you smoked at least 100 cigarettes in your entire life?" has an advantage of counting as never smokers those individuals who experimented with 1, 2, or quite a few cigarettes. Only those who have smoked at least 5 packs of cigarettes in their lifetime are counted as ever smokers. The arbitrariness of this definition reflects the lack of accepted and standardized definitions for ever smokers and never smokers. A definition of never smokers that requires only minimal or no use of tobacco may result in many individuals with extremely low exposure to cigarettes being classified as former smokers, which in general would not be biologically appropriate.

Another commonly used type of item, as in the Medical Research Council (MRC) National Survey of Health and Development (Britten 1988), for defining ever smokers is "Have you ever smoked as much as 1 cigarette a day for as long as 1 year?" This item is used by the American Thoracic Society, Division of Lung Disease in its Adult Respiratory questionnaire; however, two other choices are added— "or 20 packs of cigarettes" or "12 ounces of tobacco" (Ferris 1978). A comparable questions is "Have you ever smoked at least 5 cigarettes per week, almost every week for at least 1 year?" (Petitti, Friedman, Kahn 1981). These items that are used to classify ever smokers are based on a combination of the amount of cigarettes smoked (e.g., 365) and the duration of smoking (e.g., at least 6 or 12 months).

The particular question used to differentiate between ever smokers and never smokers can directly affect categorization of individuals. For example, Petitti, Friedman, and Kahn (1981) found that with a more specifically defined question such as "Have you ever smoked at least 5 cigarettes per week almost every week for at least 1 year?" which requires some period of "regular" smoking for an individual to be classified as an ever smoker, 128 of 252 individuals reported being never smokers. However, when assessed concurrently with another questionnaire in which regular smoking was not defined and the respondent self-defined smoking, 7 percent fewer subjects (119 of 252) reported being never smokers.

Thus, the use of more clearly defined questions, such as specifying 100 cigarettes in a lifetime, or 1 cigarette per day for 1 year, or 5 cigarettes per week for 1 year, will reduce misclassification. However, some misclassification will still occur for those individuals who smoked for relatively brief periods during their lives but cannot accurately remember how long they smoked or accurately estimate the number of cigarettes they smoked.

Attention also must be paid to defining current or former smokers. Some studies, such as the Cancer Prevention Study I (CPS-I) (Hammond and Garfinkel 1969), define current smokers as those who respond affirmatively to the question "Have you smoked within the past year?" Other studies use smoking in the past 6 months as the guideline for current smokers (Coultas et al. 1988). The criteria for questions identifying current smokers can range from having smoked in the past year, to the past 6 months, to the past week, or to an unspecified period. A few additional questions will enhance the specificity of the definitions of current smokers and former smokers. These items, or comparable ones, have been used in previous surveys, for example, the 1988 Baseline Prevalence Survey for the Community Intervention Trial for Smoking Cessation, funded by the National Cancer Institute: "At what age did you start smoking on a regular basis?"; "On the average, about how many cigarettes did you smoke per day during the last 12 months you smoked?"; and for former smokers, "When did you quit smoking cigarettes?" (recorded to exact date if possible). These items provide additional information for defining ever smokers, or stratifying by levels of exposure, and for determining the period of abstinence.

The dynamic nature of smoking cessation highlights the importance of being aware that any categorical definition of former smoker in relation to the health effects of smoking cessation will include former smokers who have been abstinent for varying periods of time. Optimally, questions on smoking history should ascertain the duration of abstinence for former smokers, and if possible, abstinence periods should be treated as continuous or categorized variables in an analysis, thus avoiding the problem of treating former smokers as a single group. However, benefits of cessation are still clearly observed in spite of the limitations of using categorical data.

The most common minimum periods of abstinence used for defining former smoking status are 24 hours, 7 days, and 30 days. The National Interagency Council on Smoking and Health (1974) recommended using a minimum of 7 days of abstinence for defining cessation. However, because of the nature of smoking, using a short abstinence period to define former smokers is not optimal in epidemiologic studies. The degree of misclassification of former smokers will depend on the minimum duration of abstinence used to define former smokers and the criterion used to consider determine relapse.

Many studies do not specify a minimum duration of abstinence for individuals classified as former smokers at a particular point in time. Data from such studies on the association of smoking cessation with health and disease outcomes must be interpreted cautiously. For example, in the reports of the Whitehall Civil Servants Study (Rose and Hamilton 1978; Rose et al. 1982), the criterion used to define abstinence is not indicated. The only information provided is that the smokers reported that "they were then smoking no cigarettes at all" (Rose and Hamilton 1978).

Regardless of the criteria used to define abstinence, the methodology for assessing smoking status, including questionnaire items, needs to be carefully described by investigators. Optimally these items should enhance the process of obtaining information regarding the duration of abstinence, making it possible to fully determine the relationship of smoking cessation to health and disease outcomes. When reviewing studies of the health effects f smoking, the definition of the former smoker must be carefully assessed, and the effect of the definition on the findings must be carefully examined.

Temporal and Frequency Issues

Studies vary according to whether smoking is assessed retrospectively or prospectively and whether a single assessment or a series of assessments is used. The category of never smokers can be assessed retrospectively, usually relying on a single assessment. Requiring subjects to reconstruct more detailed smoking histories can be very demanding. Nevertheless, simply classifying individuals as former smokers or current smokers reveals very little about the amount of smoking exposure experienced. More pertinent questions regarding exposure include "How long have you been abstinent from cigarettes?"; "At what age did you start smoking?"; "How many cigarettes did you smoke during different periods of your life?"; "How many times did you stop smoking?"; and "How long did you remain abstinent during each of these occasions?"

A series of repeated assessments can result in inconsistencies such as some individuals reporting smoking at one assessment and later reporting that they never smoked. In a followup study in England, for example, Britten (1988) found 1,296 participants aged 36 who claimed that they had never smoked. Of these, 242 (18.7 percent) previously had reported smoking less than 1 cigarette per day, and 102 (7.9 percent) previously had reported smoking at least 1 cigarette per day for at least 1 year. Of the 102 who reported previously that they had been regular smokers, 93 percent reported that the last time they had smoked was at least 10 years prior to the survey.

If the Britten study had used only one retrospective assessment of the subjects at age 36, 32.5 percent of the 1,296 subjects would have been classified as never smokers and 32.6 percent as former smokers. Assuming that reports at a young age were more accurate because memory bias was less likely to occur, the serial assessment indicates that a more accurate categorization would be 29.1 percent for never smokers and 36.5 percent for former smokers. Britten (1988) estimated that misclassification of this magnitude, when applied to a study by Friedman and colleagues (1979), would result in only a 5-percent increase from 2.41 to 2.53 in relative risks of death for former smokers compared with never smokers.

Krall and colleagues (1989) found that of 87 middle-aged adults, 87 percent accurately recalled their smoking status of 20 years earlier, but only 71 percent accurately recalled the amount that they had smoked. Furthermore, underestimation of the amount smoked was twice as common for 20 years earlier (17 vs. 9 percent) and six times more common for 32 years previously (37 vs. 6 percent). Persson and Norell (1989) found that in a random sample of 9,394 individuals in Sweden, retrospective information obtained 6 years later resulted in a strong tendency to overestimate previous cigarette consumption among individuals who had increased their smoking (69 percent overestimated) and to underestimate among individuals who had decreased their smoking (49 percent underestimated). Subjects with unchanged cigarette consumption showed the highest levels of agreement (89 percent) between original and retrospective information. Rather than reconstructing full smoking cessation histories that are subject to biased reporting, many retrospective studies rely on more limited categorization such as never, former, and current smokers.

Retrospective studies enable researchers to assess long periods of smoking abstinence without the need to observe the subjects over a long period of time, as would be necessary in prospective studies. Case–control studies, for example, can compare cases with smoking-related diseases with controls with histories of being abstinent for 10 to 20 years; in a prospective study, it may be impractical or impossible to study health consequences of cessation with more than 10 to 20 years of abstinence (Chapter 2, Part II).

Prospective studies have the potential for more reliable and valid measures of smoking status over time, especially when using a series of assessments, than do retrospective studies. In intervention trials, for example, all subjects enter the trial as current smokers. Following intensive intervention, subjects are identified as continuing smokers or former smokers (abstinent). By assessing subjects at specified intervals such as every 4 or 6 months over a series of years, especially when paired with biochemical verification (Chapter 2, see section on Biochemical Markers), researchers can reduce the measurement bias and be more confident in the reliability and validity of measures classifying continuing and former smokers and specifying length of abstinence for former smokers. In MRFIT (Ockene et al. 1990) for example, a series of 4-month followups over 6 years enabled researchers to classify participants into three categories: persistent quitters (continuous abstainers since the initial intervention), intermittent quitters (abstinent for periods of time since the initial intervention), and continuous smokers (not abstinent during any of the followup periods). Such precision in measurement is generally not possible or necessary in epidemiologic studies.

Prospective studies may use a single assessment to categorize current, former, and never smokers. These studies then prospectively examine the categories to detect differential rates of morbidity and mortality. As discussed above, the assumption that individuals will not change their smoking status maybe a flaw with such single assessments.

Improving Self-Report Measures

Ideally, assessments of smoking status need to include standardized questions to determine smoking status, that is never, current, and former smokers. For example, to be categorized as a never smoker, the necessary response would be "no" to a standard question such as, "Have you ever smoked at least 1 cigarette per day for at least 1 year?"

Whenever possible, questions should be used that allow continuous rather than dichotomous scales for response. A question such as "Do you smoke regularly?" results in a dichotomous response scale. This scale provides much less information than does a continuous scale, such as the question, "On the average, how many cigarettes do you smoke per day?" which can range from 0 to 20, 40, 60, or more. Multiple questions such as, "Have you smoked even a puff of a cigarette in the past 7 days?"; "How many cigarettes do you typically smoke each day?"; and "How many cigarettes do you typically smoke each week?" can be used to refine a category such as current smokers. Inclusion of other indices, such as biochemical markers of smoking (e.g., saliva cotinine levels), can also be used to describe smoking status.

In a followup study, measures of smoking status optimally should be repeated over multiple occasions, especially for dynamic categories like current smokers and former smokers, which are open to change over time. Repeated measures over a series of occasions provide further reliability and validity for assessments and also provide greater statistical power for detecting differences between groups. Nevertheless, studies with only a single or a few assessments of smoking behavior have been extremely informative.

Alternative Behavioral Measures

As a measure of smoking, self-report by questionnaires and interviews is the most common, the least expensive, the easiest to use, and the most feasible in epidemiologic studies (Frederiksen, Martin, Webster 1979; Pechacek, Fox et al. 1984). However, other behavioral measures have also been used in clinical studies. Because these measures are generally not used in large-scale epidemiologic studies, they will be presented only briefly in this Chapter.

Self-monitoring by the smoker, a measure of smoking commonly used in intervention studies, involves recording by paper, pencil, and mechanical counters each cigarette as it is smoked. The monitoring itself may be a reactive measure and alter the behavior, depending on the nature of the monitored behavior and motivation (Abrams and Wilson 1979; Frederiksen, Martin, Webster 1979; Lipinski et al. 1973; McFall 1978; Orleans and Shipley 1982). It is an intrusive measure that is normally restricted to small studies of high intensity. Other behavioral measures, such as direct observation, collecting and counting cigarette butts (McFall 1978), and measuring their length (Auger, Wright, Simpson 1972), are even more costly and intrusive and less appropriate for epidemiologic and large intervention studies.

Alternative types of behavioral reports for validation of smoking status include verification by an informant (Shipley 1981), by self-report measures using multiple questions about smoking behavior or status as part of the same interview or questionnaire (see above), and by sampling on multiple occasions. Examples of the latter usually involve long periods of time and often result in multiple sources of discrepancy. (See Lee 1988 for summary.)

Surrogate Assessments

In some circumstances researchers may need to obtain information from sources other than the index subjects. With some study designs, for example a case–control study of lung cancer, some subjects are unavailable to answer questions because of illness or death. In cohort studies, or intervention studies with mortality endpoints, surrogate interviews are sometimes required to assess smoking during the interval preceding death.

Failure to obtain surrogate reports can cause considerable bias in some instances. In a case–control study of oral cancer, Greenberg and coworkers (1986) obtained interviews with 112 cases (67.9 percent) and surrogate reports for 23 cases (13.9 percent). Cases needing surrogate reports had more advanced stages of disease at the time of diagnosis and were more likely to be black and less educated than cases interviewed in person. Cigarette smoking and drinking hard liquor were more common among these cases. Therefore, failure to include surrogate reports would have resulted in underestimates of the strength of association between cigarette exposure and hard liquor and the risk of oropharyngeal cancer.

Pickle, Brown, and Blot (1983) found that siblings of index subjects provided the most complete data about smoking in the subject's family of origin and early life events. Spouses and offspring supplied the most complete data about smoking history during adult life. Incomplete data generally increased with the amount of detail requested, so that there were considerably higher nonresponse rates for a detailed smoking history (approximately 50 percent) than for the history of a broad smoking status, such as never smoker (approximately 15 percent). Surrogates beyond a spouse or close relative provided much higher nonresponse rates for almost all questions in all statuses.

McLaughlin and colleagues (1987) examined the reliability of retrospective surrogate reports obtained 10 years after initial reports and compared these with retrospective self-reports using data from the NHANES-I (Cornoni-Huntley et al. 1983). Correct identification of previous smoking status was generally provided by most types of surrogates, except siblings of male decedents. The combined level of agreement for all surrogates ranged from 85 to 95 percent and was remarkably similar to that from self-reports of living subjects. Thirty-five percent of the surrogates could not provide data on when smoking began compared with 1 percent in self-reports. Surrogates who responded tended to provide a later age for starting. Surrogates did, however, provide estimates of years smoked that were comparable to the original reports. In this study, siblings and other surrogates provided less reliable reports than spouses, offspring, or parents of subjects.

Lerchen and Samet (1986) interviewed widows of lung cancer patients who had supplied their own smoking histories while alive. They found that of 77 wives of current smokers, all supplied information about the cases' cigarette smoking status (ever/never) that was in perfect agreement with the information supplied by the cases themselves. Sixty-six (86 percent) were able to supply complete responses about their husbands' smoking behavior. For those who responded, however, mean values reported by cases and their wives were not significantly different for age at which cases started smoking, years smoked, or average number of cigarettes smoked per day. Wives tended to report

20 cigarettes smoked daily even when their husbands smoked substantially more or less. Pershagen and Axelson (1982) also reported perfect agreement regarding smoker/nonsmoker status when information was obtained from a close relative (parent, wife, or child) for 14 lung cancer cases compared with information that had previously been obtained from the cases by the physician. Blot, Akiba, and Kato (1984) also interviewed next of kin in a case–control study of lung cancer among atomic bomb survivors who had previously provided information regarding their own smoking behavior while they were alive. The investigators found that only 1 percent of surrogates reported that a subject had never been a smoker while the subject reported that he or she had smoked, suggesting that the identification of never smokers by next of kin is very accurate. There was poorer agreement regarding those who smoked, with 13 percent of surrogates indicating that a subject had smoked while the subject had reported never smoking.

Sandler and Shore (1986) examined the quality of data provided by adult offspring on parents' smoking and drinking. The data were from 518 cancer cases and 518 healthy controls aged 15 to 59. When possible, mothers provided data on their own smoking and their husbands' smoking. Of 982 subjects who had lived with their natural mother, 97 percent provided data on their mothers' smoking status. Of those whose mothers reported never having smoked cigarettes, 2.7 percent were reported as ever having smoked by the adult child. Of those mothers who reported ever having smoked, 8.8 percent were reported as never smokers. Of those fathers reported by the mother as never smokers, 17.2 percent were reported by subjects as ever smokers. Of those fathers reported as ever having smoked cigarettes, 21.1 percent were reported as never smokers by their adult children. Even with the quantity of cigarettes collapsed into categories to include answers of less than 1 pack, 1 pack, and more than 1 pack, the proportion of mothers and subjects whose responses exactly agreed was 82.0 percent for mothers and 49.2 percent for fathers.

Humble, Samet, and Skipper (1984) interviewed 46 subject–spouse pairs, with 2 people in each of 38 of these pairs acting as the subject and as a surrogate for his/her spouse, thus producing 84 total subject–surrogate pairs. For the 30 current or previous cigarette smokers whose spouses gave complete smoking data regarding the subjects, the subjects reported a mean use of 17.8 cigarettes per day compared with 14.3 reported by their spouses. The difference was not significant.

Investigations indicate that useful information on smoking can be obtained in epidemiologic investigations that must rely on surrogate information (McLaughlin et al. 1987). Although greater misclassification occurs when surrogate reports are used compared with self-reports, consideration of variables such as the relationship of the informant, length of time he or she had known the case, the topic of the questions, and complexity of the data gathered from the informant can add to the validity of the data (Rogot and Reid 1975).

Nonbehavioral Measures

Methods other than self-report have been used to assess smoking status. Some researchers have expressed concern that self-report when used alone can be an inaccurate measure that underestimates the amount of cigarettes smoked (Haley and Hoffmann 1985; Marsh et al. 1988; Warner 1978) because subjects often underreport levels of cigarette consumption or misrepresent themselves as former smokers (Luepker et al. 1989; Murray and Perry 1987; Windsor and Orleans 1986; Russell 1982; Stookey et al. 1987). Underreporting also has been linked to "digit bias," that is, subjects tend to report in terms of multiples of ten and underestimate actual consumption (Pechacek, Fox et al. 1984; Vogt 1977; US DHHS 1989).

Between 1974 and 1985, estimates of U.S. cigarette consumption based on self-report accounted for only about 70 percent of consumption estimates based on cigarettes taxed and sold (Hatziandreu et al. 1989). This ratio has remained relatively stable. Most of this discrepancy is likely to be due to underreporting or a "rounding down" to the nearest multiple of a half-pack of daily cigarette consumption (Kozlowski 1986), although misreporting of smoking status may play a role as well.

Validation of self-reports with measures such as biochemical assessments represents a possible means of decreasing misclassification due to misreporting (Luepker et al. 1989; Windsor and Orleans 1986). However, some researchers note that biochemical validation techniques present different problems that also cause misclassification, thus favoring the use of self-report (Assaf et al. 1989; Crossen, Dougher, Belew 1984; Hansen, Malotte, Fielding 1985; Hatziandreu et al. 1989; Kornitzer et al. 1983; Petitti, Friedman, Kahn 1981). As noted above, sensitivity and specificity of the biochemical measures are not perfect. In addition, the procurement of biochemical measures from a large majority of self-reported quitters is not as feasible in large-scale intervention trials or observational studies as it is in smoking studies of a smaller scale and a more clinical nature. Subjects in the population samples do not have the same commitment to studies that volunteers have to clinical studies, and the former are more likely to leave the study area, which makes validation difficult (Ockene et al. 1989). Validation also requires more personal contact than is generally employed in observational or large-scale field studies, and the additional contact may not be acceptable to the subjects or feasible in the context of the study.

The section below on physiologic measures discusses methods other than behavioral measures that have been used to assess cigarette smoke exposure. These measures are then contrasted with self-report, and the varying needs for biochemical measurement among different populations are considered.

Physiologic Measures

Smoking behavior has been assessed by measuring physiologic changes that result from smoking (Pechacek, Fox et al. 1984). Smoking and smoke exposure are reflected in a variety of acute and chronic physiologic measures primarily because of the strong pharmacologic effects of nicotine. These effects include changes in heart rate, blood pressure, hand tremor, and skin temperature. Each of these measures has a wide variability under normal conditions and is affected by many factors other than smoking, thus limiting usefulness as a measure of smoking (Pechacek, Fox et al. 1984).

Biochemical Markers

Cigarette smoke is a complex mixture of chemicals, some of which are present in the tobacco leaf and some of which result from chemical reactions during either the curing process or smoking (US DHEW 1979; US DHHS 1986, 1989). Three chemical constituents of tobacco smoke, carbon monoxide (CO), hydrogen cyanide (HCN), and nicotine, pass through cigarette filters and are present in inhaled tobacco smoke in concentrations high enough to be absorbed and detected in persons who smoke. These chemicals are measurable as intact compounds or as metabolic products.

Exposure to CO can be assessed in the blood as carboxyhemoglobin (COHb) or as CO in expired alveolar air. Methods are available for measuring cotinine, the primary metabolite of nicotine, and SCN^-, a metabolite of HCN, in urine, blood, and saliva. Other measures, such as skin-surface sampling for nicotine (Nanji and Lawrence 1988) are not as well established.

Extensive reviews of the literature on the use of biochemical markers as measures of smoking status are provided by Benowitz (1983), Haley and colleagues (1986), Lee (1988), Pechacek, Fox, and colleagues (1984), and Windsor and Orleans (1986). Cummings and Richard (1988) supplied a review of optimal cutoffs for the biochemical measures discussed here. This Section is not intended to provide an indepth review of the variability and biochemical rationale for these measures and will only provide an overview of the use of biochemical assessments for smoking status.

Terminology

Sensitivity and specificity, characteristics of a test such as a biochemical assessment, are measures of validity, the extent to which the test measures truth (Fletcher, Fletcher, Wagner 1987). Typically, sensitivity and specificity are determined by comparing the test results against a reference or "gold" standard. For smoking, self-reported status has most often been used as the standard for assessing biochemical markers. The sensitivity of a biochemical test for smoking exposure is the proportion of true smokers who are classified as smokers by the biochemical test. The specificity of a biochemical test for smoking exposure is the proportion of true nonsmokers who are classified as nonsmokers by the biochemical test. A test of 100-percent sensitivity and 100-percent specificity would perfectly discriminate true smokers from true nonsmokers. However, this degree of validity is not reached by any presently available biochemical marker. In addition, the standard to which biochemical measures are compared, typically self-reported smoking status, may be of limited validity, and thereby cause apparent sensitivity and specificity to be reduced.

When continuous measures are used to test for smoking status, a cutpoint must be chosen such that those individuals whose test value exceeds the cutpoint are classified as smokers and those with values below the cutpoint are classified as nonsmokers (Cummings and Richard 1988). The level at which the cutpoint is set determines the sensitivity and specificity of the test. Lowering the cutpoint improves the sensitivity at the expense of specificity. Raising it will improve specificity at the expense of sensitivity (Cole and Morrison 1980; Browner, Newman, Cummings 1988). Selecting a cutpoint depends on the relative importance of mislabeling an actual smoker as a nonsmoker with a very insensitive but specific test versus mislabeling an actual nonsmoker as a smoker with a very sensitive but nonspecific test. This tradeoff between sensitivity and specificity is discussed in more detail elsewhere (Fletcher, Fletcher, Wagner 1987).

An important contextual issue concerns the validity with which the biochemical measure classifies individuals. When the test is applied to a population of smokers and nonsmokers, the proportion of the persons who test positive, that is, above the specified cutpoint, who are actually smokers becomes an important concern. This issue, distinct from the question of what proportion of smokers are above the cutpoint, is the crucial measure of how much misclassification occurs. This proportion, the positive predictive value of a test, depends not only on specificity and sensitivity but also on the prevalence of the condition in the population being tested (smoking in this example). The less prevalent smoking is in the screened population the lower the positive predictive value of a test (Browner, Newman, Cummings 1988).

The relative misclassification rates for smokers and nonsmokers, determined in part by the estimated prevalence of smoking in the population to which the cutpoints are applied, are particularly important in studies which use biochemical tests to verify self-reported smoking cessation (Cummings and Richard 1988; Ruth and Neaton, in press). For example, the pressure to quit smoking that is present in formal smoking cessation programs may result in a high proportion of continuing smokers who report not smoking. The use of cotinine validation in such circumstances (high prevalence of false reporting) results in a high positive predictive value, as opposed to the lower positive predictive value when the same test is applied to self-reported former smokers identified in a population-based survey (low prevalence of false reporting).

In biochemical validation studies, such as those reported in a subsequent section of this Chapter, after optimal cutpoints are set using self-report in one population as the gold standard, the biochemical marker then becomes the gold standard against which self-reported smoking status is measured in another population.

Carbon Monoxide

High concentrations of CO are present in cigarette smoke (US DHEW 1979; US DHHS 1986, 1989). Absorbed rapidly into the bloodstream during smoke inhalation, CO has a half-life of 4 to 5 hours in sedentary adults (Stewart 1975). Direct measurements of CO can be taken from exhaled alveolar air or estimated by measuring the percentage of hemoglobin combined with CO (COHb) (Stewart 1975).

Sensitivity of exhaled CO for classifying active smoking is generally in the range of 80 to 85 percent but can be affected by diurnal variability as well as other factors (Benowitz 1983). Given the short half-life of CO, levels are influenced by time of day and time elapsed since last cigarette. Measurements taken late in the day, standardized from time since last cigarette, are likely to give the best estimates of CO levels (Frederiksen and Martin 1979; Horan, Hackett, Linberg 1978; Hughes, Frederiksen, Frazier 1976). Using self-report of recency of smoking can increase sensitivity (Bauman, Koch, Bryan 1982). Sensitivity is poor for light smokers (Fortmann et al.

1984; Vogt 1982), and specificity can be reduced by exposure to CO present in the environment as a result of industrial and automobile pollution, environmental tobacco smoke, indoor combustion sources, and use of products such as marijuana (Biglan et al. 1985; Frederiksen and Martin 1979; Stewart 1975). In spite of this, only 2 to 5 percent of nonsmokers in general populations will exceed 1 percent COHb (Janzon et al. 1981; Kahn et al. 1974). Using COHb levels from a national probability sample, the Radford and Drizd (1982) reported the 95th percentile for COHb to be 1.77 percent in nonsmokers, aged 12 to 74. If a 2-percent cutpoint is applied to this sample, 3.6 percent of nonsmokers would be incorrectly classified as smokers.

Thiocyanate

High concentrations of HCN, a toxic gas, are present in cigarette smoke. However, HCN is very active chemically and is rapidly detoxified by the liver into SCN^- (Langer and Greer 1977; Boxer and Rickards 1952). Because SCN^- accumulates in body fluids, such as saliva, urine, and blood, it is used as a biochemical measure of exposure to tobacco smoke. The biologic half-life of SCN^- has been found to vary quite a bit (Bliss and O'Connell 1984) although the length of time usually noted is between 10 and 14 days (Langer and Greer 1977; Vesey 1981). Salivary SCN^- can be measured most reliably in parotid gland secretions (Shannon, Suddick, Dowd 1974); however, parotid gland secretions show some seasonal and diurnal variability (Shannon, Suddick, Dowd 1974). When serum and saliva samples are compared, the levels are 15 to 20 times higher in saliva than serum (Langer and Greer 1977; Pechacek et al. 1979; Vesey 1981). However, saliva levels are more variable (Pechacek et al. 1979).

The increment of SCN^- in light smokers is low, and there is much overlap of SCN^- levels in light smokers compared with nonsmokers (Fortmann et al. 1984; Neaton et al. 1981; Vesey et al. 1981). However, detection of light smoking in adults using SCN^- levels is better than in adolescents (Windsor et al. 1985). This is likely to be related to the fact that adolescents are often in the process of learning how to smoke and inhale, and they may not have an established pattern of smoking (Pechacek, Murray et al. 1984). For example, among younger adolescents only one-third or less could be identified on a single assessment (Hunter, Webber, Berenson 1980; Luepker et al. 1989; Pechacek, Murray et al. 1984). Specificity represents a more severe problem than sensitivity. A large number of food products are sources of either cyanogenic glycosides (e.g., almonds, bamboo shoots, sugar cane) or naturally occurring SCN^- (e.g., cauliflower, broccoli, beer) and can produce levels of SCN^- in saliva equivalent to the average levels of smokers (Langer and Greer 1977; Neaton et al. 1981; Pechacek et al. 1979; Swan et al. 1985).

The relatively low specificity and sensitivity of SCN^- testing compared with cotinine and CO make SCN^- a less useful outcome measure for smoking cessation studies (Gillies et al. 1982; Fortmann et al. 1984) unless adjustments are made using carefully collected dietary and environmental exposure data. A prime advantage of using SCN^- for biochemical validation of smoking abstinence is its long half-life compared with other biochemical measures (Fortmann et al. 1984; Steinman 1985; Murray et al. 1987;

Pechacek, Fox et al. 1984), which is of particular interest in population surveys where longer term abstinence is of concern.

Cotinine

Cotinine, a metabolic byproduct of nicotine, is distributed throughout extracellular fluid and is excreted through the kidneys and salivary glands (Benowitz 1983). About 15 to 20 percent is eliminated in the urine unchanged, and the rest is metabolized (Benowitz 1983). The half-life estimates of cotinine are variable and range from 15 to 40 hours (Carey and Abrams 1988; Knight et al. 1985; Greenberg et al. 1984; Haley and Hoffmann 1985; Haley et al. 1987; Sepkovic, Haley, Hoffmann 1986). The differences in estimated half-life for cotinine reflect not only individual differences in metabolism but also differences between smokers and nonsmokers (Haley, Sepkovic, Hoffmann 1989; Sepkovic, Haley, Hoffmann 1986; Haley et al. 1987). Cotinine levels vary with the diurnal cycle and are best assessed late in the day (Benowitz 1983). Methods are available for measuring cotinine in saliva, urine, and blood. Urinary levels have been suggested to be too variable (Pechacek, Fox et al. 1984), and plasma or serum levels appear to be the most stable (Benowitz 1983). However, sampling saliva because of ease of procurement and accuracy in classifying smokers and nonsmokers has been recommended as a useful, noninvasive method that can be applied to large-scale intervention trials (Abrams et al. 1987).

Because nicotine is unique to tobacco, cotinine is a highly valid marker for almost any tobacco use (Haley, Axelrad, Tilton 1983; Russell et al. 1981; Wald et al. 1984; Zeidenberg et al. 1977). Although nicotine has been assessed in some studies, it is recommended that cotinine be used because it has a more enduring and stable blood level (Langone, Gjika, Van Vunakis 1973). Detecting regular smokers by analysis of cotinine in blood, urine, or saliva is almost certain, and even light smokers and intermittent smokers are easily detected (Benowitz 1983; Haley, Axelrad, Tilton 1983; Paxton and Bernacca 1979; Zeidenberg et al. 1977; Carey and Abrams 1988; Williams et al. 1979). In one investigation, 95 percent of adolescent ever smokers were detected by cotinine (Williams et al. 1979). Specificity is also high; regular smokers typically have blood cotinine levels of 200 to 400 ng/mL, light smokers have 40 to 50 ng/mL, and nonsmokers are typically below 10 ng/mL. When nonsmokers are assessed, they rarely have any detectable cotinine (Benowitz 1983; Haley, Axelrad, Tilton 1983; Sepkovic and Haley 1985; Zeidenberg et al. 1977).

In comparative studies of different biochemical measures of smoking, cotinine has emerged as the measure of choice (Abrams et al. 1987; Haley, Axelrad, Tilton 1983; Jarvis et al. 1984, 1987; Knight et al. 1985; Pojer et al. 1984) because of its superior sensitivity and specificity. However, it is more expensive and more analytically complex than the other biochemical measures.

The value of biochemical measures is limited to short-term abstinence and cannot be used to document continuous abstinence in long-term studies. CO, with a half-life of 4 to 5 hours, can validate self-reports of not having smoked in the past 24 to 48 hours (Benowitz 1983). Cotinine, with a half-life of 15 to 40 hours, would have limited application for validation beyond a few days. SCN^-, with a half-life of 10 to 14 days, has been used to validate self-reports of not having smoked in the past 7 days and may be useful to validate up to 3 to 4 weeks. However, specificity of this measure is low compared with cotinine and CO.

Bogus Pipeline

The bogus pipeline, an assertion to subjects that biochemical assessments will be used to assess smoking status when they will actually only be collected but not evaluated, is used mostly in research with adolescents. One of the reasons given by researchers for continuing to use biochemical verification for at least some proportion of the total subjects is the assertion that if the subjects believe biochemical validation will occur, they will be more likely to provide valid responses to self-report measures. This "bogus pipeline effect" was first presented by Evans, Hansen, and Mittelmark (1977) from the work of Jones and Sigall (1971) concerning smoking among adolescents. It is believed that there is great pressure among adolescents to misreport smoking activities. Murray and coworkers (1987) provided an extensive review of this aspect.

Murray and Perry (1987) attempted to determine the conditions under which a bogus pipeline will be effective by manipulating conditions of anonymity. They demonstrated that a bogus pipeline for adolescents is more likely to have an effect if there is an expectation that subjects would otherwise perceive large amounts of pressure to report not smoking and there is a credible pipeline message. However, their findings suggest that an effective procedure to ensure anonymity can reduce this pressure and likewise reduce the need for the pipeline.

Contextual Issues Affecting Biochemical Assessment

The accuracy of self-report measures, the desirability for behavioral or biochemical validation of self-report, and the type of assessment needed are issues that need to be considered in the context of the type of study, the nature and size of the study sample, and possible refusal problems.

The nature of the subject sample can affect the likelihood of misreporting and therefore the desirability of validation by biochemical assessment. In Table 1, studies demonstrating misreporting rates for individuals who report cessation but who are assessed to be smokers by cotinine or nicotine measurement are classified into three types of subjects: untreated volunteer samples, intervention samples, and high-risk for disease and/or medical patients. Table 2 presents a similar classification of studies demonstrating misreporting with CO validation. The tables are adapted from Lee's work (1988) with the inclusion of additional studies. In cases where multiple cutoff criteria are recorded, the values closest to the optimal cutoff are reported. Several studies should be viewed as outliers and are noted in the tables. These studies reported unusually high rates of individuals who reported not smoking but were above the cutpoint and also employed cutoff criteria far below optimum cutpoints (Cummings and Richard 1988).

For untreated volunteer samples, the mode for individuals classified as smokers by biochemical assessment who reported not smoking is zero, and no sample exceeds 5

TABLE 1.—Measures of false reports of not smoking from studies using nicotine and cotinine as a marker

Reference	Population	Told to give up	Criterion for false reports of not smoking	% (n/N) False reports	Comments
Part I. Volunteer samples					
Russell and Feyerabend (1975)	London smokers, nonsmokers, and heavy passive smokers	No	Urinary nicotine	0 (0/27)	No overlap between range of urinary nicotine levels of smokers (N=18) and nonsmokers (N=27)
Williams et al. (1979)	Students health screening	No	Plasma cotinine	2 (2/98)	
Haley, Axelrad, Tilton (1983)	New York nonsmoking volunteers	No	Salivary or plasma cotinine	0 (0/18)	No cutpoint established; no cotinine detected in nonsmokers
Wald et al. (1984)	Nonsmokers attending BUPA[a], and Oxford colleagues	No	256 ng/mL urinary cotinine	0.9 (2/221)	Cutpoint based on distribution
Haddow, Palomaki, Knight (1986)	US women attending well-women screening	No	30 ng/mL serum cotinine 10 ng/mL serum cotinine	1.3 (3/232) 2.2 (5/232)	
Coultas et al. (1987)	New Mexico Hispanic children and adults in household survey	No	50 ng/mL salivary cotinine	3.2 (43/1,360)	46.3% of sample below age 18 yr
Lee (1987)	Representative UK sample providing saliva, without prior warning, after smoking data	No	30 ng/mL salivary cotinine 10 ng/mL salivary cotinine	2.5 (20/808) 4.2 (34/808)	
Nanji and Lawrence (1988)	Lab sample	No	1 μg/mL skin nicotine	0 (0/43)	
Pierce et al. (1987)	Sydney, Melbourne smokers	No	250 nmol/L salivary cotinine	4.0 (25/622)	

TABLE 1.—Continued

Reference	Population	Told to give up	Criterion for false reports of not smoking	% (n/N) False reports	Comments
Part II. Intervention samples					
Russell et al. (1979)	London smokers attending general practices in intervention trial	Yes	Salivary nicotine	7.1 (1/14)	No cutpoint established; length of followup not stated
Paxton (1980)	UK smokers assigned to various stop treatments	Yes	Urinary nicotine	n=2, N<60	Study began with 60 subjects; 2 false reports of not smoking detected; cutpoint not established; 6-mo followup
Jamrozik, Vessey et al. (1984)[b]	UK smokers attending general practitioners in trial of various antismoking interventions	Some groups	100 ng/mL urinary cotinine	23.9 (11/46)	If nonparticipants considered as false reports of not smoking, then 39.7% (23/58) gave erroneous reports; 1-yr followup
Russell et al. (1987)[b]	UK smokers attending general practitioners in trial of effects of brief intervention and support of a smokers' clinic	Some groups	50 μg/L urinary cotinine	38.8 (57/147)	1-yr followup
Abrams et al. (1987)	Smokers/nonsmokers in worksite cessation program	Yes	10 ng/mL salivary cotinine	9.1 (1/11)	Self-reported abstainers; 8-wk followup
Stookey et al. (1987)	Cessation study	Yes	10 ng/mL salivary cotinine	Nonsmokers 0 (0/20) Former smokers 45.1 (46/102)	Length of followup not stated

TABLE 1.—Continued

Reference	Population	Told to give up	Criterion for false reports of not smoking	% (n/N) False reports	Comments
Part III. High-risk/medical patients					
Wilcox, Hughes, Roland (1979)	Nottingham MI patients	Yes	2 µg/100 mL urinary nicotine or 10 µg/100 mL urinary cotinine	16.3 (8/49)	An additional 5 subjects had detectable levels in concentrations below the cutpoint
Jarvis et al. (1987)	Clinic outpatients	No	13.7 ng/mL serum cotinine	19 (23/121)	
		No	14.2 ng/mL salivary cotinine	18 (22/121)	
		No	49.7 ng/mL urinary cotinine	17 (21/121)	
		No	21.8 ng/mL salivary nicotine	14 (17/121)	
		No	2.3 ng/mL plasma nicotine	14 (17/121)	
		No	58.6 ng/mL urinary nicotine	16 (19/121)	
Haddow et al. (1987)	US pregnant women	No	10 ng/mL serum	4.9 (142/2,871)	Unpublished data

NOTE: n/N=number of individuals reporting not smoking but with levels of biochemical marker exceeding cutpoint divided by all individuals reporting not smoking; MI=myocardial infarction.
[a] British United Providence Association Medical Center in London.
[b] Studies classified as outliers due to low criterion cutoffs.
SOURCE: Adapted from Lee (1988).

TABLE 2.—Measures of false reports from studies using CO as a marker

Reference	Population	Told to give up	Criterion for false reports of not smoking	% (n/N) False reports	Comments
Part I. Volunteer samples					
Jones, Commins, Cernik (1972)	London taxi drivers	No	6.6% COHb	4.8 (1/21)	
Petitti, Friedman, Kahn (1981)	Californians having health checkups, 176 female twins and 91 males	No	8 ppm CO	0.6 (1/181)	
Jarvis et al. (1987)	Clinic outpatients	No No	10 ppm CO (expired air) 1.7% CO (Hb)	16 (19/121) 18 (22/121)	
Bauman, Koch, Bryan (1982)	Adolescent nonclinic setting	No	6 ppm CO (expired air) 8 ppm CO (expired air)	0 3	
Stookey et al. (1987)	Cessation study	Yes	8 ppm	0 (0/20)	
Fortmann et al. (1984)	Representative sample for cardiovascular risk study	No	8 ppm	4.2 (37/890)	
Part II. Intervention samples					
Delarue (1973)	Canadians attending voluntary antismoking clinic	Yes	2% COHb 4% COHb 6% COHb	20.6 (22/107) 9.3 (10/107) 4.7 (5/107)	1-yr followup

TABLE 2—Continued

Reference	Population	Told to give up	Criterion for false reports of not smoking	% (n/N) False reports	Comments
Ohlin, Lundh, Westling (1976)[a]	Swedish patients with smoking-related diseases attending antismoking clinic and given nicotine gum	Yes	0.8% COHb	19.2 (25/130) 32.1 (35/109)	19.2% false reports at 1-wk followup; 32.1% false reports of not smoking at 6-mo followup
Isacsson and Janzon (1976)	Swedish heavy smokers in quit-smoking research project	Yes	1% COHb	8.8 (3/34)	8–9-wk followup
Lando (1982)	US smokers in multigroup smoking cessation study	Yes	CO	0 (0/22 to 60)	1-yr followup
Malcolm et al. (1980)[a,b]	UK trial of nicotine chewing gum	Yes	1.6% COHb	41.6 (47/113)	1-mo followup
Raw et al. (1980)	UK smokers attending a smokers' clinic in comparison of psychologic treatment and use of nicotine gum	Yes	CO or COHb	0 (0/33)	1-yr followup
Lando (1981)	US smokers in multigroup smoking cessation study	Yes	CO	Between 1.4 (1/74) and 4.2 (1/24)	Not clear when 1 "deceiver" withdrew from study; 1-wk (1/74) to 1-yr (1/24) followup; abstinence status also based on reports of informants
Jarvis et al. (1982)	UK smokers attending a smokers' clinic in trial of nicotine gum	Yes	CO or COHb	0 (0/26)	1-yr followup

TABLE 2.—Continued

Reference	Population	Told to give up	Criterion for false reports of not smoking	% (n/N) False reports	Comments
Russell et al. (1987)	UK smokers attending general practitioners	Some groups	7 ppm CO	About 22	4-mo to 1-yr followup
Glasgow et al. (1984)	US worksite smoking control study	Yes	10 ppm CO	0 (0/4)	6-mo followup
Jamrozik, Fowler et al. (1984)[a]	UK smokers in trial of nicotine gum	Yes	12 ppm CO	28.0 (7/25)	6-mo followup
Clavel et al. (1985)	French trial of acupuncture and nicotine gum	Yes	5 ppm CO	0 (0/24)	Sample of study participants (N=24); 1-yr followup
Lando and McGovern (1985)	US subjects undergoing various treatments for eliminating smoking	Yes	CO	2 cases out of at most 90	Up to 2-mo followup
Richmond and Webster (1985)	Australian smokers in a general practice; randomized trial of effects of advice to give up	Test group	COHb, SCN⁻, cotinine in plasma, and reports by family and friends	5.7 (2/35)	Criteria not stated; 6-mo followup
Abrams et al. (1987)	Worksite cessation	Yes	<9 ppm CO (expired air)	11.1 (1/9)	8-wk followup
Glynn, Gruder, Jegerski (1986)	Chicago Lung Association cessation study	Yes	10 ppm CO (expired air)	15.6 (7/45)	4-wk followup
Part III. High-risk/medical patients					
Li et al. (1984)	US asbestos-exposed smokers receiving (1) behavioral counseling or (2) minimal warning	Yes	9 ppm CO	1: 22.2 (4/18) 2: 23.1 (3/13)	11-mo followup

TABLE 2.—Continued

Reference	Population	Told to give up	Criterion for false reports of not smoking	% (n/N) False reports	Comments
Vogt et al. (1977)	San Francisco Center of MRFIT	Yes	8 ppm CO	4.4 (2/45)	
Sillett et al. (1978)[a]	UK study in 2 groups: (A) survivors of MI and (B) volunteers in nicotine gum trial	Yes	1.7% COHb	A: 21.6 (11/51) B: 40.2 (33/82)	
Ronan et al. (1981)	Irish post-MI patients	Yes	1.6% COHb	8.8 (5/57)	Mean 8.6-yr followup
Research Committee of the British Thoracic Society (1983)[a]	UK patients with smoking-related diseases in 4 group intervention trials involving advice, booklet, placebo, and nicotine polacrilex gum	All groups	1.6% COHb and 73 µmol/L SCN⁻ in plasma	27 25	27% false reports rate at 6-mo followup; 25% false reports rate at 1-yr followup

NOTE: CO=carbon monoxide; n/N=number of individuals reporting not smoking but with levels of biochemical marker exceeding cutpoint divided by all individuals reporting not smoking; COHb=carboxyhemoglobin; ppm=parts/million; SCN⁻=thiocyanate; MRFIT=Multiple Risk Factor Intervention Trial; MI=myocardial infarction.
[a]Studies classified as outliers due to low criterion cutoffs.
[b]May be same group as (B) in Sillett et al. (1978).
SOURCE: Adapted from Lee (1988).

percent for either cotinine or CO. For intervention studies, values are typically 2 to 5 percent for cotinine and 0 to 10 percent for CO. High risk/medical samples appear to have the highest rates of misclassification of former smokers with the rates exceeding 20 percent. For example, as shown in Table 1, Jarvis and colleagues (1987) reported very low rates (1 percent) of false reporting in vascular patients who were not advised to quit compared with the rate in high-risk patients who were advised to quit (17 percent). It is likely that the pressure to stop smoking influenced the accuracy of patient reporting.

Observation studies in which no intervention occurs, or intervention studies in which there is minimal intervention or interaction with smokers, are less likely to prompt false reports of smoking cessation than studies in which intensive intervention does occur. In the former types of studies, in which no or low-intensity intervention occurred, there was a much lower prevalence of subjects reporting a 24-hour quit attempt during the past 6 months or current abstinence (Prochaska et al. 1985) than in intensive intervention studies, making misreporting less likely. A greater tendency to misreport in no or low-intensity intervention studies might occur with adolescents, for whom pressures to report not smoking may be omnipresent (Pechacek, Murray et al. 1984; Chapter 2, see section on Bogus Pipeline). A similar pressure might occur in some other instances, such as worksites in which a ban has been placed on smoking, where no intervention occurs but there may still be pressure on individuals to misreport. However, no studies have looked at the possibility of misreporting in such instances. The context in which the study takes place is likely to influence the degree of misreporting. Data currently being collected from smoking cessation programs in a wide variety of contexts may help to clarify this issue.

Clinic interventions and intensive interventions, on the other hand, typically ask participants to set a quit date. Close relationships are developed with the counselors, and self-reports of quitting are often given initially in a peer group. Under these higher demand conditions, biochemical verification may be needed to decrease the misreporting of current smokers as former smokers. For example, in MRFIT, special intervention subjects claiming to be former smokers at followup examinations had mean SCN^- levels between those of never smokers and continuing smokers (Ockene et al. 1982). Similar discrepancies between reported and validated cessation rates did not occur for the usual care men who had not received intensive intervention.

The use of biochemical tests for validating self-reports in epidemiologic studies has a number of limitations. The tests do not have perfect sensitivity and specificity; their half-lives do not necessarily fit the timeframe to be covered; and not all subjects are willing to provide the necessary samples for assessment. A very sensitive test may misclassify subjects as smokers if they have heavy passive smoke exposure (DiGuisto and Eckhard 1986; Haddow, Palomaki, Knight 1986; Haley et al. 1989; Jarvis et al. 1985), smoke occasionally (i.e., 1 or 2 cigarettes on isolated occasions) (Williams et al. 1979), and/or use nicotine in some other form, such as nicotine polacrilex gum or smokeless tobacco (Cohen et al. 1988; Slattery et al. 1989). Biochemical markers are also limited because they assess relatively short-term cessation (less than 2 weeks), and in studies concerned with the impact of cessation on health, there is more interest in evaluating consequences of long-term cessation.

In large-scale studies, use of biochemical assessments is generally not feasible; thus, mandatory use of such assessments and subsequent classification of refusers as smokers (as suggested by some investigators involved in clinical intervention studies e.g., Windsor and Orleans 1986) would result in an unacceptable distortion of the outcome data. In addition, some subjects may drop out if validation is required. The effect of lost subjects on study results may be difficult to estimate. In contexts other than intensive intervention trials, self-reported smoking status at the time of measurement and concurrent biochemical assessment have been demonstrated to be highly concordant (Fortmann et al. 1984; Petitti, Friedman, Kahn 1981) (Tables 1 and 2). This high concordance supports the use of self-report as a valid measure of smoking status in observation studies of the health effects of smoking cessation.

PART II. ASSESSING THE CONSEQUENCES OF SMOKING CESSATION

Study Designs Used to Assess the Consequences of Cessation

Overview of Study Design

Most evidence on the health benefits of smoking cessation derives from studies of human populations and not from animal studies or other types of research. Research on humans can be classified as experimental (the investigator assigns subjects to be exposed or not exposed to the risk factors or preventive factors of interest) or observational (the investigator does not determine whether subjects are exposed or not exposed to the factors of interest; exposure reflects the subjects' choices or some other process). Intervention studies include randomized or nonrandomized community-based investigations and clinical trials. The clinical trial, involving randomization of subjects to be exposed or not exposed to an intervention, has been used to investigate the effects of smoking cessation in patient groups and in populations. The observational designs include the ecologic study, the cross-sectional study, the cohort study, and the case–control study.

The biases potentially affecting these studies can be broadly classified as selection bias, information bias, and confounding bias (Table 3) (Kleinbaum, Kupper, Morgenstern 1982). Selection bias refers to distortion of an exposure–disease relationship by the mechanism through which subjects are selected. Information bias arises from the incorrect categorization of subjects as exposed or not exposed or as diseased or not diseased. The resulting misclassification of subjects on exposure or disease status may occur in a random or nonrandom fashion (Chapter 2, Part I). Confounding bias refers to the distortion of the apparent effect of an exposure on risk caused by association with other factors that affect outcome (Last 1988). In the subsequent review of the study designs used to assess the benefits of smoking cessation, sources of bias most relevant to each design are highlighted.

TABLE 3.—Examples of potential methodologic problems in investigating the health consequences of smoking cessation

Problem	Consequences
Current smokers developing symptoms of disease quit smoking	Apparent benefits of cessation are reduced
Self-reported former smokers are actually smoking (information bias)	Apparent benefits of cessation are reduced
Former smokers tend to have smoked less than persistent smokers (confounding bias)	Failure to account for the difference may exaggerate the apparent benefits of cessation
Former smokers tend to have a healthier lifestyle than persistent smokers (confounding bias)	Failure to account for the difference may exaggerate the apparent benefits of cessation
Smoking practices and the presence of smoking-related diseases affect participation in studies (selection bias)	Apparent benefits of cessation may be increased or decreased
Small number of subjects in a study	A beneficial effect of cessation may not reach statistical significance

Ecologic Studies

Ecologic studies represent a descriptive approach for examining the relation between risk factors and disease. Groups, rather than individuals, are the unit of analysis in ecologic studies. For example, changes in lung cancer mortality rates for selected countries have been examined for correlation with changes in measures of smoking for those countries, such as the percentage of smokers or per capita cigarette consumption (US PHS 1964; Cairns 1975; Cummings 1984; Doll and Peto 1981). Ecologic studies often have the advantage of being performed inexpensively and feasibly by using already available data. This design has well-described limitations related to the estimation of exposure and control of confounding, and may yield seriously biased data on exposure–disease relationships (Kleinbaum, Kupper, Morgenstern 1982; Rothman 1986).

Cross-Sectional Studies

In a cross-sectional or prevalence study, exposure and outcome are assessed at the same point in time among individuals in a population. Because cross-sectional studies measure exposure and outcome variables simultaneously, the true temporal relation between exposure and disease may be obscured (Rothman 1986). However, cross-sectional studies can be readily performed and have supplied much of the evidence on smoking cessation and nonmalignant respiratory diseases (Chapter 7).

Cross-sectional studies may be affected by selection bias. Because cigarette smoking is a strong cause of disease and death, groups studied cross-sectionally may not accurately reflect the natural history of smoking, smoking cessation, and the development of smoking-related illness. The proportion of heavier smokers and more susceptible smokers may be reduced compared with the original birth cohorts giving rise to the cross-sectional study population (McLaughlin et al. 1987). Former smokers who stopped because of the development of disease may be underrepresented, whereas those who stopped to reduce the risk of illness may be overrepresented.

Information bias is also of potential importance in cross-sectional studies. Preexisting conditions in survey participants may affect recall of past smoking or may alter the approach used by interviewers to gather smoking information. However, as summarized in Tables 1 and 2, cross-sectional surveys generally demonstrate low rates of misreporting of smoking status when compared with cotinine and CO levels.

As mentioned previously, a single observation on smoking behavior may lead to misclassification of smokers because of the dynamic nature of smoking behavior. Former smokers are typically a heterogeneous group with periods of abstinence ranging from days to years. For example, in the 1986 Adult Use of Tobacco Survey (US DHHS 1989), the subjects' responses were classified in 10 categories, 4 of which included former smokers. Of the former smokers, 12.5 percent had quit within the past 3 months, 7.8 percent had quit in the past 3 to 12 months, 22.3 percent had quit in the past 1 to 5 years, and 57.4 percent had quit 5 or more years earlier.

Cohort Studies

In a cohort study, the subjects are selected on the basis of exposure status (e.g., smoking behavior) and observed for development of disease. Observation may be forward in time (prospective), backward in time (historical or retrospective), or both. Correct conclusions can usually be made about the temporal relation between exposure (smoking cessation) and outcome (reduction of morbidity or mortality). With the cohort design, multiple health outcomes can be considered simultaneously. For example, the CPS-I and CPS-II conducted by the American Cancer Society (ACS) examined the effect of smoking behavior on total mortality and specific causes of death.

In a study of smoking cessation, selection bias could affect the findings of cohort studies if subjects lost to observation were more or less likely to benefit from smoking cessation than subjects remaining under observation (Greenland 1977). For intervention studies and cohort studies, the rate of subject loss provides an index of the potential selection bias.

In a cohort study of smoking cessation, some misclassification of exposure may be introduced if the classification of smoking status is based on a single assessment. Although the categorization of smoking status may be correct at the time the information is collected, inevitably some former smokers will resume smoking and some current smokers will stop. The extent of the resulting error will increase with the duration of followup. The resulting misclassification will tend to underestimate the effects of quitting because those who relapse to become current smokers would not be expected to experience beneficial effects attributable to quitting.

For example, in ACS CPS-I involving nearly 1 million people, Hammond and Garfinkel (1969) studied changes in smoking status over a 2-year period. Male former cigarette smokers in 1959–60 who reported that they were smoking in 1961–62 varied according to duration of prolonged abstinence reported in the 1959–60 survey. For respondents abstinent less than 1 year in 1959–60, 37.3 percent reported smoking 2 years later; of those reporting abstinence for 1 to 2 years, 19.1 percent were smoking 2 years later; and of those reporting abstinence of more than 2 years, 4.6 percent were smoking 2 years later. For all males who were former smokers in 1959–60, 11.3 percent reported smoking 2 years later. For all female former smokers in 1959–60, 6 percent reported smoking 2 years later. In the U.S. Veterans Study (Rogot and Murray 1980; Kahn 1966), male veterans in a cohort of 248,846 were classified based on responses to questionnaires administered in 1954 or in 1957 (if the 1954 questionnaire was not returned) and then followed for 16 years to determine the relationship between tobacco use and mortality. Undoubtedly, many of the original current smokers became former smokers as a result of the strong trend of smoking cessation among U.S. males during the followup period (US DHHS 1989).

Repeated assessment of smoking status in a cohort study can mitigate misclassification due to changes in smoking status over time (Chapter 2, Part I). Repeated measures are often feasibly made in cohort studies to minimize the effects of misclassification. Alternatively, validation substudies can be conducted within the cohort to quantify misclassification errors (Greenland 1988).

Case–Control Studies

Case–control studies involve selection of study subjects based on the presence (cases) or absence (controls) of a disease. Exposure and other attributes of cases and controls (e.g., smoking status or lifetime cigarette consumption) are then measured. The groups are compared with respect to the proportion having the attribute of interest to calculate the exposure odds ratio, which estimates the relative risk associated with exposure. Case–control studies can generally be conducted in less time than cohort studies or intervention studies and are less expensive to perform. Case–control studies are well suited for evaluation of diseases with low incidence rates.

Case–control analyses may be affected by information bias and selection bias. Case–control studies are prone to information bias if lifetime exposure histories are collected by interview (Schlesselman 1982). Retrospective lifetime histories of smoking or other exposures obtained from ill or elderly subjects may introduce misclassification. Similarly, studies that rely on reports from surrogates to assess smoking may misclassify exposure. If individuals classified as cases recall more accurately or less accurately than those classified as controls, differential misclassification results (Gordis 1982). Differential misclassification may also be introduced if respondents deliberately falsify answers or if interviewers differentially gather information from cases and controls (interviewer bias); interviewers not blinded to case–control status may probe more intensely for a putative causal exposure in cases than in controls (Sackett 1979). Blinding is often not feasible, and meticulous attention must be directed to training interviewers and to designing questionnaires to remove the possibility of interviewer bias. Although selection bias may affect any case–control study that is not population-based, it is unlikely to be of particular importance in most case–control studies of smoking cessation.

Intervention Trials

Intervention trials are designed to test a hypothesized cause–effect relationship or the benefits of a preventive program by modifying the putative causal or preventive factor and measuring the effect on relevant outcome measures. Intervention trials may be directed at individuals or groups, such as communities. Regardless of the unit of observation, the trials may be conducted with (e.g., a clinical trial) or without randomization to the intervention.

Clinical trials are most commonly used to assess therapeutic interventions, but this design has also been used to evaluate preventive interventions, such as smoking cessation. A clinical trial includes one or more comparison groups in which subjects receive the control intervention; subjects are randomly assigned to the treatment and comparison groups to ensure that the groups are comparable with respect to characteristics potentially affecting the outcomes of interest. Individuals or groups such as communities can be the units of randomization. Within the limits of chance, random assignment makes the intervention and control groups similar at the onset of study.

Although widely used to test smoking cessation methods, clinical trials have been used infrequently to assess the health benefits of smoking cessation. In comparison with observation studies, the clinical trial design offers the potential for eliminating or more tightly controlling bias from the selection of subjects and from confounding. However, for many health outcomes, both a large sample size and a lengthy followup period may be needed to have sufficient statistical power. Moreover, in a study of smoking cessation, the power of the trial also depends on the extent of the reduction in smoking in the intervention group, in comparison with the control group. In the reported smoking intervention trials, only a minority of participants attained continuous or prolonged abstinence following most cessation interventions (Hunt, Barnett, Branch 1971; Hunt and Bespalec 1973; Ockene et al. 1990). Even with intensive, prolonged interventions, as in MRFIT, only 42 percent of smokers within the special intervention group were not smoking at 6-year followup, and only 26 percent of baseline smokers had been continuously abstinent from cigarettes over this prolonged period (Ockene et al. 1990).

Only a few clinical trials provide information relevant to the health benefits of cessation (Chapter 3). In the Whitehall Civil Servants Study (Rose et al. 1982), the investigators randomly intervened in smoking with advice from a physician in a group of men at high risk for cardiopulmonary disease. In MRFIT, smoking intervention was one component of the risk factor intervention program directed at the special intervention group (MRFIT Research Group 1982).

In most clinical trials that assess the effect of cessation on disease outcomes, such as the Whitehall Civil Servants Study (Rose et al. 1982), the investigators did not monitor longitudinally the persistence of quitting or levels of biochemical markers. The only clinical trial that has provided these measures is MRFIT (Ockene et al. 1990). Although maintained cessation rates were significantly greater in the special intervention than in the usual care group, to date the difference has not been large enough to provide adequate statistical power to assess the effect of smoking cessation alone on differences in morbidity and mortality between the intervention and control groups (Chapter 3). However, MRFIT was designed as a multifactor trial and did not assess the impact of smoking cessation alone. Because MRFIT results indicated the greatest difference in smoking cessation between special intervention and usual care subjects compared with any other clinical trial and still lacked the power to detect outcome differences from smoking cessation, it is unlikely that smaller trials would have sufficient power to demonstrate an effect of cessation on morbidity and mortality (Chapter 3) (US DHHS 1983).

Compared with observational studies which place few demands directly on subjects, the use of interventions for smoking cessation in clinical trials increases the probability of misreporting smoking status at postintervention followup because of the expectations of the participants and the investigators. Typical periodic followup in clinical trials, however, reduces the chances of misclassification related to relapses or to delayed action to quit smoking—phenomena that are often not adequately recorded in observational studies. Routine followup also allows for more accurate measurements of the duration of prolonged or continuous abstinence and the opportunity to validate with biochemical testing.

Intervention trials other than clinical trials also provide information on the health consequences of smoking cessation. A number of studies are in progress involving interventions of varying intensity within a community. The North Karelia project conducted in Finland is such a community trial; a comprehensive, community-based intervention program was conducted to reduce cardiovascular disease (CVD) (Tuomilehto et al. 1986). Mortality rates in North Karelia were compared with those in other areas of Finland.

Methodologic Issues

Introduction

Epidemiologic studies have been the principal source of information on the health benefits of smoking cessation. Although the resulting data have provided strong evidence for the benefits of cessation, the data need to be interpreted with consideration of potential sources of bias and of other methodologic issues. This Section considers the methodologic issues potentially affecting interpretation of studies of the health consequences of smoking cessation. The criteria for causality have served as a basis for evaluating all of the evidence relevant to a particular association (US PHS 1964; US DHHS 1982, 1989). However, associations found in individual studies must also be assessed carefully. In any epidemiologic or clinical study, association may result by chance, as the result of bias, or through a causal mechanism. Thus, this Section presents an overview of statistical considerations relevant to studies of smoking cessation and the most prominent sources of bias in such studies—information bias and confounding bias. It also considers the potentially complex problem of analyzing data on the effects of smoking cessation.

Statistical Considerations

Statistical significance testing addresses the likelihood that an observed association has occurred by chance if, in fact, exposure and disease are unassociated (the null hypothesis). By convention, probability (p) values less than 0.05 are generally accepted as "statistically significant"; that is, chance is considered an unlikely explanation for the association. For example, if the p value is less than 0.05, the probability that chance explains the association is less than 5 percent. Confidence intervals describe the range of effects compatible with the data at some specified level of probability, for example 95 percent.

Some studies find associations that do not attain statistical significance. "Negative" investigations must be interpreted in the context of an investigation's sample size; a small sample size may not provide sufficient information to test associations in the range of interest. Such small sample sizes often provide inadequate statistical power to test for the anticipated effects of smoking cessation, and such studies are uninformative as a result. In interpreting associations not achieving statistical significance, confidence limits describe the range of effect compatible with the data.

Bias

In any epidemiologic study, associations may be affected by bias. Biases from misclassification and from confounding need to be considered in interpreting the findings of studies of the consequences of smoking cessation. This Section focuses on the effects of these biases in studies of smoking cessation.

Categorizing the dynamic process of smoking cessation poses a substantial challenge to epidemiologic researchers (Chapter 2, Part I). Moreover, subjects may not accurately report their own smoking behavior, and reliance on surrogate sources of information on smoking, as may be necessary in case–control studies, may also introduce error.

The consequences of misclassification in observation studies have received substantial consideration in the epidemiologic literature (Copeland et al. 1977; Greenland 1980; Fleiss 1981; Kleinbaum, Kupper, Morgenstern 1982; Schlesselman 1982; Rothman 1986). Misclassification can occur in classifying either exposure or outcome. Only exposure misclassification, that is smoking status, will be considered in this Section (Chapter 2, Part I).

Misclassification may be classified as nondifferential (or random) or as differential; both types of misclassification are potentially relevant to studies of smoking cessation. Nondifferential misclassification occurs randomly in relation to disease or outcome status, whereas differential misclassification affects exposure information in a pattern that varies with outcome status. For example, differential misclassification would occur in a case–control study of lung cancer if cases tended to minimize the extent of past smoking in comparison with the information given by controls; elderly cases and controls might introduce nondifferential misclassification from errors in recall of past smoking.

The consequences of nondifferential and differential misclassification have been addressed in the epidemiologic literature. Bross (1954) is credited with demonstrating that random misclassification in a 2x2 contingency table diminishes an association that exists between two variables; in general for such cross-classified data, nondifferential misclassification of exposure biases toward the null value, indicating no effect of eposure (Rothman 1986). For exposures classified into three or more levels, the consequencs of nondifferential misclassification are not exclusively directed toward reducing the degree of association. Differential misclassification may either strengthen or weaken associations, depending on the direction of the bias in reporting exposure (Kleinbaum, Kupper, Morgenstern 1982; Rothman 1986).

The information presented in prior sections of this Cnapter describes the directions that bias may take and allows some generalizations. First, some degree of nondifferential misclassification may affect studies of active smoking and of smoking cessation; the extent of misclassification depends on the type of information collected, the choice of respondents (index subject or surrogate), and the health and age of the respondents. Second, because disease is present at the time of interview, nondifferential misclassification is particularly likely to affect exposure information collected in cross-sectional studies and case–control studies, but little empirical evidence is available. Third, because of the dynamic nature of smoking cessation, some current and former smokers will be misclassified in cohort studies and clinical trials unless smoking behaviors are measured with sufficient frequency during followup.

For example, MRFIT data illustrate the potential for misclassification of current and former smokers as smoking status changes over time if smoking status is not longitudinally assessed (Ockene et al. 1990). The usual care group included 4,091 smokers at baseline with 12.7 percent reporting quitting by the first annual followup visit. Of those first-year quitters, only about half or 6.3 percent of all usual care smokers maintained abstinence for the entire 6-year followup period ("continued stoppers"). However in each year of followup, additional smokers quit ("new stoppers") at a maximum rate of 7.5 percent between the first and second years, decreasing to the lowest rate of 4.2 percent between the fifth and sixth years. Simultaneously, smokers who quit and relapsed during the trial succeeded in quitting in subsequent followup periods ("recycled stoppers"). Recycled stoppers increased from 5.3 percent of the usual care baseline smokers in the third year to 15.3 percent at the end of the sixth year. By the sixth year of the study, 25.8 percent of the usual care group were classified as former smokers; 6.3 percent stopped during the first year and maintained abstinence for the remaining 6-year followup period; 15.3 percent stopped, relapsed, and stopped again; and 4.2 percent stopped for the first time in the last year of followup. Although the usual care group is not representative of adult male smokers, these data illustrate the dynamics of smoking behavior and the potential for misclassification.

Incorrect categorization of some current smokers as former smokers and of some former smokers as current smokers, if nondifferential, would tend to reduce the apparent benefit of smoking cessation, as disease occurrence is reduced in the category of apparent current smokers by the inclusion of former smokers and is increased in the category of apparent former smokers by the inclusion of current smokers. Stratification by the duration of abstinence may provide some control of this type of misclassification.

The category of never smokers in an epidemiologic study may include some persons who smoked in the past (Britten 1988; Persson and Norell 1989). In general, former smokers who reported themselves as never smokers consumed fewer cigarettes than those correctly categorizing themselves as former smokers. Nevertheless, the bias resulting from the inclusion of some former smokers in the category of never smokers would tend to reduce the apparent benefit of cessation when former smokers are compared with never smokers.

The consequences of misclassification must be considered in the context of the disease under investigation. For example, in studying lung cancer and smoking cessation, the failure of long-term former smokers to report a brief period of relapse has little relevance. In contrast, unreported periods of relapse would be relevant in assessing smoking cessation and occurrence of myocardial infarction or of respiratory symptoms, conditions for which cessation has some short-term benefit.

Bias from confounding is also of concern in studies of the health consequences of smoking cessation. Former smokers tend to differ from continuing smokers in the earlier intensity of cigarette smoking and in other aspects of lifestyle that may determine disease risk. Former smokers tend to have smoked fewer cigarettes per day and to have started smoking at an older age than continuing smokers (Friedman et al. 1979; Garvey et al. 1983; Myers et al. 1987; Volume Appendix). Thus, at any age, former smokers have had less cumulative exposure to cigarette smoke, on average, than continuing smokers. Failure to account appropriately for differences in cumulative exposure between former smokers and continuing smokers may exaggerate the benefits of cessation. Misclassification of smoking measures may limit the degree to which confounding can be controlled (Greenland 1980; Rothman 1986).

Other differences between former smokers and current smokers may also influence disease risk. Former smokers are more likely to be of higher socioeconomic status than continuing smokers and tend to follow a healthier lifestyle than persistent smokers (Chapter 11 and Volume Appendix). Former smokers generally drink less alcohol and less coffee, are more physically active, and experience less stress, although their relative body weight tends to be greater (Friedman et al. 1979; Kaprio and Koskenvuo 1988; Chapters 10 and 11). However, some persons may stop smoking because a personal combination of risk factors places them at increased risk for disease. In the British Regional Heart Study, former smokers had higher blood pressure and total serum cholesterol at entry than current or never smokers (Cook et al. 1986).

In fact, observed mortality rates for many diseases have been higher for former smokers than current smokers during the first few years following cessation. Persons with symptoms of incipient illness or with newly diagnosed illness may stop smoking (Hammond and Garfinkel 1966). Consequently, mortality rates for former smokers immediately following cessation may exceed those for current smokers.

In studies of the effect of cessation on the course of established disease, consideration must be given to the severity of the underlying disease in former smokers and persistent smokers. For example, in a study of mortality following myocardial infarction, persons who quit smoking were at greater risk for death than those who did not quit because of more severe underlying disease (Vlietstra et al. 1986; Hermanson et al. 1988).

Analytic Issues in Observation Studies

Complex associations among disease risk, age, and duration of active smoking and abstinence further complicate assessment of the health consequences of cessation. Analytic approaches should represent these relationships in a biologically appropriate fashion. The risks of many cigarette-related diseases (e.g., cancer, CVD, and chronic obstructive pulmonary disease) increase with age (Figure 2). Following cessation, disease risk may change in diverse patterns, depending on the disease-specific mechanisms through which cessation alters disease occurrence. Disease risk may be unaltered (Curve A), decline quickly or slowly compared with that for never smokers (Curve C), or decline to a level between that of never and persistent smokers (Curve B) (Figure 2). Comparing the disease risk for former smokers with the risk for persistent

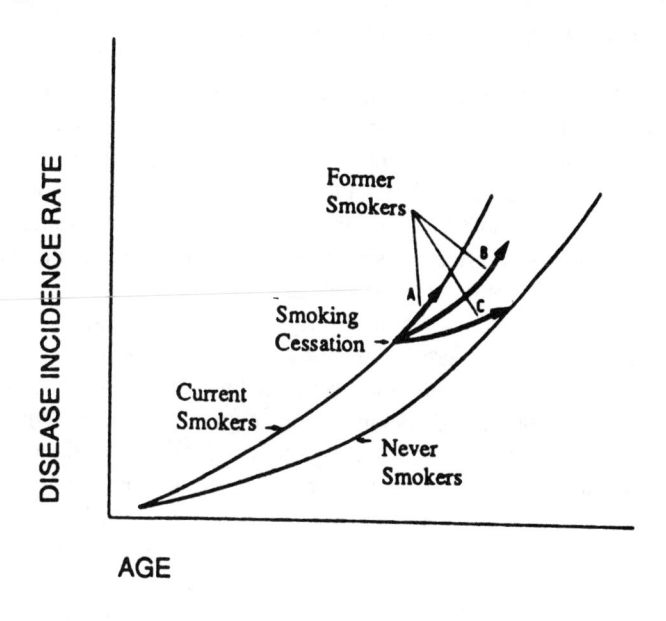

FIGURE 2.—Hypothetical examples of disease incidence rates for current, former, and never smokers, by age

smokers describes the disease burden removed by cessation; whenever possible, this Report provides this comparison. For many diseases, risks for former smokers do not revert to those for never smokers. Relative risks for former smokers compared with never smokers describe the persisting consequences of past active smoking.

Thus, in studies concerning the consequences of smoking cessation, the analytic focus is on describing disease incidence after cessation in relation to either the incidence of disease in never smokers or in smokers who do not stop smoking. Interest centers on addressing several questions: In a population that started smoking at a given age, smoked at the same rate, and then quit at a given age, how does the disease rate evolve as a function of time since quitting? In particular, how does the disease rate compare with that of a population of lifelong nonsmokers of the same age or with that of a population of smokers who continue to smoke at the same rate? How does the disease rate after cessation depend on such factors as duration of smoking, number of cigarettes smoked daily, age at starting, or other factors? These analytic questions are generally addressed by estimating either the attributable risk (the difference between the risks for exposed and nonexposed) or the relative risk (the ratio of the risks in exposed and nonexposed) and comparing former smokers with either never smokers or current smokers.

A cohort study that observed subjects from birth to death could supply the data requisite for meeting these analytic goals. Observations could be made concerning the age at starting smoking, the amount smoked, the age at stopping smoking, the duration of time since stopping smoking, and the occurrence of disease. Incidence rates could be calculated and the attributable risk or relative risk considered as a function of time since quitting. To assess the effects of such factors as duration or amount of smoking, smoking cohorts with different durations and rates could be analyzed.

Typically, however, cohort studies enroll subjects at various ages, and the smoking histories of the subjects span a broad range of ages at starting smoking, durations of smoking, amounts of smoking, ages at stopping smoking, and ages at observation. In analyzing data from a cohort study, stratification and multivariate modeling are used to describe the disease occurrence in former smokers in relation to the time interval since cessation. New statistical methods have facilitated the analysis of longitudinal data on cancer and other diseases (Breslow and Day 1987; Thomas 1988). The analytic approach should provide control for the effect of changing disease risk with increasing age; as duration of smoking abstinence increases, age and disease risk should be compared with that of never or current smokers in the same age stratum.

However, some analytic approaches may introduce overadjustment for the time-related dimensions of smoking history and of age and obscure the benefits of cessation. Age at starting smoking, age at observation, duration of smoking, and duration of abstinence are interdependent; specification of any three of these variables fixes the fourth. Assuming that current and former smokers of a given attained age started smoking at about the same age, the duration of smoking among former smokers must be less than for current smokers. Thus, adjustment for duration of smoking in comparing current and former smokers is incorrect. Methods that attempt to allow each of these four time-dependent factors to vary freely are inappropriate and provide biased descriptions of the variation in risk following cessation (Brown and Chu 1987).

Data from case–control studies can be used for the same analytic objectives. Information on age at starting to smoke, duration of smoking, duration of abstinence, and number of cigarettes smoked can be obtained retrospectively. Conventional analytic methods enable calculation of odds ratios by time since quitting, which estimate the ratios of incidence rates; the reference group for former smokers can be either never smokers or current smokers.

Risk of disease for former smokers changes because exposure to active smoking ceases; for some diseases, the exposure of interest in assessing the health consequences of cessation is the subsequent tobacco exposure experienced by continuing users but avoided by former smokers. Some analytic methods may not address adequately this avoided exposure. For example, using variables for cumulative exposure combines the additional exposure for the continuing smoker with the consumption to the point of cessation for the abstinent smoker. If repair processes affect disease risk after cessation, then the interval of abstinence is also a relevant exposure parameter. Thus, regardless of the type of data analyzed, the method of analysis should properly represent the underlying biologic process.

SUMMARY

Correct classification of smoking status is important to determine accurately the effects of cessation. Smoking cessation is a dynamic process in which smokers progress through a series of stages in an effort to quit smoking. These stages have been labeled differently by various investigators. The model generating the most research refers to the stages as precontemplation, contemplation, action, and maintenance and/or relapse. Very few smokers progress through these stages linearly, because most smokers relapse and recycle through the stages three or four times before attaining long-term maintenance.

Four common types of studies for assessing the health consequences of smoking cessation are vulnerable to various sources of information bias leading to misclassification of smoking status. Cross-sectional surveys have a relatively low frequency of misreporting; however, recall of duration of abstinence is vulnerable to error. A case–control study, because of its retrospective nature, is possibly more likely to have misreporting of smoking status in diseased cases than in nondiseased controls. Cohort studies are likely to have low rates of misreporting of initial smoking status but high rates of misclassification due to changes in smoking status over time. Clinical trials are likely to have high rates of misreporting for subjects receiving intensive clinical interventions. However, such trials should have relatively little misclassification of smoking status over time and provide more accurate assessment of duration of abstinence when regular followups are maintained.

Misclassification of smokers as former smokers will have the effect of underestimating the benefits of smoking cessation when a true effect exists. The extent of the bias is proportional to the degree of misclassification. Any specificity added to measurement by validation measures will diminish the misclassification bias.

CONCLUSIONS

1. Most former smokers have cycled several times through the process of smoking cessation and relapse before attaining long-term abstinence. Any static measure of smoking status is thus a simplification of a dynamic process.

2. In studies of the health effects of smoking cessation, persons classified as former smokers may include some current smokers. Consequently, the health benefits of smoking cessation are likely to be underestimated.

3. In contexts other than intervention trials, self-reported smoking status at the time of measurement and concurrent biochemical assessment are highly concordant. This high concordance supports self-report as a valid measure of smoking status in observational studies of the health effects of smoking cessation.

References

ABRAMS, D.B., FOLLIC, M.J., BIENER, L., CAREY, K.B., HITTI, J. Saliva cotinine as a measure of smoking status in field settings. *American Journal of Public Health* 77(7):846–848, July 1987.

ABRAMS, D.B., WILSON, G.T. Self-monitoring and reactivity in the modification of cigarette smoking. *Journal of Consulting and Clinical Psychology* 47(2):243–251, 1979.

ASSAF, A.R., MCKENNEY, J.L., BANSPACH, S.W., CARLETON, R.A. Validation of self-reported smoking practices. Paper presented at the 10th Annual Convention of the Society of Behavioral Medicine, April 1989.

AUGER, T.J., WRIGHT, E. JR., SIMPSON, R.H. Posters as smoking deterrents. *Journal of Applied Psychology* 56(2):169–171, April 1972.

BAUMAN, K.E., KOCH, G.G., BRYAN, E.S. Validity of self-reports of adolescent cigarette smoking. *International Journal of the Addictions* 17(7):1131–1136, 1982.

BENOWITZ, N.L. The use of biologic fluid samples in assessing tobacco smoke consumption. In: Grubowski, J., Bell, C.S. (eds.) *Measurement in the Analysis and Treatment of Smoking Behavior*. NIDA Research Monograph 48. U.S. Department of Health and Human Services, Public Health Service, Alcohol, Drug Abuse, and Mental Health Administration, National Institute on Drug Abuse. 1983, pp. 6–26.

BIGLAN, A., GALLISON, C., ARY, D., THOMPSON, R. Expired air carbon monoxide and saliva thiocyanate: Relationships to self-reports of marijuana and cigarette smoking. *Addictive Behaviors* 10(2):137–144, 1985.

BLISS, R.E., O'CONNELL, K.A. Problems with thiocyanate as an index of smoking status: A critical review with suggestions for improving the usefulness of biochemical measures in smoking cessation research. *Health Psychology* 3(6):563–581, 1984.

BLOT, W.J., AKIBA, S., KATO, H. Ionizing radiation and lung cancer: A review including preliminary results from a case-control study among A-bomb survivors. In: Prentice, R.L., Thompson, D.J. (eds.) *Atomic Bomb Survivor Data: Utilization and Analysis*. Philadelphia: Siam Institute for Mathematics and Society, 1984.

BOXER, G.E., RICKARDS, J.C. Studies on the metabolism of the carbon of cyanide and thiocyanate. *Archives of Biochemistry and Biophysics* 39(1):7–26, July 1952.

BRESLOW, N.E., DAY, N.E. *Statistical Methods in Cancer Research. Volume II—The Design and Analysis of Cohort Studies*. IARC Scientific Publications No. 82, International Agency for Research on Cancer, Lyon, France, 1987.

BRITTEN, N. Validity of claims to lifelong non-smoking at age 36 in a longitudinal study. *International Journal of Epidemiology* 17(3):525–529, 1988.

BROSS, I.D.J. Misclassification in 2x2 tables. *Biometrics* 10:478–486, 1954.

BROWN, C.C., CHU, K.C. Use of multistage models to infer stage affected by carcinogenic exposure: Example of lung cancer and cigarette smoking. *Journal of Chronic Diseases* 40(Supplement 2):171S–179S, 1987.

BROWNELL, K.D., MARLATT, G.A., LICHTENSTEIN, E., WILSON, G.T. Understanding and preventing relapse. *American Psychologist* 41(7):765–782, July 1986.

BROWNER, W.S., NEWMAN, T.B., CUMMINGS, S.R. Designing a new study. III. Diagnostic tests. In: Hulley, S., Cummings, S. (eds.) *Designing a New Study*. 1988, Chapter 9.

CAIRNS, J. The cancer problem. *Scientific American* 233(5):64–72, 77–78, November 1975.

CAREY, K.B., ABRAMS, D.B. Properties of saliva cotinine in young adult light smokers. *American Journal of Public Health* 78(7):842–843, July 1988.

CLAVEL, F., BENHAMOU, S., COMPANY-HUERTAS, A., FLAMANT, R. Helping people to stop smoking: Randomised comparison of groups being treated with acupuncture and nicotine gum with control group. *British Medical Journal* 291(6508)1538–1539, November 30, 1985.

COHEN, S., LICHTENSTEIN, E., PROCHASKA, J.O., ROSSI, J.S., GRITZ, E.R., CARR, C.R., ORLEANS, C.T., SCHOENBACH, V.J., BIENER, L., ABRAMS, D., DICLEMENTE, C., CURRY, S., MARLATT, G.A., CUMMINGS, K.M., EMONT, S.L., GIOVINO, G., OSSIP-KLEIN, D. Debunking myths about self-quitting. Evidence from 10 prospective studies of persons who attempt to quit smoking by themselves. *American Psychologist* 44(11):1355–1365, November 1989.

COHEN, S.J., KATZ, B.P., DROOK, C.A., CHRISTEN, A.G., MCDONALD, J.L., OLSON, B.L., CLOYS, L.A., STOOKEY, G.K. Overreporting of smokeless tobacco use by adolescent males. *Journal of Behavioral Medicine* 11(4):383–393, August 1988.

COLE, P., MORRISON, A.S. Basic issues in population screening for cancer. *Journal of the National Cancer Institute* 64(5):1263–1272, May 1980.

COOK, D.G., POCOCK, S.J., SHAPER, A.G., KUSSICK, S.J. Giving up smoking and the risk of heart attacks. A report from the British Regional Heart Study. *Lancet* 2(8520):1376–1380, December 13, 1986.

COPELAND, K.T., CHECKOWAY, H., MCMICHAEL, A.J., HOLBROOK, R.H. Bias due to misclassification in the estimation of relative risk. *American Journal of Epidemiology* 105(5):488–495, May 1977.

CORNONI-HUNTLY, J., BARBANO, H.E., BRODY, J.A., COHEN, B., FELDMAN, J.J., KLEINMAN, J.C., MADANS, J. National Health and Nutrition Examination I Epidemiology Follow-up Survey. *Public Health Reports* 98:245–251, 1983.

COULTAS, D.B., HOWARD, C.A., PEAKE, G.T., SKIPPER, B.J., SAMET, J.M. Salivary cotinine levels and involuntary tobacco smoke exposure in children and adults in New Mexico. *American Review of Respiratory Disease* 136(2):305–309, 1987.

COULTAS, D.B., HOWARD, G.A., PEAKE, G.T., SKIPPER, B.J., SAMET, J.M. Discrepancies between self-reported and validated cigarette smoking in a community survey of New Mexico Hispanics. *American Review of Respiratory Disease* 137:810–814, 1988.

CROSSEN, J.R., DOUGHER, M.J., BELEW, J. Comparison of reactive and non-reactive measures of smoking cessation at follow-up. *Addictive Behaviors* 9(3):295–298, 1984.

CUMMINGS, K.M. Changes in the smoking habits of adults in the United States and recent trends in lung cancer mortality. *Cancer Detection and Prevention* 7:125–134, 1984.

CUMMINGS, S.R., RICHARD, R.J. Optimum cutoff points for biochemical validation of smoking status. *American Journal of Public Health* 78(5):574–575, May 1988.

DELARUE, N.C. A study in smoking withdrawal. *Canadian Journal of Public Health* 64(Supplement):S5–S19, March–April 1973.

DICLEMENTE, C.C., PROCHASKA, J.O. Self-change and therapy change of smoking behavior: A comparison of processes of change in cessation and maintenance. *Addictive Behaviors* 7(2):133–142, 1982.

DIGIUSTO, E., ECKHARD, I. Some properties of saliva cotinine measurements in indicating exposure to tobacco smoking. *American Journal of Public Health* 76(10):1245–1246, October 1986.

DOLL, R., PETO, R. The causes of cancer: Quantitative estimates of avoidable risks of cancer in the United States today. *Journal of the National Cancer Institute* 66(6):1191–1308, June 1981.

EVANS, R.I., HANSEN, W.B., MITTELMARK, M.B. Increasing the validity of self-reports of smoking behavior in children. *Journal of Applied Psychology* 62(4):521–523, April 1977.

FERRIS, B.G. Epidemiology standardization project. *American Review of Respiratory Disease* 118(Supplement 6):1–120, 1978.

FLEISS, J.L. *Statistical Methods for Rates and Proportions*, Second Edition. New York: John Wiley and Sons, 1981.

FLETCHER, R.H., FLETCHER, S.W., WAGNER, E.H. *Clinical Epidemiology: The Essentials*, Second Edition. Baltimore: Williams and Wilkins, 1988.

FORTMANN, S.P., ROGERS, T., VRANIZAN, K., HASKELL, W.L., SOLOMON, D.S., FARQUHAR, J.W. Indirect measures of cigarette use: Expired-air carbon monoxide versus plasma thiocyanate. *Preventive Medicine* 13(1):127–135, January 1984.

FREDERIKSEN, L.W., MARTIN, J.E. Carbon monoxide and smoking behavior. *Addictive Behaviors* 4(1):21–30, 1979.

FREDERIKSEN, L.W., MARTIN, J.E., WEBSTER, J.S. Assessment of smoking behavior. *Journal of Applied Behavioral Analysis* 12(4):653–664, Winter 1979.

FRIEDMAN, G.D., SIEGELAUB, A.B., DALES, L.G., SELTZER, C.C. Characteristics predictive of coronary heart disease in ex-smokers before they stopped smoking: Comparison with persistent smokers and nonsmokers. *Journal of Chronic Diseases* 32:175–190, 1979.

GARVEY, A.J., BOSSÉ, R., GLYNN, R.J., ROSNER, B. Smoking cessation in a prospective study of healthy adult males: Effects of age, time period, and amount smoked. *American Journal of Public Health* 73(4):446–450, April 1983.

GARVEY, A.J., HEINOLD, J.W., ROSNER, B. Self-help approaches to smoking cessation: A report from the normative aging study. *Addictive Behaviors* 14:23–33, 1989.

GILLIES, P.A., WILCOX, B., COATES, C., KRISTMUNDSDOTTIR, F., REID, D.J. Use of objective measurement in the validation of self-reported smoking in children aged 10 and 11 years: Saliva thiocyanate. *Journal of Epidemiology and Community Health* 36(3):205–208, 1982.

GLASGOW, R.E., KLESGES, R.C., GODDING, P.R., VASEY, M.W., O'NEILL, H.K. Evaluation of a worksite-controlled smoking program. *Journal of Consulting and Clinical Psychology* 52(1):137–138, February 1984.

GLYNN, S.M., GRUDER, C.L., JEGERSKI, J.A. Effects of biochemical validation of self-reported cigarette smoking on treatment success and on misreporting abstinence. *Health Psychology* 5(2):125–136, 1986.

GORDIS, L. Should dead cases be matched to dead controls? *American Journal of Epidemiology* 115(1):1–5, January 1982.

GREENBERG, R.A., HALEY, N.J., ETZEL, R.A., LODA, F.A. Measuring the exposure of infants to tobacco smoke. Nicotine and cotinine in urine and saliva. *New England Journal of Medicine* 310(17):1075–1078, April 26, 1984.

GREENBERG, R.S., LIFF, J.M., GREGORY, H.R., BROCKMAN, J.E. The use of interviews with surrogate respondents in a case–control study of oral cancer. *Yale Journal of Biology and Medicine* 59(5):497–504, September–October 1986.

GREENLAND, S. Response and follow-up bias in cohort studies. *American Journal of Epidemiology* 106(3):184–187, September 1977.

GREENLAND, S. The effect of misclassification in the presence of covariates. *American Journal of Epidemiology* 112(4):564–569, October 1980.

GREENLAND, S. Statistical uncertainty due to misclassification: Implications for validation substudies. *Journal of Clinical Epidemiology* 41(12):1167–1174, 1988.

HADDOW, J.E., KNIGHT, G.J., PALOMAKI, G.E., KLOZA, E.M., WALD, N.J. Cigarette consumption and serum cotinine in relation to birthweight. *British Journal of Obstetrics and Gynaecology* 94(7):678–681, July 1987.

HADDOW, J.E., PALOMAKI, G.E., KNIGHT, G.J. Use of serum cotinine to assess the accuracy of self reported non-smoking. (Letter.) *British Medical Journal* 293(6557):1306, November 15, 1986.

HALEY, N.J., AXELRAD, C.M., TILTON, K.A. Validation of self-reported smoking behavior: Biochemical analyses of cotinine and thiocyanate. *American Journal of Public Health* 73(10):1204–1207, October 1983.

HALEY, N.J., COLOSIMO, S.G., AXELRAD, C.M., HARRIS, R., SEPKOVIC, D.W. Biochemical validation of self-reported exposure to environmental tobacco smoke. *Environmental Research* 49(1):127–135, June 1989.

HALEY, N.J., HOFFMANN, D. Analysis for nicotine and cotinine in hair to determine cigarette smoker status. *Clinical Chemistry* 31(10):1598–1600, October 1985.

HALEY, N.J., SEPKOVIC, D.W., LOUIS, E., HOFFMANN, D. Absorption and elimination of nicotine by smokers, nonsmokers, and chewers of nicotine gum. In: Rand, R.J., Thurau, K. (eds.) *The Pharmacology of Nicotine*, ICSU Symposium Series 9, Washington, DC: IRL Press, 1987, pp. 20–21.

HALEY, N.J., SEPKOVIC, D.W., HOFFMANN, D. Elimination of cotinine from body fluids: Disposition in smokers and nonsmokers. *American Journal of Public Health* 79(8):1046–1048, August 1989.

HAMMOND, E.C., GARFINKEL, L. The influence of health on smoking habits. In: Haenszel, W. (ed.) *Epidemiological Approaches to the Study of Cancer and Other Chronic Diseases*. NCI Monograph No. 19. U.S. Department of Health, Education, and Welfare, Public Health Service, National Cancer Institute, January 1966, pp. 269–285.

HAMMOND, E.C., GARFINKEL, L. Coronary heart disease, stroke and aortic aneurysm. Factors in etiology. *Archives of Environmental Health* 19:167–182, August 1969.

HANSEN, W.B., MALOTTE, C.K., FIELDING, J.E. The bogus pipeline revisited: The use of the threat of detection as a means of increasing self-reports of tobacco use. *Journal of Applied Psychology* 70(4):789–792, November 1985.

HATZIANDREU, E.J., PIERCE, J.P., FIORE, M.C., GRISE, V., NOVOTNY, T.E., DAVIS, R.M. The reliability of self-reported cigarette consumption in the United States. *American Journal of Public Health* 79(8):1020–1023, August 1989.

HERMANSON, B., OMENN, G.S., KRONMAL, R.A., GERSH, B.J. Beneficial six-year outcome of smoking cessation in older men and women with coronary artery disease. Results from the CASS Registry. *New England Journal of Medicine* 319(21):1365–1369, November 24, 1988.

HORAN, J.J., HACKETT, G., LINBERG, S.E. Factors to consider when using expired air carbon monoxide in smoking assessment. *Addictive Behaviors* 3(1):25–28, 1978.

HORN, D. A model for the study of personal choice health behaviour. *International Journal of Health Education* 19:89–98, 1976.

HUGHES, G.H., HYMOWITZ, N., OCKENE, J.K., SIMON, N., VOGT, T.M. The Multiple Risk Factor Intervention Trial (MRFIT). V. Intervention on smoking. *Preventive Medicine* 10(4):476–500, July 1981.

HUGHES, J., FREDERIKSEN, L., FRAZIER, M. A carbon monoxide analyzer for measurement of smoking behavior. *Behavior Therapy* 9:293–296, 1976.

HUMBLE, C.G., SAMET, J.M., SKIPPER, B.E. Comparison of self- and surrogate-reported dietary information. *American Journal of Epidemiology* 119(1):86–98, 1984.

HUNT, W.A., BARNETT, L.W., BRANCH, L.G. Relapse rates in addiction programs. *Journal of Clinical Psychology* 27(4):455–456, October 1971.

HUNT, W.A., BESPALEC, D.A. An evaluation of current methods of modifying smoking behavior. *Journal of Clinical Psychology* 30:431–438, 1973.

HUNTER, S.M., WEBBER, L.S., BERENSON, G.S. Cigarette smoking and tobacco usage behavior in children and adolescents: Bogalusa Heart Study. *Preventive Medicine* 9(6):701–712, November 1980.

ISACSSON, S.-O., JANZON, L. Results of a quit-smoking research project in a randomly selected population. *Scandinavian Journal of Social Medicine* 4:25–29, 1976.

JAMROZIK, K., FOWLER, G., VESSEY, M., WALD, N. Placebo controlled trial of nicotine chewing gum in general practice. *British Medical Journal* 289(6448):794–797, September 29, 1984.

JAMROZIK, K., VESSEY, M., FOWLER, G., WALD, N., PARKER, G., VAN VUNAKIS, H. Controlled trial of three different antismoking interventions in general practice. *British Medical Journal* 288(6429):1499–1503, May 19, 1984.

JANZON, L., LINDELL, S.-E., TRELL, E., LARME, P. Smoking habits and carboxyhaemoglobin. A cross-sectional study of an urban population of middle-aged men. *Journal of Epidemiology and Community Health* 35(4):271–273, December 1981.
JARVIS, M., TUNSTALL-PEDOE, H., FEYERABEND, C., VESEY, C., SALLOOJEE, Y. Biochemical markers of smoke absorption and self reported exposure to passive smoking. *Journal of Epidemiology and Community Health* 38(4):335–339, December 1984.
JARVIS, M., TUNSTALL-PEDOE, H., FEYERABEND, C., VESEY, C., SALOOJEE, Y. Comparison of tests used to distinguish smokers from nonsmokers. *American Journal of Public Health* 77(11):1435–1438, November 1987.
JARVIS, M.J., RAW, M., RUSSELL, M.A.H., FEYERABEND, C. Randomised controlled trial of nicotine chewing-gum. *British Medical Journal* 285(6341):537–540, August 21, 1982.
JARVIS, M.J., RUSSELL, M.A.H., FEYERABEND, C., EISER, J.R., MORGAN, M. Passive exposure to tobacco smoke: Saliva cotinine concentrations in a representative population sample of nonsmoking schoolchildren. *British Medical Journal* 291(6500):927–929, October 5, 1985.
JONES, E.E., SIGALL, H. The bogus pipeline: A new paradigm for measuring affect and attitude. *Psychological Bulletin* 76:349–364, 1971.
JONES, R.D., COMMINS, B.T., CERNIK, A.A. Blood lead and carboxyhaemoglobin levels in London taxi drivers. *Lancet* 2:302–303, August 12, 1972.
KAHN, A., RUTLEDGE, R.B., DAVIS, G.L., ALTES, J.A., GANTNER, G.E., THORNTON, C.A., WALLACE, N.D. Carboxyhemoglobin sources in the metropolitan St. Louis population. *Archives of Environmental Health* 29(3):127–135, September 1974.
KAHN, H.A. The Dorn study of smoking and mortality among U.S. veterans: Report on eight and one-half years of observations. In: Haenszel, W. (ed.) *Epidemiological Approaches to the Study of Cancer and Other Chronic Diseases*, NCI Monograph No. 19. U.S. Department of Health, Education, and Welfare, Public Health Service, National Cancer Institute, January 1966, pp. 1–125.
KAPRIO, J., KOSKENVUO, M. A prospective study of psychological and socioeconomic characteristics, health behavior and morbidity in cigarette smokers prior to quitting compared to persistent smokers and non-smokers. *Journal of Clinical Epidemiology* 41(2):139–150, 1988.
KIRSCHT, J.P., JANZ, N.K., BECKER, M.H., ERAKER, S.A., BILLI, J.E., WOOLLISCROFT, J.O. Beliefs about control of smoking and smoking behavior: A comparison of different measures in different groups. *Addictive Behaviors* 12(2):205–208, 1987.
KLEINBAUM, D.G., KUPPER, L.L., MORGENSTERN, H. *Epidemiologic Research: Principles and Quantitative Methods*. Belmont, California: Lifetime Learning Publications, 1982.
KNIGHT, G.J., WYLIE, P., HOLMAN, M.S., HADDOW, J.E. Improved radioimmunoassay for cotinine by selective removal of bridge antibodies. *Clinical Chemistry* 31(1):118–121, January 1985.
KORNITZER, M., VANHEMELDONCK, A., BOURDOUX, P., DE BACKER, G. Belgian heart disease prevention project: Comparison of self-reported smoking behaviour with serum thiocyanate concentrations. *Journal of Epidemiology and Community Health* 37(2):132–136, June 1983.
KOZLOWSKI, L.T. Pack size, reported smoking rates and public health. *American Journal of Public Health* 76(11):1337–1338. November 1986.
KRALL, E.A., VALADIAN, I., DWYER, J.T., GARDNER, J. Accuracy of recalled smoking data. *American Journal of Public Health* 79(2):200–206, February 1989.
LANDO, H.A. Effects of preparation, experimenter contact, and a maintained reduction alternative on a broad-spectrum program for eliminating smoking. *Addictive Behaviors* 6:123–133, 1981.

LANDO, H.A. A factorial analysis of preparation, aversion, and maintenance in the elimination of smoking. *Addictive Behaviors* 7:143–154, 1982.

LANDO, H.A., MCGOVERN, P.G. Nicotine fading as a nonaversive alternative in a broad-spectrum treatment for eliminating smoking. *Addictive Behaviors* 10:153–161, 1985.

LANGER, P., GREER, M.A. *Antithyroid Substances and Naturally Occurring Goitrogens*. Basel: S. Karger, 1977.

LANGONE, J.J., GJIKA, H.B., VAN VUNAKIS, H. Nicotine and its metabolites. Radioimmunoassays for nicotine and cotinine. *Biochemistry* 12(24):5025–5030, November 20, 1973.

LAST, J.M. (ed.) *A Dictionary of Epidemiology*, Second Edition. New York: Oxford University Press, 1988.

LEE, P.N. Passive smoking and lung cancer association: A result of bias? *Human Toxicology* 6:517–524, 1987.

LEE, P.N. *Misclassification of Smoking Habits and Passive Smoking. A Review of the Evidence*. Berlin: Springer-Verlag, 1988.

LERCHEN, M.L., SAMET, J.M. An assessment of the validity of questionnaire responses provided by a surviving spouse. *American Journal of Epidemiology* 123(3):481–489, March 1986.

LI, V.C., KIM, Y.J., EWART, C.K., TERRY, P.B., CUTHIE, J.C., WOOD, J., EMMETT, E.A., PERMUTT, S. Effects of physician counseling on the smoking and behavior of asbestos-exposed workers. *Preventive Medicine* 13(5):462–476, September 1984.

LICHTENSTEIN, E., BROWN, R.A. Smoking cessation methods: Review and recommendations. In: Miller, W.R. (ed.) *The Addictive Behaviors: Treatment of Alcoholism, Drug Abuse, Smoking and Obesity*. New York: Pergamon Press, 1980.

LIPINSKI, D., BLACK, J.L., NELSON, R.O., CIMINERO, A.R. Influence of motivational variables on the reactivity and reliability of self-recording. *Journal of Consulting and Clinical Psychology* 43(5):637–646, October 1973.

LUEPKER, R.V., PALLONEN, U.E., MURRAY, D.M., PIRIE, P.L. Validity of telephone surveys in assessing cigarette smoking in young adults. *American Journal of Public Health* 79(2):202–204, February 1989.

MALCOLM, R.E., SILLET, R.W., TURNER, J.A.M.C.M., BALL, K.P. The use of nicotine chewing gum as an aid to stopping smoking. *Psychopharmacology* 70(3):295–296, 1980.

MARLATT, G.A., CURRY, S., GORDON, J.R. A longitudinal analysis of unaided smoking cessation. *Journal of Consulting and Clinical Psychology* 56(5):715–720, October 1988.

MARLATT, G.A., GORDON, J.R. *Relapse Prevention: Maintenance Strategies in the Treatment of Addictive Behaviors*. New York: Guilford Press, 1985.

MARSH, G.M., SACHS, D.P.L., CALLAHAN, C., LEVITON, L.C., RICCI, E., HENDERSON, V. Direct methods of obtaining information on cigarette smoking in occupational studies. *American Journal of Industrial Medicine* 13:71–103, 1988.

MCFALL, R.M. Smoking-cessation research. *Journal of Consulting and Clinical Psychology* 46(4):703–712, August 1978.

MCLAUGHLIN, J.K., DIETZ, M.S., MEHL, E.S., BLOT, W.J. Reliability of surrogate information on cigarette smoking by type of informant. *American Journal of Epidemiology* 126(1):144–146, July 1987.

MULTIPLE RISK FACTOR INTERVENTION TRIAL RESEARCH GROUP. Multiple Risk Factor Intervention Trial. Risk factor changes and mortality results. *Journal of the American Medical Association* 248(12):1465–1477, September 24, 1982.

MURRAY, D.M., O'CONNELL, C.M., SCHMID, L.A., PERRY, C.L. The validity of smoking self-reports by adolescents: A reexamination of the bogus pipeline procedure. *Addictive Behaviors* 12(1):7–15, 1987.

MURRAY, D.M., PERRY, C.L. The measurement of substance use among adolescents: When is the "bogus pipeline" method needed? *Addictive Behaviors* 12(3):225-233, 1987.

MYERS, A.H., ROSNER, B., ABBEY, H., WILLET, W., STAMPFER, M.J., BAIN, C., LIPNICK, R., HENNEKENS, C., SPEIZER, F. Smoking behavior among participants in the Nurses' Health Study. *American Journal of Public Health* 77(5):628-630, May 1987.

NANJI, A.A., LAWRENCE, A.H. Skin surface sampling for nicotine: A rapid, noninvasive method for identifying smokers. *International Journal of the Addictions* 23(11):1207-1210, 1988.

NATIONAL INTERAGENCY COUNCIL ON SMOKING AND HEALTH. *Guidelines for Research on the Effectiveness of Smoking Cessation Programs: A Committee Report.* Chicago: American Dental Association, October 1974, pp. 46.

NEATON, J.D., BROSTE, S., COHEN, L., FISHMAN, E.L., KJELSBERG, M.O., SCHOENBERGER, J. The Multiple Risk Factor Intervention Trial (MRFIT). VII. A comparison of risk factor changes between the two study groups. *Preventive Medicine* 10(4):519-543, July 1981.

OCKENE, J.K., HYMOWITZ, N., SEXTON, M., BROSTE, S.K. Comparison of patterns of smoking behavior change among smokers in the Multiple Risk Factor Intervention Trial (MRFIT). *Preventive Medicine* 11:621-638, 1982.

OCKENE, J.K., KRISTELLE, J.K., GOLDBERG, R., OCKENE, I., BARRETT, S., MERRIAM, P. A smoking intervention in patients with coronary artery disease: Results of a randomized clinical trial. Presented at Society of Behavioral Medicine, San Francisco, California, April 1989.

OCKENE, J.K., KULLER, L.H., SVENDSEN, K.H., MEILAHN, E. The relationship of smoking cessation to coronary heart disease and lung cancer in the Multiple Risk Factor Intervention Trial (MRFIT). *American Journal of Public Health* 80(8):954-958, August 1990.

OHLIN, P., LUNDH, B., WESTLING, H. Carbon monoxide blood levels and reported cessation of smoking. *Psychopharmacology* 49:263-265, 1976.

ORLEANS, C.S., SHIPLEY, R.H. Assessment in smoking cessation research: Some practical guidelines. In: Keefe, F.J., Blumenthal, J.A. (eds.) *Assessment Strategies in Behavioral Medicine.* New York: Grune and Stratton, 1982.

PAXTON, R. The effects of a deposit contract as a component in a behavioural programme for stopping smoking. *Behaviour Research and Therapy* 18:45-50, 1980.

PAXTON, R., BERNACCA, G. Urinary nicotine concentrations as a function of time since last cigarette: Implications for detecting faking in smoking clinics. *Behavior Therapy* 10:523-528, 1979.

PECHACEK, T.F., FOX, B.H., MURRAY, D.M., LUEPKER, R.V. Review of techniques for measurement of smoking behavior. In: Matarazzo, J.D., Weiss, S.M., Herd, J.A., Miller, N.E. (eds.) *Behavioral Health: A Handbook of Health Enhancement and Disease Prevention.* New York: John Wiley and Sons, 1984, pp. 729-754.

PECHACEK, T.F., LUEPKER, R., JACOBS, D., FRASER, G., BLACKBURN, H. Effect of diet and smoking on serum and saliva thiocyanates. *Cardiovascular Disease Epidemiology Newsletter* 27:96, 1979.

PECHACEK, T.F., MURRAY, D.M., LUEPKER, R.V., MITTELMARK, M.B., JOHNSON, C.A., SHUTZ, J.M. Measurement of adolescent smoking behavior: Rationale and methods. *Journal of Behavioral Medicine* 7(1):123-140, March 1984.

PERSHAGEN, G., AXELSON, O. A validation of questionnaire information on occupational exposure and smoking. *Scandinavian Journal of Work, Environment and Health* 8(1):24-28, 1982.

PERSSON, P.G., NORELL, S.E. Retrospective versus original information on cigarette smoking. Implications for epidemiologic studies. *American Journal of Epidemiology* 130(4):705–712, October 1989.

PETITTI, D.B., FRIEDMAN, G.D., KAHN, W. Accuracy of information on smoking habits provided on self-administered research questionnaires. *American Journal of Public Health* 71(3):308–311, March 1981.

PICKLE, L.W., BROWN, L.M., BLOT, W.J. Information available from surrogate respondents in case–control interview studies. *American Journal of Epidemiology* 118(1):98–108, July 1983.

PIERCE, J.P., DWYER, T., DIGIUSTO, E., CARPENTER, T., HANNAM, C., AMIN, A., YONG, C., SARFATY, G., SHAW, J., BURKE, N., QUIT FOR LIFE STEERING COMMITTEE. Cotinine validation of self-reported smoking in commercially run community surveys. *Journal of Chronic Diseases* 40(7):689–695, 1987.

POJER, R., WHITFIELD, J.B., POULOS, V., ECKARD, I.F., RICHMOND, R., HENSLEY, W.J. Carboxyhemoglobin, cotinine, and thiocyanate assay compared for distinguishing smokers from non-smokers. *Clinical Chemistry* 30(8):1377–1380, 1984.

PROCHASKA, J., DICLEMENTE, C.C. *The Transtheoretical Approach: Crossing Traditional Boundaries of Therapy.* Pacific Grove, California: Brooks/Cole Publishing Company, 1984.

PROCHASKA, J., VELICER, W., DICLEMENTE, C., GUADAGNOLI, E., ROSSI, J. Patterns of change: Dynamic typology applied to smoking cessation. *Multivariate Behavioral Research*, in press.

PROCHASKA, J.O., DICLEMENTE, C.C. Stages and processes of self-change of smoking: Toward an integrative model of change. *Journal of Consulting and Clinical Psychology* 51(3):390–395, 1983.

PROCHASKA, J.O., DICLEMENTE, C.C. Toward a comprehensive model of change. In: Miller, W., Heather, N. (eds.) *Treating Addictive Behaviors. Processes of change.* New York: Plenum Press, 1986, pp. 3–27.

PROCHASKA, J.O., DICLEMENTE, C.C., VELICER, W.F., GINPIL, S., NORCROSS, J.C. Predicting change in smoking status for self-changers. *Addictive Behaviors* 10:395–406, 1985.

RADFORD, E.P., DRIZD, T.A. Blood carbon monoxide levels in persons 3–74 years of age: United States, 1976–80. National Center for Health Statistics. In: *Vital and Health Statistics No. 76*, DHHS Publication No. (PHS) 82-1250, March 17, 1982.

RAW, M., JARVIS, M.J., FEYERABEND, C., RUSSELL, M.A.H. Comparison of nicotine chewing-gum and psychological treatments for dependent smokers. *British Medical Journal* 281:481–482, 1980.

RESEARCH COMMITTEE OF THE BRITISH THORACIC SOCIETY. Comparison of four methods of smoking withdrawal in patients with smoking related diseases. *British Medical Journal* 286(6366):595–597, February 1983.

RICHMOND, R., WEBSTER, I. Evaluation of general practitioners' use of a smoking intervention programme. *International Journal of Epidemiology* 14(3):396–401, 1985.

ROGOT, E., MURRAY, J.L. Smoking and causes of death among U.S. veterans: 16 years of observation. *Public Health Reports* 95(3):213–222, May–June 1980.

ROGOT, E., REID, D.D. The validity of data from next-of-kin in studies of mortality among migrants. *International Journal of Epidemiology* 4(1):51–54, 1975.

RONAN, G., RUANE, P., GRAHAM, I.M., HICKEY, N., MULCAHY, R. The reliability of smoking history amongst survivors of myocardial infarction. *British Journal of Addiction* 76:425–428, 1981.

ROSE, G., HAMILTON, P.J. A randomised controlled trial of the effect on middle-aged men of advice to stop smoking. *Journal of Epidemiology and Community Health* 32(4):275–281, December 1978.

ROSE, G., HAMILTON, P.J.S., COLWELL, L., SHIPLEY, M.J. A randomised controlled trial of anti-smoking advice: 10-year results. *Journal of Epidemiology and Community Health* 36(2):102–108, June 1982.

ROSEN, T.J., SHIPLEY, R.H. A stage analysis of self-initiated smoking reductions. *Addictive Behaviors* 8(3):263–272, 1983.

ROTHMAN, K.J. *Modern Epidemiology.* Boston: Little, Brown and Company, 1986.

RUSSELL, M. Cigarette consumption and biochemical measures of smoke intake. (Letter.) *British Medical Journal* 285(6340):507–508, August 14, 1982.

RUSSELL, M.A.H., FEYERABEND, C. Blood and urinary nicotine in non-smokers. *Lancet* 1(7900):179–181, January 25, 1975.

RUSSELL, M.A.H., JARVIS, M.J., DEVITT, G., FEYERABEND, C. Nicotine intake by snuff users. *British Medical Journal* 283(6295):814–817, September 26, 1981.

RUSSELL, M.A.H., STAPLETON, J.A., JACKSON, P.H., HAJEK, P., BELCHER, M. District programme to reduce smoking: Effect of clinic supported brief intervention by general practitioners. *British Medical Journal* 295(6608):1240–1244, November 14, 1987.

RUSSELL, M.A.H., WILSON, C., TAYLOR, C., BAKER, C.D. Effect of general practitioners' advice against smoking. *British Medical Journal* 2:231–235, July 28, 1979.

RUTH, K., NEATON, J. Evaluation of two biological markers of tobacco exposure used in the MRFIT. *Preventive Medicine*, in press.

SACKETT, D.L. Bias in analytic research. *Journal of Chronic Diseases* 32(1–2):51–63, 1979.

SANDLER, D.P., SHORE, D.L. Quality of data on parents' smoking and drinking provided by adult offspring. *American Journal of Epidemiology* 124(5):768–778, November 1986.

SCHACHTER, S. Recidivism and self-cure of smoking and obesity. *American Psychologist* 37(4):436–444, April 1982.

SCHLESSELMAN, J.J., STOLLEY, P.D. *Case Control Studies: Design, Conduct, Analysis.* Monographs in Epidemiology and Biostatistics: No. 2 New York: Oxford University Press, 1982.

SEPKOVIC, D.W., HALEY, N.J. Biomedical applications of cotinine quantitation in smoking related research. *American Journal of Public Health* 75(6):663–665, June 1985.

SEPKOVIC, D.W., HALEY, N.J., HOFFMANN, D. Elimination from the body of tobacco products by smokers and passive smokers. (Letter.) *Journal of the American Medical Association* 256(7):863, August 1986.

SHANNON, I., SUDDICK, R., DOWD, F. JR. Saliva: Composition and secretion. In: Meyers, H. (ed.) *Monographs in Oral Science*, Volume 2. New York: S. Karger, 1974.

SHIPLEY, R.H. Maintenance of smoking cessation. Effects of follow-up letters, smoking motivation, muscle tension and health locus of control. *Journal of Consulting and Clinical Psychology* 49(6):982–984, December 1981.

SHUMAKER, S.A., GRUNBERG, N.E. Proceedings of the National Working Conference on Smoking Relapse. *Health Psychology* 5(Supplement):1–99, 1986.

SILLETT, R.W., WILSON, M.B., MALCOLM, R.E., BALL, K.P. Deception among smokers. *British Medical Journal* 2:1185–1186, October 28, 1978.

SLATTERY, M.L., HUNT, S.C., FRENCH, T.K., FORD, M.H., WILLIAMS, R.R. Validity of cigarette smoking habits in three epidemiologic studies in Utah. *Preventive Medicine* 18:11–19, 1989.

STEINMAN, G.D. Thiocyanate vs. cotinine as a marker to identify smokers. (Letter.) *Clinical Chemistry* 31(8):1406, August 1985.

STEWART, R.D. The effect of carbon monoxide on humans. *Annual Review of Pharmacology* 15:409–425, 1975.

STOOKEY, G.K., KATZ, B.P., OLSON, B.L., DROOK, C.A., COHEN, S.J. Evaluation of biochemical validation measures in determination of smoking status. *Journal of Dental Research* 66(10):1597–1601, 1987.

SWAN, G.E., PARKER, S.D., CHESNEY, M.A., ROSENMAN, R.H. Reducing the confounding effects of environment and diet on saliva thiocyanate values in ex-smokers. *Addictive Behaviors* 10(2):187–190, 1985.

THOMAS, D.C. Models for exposure-time-response relationships with applications to cancer epidemiology. *Annual Review of Public Health* 9:451–482, 1988.

TUOMILEHTO, J., GEBOERS, J., SALONEN, J.T., NISSINEN, A., KUULASMAA, K., PUSKA, P. Decline in cardiovascular mortality in North Karelia and other parts of Finland. *British Medical Journal* 293:1068–1071, October 25, 1986.

U.S. DEPARTMENT OF HEALTH AND HUMAN SERVICES. *The Health Consequences of Smoking: Cancer. A Report of the Surgeon General.* U.S. Department of Health and Human Services, Public Health Service, Office on Smoking and Health. DHHS Publication No. (PHS) 82-50179, 1982.

U.S. DEPARTMENT OF HEALTH AND HUMAN SERVICES. *The Health Consequences of Smoking: Cardiovascular Disease. A Report of the Surgeon General.* U.S. Department of Health and Human Services, Public Health Service, Office on Smoking and Health. DHHS Publication No. (PHS) 84-50204, 1983.

U.S. DEPARTMENT OF HEALTH AND HUMAN SERVICES. *The Health Consequences of Involuntary Smoking. A Report of the Surgeon General.* U.S. Department of Health and Human Services, Public Health Service, Centers for Disease Control. DHHS Publication No. (CDC) 87-8398, 1986.

U.S. DEPARTMENT OF HEALTH AND HUMAN SERVICES. *Reducing the Health Consequences of Smoking: 25 Years of Progress. A Report of the Surgeon General.* U.S. Department of Health and Human Services, Public Health Service, Centers for Disease Control, Center for Chronic Disease Prevention and Health Promotion, Office on Smoking and Health. DHHS Publication No. (CDC) 89-8411, 1989.

U.S. DEPARTMENT OF HEALTH, EDUCATION, AND WELFARE. *Smoking and Health. A Report of the Surgeon General.* U.S. Department of Health, Education, and Welfare, Public Health Service, Office of the Assistant Secretary for Health, Office on Smoking and Health. DHEW Publication No. (PHS) 79-50066, 1979.

U.S. PUBLIC HEALTH SERVICE. *Smoking and Health. Report of the Advisory Committee to the Surgeon General of the Public Health Service.* U.S. Department of Health, Education, and Welfare, Public Health Service, Center for Disease Control. PHS Publication No. 1103, 1964.

VESEY, C. Thiocyanates and cigarette consumption. In: Greenlaugh, R.M. (ed.) *Smoking and Arterial Disease.* London: Pitman Press, 1981.

VLIETSTRA, R.E., KRONMAL, R.A., OBERMAN, A., FRYE, R.L., KILLIP, T. III. Effect of cigarette smoking on survival of patients with angiographically documented coronary artery disease. Report from the CASS Registry. *Journal of the American Medical Assocation* 255(8):1023–1027, February 28, 1986.

VOGT, T.M. Smoking behavioral factors as predictors of risks. In: Jarvik, M.E., Cullen, J.W., Gritz, E.R., Vogt, T.M., West, L.J. (eds.) *Research on Smoking Behavior.* NIDA Research Monograph 17. U.S. Department of Health, Education, and Welfare, Public Health Service, Alcohol, Drug Abuse, and Mental Health Administration, National Institute on Drug Abuse. DHEW Publication No. (ADM) 78-581, December 1977, pp. 98–110.

VOGT, T.M. Questionnaires vs. biochemical measures of smoking exposure. (Letter.) *American Journal of Public Health* 72(1):93, January 1982.

VOGT, T.M., SELVIN, S., WIDDOWSON, G., HULLEY, S.B. Expired air carbon monoxide and serum thiocyanate as object measures of cigarette exposure. *American Journal of Public Health* 67(6):545–549, June 1977.

WALD, N.J., BOREHAM, J., BAILEY, A., RICHIE, C., HADDOW, J.E., KNIGHT, G. Urinary cotinine as marker of breathing other people's tobacco smoke. (Letter.) *Lancet* 1(8370):230–231, January 28, 1984.

WARNER, K.E. Possible increases in the underreporting of cigarette consumption. *Journal of the American Statistical Association* 73(362):314–318, June 1978.

WILCOX, R.G., HUGHES, J., ROLAND, J. Verification of smoking history in patients after infarction using urinary nicotine and cotinine measurements. *British Medical Journal* 2:1026–1028, October 27, 1979.

WILLIAMS, C.L., ENG, A., BOTVIN, G.J., HILL, P., WYNDER, E.L. Validation of students' self-reported cigarette smoking status with plasma cotinine levels. *American Journal of Public Health* 69(12):1272–1274, December 1979.

WINDSOR, R.A., CUTTER, G., MORRIS, J., REESE, T., MANZELLA, B., BARTLETT, E.E., SAMUELSON, G., SPANOS, P. The effectiveness of smoking cessation methods for smokers in public health maternity clinics: A randomized trial. *American Journal of Public Health* 75(12):1389–1392, December 1985.

WINDSOR, R.A., ORLEANS, C.T. Guidelines and methodological standards for smoking cessation intervention research among pregnant women: Improving the science and art. *Health Education Quarterly* 13(2):131–161, Summer 1986.

ZEIDENBERG, P., JAFFE, J.H., KANZLER, M., LEVITT, M.D., LANGONE, J.J., VAN VANAKIS, H. Nicotine: Cotinine levels in blood during cessation of smoking. *Comprehensive Psychiatry* 18(1):93–101, January–February 1977.

CHAPTER 3
SMOKING CESSATION AND OVERALL MORTALITY AND MORBIDITY

CONTENTS

Introduction 75
Smoking Cessation and Overall Mortality in Cohort Studies 75
Smoking Cessation and Overall Mortality in Intervention Studies 84
Smoking Cessation and Medical Care Utilization 87
    Population Projections 87
    Observational Studies 87
Smoking Cessation and Health Status 87
Conclusions 92
Chapter 3 Appendix 93
References 99

INTRODUCTION

The overall risk of mortality among smokers has been discussed in several prior reports of the Surgeon General (US PHS 1964, 1969; US DHEW 1979; US DHHS 1989). The 1989 Report estimated that approximately 390,000 Americans died in 1985 from diseases attributable to smoking (US DHHS 1989). Another source (Mattson, Pollack, Cullen 1987) estimated that 36 percent of heavy smokers aged 35 will die before age 85, and 28 percent before age 75, from a disease caused by smoking. Prior reports of the Surgeon General (US PHS 1968; US DHEW 1979; US DHHS 1989) have reviewed the association of smoking with overall morbidity, concluding that overall morbidity is increased among smokers. Quantitative estimates of the amount of morbidity attributable to smoking vary because of differences in the measures of morbidity used.

Data from the aggregate of studies of overall mortality and morbidity among smokers and former smokers show that smoking causes increased risk of morbidity and mortality. However, the temporal pattern of the reduced all-cause mortality after quitting and the effects on mortality risk of quitting at various ages have not been fully described. In addition, questions about the benefits of smoking cessation for mortality have arisen because of the results of studies involving interventions to promote smoking cessation. The association of smoking with medical care utilization is a topic that has not been addressed in detail in previous reports of the Surgeon General.

This Chapter reviews studies of overall mortality among former smokers, with particular attention to the temporal pattern of decline in mortality after quitting and the association of age at quitting with decline in mortality. Overall mortality in intervention studies that include smoking cessation is discussed with attention to problems of inferring the benefits of smoking cessation for the individual from these studies. Studies of medical care utilization by and health status of former smokers are described.

SMOKING CESSATION AND OVERALL MORTALITY IN COHORT STUDIES

Table 1 summarizes the results of major cohort studies comparing overall mortality among never, current, and former smokers. The studies consistently showed a substantially lower risk of mortality among former smokers in comparison with continuing smokers. Compared with continuing smokers, former smokers had a progressive decline in mortality risk as duration of abstinence increased, although risk in some studies was increased for 1 to 3 years after cessation, almost certainly because some people quit due to ill health (Chapter 2).

The durations of abstinence required for former smokers to reach the mortality risk of never smokers differ among studies. The American Cancer Society (ACS) study of 1 million American volunteers (Hammond 1966), also known as the 25-State Study and as the Cancer Prevention Study I (ACS CPS-I), found that after 10 years, mortality rates among former smokers of fewer than 20 cigarettes per day reached levels equivalent to those of never smokers. Among former smokers of 20 cigarettes or more per day,

TABLE 1.—Summary of longitudinal studies of overall mortality ratios relative to never smokers among male current and former smokers according to duration of abstinence (when reported)

Study		Current smokers	Former smokers Duration of abstinence (yr)				
			All	1–4	5–9	10–15	>15
British Physicians[a] (Doll and Peto 1976)		1.8	1.5	1.5	1.5	1.3	1.1
ACS CPS-I[b] (Hammond 1966)	1–19 cig/day	1.72		1.44	1.34	1.01	1.47
	20–39 cig/day	1.92		1.96	1.48	1.31	1.22
U.S. Veterans[c] (Kahn 1966)	10–20 cig/day	1.82			1.87	1.24	
	21–39 cig/day	2.04			2.08	1.88	
Swedish study (Carstensen, Pershagen, Eklund 1987)	1–7 g/day[d]	1.21	1.08				
	8–15 g/day[d]	1.35					
	>15 g/day[d]	1.70					
				<5	≥5		
Australian petrochemical workers[e] (Christie et al. 1987)	1–19 cig/day	1.45		1.60	0.93		
	20–29 cig/day	2.09		1.55	0.90		
	≥30 cig/day	2.10		1.58	0.92		
Framingham[a] (Gordon, Kannel, McGee 1974)		1.47	0.84				

TABLE 1.—Continued

Study	Current smokers	Former smokers All durations	
		Temporary quitters	Persistent quitters
California HMO[f] (Friedman et al. 1981)	1.82	1.51	1.13

NOTE: All mortality ratios are relative to never smokers. ACS CPS-I=American Cancer Society Cancer Prevention Study I; HMO=Health Maintenance Organization.
[a]Age-adjusted.
[b]Aged 50–74.
[c]Aged 54–64.
[d]Tobacco consumption in g/day.
[e]Former smokers are those with sustained abstinence.
[f]Persistent quitters are those with sustained abstinence.

mortality risk was still higher than that of never smokers even after 10 years of abstinence.

The more recent ACS study, ACS CPS-II, is designed similarly to CPS-I. Researchers enlisted 77,000 volunteers, who then solicited their friends, neighbors, and relatives to participate in the study. Those enrolled completed a four-page confidential questionnaire on medical history, health behaviors, medication use, and occupational exposures (Stellman and Garfinkel 1986; Garfinkel and Stellman 1988). A total of 521,555 men and 658,748 women were enrolled; 4-year followup data (1982–86) on the cohort were included in the 1989 Surgeon General's Report (US DHHS 1989).

In this Report, mortality rates for all causes of death from the ACS CPS-II were calculated using updated data for the same 4-year followup period (Table 2). Rates were calculated by gender in 5-year age groups for current and former smokers according to level of cigarette consumption (1–20 cig/day, ≥21 cig/day for males; 1–19 cig/day, ≥20 cig/day for females). Rates for former smokers were further stratified by years since smoking cessation (<1, 1–2, 3–5, 6–10, 11–15, and ≥16). Slightly different strata were used for men and women with respect to daily cigarette consumption in order to provide suitable distributions of subjects across categories of smokers and ex-smokers.

TABLE 2.—Overall mortality ratios among current and former smokers, relative to never smokers, by sex and duration of abstinence at date of enrollment, ACS CPS-II

	Current smokers	Former smokers Duration of abstinence at enrollment (yr)					
		<1	1–2	3–5	6–10	11–15	≥16
Males							
1–20 cig/day	2.22	2.49	2.38	2.03	1.63	1.38	1.06
≥21 cig/day	2.43	2.77	2.64	2.25	2.04	1.77	1.27
Females							
1–19 cig/day	1.60	1.58	1.96	1.41	1.14	1.10	1.01
≥20 cig/day	2.10	3.39	2.58	2.03	1.60	1.38	1.15

	Current smokers	Former smokers excluding those with cancer, heart disease, or stroke and those "sick" at interview Duration of abstinence at enrollment (yr)					
		<1	1–2	3–5	6–10	11–15	≥16
Males							
1–20 cig/day	2.34	2.06	2.05	1.89	1.48	1.29	1.01
≥21 cig/day	2.73	1.85	2.15	1.90	1.77	1.65	1.19
Females							
1–19 cig/day	1.82	0.76	1.26	1.42	1.01	1.09	1.00
≥20 cig/day	2.46	3.33	2.15	1.44	1.46	1.18	0.95

NOTE: Mortality ratios are relative to those of never smokers. ACS CPS-II=American Cancer Society Cancer Prevention Study II.
SOURCE: Unpublished tabulations, American Cancer Society.

In this analysis, subjects who had quit smoking were assigned to the duration of abstinence category appropriate for when they enrolled in the study. This method of assignment tends to blunt the rate of decline of mortality risk according to duration of abstinence when compared with never smokers because former smokers do not change categories as duration of abstinence lengthens. No attempt was made in this study to determine smoking status after enrollment, and persons who had quit at enrollment but had resumed smoking were still considered former smokers. Likewise, persons who smoked at enrollment but subsequently quit remain assigned to the current smoker category. This probably leads to some degree of misclassification and affects relative risk estimates (Chapter 2).

Like ACS CPS-I and other cohort studies, mortality ratios were substantially lower among former smokers than continuing smokers for all durations of abstinence except that of 1 to 3 years. With the exclusion of those subjects who had a history of cancer, heart disease, or stroke and those who said they were "sick" at the time of recruitment, mortality ratios were lower among former than continuing smokers for all durations of abstinence, among males at all prior levels of cigarette consumption, and among females who smoked fewer than 20 cigarettes per day before they quit.

The difference in the pattern of decline in overall mortality between all subjects and the subset of subjects who were healthy at recruitment provides strong evidence that recent quitters disproportionately include those who have quit because they are ill. In contrast with ACS CPS-I, which was conducted in the early 1960s, mortality ratios among both heavy and light smokers in ACS CPS-II remained substantially elevated in comparison with those of never smokers 10 years after quitting. This increase was evident in all subjects and in the subset of subjects who did not have a history of cancer, heart disease, or stroke and who did not state that they were "sick" when recruited. Sixteen years after quitting, the mortality risk among male former smokers of fewer than 21 cigarettes reached that of never smokers but remained elevated among former smokers of 21 cigarettes or more. Among female former smokers in both categories, mortality was comparable with that of never smokers after 16 years of abstinence.

The results of ACS CPS-II are broadly in agreement with those of the British Physicians Study (Doll and Peto 1976; Doll and Hill 1964a,b) and the U.S. Veterans Study (Kahn 1966; Rogot and Murray 1980). In both, the overall mortality risk among former smokers remained elevated in comparison with that of never smokers up to 15 years after quitting, although the risk was substantially less than among continuing smokers.

An Australian study of petrochemical workers (Christie et al. 1987) appears to differ from the other cohort studies in finding that overall mortality risk among former smokers reached that of never smokers 5 years after quitting. This study is unique in that subjects classified as former smokers were all persistent abstainers.

The differences among other studies in estimates of the duration of abstinence needed for a former smoker to have the same overall mortality risk as a never smoker are likely to be due to other smoking-related factors, such as age at smoking initiation, that differ among study populations and over time (Chapter 2). Irrespective of the duration of abstinence needed to reach the mortality risk of never smokers, former smokers have substantially lower mortality when compared with continuing smokers.

For three representative age groups (50–54, 60–64, and 70–74 yr), Figure 1 shows the relative risk of death among current and former smokers compared with never smokers based on recent ACS CPS-II data for the subjects who did not have cancer, heart disease, or stroke and were not "sick" at recruitment. Complete data from ACS CPS-II on mortality in current, former, and never smokers aged 50–74 years are presented in Table 7 of the Chapter Appendix. Data are not presented for those aged less than 45 years and greater than 80 years because there were fewer than 10 deaths in almost all of the categories of former smokers. In each of the age subgroups shown in Figure 1, among both sexes and among former light and heavy smokers, mortality risk relative to continuing smokers decreased with increasing duration of abstinence.

Using a method described by Kleinbaum, Kupper, and Morgenstern (1982), the data from ACS CPS-II were also used to estimate the effects of quitting at various ages on the cumulative risk of total mortality in a fixed interval after cessation. Several assumptions have been made in conjunction with CPS-II age-specific mortality data in order to estimate as many as 16.5 years' risk of death from all causes for individuals who continue to smoke and those who stop smoking. The first assumption is that age-specific mortality rates measured from 1982–86 CPS-II data remain constant for the next 16.5 years. The first category of smoking cessation is 1–2 years; that is, the individual gave up smoking 1 to 2 years ago. It is assumed that, on average, respondents in the 1–2-year category gave up smoking 1.5 years ago. Similarly, for the cessation categories 3–5, 6–10, and 11–15 years, the average durations of abstinence are 4, 8, and 13 years, respectively. It is further assumed that respondents are exposed to the age-specific mortality rates of the age interval in which quitting occurs for 1.5 years and to each of the next three age intervals for 5 years each, making a total of 16.5 years. For example, a quitter of the 40–44-year interval would be exposed to the age-specific mortality rates of the 40–44-year-olds for 1.5 years, to those of 45–49-year-olds for 5 years, to those of 50–54-year-olds for 5 years, and to 55–59-year-olds for 5 years.

The results of this analysis, presented in Table 3 and in greater detail in Table 8 of the Chapter Appendix, show that the benefits of cessation for total mortality extend to quitting at older ages. For example, a healthy man aged 60–64 years who smokes 21 cigarettes or more per day is estimated to have a chance of dying in the next 16.5 years of 56 percent if he continues to smoke and 51 percent if he quits. Quitting smoking at younger ages confers even greater proportionate increases in survival (see Figure 2 of the Chapter Appendix).

Framingham investigators recently analyzed data from their cohort (D'Agostino et al. 1989) and also found that the benefits of quitting apply to those who quit at more advanced ages. These researchers estimated that mean additional life expectancy for those who quit at ages 35 to 39 was 5.1 years for males and 3.2 years for females. For those who quit at ages 65 to 69, additional life expectancy was estimated to be 1.3 years for males and 1.0 year for females.

As discussed in detail in Chapter 2 and other chapters, smokers differ from nonsmokers in a variety of social, behavioral, and psychological characteristics, and successful quitters differ from those who continue to smoke (Rode, Ross, Shephard 1972; Blair et al. 1980; Haines, Imeson, Meade 1980; McManus and Weeks 1982; Billings and Moos 1983; Gottlieb 1983; Brod and Hall 1984; Seltzer and Oechsli 1985;

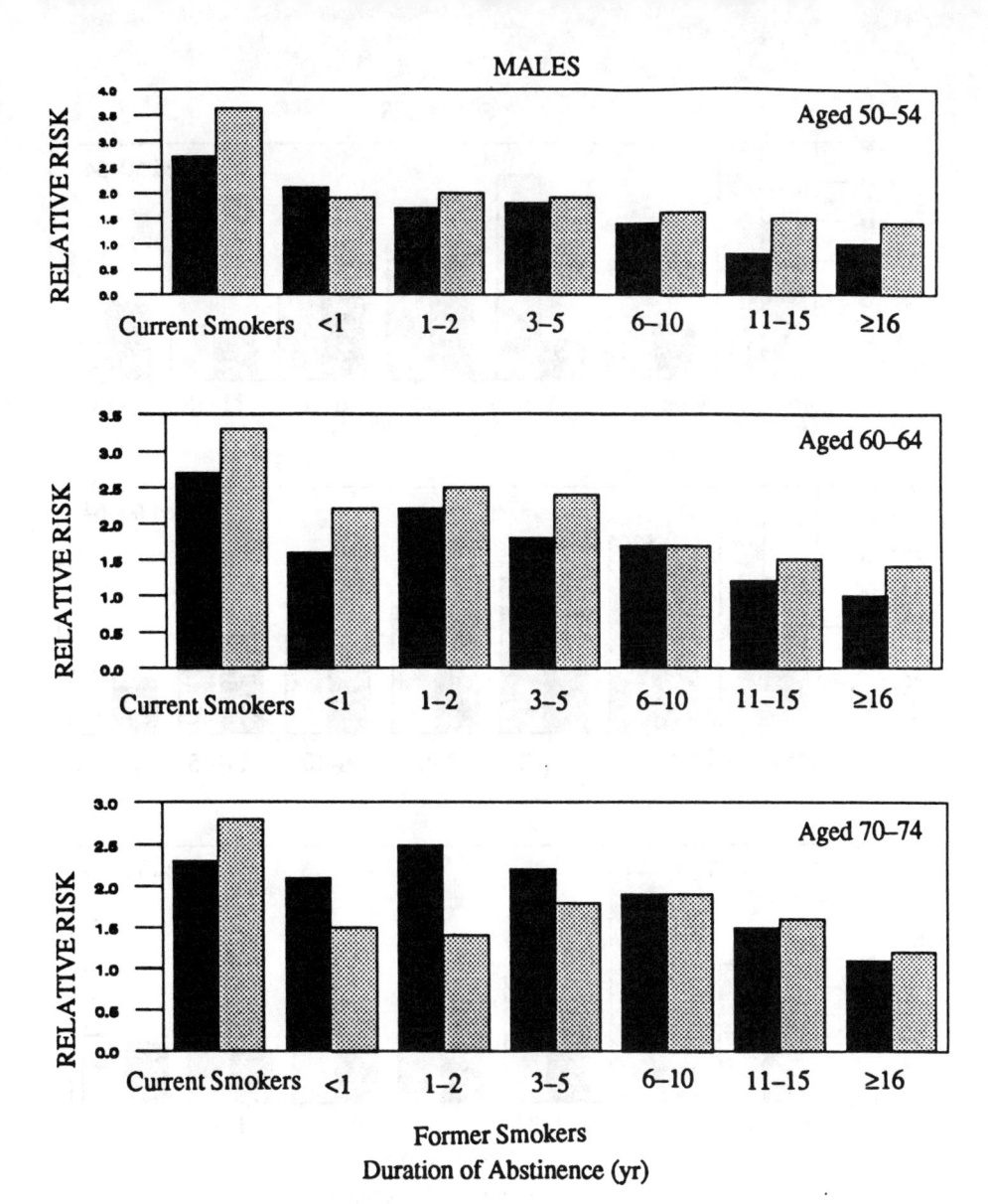

FIGURE 1.—Compared with never smokers, relative risk of mortality in current and former smokers aged 50–54, 60–64, and 70–74 at enrollment, by amount smoked and duration of abstinence

SOURCE: Unpublished tabulations, American Cancer Society.

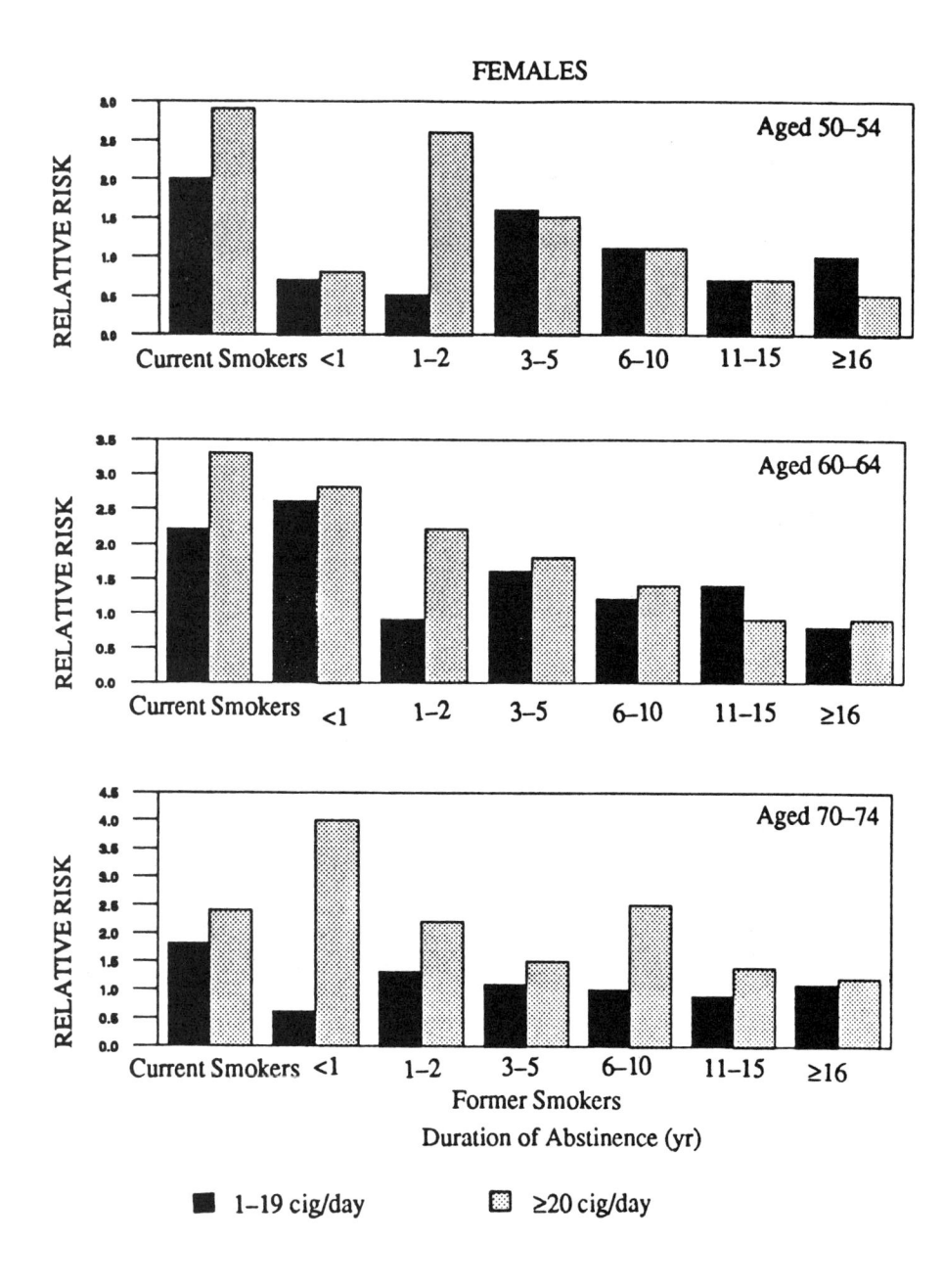

FIGURE 1. (Continued)—Compared with never smokers, relative risk of mortality in current and former smokers aged 50–54, 60–64, and 70–74 at enrollment, by amount smoked and duration of abstinence

SOURCE: Unpublished tabulations, American Cancer Society.

TABLE 3.—Estimated probability of dying in the next 16.5-year interval for quitting at various ages compared with never smoking and continuing to smoke, by amount smoked and sex

	Males				
Age at quitting or at start of interval	Never smokers	1–20 cig/day		≥21 cig/day	
		Continuing smokers	Former smokers	Continuing smokers	Former smokers
40–44	0.05	0.11	0.05	0.14	0.07
45–49	0.07	0.18	0.10	0.22	0.11
50–54	0.11	0.27	0.17	0.31	0.21
55–59	0.18	0.39	0.28	0.46	0.33
60–64	0.30	0.54	0.46	0.56	0.51
65–69	0.46	0.68	0.59	0.67	0.64
70–74[a]	0.40	0.61	0.55	0.58	0.52

	Females				
Age at quitting or at start of interval	Never smokers	1–19 cig/day		≥20 cig/day	
		Continuing smokers	Former smokers	Continuing smokers	Former smokers
40–44	0.03	0.06	0.03	0.08	0.04
45–49	0.04	0.09	0.06	0.13	0.05
50–54	0.07	0.14	0.07	0.19	0.09
55–59	0.11	0.21	0.12	0.27	0.15
60–64	0.18	0.30	0.19	0.38	0.32
65–69	0.30	0.46	0.39	0.52	0.32
70–74[a]	0.26	0.41	0.27	0.45	0.31

NOTE: Based on American Cancer Society Cancer Prevention Study II data for persons without a history of cancer, heart disease, or stroke who were not "sick" at enrollment.

[a] Estimates for quitting at this age are estimates of the probability of dying in the next 12.5-yr interval.

SOURCE: Unpublished tabulations, American Cancer Society.

Kaprio and Koskenvuo 1988). These differences may exist among adolescents prior to initiation of smoking (Seltzer and Oechsli 1985). For these reasons, interpretations of studies comparing these self-selected groups (never smokers, smokers, and quitters) must consider the problem of confounding (Chapter 2). Misclassification, which is discussed in detail in Chapter 2, also must be considered. However, studies of smoking cessation predominantly misclassify persons who are still smoking cigarettes as former smokers, and this would tend to obscure the benefits of cessation in comparison with continued smoking. Further, although the possibility of uncontrolled confounding needs to be considered in epidemiologic studies of smoking cessation and mortality, the totality of data must be interpreted with consideration of its consistency. To account for the evidence of a benefit of quitting that derives from nonexperimental cohort studies, confounders would need to be distributed quite differently among current and former smokers and would need to be strong predictors of mortality. There is no substantial evidence that this is the case.

SMOKING CESSATION AND OVERALL MORTALITY IN INTERVENTION STUDIES

Five studies, four of which were randomized trials, evaluated overall mortality in relation to interventions that included smoking cessation as a component. The results of these studies are summarized in Table 4.

TABLE 4.—Summary of overall mortality ratios in intervention studies in which smoking cessation was a component

Study	Intervention	Subjects (age)	Difference in smoking	Mortality ratio
Whitehall Civil Servants[a] (Rose et al. 1982)	Smoking	Males (40–59)	–14%[b]	0.98
North Karelia (Tuomilehto et al. 1986)	Smoking, BP, diet	Both sexes (35–64)	Males –4%[b] Females –3%[b]	1.00[c] (males) 0.94[c] (females)
Oslo[a] (Hjermann et al. 1981)	Smoking, BP, diet	Males (40–59)	–4 cig/day[b]	0.68[d]
WHO[a] (WHO European Collaborative Group 1983)	Smoking, BP, diet	Males (40–59)	–8.9%	0.97[d]
MRFIT[a] (MRFIT Research Group 1982, 1990)	Smoking, BP, diet	Males (35–57)	–13%[b]	1.02[d] (7 yr) 0.92 (10.5 yr)

NOTE: BP=blood pressure; WHO=World Health Organization; MRFIT=Multiple Risk Factor Intervention Trial.
[a]Randomized trial.
[b]Intervention minus control.
[c]Change in mortality in rest of Finland/change in mortality in North Karelia.
[d]Mortality in intervention/mortality in control.

Only one study examined smoking intervention alone (Rose and Hamilton 1978; Rose et al. 1982). Of 1,445 male smokers, aged 40 to 59 and at high risk of coronary heart disease (CHD) or chronic bronchitis, 714 were randomly assigned to an intervention group and 731 to a normal care group. Men in the intervention group were given individual advice to quit smoking, and if interested in quitting, up to four additional visits over 12 months. At the 9-year followup, 55 percent of responders in the intervention reported abstinence compared with 41 percent in the normal care group. After 10 years of followup, there were 123 deaths in the intervention group and 128 in the normal care group. The proportionate difference in total mortality between the intervention group and normal care group (–2 percent) was not statistically significant, but the confidence interval was wide (–22 percent to +23 percent). There were 81 smoking-related deaths in the intervention group and 92 in the normal care group. The proportionate difference in smoking-related deaths was –9 percent. Again the confidence interval was wide (–31 percent to +20 percent). Twenty percent of the men in the intervention group who quit smoking cigarettes took up pipe or cigar smoking compared with 3 percent of the men in the normal care group, and to the extent that pipe and cigar smoking are mortality risk factors, any benefit of cessation of cigarette smoking is obscured.

This trial is largely uninformative as to the benefit or lack of benefit of smoking cessation for total mortality because of the small number of subjects. The trial was further compromised by the relatively poor compliance of the subjects with the intervention; the net reduction in mean cigarette consumption over the 10 years of the followup among the intervention group compared with the normal care group was only 7.6 cigarettes per day.

Other intervention studies that allow assessment of the relation of smoking cessation to overall mortality have involved multiple interventions aimed at reducing several different factors for CHD. The ability to draw conclusions about the effect of smoking cessation on overall mortality from these studies is quite limited for this reason.

The North Karelia study targeted a region of Finland that had the world's highest CHD death rate at the time of the study's initiation (Tuomilehto et al. 1986) and was aimed at modifying smoking, cholesterol levels, and blood pressure. The rest of Finland was used for comparison. In the 10 years after initiation of an aggressive risk reduction program, there was a 35-percent decrease in smoking in North Karelia compared with a 2-percent reduction in the rest of Finland (Salonen et al. 1989). Blood pressure and cholesterol levels did not change significantly in the intervention area compared with the rest of Finland. Total mortality in the intervention area in the 10 years after the start of the study declined more rapidly than in the rest of Finland, although the difference in the rate of decline in overall mortality was not statistically significant.

For at least two reasons, interpretation of the North Karelia study is problematic with respect to the effect of smoking cessation on overall mortality. First, the study was nonexperimental, with conclusions based on a comparison of total mortality in the study area with that of Finland. During the study period, overall mortality also declined in the rest of Finland, perhaps because of secular changes in other factors related to mortality and to changes in medical care (Salonen et al. 1989). Second, the study was not designed to investigate smoking cessation alone. Because of the mixing of interventions for three CHD risk factors, it was difficult to isolate the impact of the smoking cessation component.

The Oslo study (Hjermann 1980; Hjermann et al. 1981; Holme 1982) involved 1,232 normotensive men at high risk for CHD because of their smoking behavior and cholesterol levels. The men were randomly assigned either to receive interventions aimed at reducing both CHD risk factors or to a control group. Tobacco consumption, including pipe and cigar smoking, fell 45 percent more in the intervention group than in the control group.

There was also a mean difference of 13 percent in serum cholesterol between the intervention and control groups over 5 years (Hjermann et al. 1981). The study was small, and it was not designed to examine total mortality endpoints; only 42 deaths were observed. Nevertheless, the mortality rate in the intervention group was one-third lower than in the control group (one-sided p value=0.12). Because there were changes in both smoking and cholesterol levels, the difference in mortality cannot be attributed entirely to smoking cessation.

The World Health Organization (WHO) European Collaborative Group conducted an intervention study in factories in four European countries (WHO European Collaborative Group 1983). The study involved random allocation of 66 factories that employed 49,781 men aged 40 to 59 to an intervention program targeting smoking, cholesterol level, and blood pressure or to a control group. After 4 years, the net reduction in mean cigarettes per day in the intervention factories was 8.9 percent (WHO European Collaborative Group 1983). At 6 years, overall mortality in the intervention factories was 4.04 percent; in the control factories, it was 4.15. The difference was not statistically significant.

The Multiple Risk Factor Intervention Trial (MRFIT) was a randomized study of more than 12,000 American men, aged 35 to 57 at entry, who were at high risk for CHD on the basis of their smoking behavior, blood pressure, and cholesterol levels (MRFIT Research Group 1982). Men in the special intervention group received an intensive intervention aimed at reducing blood pressure and cholesterol and encouraging smoking cessation. Men in the usual care group were referred to their physicians and examined annually. The interventions continued over the entire course of the study. At 6 years, 44.4 percent of special intervention smokers and 25.8 percent of the usual care smokers reported cessation. In the 7-year followup data reported in 1982, there was no difference in total mortality between the special intervention and usual care groups (MRFIT Research Group 1982). However, in the 10.5-year followup data of MRFIT participants, overall mortality for the special intervention participants was 7.7 percent lower than for the usual care group (one-sided p value=0.10; 90-percent confidence interval (CI), −16.6 to +2.3) (MRFIT Research Group 1990).

A subgroup of MRFIT special intervention participants, who were hypertensive, had resting electrocardiogram abnormalities, and comprised 31 percent of the special intervention group, may have suffered excess mortality as a result of an unanticipated adverse effect of one of the antihypertensive drugs (Cutler, MacMahon, Furberg 1989). This has recently been suggested as an explanation for the absence of an overall difference in mortality between the special intervention and usual care groups at the 7-year followup (MRFIT Research Group, submitted for publication). Furthermore, Ockene and coworkers (1990) recently reported that at 10.5 years, MRFIT participants who quit smoking had significantly lower death rates than those who continued to smoke in both special intervention and usual care groups. Most important, like the other multifactor intervention trials, it is difficult to infer a benefit or a lack of benefit of smoking cessation for total mortality from this study.

In summary, studies involving smoking cessation interventions include a randomized trial in which smoking cessation was the sole intervention and three intervention studies in which it was a component. The small size of the former and the mixing of a smoking intervention with other interventions in the latter make it impossible to reach conclusions about the benefits of smoking cessation from these studies alone; however, nonintervention (i.e., cohort) studies described in the previous Section clearly indicate a benefit of smoking cessation on overall mortality.

SMOKING CESSATION AND MEDICAL CARE UTILIZATION

Population Projections

The relationship between smoking cessation and medical care utilization is a complex issue. Data on differential disease and mortality rates comparing smokers and abstainers are abundant, and many investigators have used these data to project the savings in dollars attributable to smoking cessation (Weinkam, Rosenbaum, Sterling 1987; Leu and Schaub 1983; Luce and Schweitzer 1978; Oster, Colditz, Kelly 1984). Generally, these projections produce results that depend on the many assumptions of the models that create them. For example, Luce and Schweitzer (1978) projected that the total 1976 dollar cost of smoking in the United States was about $27.5 billion and that excess medical care costs accounted for about $8.2 billion of those costs. Weinkam, Rosenbaum, and Sterling (1987) and Leu and Schaub (1983), both using population simulation approaches, concluded that smoking does not, over a lifetime, lead to increased medical care utilization. This is because the short-term higher levels of utilization of smokers are approximately balanced by shorter longevity and the resulting reduced need for medical care.

Oster, Colditz, and Kelly (1984) used population projections to estimate the medical care costs of smoking and the proportion of those costs that are potentially recoverable depending on the age at which smoking is given up and the level of smoking prior to quitting. Male light smokers (<1 pack/day) who quit between ages 35 and 39 were estimated to recover about 59 percent of their lifetime excess medical care costs. Even if quitting was delayed until ages 75 to 79, light smokers were estimated to recover one-third of the costs. For heavy smokers, quitting earlier was estimated to have somewhat more benefit. For both sexes and all levels of smoking, medical care cost savings from smoking cessation were estimated to be substantial.

Observational Studies

Table 5 summarizes studies that directly measured utilization of medical services by current smokers, former smokers, and never smokers. These studies suggest that smoking is associated with higher utilization of hospital services and that former smokers experienced a brief period of increased utilization of hospital services just after quitting followed by declines in utilization to levels of never smokers. Modest increases in outpatient utilization by smokers are to some degree offset by a decreased propensity to use preventive care services (Marsden, Bray, Herbold 1988; Vogt and Schweitzer 1985; Oakes et al. 1974).

SMOKING CESSATION AND HEALTH STATUS

Table 6 summarizes studies of smoking cessation and health status. The variety of measures used makes direct comparison across studies problematic. Furthermore, in most cases, only a comparison of measures for never, current, and former smokers is available. Because some smokers quit due to illness and because most studies fail to

TABLE 5.—Summary of studies of medical care utilization among smokers and former smokers

Reference	Population	Measure of medical care utilization	Results
Ashford (1973)	75,500 residents of Exeter	Physician visits, home visits, hospitalization	No consistent differences in any measure of utilization between former smokers and current smokers.
Oakes et al. (1974)	2,557 HMO members in California	Physician visits, hospitalization	Male former smokers have more physician visits than current smokers; female former smokers have more physician visits than current smokers. Male former smokers are less likely than current smokers to be hospitalized; hospitalization among female former smokers compared with current smokers varies with age.
Marsden, Bray, Herbold (1988)	1985 worldwide survey of alcohol and drug use by military personnel	Physician visits, days hospitalized	Physician visits[a] / Days hospitalized[a]: Nonsmokers 2.41 / 0.64; Smokers ≤0.5 ppd 2.37 / 0.82; 1 ppd 2.56 / 0.68; ≥1.5 ppd 3.16 / 0.99
Vogt and Schweitzer (1985)	2,582 HMO members in Oregon	Days hospitalized, physician visits	Former smokers have lower mean number of hospital days than current smokers after adjustment for age, sex, duration of membership, and alcohol use. Total physician visits are higher among former smokers than current smokers after adjustment for age, sex, duration of membership, and alcohol use.
Newcomb and Bentler (1987)	654 adults aged 21–24, in Los Angeles	Nights hospitalized, physician visits	Adolescent smoking is related to spending more nights in the hospital and having more physician visits for illness during early adulthood.
Freeborn et al. (1990)	312 adults aged ≥65 in an HMO in Oregon	Ambulatory care use	Smokers consistently are more often in upper tertile of care utilization.

NOTE: ppd=packs/day; HMO=Health Maintenance Organization.
[a]Mean.

identify the reasons for quitting, the relation between quitting and health status may be obscured in studies that classify persons as former and current smokers (Chapter 2). A few studies differentiate between short-term abstainers (<1 yr) and long-term abstainers (>1 yr), and these studies are highlighted.

Data from the National Center for Health Statistics (US DHHS 1980) suggest that former smokers have fewer illness days than continuing smokers, particularly among younger women. Gallop (1989) found that former smokers have absentee rates between those of current smokers and never smokers.

Segovia, Bartlett, and Edwards (1989) conducted a telephone survey of 3,300 adults and found a strong relation between smoking status and the reporting of good health. Persons who had quit smoking for more than 1 year reported good health with about the same frequency as persons who smoked only 1 to 5 cigarettes per day, whereas those who had quit for less than 1 year reported good health at a frequency comparable with smokers of 16 to 20 cigarettes per day. Balarajan, Yuen, and Bewley (1985) examined the associations among various levels of smoking, recent and former cessation, and presence of acute and chronic illness, medical office visits, and doctor consultations. Current smokers had a higher prevalence of acute and chronic illness, and rates varied in relation to the amount smoked. Former smokers who had quit in the year prior to the survey had higher rates of illness compared with continuing smokers, and former smokers who quit more than 1 year prior to the survey had rates between those of never smokers and smokers of 20 cigarettes or more per day.

Reed (1983) found no difference in general physical health status between current, former, and never smokers, not otherwise defined. Seidell and colleagues (1986) examined the number of reported health complaints, out of an inventory of 51 possible complaints, by smoking status and found that male, but not female, former smokers reported fewer health complaints than smokers.

Astrand and Isacsson (1988) found that male employees of a pulp and paper plant who smoked retired at an earlier age than nonsmokers. Data from the 1979 National Health Interview Survey indicate that smokers have more restricted activity days, more bed disability days, more hospital days, more physician visits, and an increased probability of being unable to work or keep house, than nonsmokers (Rice, Hodgson, Sinsheimer 1986). Analyses of data for the 1976–80 Health Interview Surveys showed that smokers have a 55 to 75 percent excess in days with respiratory conditions associated with reduced activity (Ostro 1989). Smokers experience more school absences (Charlton and Blair 1989; Alexander and Klassen 1988) and work absenteeism (Andersson and Malmgren 1986; Coughlin 1987; Hendrix and Taylor 1987; Gallop 1989) than do never smokers. None of these studies reported information on former smokers.

These studies are extremely heterogeneous, with some methodologic shortcomings (Chapter 2). Furthermore, smoking is associated with other behaviors that may affect health (Pearson et al. 1987; Stephens 1986), and the studies do not adjust for changes in other risk variables, such as increased exercise, that might be associated with smoking cessation. Taken together, however, the studies are consistent with the hypothesis that smoking cessation produces improvements in health status. This conclusion is evident particularly when considering that smoking-related morbidity is a powerful motivation to quit smoking and that recent quitters are likely to be sicker than continuing smokers.

TABLE 6.—Relation of smoking cessation to various measures of general health status

Reference	Population	Health status measure	Current smokers	Former smokers	Never smokers
US DHHS (1985)	Representative sample of US population	Days of work lost due to illness	Females ≥20 yr 1.00[a] 20–44 yr 1.00[a] 45–64 yr 1.00[a] Males ≥20 yr 1.00[a] 20–44 yr 1.00[a] 45–64 yr 1.00[a]	0.82[b] 0.79 0.91 1.03[b] 0.92 1.05	0.86[b] 0.79 1.00 0.79[b] 0.86 0.66
Reed (1983)	450 employees offered subscription to an HMO	General physical health status	0.50[c]	0.52[c]	0.49[c]
Balarajan, Yuen, Bewley (1985)	Household survey of residents of Great Britain	Self-report of illness and physician visits	Cig/day 1–9 10–19 ≥20 Chronic illness 1.07[d] 1.31[d] 1.76[d] Acute illness 1.03 1.09 1.29 Outpatient visit 1.46 1.46 1.43 Physician 1.12 1.08 1.09 consultation	Quit Quit ≥1 yr <1 yr 1.43[d] 1.26[d] 1.11 1.48 1.40 1.25 1.19 1.47	1.0[a] 1.0[a] 1.0[a] 1.0[a]
Seidell et al. (1986)	1,245 persons in a morbidity registry	Number of health complaints	Cig/day <10 ≥10 Females 9.6 11.6 Males 9.0 9.6	10.2 6.8	9.0 7.3

TABLE 6.—Continued

Reference	Population	Health status measure	Results				
			Current smokers			Former smokers		Never smokers
			Cig/day			Quit ≤1 yr	Quit >1 yr	
			11–15	21–25	>31			
Segovia, Bartlett, Edwards (1989)	Telephone survey of representative sample US adults	Self-report of "good health"	4.18[e]	2.00[e]	1.46[e]	3.42[e]	5.13[e]	6.14[e]
Gallop (1989)	Workers in the pulp/paper industry	Work absences	1.25[f]			1.09[f]		1.00[e]

[a]Referrent.
[b]Ratio compared with current smokers.
[c]Mean ridit score adjusted for age and sex.
[d]Odds ratio compared with never smokers and adjusted for age, sex, and socioeconomic status.
[e]Log odds of self-report of good health.
[f]Ratio of absences compared with never smokers.

CONCLUSIONS

1. Former smokers live longer than continuing smokers, and the benefits of quitting extend to those who quit at older ages. For example, persons who quit smoking before age 50 have one-half the risk of dying in the next 15 years compared with continuing smokers.

2. Smoking cessation at all ages reduces the risk of premature death.

3. Among former smokers, the decline in risk of death compared with continuing smokers begins shortly after quitting and continues for at least 10 to 15 years. After 10 to 15 years of abstinence, risk of all-cause mortality returns nearly to that of persons who never smoked.

4. Former smokers have better health status than current smokers as measured in a variety of ways, including days of illness, number of health complaints, and self-reported health status.

CHAPTER 3 APPENDIX

TABLE 7.—Age- and sex-specific mortality rates among never smokers, continuing smokers, and former smokers by amount smoked and duration of abstinence at time of enrollment for subjects in ACS CPS–II study who did not have a history of cancer, heart disease, or stroke and were not sick at enrollment

Males

			Former smokers (1–20 cig/day)					
				Duration of abstinence (yr)				
Age	Never smokers	Current smokers	<1	1–2	3–5	6–10	11–15	≥16
45–49	186.0	439.2	234.4	365.8	159.6	216.9	167.4	159.5
50–54	255.6	702.7	544.7	431.0	454.8	349.7	214.0	250.4
55–59	448.9	1,132.4	945.2	728.8	729.4	590.2	447.3	436.6
60–64	733.7	1,981.1	1,177.7	1,589.2	1,316.5	1,266.9	875.6	703.0
65–69	1,119.4	3,003.0	2,244.9	3,380.3	2,374.9	1,820.2	1,669.1	1,159.2
70–74	2,070.5	4,697.5	4,255.3	5,083.0	4,485.0	3,888.7	3,184.3	2,194.9
75–79	3,675.3	7,340.6	5,882.4	6,597.2	7,707.5	4,945.1	5,618.0	4,128.9

Males

		Former smokers (≥21 cig/day)					
			Duration of abstinence (yr)				
Age	Current smokers	<1	1–2	3–5	6–10	11–15	≥16
45–49	610.0	497.5	251.7	417.5	122.6	198.3	193.4
50–54	915.6	482.8	500.7	488.9	402.9	393.9	354.3
55–59	1,391.0	1,757.1	953.5	1,025.8	744.0	668.5	537.8
60–64	2,393.4	1,578.4	1,847.2	1,790.1	1,220.7	1,100.0	993.3
65–69	3,497.9	2,301.8	3,776.6	2,081.0	2,766.4	2,268.1	1,230.7
70–74	5,861.3	3,174.6	2,974.0	3,712.9	3,988.8	3,268.6	2,468.9
75–79	6,250.0	4,000.0	4,424.8	7,329.8	6,383.0	7,666.1	5,048.1

TABLE 7.—Continued

Females

Age	Never smokers	Current smokers	Former smokers (1–19 cig/day) Duration of abstinence (yr)				
			<1	1–2	3–5	6–10	11–15	≥16
45–49	125.7	225.6	0	433.9	212.0	107.2	135.9	91.0
50–54	177.3	353.8	116.8	92.1	289.5	200.9	121.3	172.1
55–59	244.8	542.8	287.4	259.5	375.9	165.8	202.2	247.2
60–64	397.7	858.0	1,016.3	365.0	650.9	470.8	570.6	319.7
65–69	692.1	1,496.2	1,108.0	1,348.5	1,263.2	864.8	586.6	618.0
70–74	1,160.0	2,084.8	645.2	1,483.1	1,250.0	1,126.3	1,070.5	1,272.1
75–79	2,070.8	3,319.5	0	2,580.6	2,590.7	3,960.4	1,666.7	1,861.5

Females

Age	Current smokers	Former smokers (≥20 cig/day) Duration of abstinence (yr)				
		<1	1–2	3–5	6–10	11–15	≥16
45–49	277.9	266.7	102.7	178.6	224.7	142.1	138.8
50–54	517.9	138.7	466.8	270.1	190.2	116.8	83.0
55–59	823.5	473.6	602.0	361.0	454.5	412.2	182.1
60–64	1,302.9	1,114.8	862.1	699.6	541.7	373.1	356.4
65–69	1,934.9	2,319.6	1,250.0	1,688.0	828.7	797.9	581.5
70–74	2,827.0	4,635.8	2,517.2	1,687.3	2,848.7	1,621.2	1,363.4
75–79	4,273.1	2,409.6	5,769.2	3,125.0	2,978.7	2,803.7	2,195.4

NOTE: Mortality rates are per 100,000 persons. ACS CPS-II=American Cancer Society Cancer Prevention Study II.
SOURCE: Unpublished tabulations, American Cancer Society.

TABLE 8.—Estimated probability of dying in the next 16.5-year interval (95% CI) for quitting at various ages compared with never smoking and continuing to smoke, by amount smoked and sex

Males

Age at quitting or at start of interval	Never smokers	1–20 cig/day Continuing smokers	1–20 cig/day Former smokers	≥21 cig/day Continuing smokers	≥21 cig/day Former smokers
40–44	0.05 (0.04–0.05)	0.11 (0.10–0.12)	0.05 (0.04–0.06)	0.14 (0.13–0.15)	0.07 (0.06–0.09)
45–49	0.07 (0.07–0.08)	0.18 (0.17–0.19)	0.10 (0.08–0.11)	0.22 (0.21–0.23)	0.11 (0.10–0.13)
50–54	0.11 (0.11–0.12)	0.27 (0.26–0.28)	0.17 (0.15–0.19)	0.31 (0.30–0.33)	0.21 (0.18–0.23)
55–59	0.18 (0.17–0.19)	0.39 (0.38–0.41)	0.28 (0.25–0.31)	0.46 (0.43–0.48)	0.33 (0.30–0.37)
60–64	0.30 (0.28–0.31)	0.54 (0.52–0.57)	0.46 (0.42–0.50)	0.56 (0.51–0.61)	0.51 (0.48–0.57)
65–69	0.46 (0.43–0.48)	0.68 (0.64–0.72)	0.59 (0.51–0.67)	0.67 (0.57–0.78)	0.64 (0.51–0.77)
70–74[a]	0.40 (0.38–0.43)	0.61 (0.56–0.65)	0.55 (0.45–0.64)	0.58 (0.44–0.71)	0.51 (0.32–0.72)

Females

Age at quitting or at start of interval	Never smokers	1–19 cig/day Continuing smokers	1–19 cig/day Former smokers	≥20 cig/day Continuing smokers	≥20 cig/day Former smokers
40–44	0.03 (0.03–0.03)	0.06 (0.05–0.06)	0.03 (0.02–0.04)	0.08 (0.08–0.09)	0.04 (0.03–0.05)
45–49	0.04 (0.04–0.04)	0.09 (0.08–0.09)	0.06 (0.04–0.07)	0.13 (0.12–0.13)	0.05 (0.04–0.07)
50–54	0.07 (0.06–0.07)	0.14 (0.13–0.15)	0.07 (0.05–0.09)	0.19 (0.18–0.20)	0.09 (0.07–0.11)
55–59	0.11 (0.11–0.11)	0.21 (0.19–0.22)	0.13 (0.09–0.16)	0.27 (0.25–0.29)	0.15 (0.12–0.19)
60–64	0.18 (0.18–0.19)	0.30 (0.27–0.33)	0.19 (0.13–0.25)	0.38 (0.34–0.41)	0.32 (0.24–0.39)
65–69	0.30 (0.29–0.31)	0.46 (0.41–0.52)	0.39 (0.26–0.52)	0.52 (0.45–0.59)	0.32 (0.17–0.47)
70–74[a]	0.26 (0.25–0.27)	0.41 (0.35–0.47)	0.27 (0.09–0.46)	0.45 (0.37–0.53)	0.31 (0.13–0.50)

NOTE: Based on American Cancer Society Cancer Prevention Study II data for persons without a history of cancer, heart disease, or stroke who were not "sick" at enrollment. CI=confidence interval.
[a] Estimates for quitting at this age are estimates of the probability of dying in the next 12.5-yr interval.
SOURCE: Unpublished tabulations, American Cancer Society.

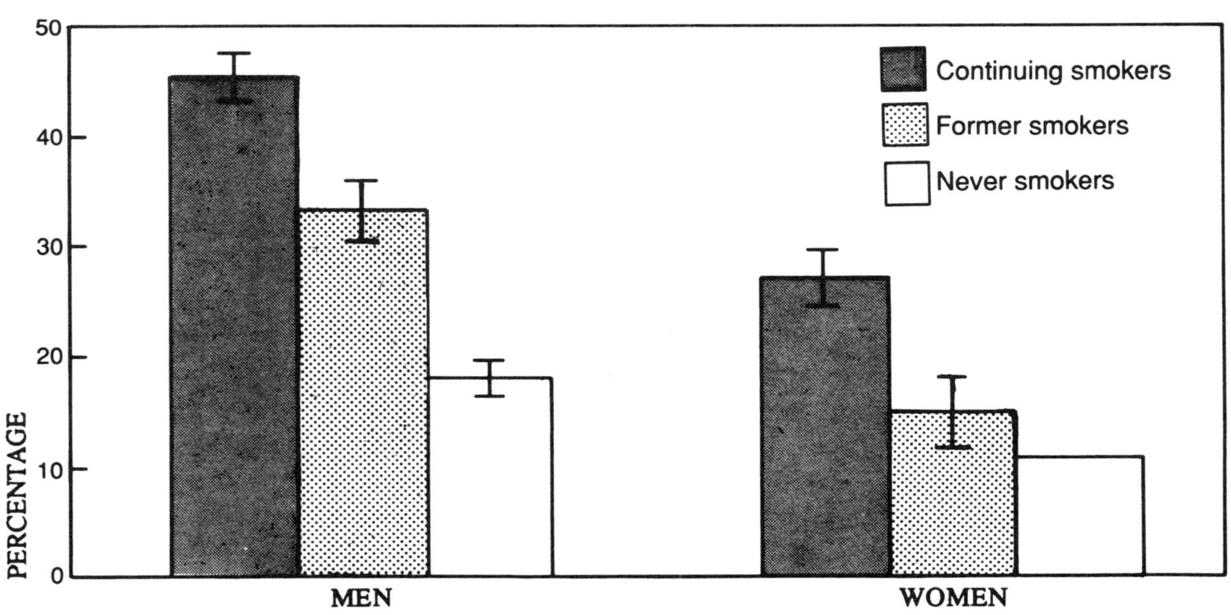

FIGURE 2.—**Estimated probability of dying in the next 16.5-yr interval for quitting at ages 55–59 compared with never smoking and continuing to smoke, by sex**

NOTE: Continuing and former smokers include only those smoking ≥21 (men) or ≥20 (women) cig/day. Vertical bars represent 95% CI; the interval for female never smokers is not shown because it is extremely narrow (11–11%). Based on American Cancer Society Cancer Prevention Study II data for persons without a history of cancer, heart disease, or stroke who were not "sick" at enrollment.

SOURCE: Unpublished tabulations, American Cancer Society, (see Table 8).

References

ALEXANDER, C.S., KLASSEN, A.C. Drug use and illnesses among eighth grade students in rural schools. *Public Health Reports* 103(4):394–399, July–August 1988.

AMERICAN CANCER SOCIETY. Unpublished tabulations.

ANDERSSON, G., MALMGREN, S. Risk factors and reported sick leave among employees of Saab-Scania, Linkoping, Sweden, between the ages of 50 and 59. *Scandinavian Journal of Social Medicine* 14(1):25–30, 1986.

ASHFORD, J.R. Smoking and the use of the health services. *British Journal of Preventive and Social Medicine* 27(1):8–17, February 1973.

ASTRAND, N.-E., ISACSSON, S.-O. Back pain, back abnormalities, and competing medical, psychological, and social factors as predictors of sick leave, early retirement, unemployment, labour turnover and mortality: A 22 year follow up of male employees in a Swedish pulp and paper company. *British Journal of Industrial Medicine* 45(6):387–395, June 1988.

BALARAJAN, R., YUEN, P., BEWLEY, B.R. Smoking and state of health. *British Medical Journal* 291(6510):1682, December 14, 1985.

BILLINGS, A.G., MOOS, R.H. Social–environmental factors among light and heavy cigarette smokers: A controlled comparison with nonsmokers. *Addictive Behaviors* 8(4):381–391, 1983.

BLAIR, A., BLAIR, S.N., HOWE, H.G., PATE, R.R., ROSENBERG, M., PARKER, G.M., PICKLE, L.W. Physical, psychological, and sociodemographic differences among smokers, ex-smokers, and nonsmokers in a working population. *Preventive Medicine* 9(6):747–759, November 1980.

BROD, M., HALL, S.M. Joiners and non-joiners in smoking treatment: A comparison of psychosocial variables. *Addictive Behaviors* 9(2):217–221, 1984.

CARSTENSEN, J.M., PERSHAGEN, G., EKLUND, G. Mortality in relation to cigarette and pipe smoking: 16 years' observation of 25,000 Swedish men. *Journal of Epidemiology and Community Health* 41:166–172, 1987.

CHARLTON, A., BLAIR, V. Absence from school related to children's and parental smoking habits. *British Medical Journal* 298(6666):90–92, January 14, 1989.

CHRISTIE, D., ROBINSON, K., GORDON, I., WEBLEY, C., BISBY, J. Current mortality in the Australian petroleum industry: The healthy-worker effect and the influence of life-style factors. *Medical Journal of Australia* 147(5):222, 224–225, September 7, 1987.

COUGHLIN, S.M. Prevalence of smoking at a large sugar cane plantation in Hawaii. *Hawaii Medical Journal* 46(12):468–473, December 1987.

CUTLER, J.A., MACMAHON, S.W., FURBERG, C.D. Controlled clinical trials of drug treatment for hypertension: A review. *Hypertension* 13(5, Part 2):136–144, May 1989.

D'AGOSTINO, R.B., KANNEL, W.B., BELANGER, A.J., SYTKOWSKI, P.A. Trends in CHD and risk factors at age 55–64 in the Framingham Study. *International Journal of Epidemiology* 18(3, Supplement 1):S67–S72, 1989.

DOLL, R., HILL, A.B. Mortality in relation to smoking: Ten years' observations of British doctors. *British Medical Journal* 1(5395):1399–1410, May 30, 1964a.

DOLL, R., HILL, A.B. Mortality in relation to smoking: Ten years' observations of British doctors. *British Medical Journal* 1(5396):1410–1467, June 6, 1964b.

DOLL, R., PETO, R. Mortality in relation to smoking: 20 years' observations of male British doctors. *British Medical Journal* 2:1525–1536, December 25, 1976.

FREEBORN, D.K., MULLOOLY, J.P., POPE, C.R., MCFARLAND, B.H. Smoking and consistently high use of medical care among older HMO members. *American Journal of Public Health* 80(5):603–605, May 1990.

FRIEDMAN, G.D., PETITTI, D.B., BAWOL, R.D., SIEGELAUB, A.B. Mortality in cigarette smokers and quitters. *New England Journal of Medicine* 304(23):1407–1410, June 4, 1981.

GALLOP, B. Sickness absenteeism and smoking. (Letter.) *New Zealand Medical Journal* 102(863):112, March 8, 1989.

GARFINKEL, L., STELLMAN, S.D. Smoking and lung cancer in women: Findings in a prospective study. *Cancer Research* 48(23):6951–6955, December 1, 1988.

GORDON, T., KANNEL, W.B., MCGEE, D. Death and coronary attacks in men after giving up cigarette smoking. *Lancet* 1345–1348, December 7, 1974.

GOTTLIEB, N.H. The determination of smoking types: Evidence for a sociological-pharmacological continuum. *Addictive Behaviors* 8(1):47–51, 1983.

HAINES, A.P., IMESON, J.D., MEADE, T.W. Psychoneurotic profiles of smokers and non-smokers. *British Medical Journal* 280(6229):1422, June 14, 1980.

HAMMOND, E.C. Smoking in relation to the death rates of one million men and women. In: Haenszel, W. (ed.) *Epidemiological Approaches to the Study of Cancer and Other Chronic Diseases.* NCI Monograph 19. U.S. Department of Health, Education, and Welfare, Public Health Service, National Cancer Institute, January 1966, pp. 127–204.

HENDRIX, W.H., TAYLOR, G.S. A multivariate analysis of the relationship between cigarette smoking and absence from work. *American Journal of Health Promotion* 2(2):5–11, Fall 1987.

HJERMANN, I. Smoking and diet intervention in healthy coronary high risk men. Methods and 5-year follow-up of risk factors in a randomized trial. The Oslo Study. *Journal of the Oslo City Hospitals* 30(1):3–17, January 1980.

HJERMANN, I., HOLME, I., VELVE BYRE, K., LEREN, P. Effect of diet and smoking intervention on the incidence of coronary heart disease. *Lancet* 2(8259):1303–1310, December 12, 1981.

HOLME, I. On the separation of the intervention effects of diet and antismoking advice on the incidence of major coronary events in coronary high risk men. The Oslo Study. *Journal of the Oslo City Hospitals* 32(3/4):31–54, March–April 1982.

KAHN, H.A. The Dorn study of smoking and mortality among U.S. veterans: Report on eight and one-half years of observation. In: Haenszel, W. (ed.) *Epidemiological Approaches to the Study of Cancer and Other Chronic Diseases.* NCI Monograph 19. U.S. Department of Health, Education, and Welfare, Public Health Service, National Cancer Institute, January 1966, pp. 1–125.

KAPRIO, J., KOSKENVUO, M. A prospective study of psychological and socioeconomic characteristics, health behavior and morbidity in cigarette smokers prior to quitting compared to persistent smokers and non-smokers. *Journal of Clinical Epidemiology* 41(2):139–150, 1988.

KLEINBAUM, D.G., KUPPER, L.L., MORGENSTERN, H. *Epidemiologic Research.* Belmont, California: Lifetime Learning Publications, 1982.

LEU, R.E., SCHAUB, T. Does smoking increase medical care expenditure? *Social Science and Medicine* 17(23):1907–1914, 1983.

LUCE, B.R., SCHWEITZER, S.O. Smoking and alcohol abuse: A comparison of their economic consequences. *New England Journal of Medicine* 298(10):569–571, March 9, 1978.

MARSDEN, M.E., BRAY, R.M., HERBOLD, J.R. Substance use and health among U.S. military personnel: Findings from the 1985 worldwide survey. *Preventive Medicine* 17(3):366–376, May 1988.

MATTSON, M.E., POLLACK, E.S., CULLEN, J.W. What are the odds that smoking will kill you? *American Journal of Public Health* 77(4):425–431, April 1987.

MCMANUS, I.C., WEEKS, S.J. Smoking, personality and reasons for smoking. *Psychological Medicine* 12(2):349–356, May 1982.

MULTIPLE RISK FACTOR INTERVENTION TRIAL RESEARCH GROUP. Multiple Risk Factor Intervention Trial. Risk factor changes and mortality results. *Journal of the American Medical Association* 248(12):1465–1477, September 24, 1982.

MULTIPLE RISK FACTOR INTERVENTION TRIAL RESEARCH GROUP. Mortality rates after 10.5 years for participants in the Multiple Risk Factor Intervention Trial. Findings related to *a priori* hypotheses of the trial. *Journal of the American Medical Association* 263(13):1795–1801, April 4, 1990.

MULTIPLE RISK FACTOR INTERVENTION TRIAL RESEARCH GROUP. 10.5 year mortality for participants in the Multiple Risk Factor Intervention Trial. Findings for subgroups with hypertension at baseline. Submitted for publication.

NEWCOMB, M.D., BENTLER, P.M. The impact of late adolescent substance use on young adult health status and utilization of health services: A structural-equation model over four years. *Social Science and Medicine* 24(1):71–82, 1987.

OAKES, T.W., FRIEDMAN, G.D., SELTZER, C.C., SIEGELAUB, A.B., COLLEN, M.F. Health service utilization by smokers and nonsmokers. *Medical Care* 12(11):958–966, November 1974.

OCKENE, J.K., KULLER, L.H., SVENDSEN, K.H., MEILAHN, E. The relationship of smoking cessation to coronary heart disease and lung cancer in the Multiple Risk Factor Intervention Trial (MRFIT). *American Journal of Public Health* 80(8):954–958, August 1990.

OSTER, G., COLDITZ, G.A., KELLY, N.L. The economic costs of smoking and benefits of quitting for individual smokers. *Preventive Medicine* 13(4):377–389, July 1984.

OSTRO, B.D. Estimating the risks of smoking, air pollution, and passive smoke on acute respiratory conditions. *Risk Analysis* 9(2):189–196, 1989.

PEARSON, D.C., GROTHAUS, L.C., THOMPSON, R.S., WAGNER, E.H. Smokers and drinkers in a health maintenance organization population: Lifestyles and health status. *Preventive Medicine* 16(6):783–795, November 1987.

REED, W.L. Physical health status as a consequence of health practices. *Journal of Community Health* 8(4):217–228, Summer 1983.

RICE, D.P., HODGSON, T.A., SINSHEIMER, P. The economic costs of the health effects of smoking, 1984. *Milbank Quarterly* 64(4):489–547, 1986.

RODE, A., ROSS, R., SHEPHARD, R.J. Smoking withdrawal programme. Personality and cardiorespiratory fitness. *Archives of Environmental Health* 24(1):27–36, January 1972.

ROGOT, E., MURRAY, J.L. Smoking and causes of death among U.S. veterans: 16 years of observation. *Public Health Reports* 95(3):213–222, May–June 1980.

ROSE, G., HAMILTON, P.J. A randomised controlled trial of the effect on middle-aged men of advice to stop smoking. *Journal of Epidemiology and Community Health* 32(4):275–281, December 1978.

ROSE, G., HAMILTON, P.J.S., COLWELL, L., SHIPLEY, M.J. A randomised controlled trial of anti-smoking advice: 10-year results. *Journal of Epidemiology and Community Health* 36(2):102–108, June 1982.

SALONEN, J.T., TUOMILEHTO, J., NISSINEN, A., KAPLAN, G.A., PUSKA, P. Contribution of risk factor changes to the decline in coronary incidence during the North Karelia project: A within community analysis. *International Journal of Epidemiology* 18(3):595–601, September 1989.

SEGOVIA, J., BARTLETT, R.F., EDWARDS, A.C. The association between self-assessed health status and individual health practices. *Canadian Journal of Public Health* 80(1):32–37, January–February 1989.

SEIDELL, J.C., BAKX, K.C., DEURENBERG, P., BUREMA, J., HAUTVAST, J.G., HUYGEN, F.J. The relation between overweight and subjective health according to age, social class, slimming behavior and smoking habits in Dutch adults. *American Journal of Public Health* 76(12):1410–1415, December 1986.

SELTZER, C.C., OECHSLI, F.W. Psychosocial characteristics of adolescent smokers before they started smoking: Evidence of self-selection. A prospective study. *Journal of Chronic Diseases* 38(1):17–26, 1985.

STELLMAN, S.D., GARFINKEL, L. Smoking habits and tar levels in a new American Cancer Society prospective study of 1.2 million men and women. *Journal of the National Cancer Institute* 76(6):1057–1063, June 1986.

STEPHENS, T. Health practices and health status: Evidence from the Canada Health Survey. *American Journal of Preventive Medicine* 2(4):209–215, July–August 1986.

TUOMILEHTO, J., GEBOERS, J., SALONEN, J.T., NISSINEN, A., KUULASMAA, K., PUSKA, P. Decline in cardiovascular mortality in North Karelia and other parts of Finland. *British Medical Journal* 293:1068–1071, October 25, 1986.

U.S. DEPARTMENT OF HEALTH AND HUMAN SERVICES. *The Health Consequences of Smoking for Women. A Report of the Surgeon General.* U.S. Department of Health and Human Services, Public Health Service, Office of the Assistant Secretary for Health, Office on Smoking and Health, 1980.

U.S. DEPARTMENT OF HEALTH AND HUMAN SERVICES. *The Health Consequences of Smoking: Cancer and Chronic Lung Disease in the Workplace. A Report of the Surgeon General.* U.S. Department of Health and Human Services, Public Health Service, Office on Smoking and Health. DHHS Publication No. (PHS) 85-50207, 1985.

U.S. DEPARTMENT OF HEALTH AND HUMAN SERVICES. *Reducing the Health Consequences of Smoking: 25 Years of Progress. A Report of the Surgeon General.* U.S. Department of Health and Human Services, Public Health Service, Centers for Disease Control, Center for Chronic Disease Prevention and Health Promotion, Office on Smoking and Health. DHHS Publication No. (CDC) 89-8411, 1989.

U.S. DEPARTMENT OF HEALTH, EDUCATION, AND WELFARE. *Smoking and Health, A Report of the Surgeon General.* U.S. Department of Health, Education, and Welfare, Public Health Service, Office of the Assistant Secretary for Health, Office on Smoking and Health. DHEW Publication No. (PHS) 79-50066, 1979.

U.S. PUBLIC HEALTH SERVICE. *Smoking and Health. Report of the Advisory Committee to the Surgeon General of the Public Health Service.* U.S. Department of Health, Education, and Welfare, Public Health Service, Center for Disease Control. PHS Publication No. 1103, 1964.

U.S. PUBLIC HEALTH SERVICE. *The Health Consequences of Smoking. A Public Health Service Review: 1967.* U.S. Department of Health, Education, and Welfare, Public Health Service, Health Services and Mental Health Administration. PHS Publication No. 1696, revised 1968.

U.S. PUBLIC HEALTH SERVICE. *The Health Consequences of Smoking. 1969 Supplement to the 1967 Public Health Service Review.* U.S. Department of Health, Education, and Welfare, Public Health Service. DHEW Publication No. 1969-2 (Supplement), 1969.

VOGT, T.M., SCHWEITZER, S.O. Medical costs of cigarette smoking in a health maintenance organization. *American Journal of Epidemiology* 122(6):1060–1066, December 1985.

WEINKAM, J.J., ROSENBAUM, W., STERLING, T.D. Smoking and hospital utilization. *Social Science and Medicine* 24(11):983–986, 1987.

WORLD HEALTH ORGANIZATION EUROPEAN COLLABORATIVE GROUP. Multifactorial trial in the prevention of coronary heart disease. 3. Incidence and mortality results. *European Heart Journal* 4:141–147, 1983.

CHAPTER 4
SMOKING CESSATION AND RESPIRATORY CANCERS

CONTENTS

Lung Cancer 107
   Pathophysiologic Framework 107
      Smoking and Histopathology of the Airways 108
      Other Changes 109
   Smoking Cessation and Lung Cancer Risk 110
      Pattern of Changing Risk After Cessation 110
      Effect of Antecedent Smoking History 122
         Duration of Smoking 122
         Daily Cigarette Consumption 124
         Inhalation Practices 124
         Different Tobacco Products 124
         Effect of Age at Cessation 125
   Multistage Modeling 126
   Cessation After Developing Disease 129
   Cessation After Diagnosis of Lung Cancer 129

Laryngeal Cancer 131
   Pathophysiologic Framework 131
   Smoking Cessation and Laryngeal Cancer Risk 131

Conclusions 135

References 137

LUNG CANCER

Epidemiologic studies have provided overwhelming evidence for a causal association of cigarette smoking with lung cancer (US PHS 1964; US DHEW 1979; US DHHS 1989). The plausibility of this association is supported by the presence of numerous carcinogens in tobacco smoke. Compared with the risk among never smokers, the risk of lung cancer for smokers may be increased twentyfold or more for heavy smokers (US DHHS 1989). Risk of lung cancer increases with the number of cigarettes smoked daily and the duration of cigarette smoking; risk declines after cessation (US DHHS 1982, 1989). For example, in an analysis of data from the British Physicians Study, Doll and Peto (1978) indicated that among subjects who persisted in smoking, lung cancer incidence increased with the fourth or fifth power of the duration of smoking and with approximately the square of daily cigarette consumption. In 1985, estimated attributable risks of lung cancer from cigarette smoking were 90 percent for males and 79 percent for females in the United States (US DHHS 1989).

This Section considers the effects of cigarette smoking on the epithelium of the airways of the lungs, the site from which most lung cancers stem, and the evolution of the smoking-related changes after cessation. The epidemiologic evidence on lung cancer risk after smoking cessation is comprehensively reviewed; the change in risk over time following cessation is described; and factors modifying the effect of cessation are considered. The Section includes discussion of the application of multistage modeling to data on smoking cessation.

Pathophysiologic Framework

Previous Surgeon General's reports have provided extensive reviews on carcinogenic components of tobacco smoke and on experimental carcinogenesis with tobacco smoke (US DHEW 1979; US DHHS 1982, 1986). Tobacco smoke contains numerous carcinogenic agents with both initiating and promoting activity. Although the specific mechanisms of respiratory tract carcinogenesis by tobacco smoke are not yet fully characterized, the plausibility of the smoking–lung cancer relation has been considered to be well supported by the available information (US PHS 1964; US DHHS 1982).

Carcinogenesis in the respiratory tract is widely considered to be a multistep process involving sequential changes in a cell from the normal to the malignant state. Extensive experimental and human evidence is consistent with the multistage hypothesis, and application of the new molecular and cellular biology techniques to the study of lung cancer is providing further insights into the genetic mechanisms underlying the development of this disease (Birrer and Minna 1988). Experiments with animals have shown that agents may initiate or promote cancer. In animal experiments involving a sequence of exposures to agents, those agents that cause cancer when administered initially are referred to as initiators, whereas agents that promote the growth of initiated cells are referred to as promoters.

Diverse multistep models of carcinogenesis have been developed (Farber 1984). The age–incidence patterns for epithelial cancers such as lung cancer, which show that the rates usually increase as a power of age, are also consistent with a multistage process

(Doll 1971; Doll and Peto 1978; Peto 1984; Day 1984). The bronchial epithelia of sustained smokers show a progression of abnormality (Saccomanno et al. 1974). The pseudostratified, ciliated epithelium becomes metaplastic and then dysplastic. Carcinoma in situ may develop and eventually become invasive (McDowell, Harris, Trump 1982). To the extent that cigarette smoking affects late as well as early stages in this process, smoking cessation would be expected to have beneficial consequences on lung cancer incidence. The epidemiologic evidence provides strong support for the anticipated benefits of smoking cessation.

Cigarette smoking is associated with changes in the large and small airways, in the respiratory epithelium and parenchyma, and in the numbers, type, and functional capacities of inflammatory cells. The reversibility of these changes after smoking cessation is germane to respiratory carcinogenesis and to the health consequences of smoking cessation. This Section focuses on studies that have examined the effect of smoking on the respiratory epithelium and on the cells in the lungs of current, former, and never smokers. Additional relevant information is reviewed in Chapter 7 and in previous reports of the Surgeon General (US DHHS 1984, 1986).

Smoking and Histopathology of the Airways

Extensive histopathologic evidence is available on the effects of smoking on the airways of the lung. The association between smoking and premalignant changes in the bronchial epithelium has been addressed by many investigators (US DHHS 1982). Based on sequential examinations of exfoliative cytologic specimens from uranium miners over a period of many years, Saccomanno and colleagues (1974) reported evidence of squamous metaplasia progressing through increasing atypia to carcinoma in situ and invasive bronchogenic carcinoma. Detailed observations have been made on the histopathology of lung specimens obtained at autopsy (Auerbach et al. 1957, 1962a,b, 1963, 1964, 1972; Auerbach, Garfinkel, Hammond 1974).

In 1962, Auerbach and coworkers (1962a) reported that the frequency and intensity of epithelial changes increased with the number of cigarettes smoked daily. In addition, these investigators assessed changes following smoking cessation in postmortem bronchial epithelial specimens from 72 ex-smokers and controls matched individually with 2 controls per case (Auerbach et al. 1962b). One control was a current smoker matched with an ex-smoker on age, occupation, residence, and smoking history. The second control was a lifetime nonsmoker also matched with an ex-smoker on age, occupation, and residence. Some type of epithelial abnormality was found in 98 percent of histologic sections from current smokers, 67 percent from ex-smokers, but only 26 percent from never smokers. This pattern persisted for many specific types of epithelial abnormalities including absence of ciliated cells, presence of atypical cells, and presence of hyperplasia and goblet cells in glands (Table 1). The occurrence of unciliated atypical cells, the most severe change before invasive carcinoma, was similar among ex-smokers and never smokers but was considerably greater among current smokers. The number of cells with atypical nuclei was reported to decrease with increasing number of years since smoking cessation. When current smokers were matched with former smokers of the same age at time of cessation, former smokers

TABLE 1.—Histologic changes (%) in bronchial epithelium by smoking status

	Smoking status		
	Current smokers	Ex-smokers	Never smokers
Sections with 1 or more epithelial lesions	97.8	66.6	25.7
Cilia present on 3 or more cell rows	92.7	57.3	12.1
Cilia absent	20.5	15.1	14.8
Atypical cells present	93.2	6.0	1.2
Unciliated atypical cells	19.0	0.9	0.1

SOURCE: Auerbach et al. (1962b).

showed fewer lesions, suggesting that the number of lesions decreased rather than merely failed to increase after cessation of smoking.

Auerbach and colleagues (1964) also reported that among cigarette smokers, there was a high degree of association between all types of histologic changes in the bronchi and in the lung parenchyma. However, the lungs of ex-smokers were more similar to those of never smokers than to those of current smokers with respect to cells with atypical nuclei. In this study of 46 ex-smokers, 32 had few atypical cells in their bronchial epithelium. Auerbach and associates (1964) suggested that with cessation of smoking, cells with atypical nuclei gradually disappeared from the bronchial epithelium and were replaced with normal cells.

Other Changes

Several reports have described levels of DNA adducts formed by the combination of chemical carcinogens or their metabolites with DNA in the tissues of never, former, and current smokers. Decline of DNA adduct levels in human lungs after smoking cessation has been reported by Phillips and coworkers (1988). These investigators utilized autoradiographs of chromatograms of ^{32}P-postlabeled digests of DNA from lungs of current, former, and never smokers. A linear relationship was observed between number of cigarettes smoked per day and DNA adduct levels (Pearson correlation coefficient, r=0.72, p<0.001). In addition, ex-smokers who had quit smoking 1 to 3 months previously had adduct levels typical of the current smokers (12–14 adducts/10^8 nucleotides), whereas those who had not smoked for 5 years or more had adduct levels similar to those of never smokers (1.7–4.9 adducts/10^8 nucleotides). These investigators suggested that the reduced risk of lung cancer among ex-smokers may be due to loss of the promutagenic lesions that initiate the process, in addition to late-stage effects.

Randerath and colleagues (1989) also used a ^{32}P-postlabeling assay to study DNA damage in relation to cigarette smoking. Adduct profiles and levels were determined in nontumorous surgical specimens taken from patients with lung or laryngeal cancer.

Characteristic profiles were found in the laryngeal and lung tissues; levels of adducts tended to increase with the amount of cumulative smoking. The study included only three long-term former smokers with duration of abstinence ranging from 10 to 14 years. These subjects had low levels of adducts compared with current smokers.

Smoking Cessation and Lung Cancer Risk

Pattern of Changing Risk After Cessation

Numerous cohort and case–control studies have documented a reduction in the relative risk of lung cancer among former smokers compared with current smokers. The findings of selected studies are presented in Table 2. Former smokers in these studies experienced a 10- to 800-percent increase in risk of lung cancer compared with never smokers; however, compared with current smokers, former smokers showed a 20- to 90-percent reduction in risk.

The relative risk estimates provided in Table 2 group former smokers with varying durations of abstinence from smoking. However, the number of years since cessation has a strong effect on risk of lung cancer among former smokers; in studies assessing risk by duration of abstinence, the reduced risk has been evident within 5 years of cessation compared with continued smoking, and the benefit of cessation has increased as the duration of abstinence lengthened. However, in most of the studies, the risk of lung cancer among former smokers remained elevated above the risk among never smokers, even in the longest periods of abstinence evaluated. In many studies, risks among former smokers were higher than among continuing smokers during the first few years after stopping smoking. This pattern of risk reflects cessation by individuals who quit smoking because of symptoms and illness before the clinical diagnosis of lung cancer (Chapter 2; Haenszel, Loveland, Sirken 1962; Doll and Hill 1964; Kahn 1966).

Table 3 summarizes standardized mortality ratios of lung cancer among former smokers by years of abstinence, as reported in five cohort studies: British physicians, U.S. veterans, Japanese males, and the American Cancer Society Cancer Prevention Studies, ACS CPS-I and ACS CPS-II. These studies varied in the length of followup, the extent of information obtained on smoking history, and the number of lung cancer cases. Compared with never smokers, former smokers who had been abstinent for 10 to 20 years or more showed a varying extent of risk reduction among the studies. In the British Physicians Study, U.S. Veterans Study, and ACS CPS-II, former smokers who had been abstinent for 15 years or more showed an 80- to 90-percent reduction in risk compared with current smokers. The percentage reduction in risk was slightly lower among the Japanese cohort and higher in ACS CPS-I.

Results from selected case–control studies are shown in Table 4. As in the cohort studies, former smokers who had been abstinent the longest experienced increased risk compared with never smokers, but substantially reduced risk in most studies compared with current smokers.

Thus, reduction in risk of lung cancer after smoking cessation has been observed in numerous cohort and case–control studies conducted in the United Kingdom (Doll and Peto 1976; Alderson, Lee, Wang 1985), the United States (Kahn 1966; Hammond 1966;

TABLE 2.—Relative risks of lung cancer among never, former, and current smokers in selected epidemiologic studies

Reference	Population	Subgroup	Never smokers	Former smokers 1–19 cig/day	Former smokers ≥20 cig/day	Current smokers 1–19 cig/day	Current smokers ≥20 cig/day
Hammond (1966)	ACS CPS-I		1.0	2.0	7.9	6.5	13.7
Kahn (1966)	US veterans		1.0	4.7		10.9	
Canadian Department of National Health and Welfare (1966)	Canadian males		1.0	6.1		14.9	
Cederlof et al. (1975)		Males	1.0	6.1		7.8	
		Females	1.0	1.5		4.5	
Doll and Peto (1976)	British male physicians		1.0	4.3		10.4	
Doll et al. (1980)	British female physicians		1.0	3.3		6.4[a]	
Wigle, Mao, Grace (1980)	Alberta (Canada) cancer patients	Males	1.0	6.5		10.4	
		Females	1.0	2.1		5.2	
Wu et al. (1985)	Los Angeles (CA) whites	Squamous	1.0	7.7		35.3	
		Adenocarcinoma	1.0	1.2		4.1	
Carstensen, Pershagen, Eklund (1987)	Swedish males		1.0	1.1		7.5[b]	
ACS (unpublished tabulations)	ACS CPS-II	Males	1.0	8.9		21.3	
		Females	1.0	4.8		12.1	

NOTE: ACS CPS-I and II=American Cancer Society Cancer Prevention Studies I and II.
[a] 15–24 cig/day.
[b] 8–15 cig/day.

TABLE 3.—Lung cancer mortality ratios among never, current, and former smokers by number of years since stopped smoking (relative to never smokers), prospective studies

Reference	Population	Smoking status and yr since stopped smoking	Mortality ratios (N)[a]	Comments
Doll and Peto (1976)	British male physicians	Never smokers	1.0 (7)	1951–71, 20-yr followup; data on former smokers in summary form
		Current smokers	15.8 (123)	
		Former smokers		
		1–4	16.0 (15)	
		5–9	5.9 (12)	
		10–14	5.3 (9)	
		≥15	2.0 (7)	
Rogot and Murray (1980)	US veterans[b]	Current smokers	11.3 (2,609)	1954–69, 16-yr followup
		Former smokers		
		1–4	18.8 (47)	
		5–9	7.7 (86)	
		10–14	4.7 (100)	
		15–19	4.8 (115)	
		≥20	2.1 (123)	
US DHHS (1982)	Japanese males	Current smokers	3.8	
		Former smokers		
		1–4	4.7	
		5–9	2.5	
		≥10	1.4	

TABLE 3.—Continued

Reference	Population	Smoking status and yr since stopped smoking	Mortality ratios (N)[a]		Comments
			1–19 cig/day	≥20 cig/day	
Hammond (1966)	ACS CPS-I males				1959–63, 3.5-yr followup, men aged 50–69
		Never smokers	1.0 (32)	1.0 (32)	
		Current smokers	6.5 (8.0)	13.7 (351)	
		Former smokers			
		<1	7.2 (3)	29.1 (33)	
		1–4	4.6 (5)	12.0 (33)	
		5–9	1.0 (1)	7.2 (22)	
		≥10	0.4 (1)	1.1 (5)	
			1–20 cig/day	≥21 cig/day	
ACS (unpublished tabulations)	ACS CPS-II males	Never smokers	1.0 (81)	1.0 (81)	
		Current smokers	18.8 (608)	26.9 (551)	
		Former smokers			
		<1	26.7 (33)	50.7 (64)	
		1–2	22.4 (71)	33.2 (117)	
		3–5	16.5 (82)	20.9 (96)	
		6–10	8.7 (80)	15.0 (106)	
		11–15	6.0 (69)	12.6 (95)	
		≥16	3.1 (144)	5.5 (112)	

TABLE 3.—Continued

Reference	Population	Smoking status and yr since stopped smoking	Mortality ratios (N)[a]		Comments
			1–19 cig/day	≥20 cig/day	
ACS (unpublished tabulations)	ACS CPS-II females	Never smokers	1.0 (181)	1.0 (181)	
		Current smokers	7.3 (145)	16.3 (434)	
		Former smokers			
		<1	7.9 (5)	34.3 (31)	
		1–2	9.1 (13)	19.5 (42)	
		3–5	2.9 (7)	14.6 (42)	
		6–10	1.0 (4)	9.1 (32)	
		11–15	1.5 (6)	5.9 (20)	
		≥16	1.4 (23)	2.6 (18)	

NOTE: ACS CPS-I and -II=American Cancer Society Cancer Prevention Studies I and II.
[a] Number of observations.
[b] Includes data only for ex-cigarette smokers who stopped for reasons other than physician's order.

TABLE 4.—Relative risks of lung cancer among former smokers, by number of years since stopped smoking, and current smokers, from selected case–control studies

Reference	Population	Definition of former smoker	Smoking status and yr since stopped	Results	Adjustment[a]
Graham and Levin (1971)	New York	At hospital admission	Never smokers Current smokers Former smokers 　0–0.5 　>0.5–1 　>1–3 　>3–10 　>10	Males 1.0 8.8 42.2 23.3 10.0 3.3 1.3	Crude
Wigle, Mao, Grace (1980)	Alberta, Canada, cancer patients	At interview	Never smokers Current smokers Former smokers 　<2 　2–9 　10–14 　≥15	Males　Females 0.1　　0.2 1.0　　1.0 2.4　　0.9 0.7　　0.5 0.7　　0.5 0.2　　0.4	Age and cumulative smoking
Correa et al. (1984)	Louisiana	NR	Never smokers Current smokers Former smokers 　3–5 　6–20 　>20	Males and females 1.0 12.6 7.7 7.0 3.9	Sex and age

TABLE 4.—Continued

Reference	Population	Definition of former smoker	Smoking status and yr since stopped	Results		Adjustment[a]
				Males	Females	
Alderson, Lee, Wang (1985)	United Kingdom	At hospital admission	Never smokers	0.1	0.2	Age
			Current smokers	1.0	1.0	
			Former smokers			
			1–3	1.8	2.1	
			5–10	0.4	0.7	
			>10	0.3	0.3	
				Males	Females	
Gao et al. (1988)	Shanghai	NR	Never smokers	1.0	1.0	Age and education
			Current smokers	3.9	2.9	
			Former smokers			
			1–4	6.9	7.2	
			5–9	3.1	3.9	
			≥10	1.1	2.2	
				Males		
Higgins, Mahan, Wynder (1988)	6 US cities	At least 1 yr at time of interview	Never smokers	1.0		
			Former smokers			
			<10	11.9		
			10–19	6.1		
			20–29	3.7		
			≥30	1.9		
				Males	Females	
Joly, Lubin, Caraballoso (1983)	Cuba	NR	Current smokers	1.0	1.0	Duration of smoking
			Former smokers			
			1–4	1.2	2.0	
			≥5	0.6	0.9	

TABLE 4.—Continued

Reference	Population	Definition of former smoker	Smoking status and yr since stopped	Results		Adjustment[a]
Lubin et al. (1984a)	European case–control study	At interview	Current smokers Former smokers 1–4 5–9 10–14 15–19 20–24 ≥25	Males 1.0 1.1 0.7 0.6 0.4 0.4 0.3	Females 1.0 0.9 0.7 0.4 0.5 0.5 0.3	Duration of smoking
Pathak et al. (1986)	New Mexico	At least 1 yr before interview	Current smokers Former smokers 5 10 20	Males ≤65 1.0 0.5 0.2 0.1	>65 1.0 0.7 0.5 0.3	Number of cig/day
Damber and Larsson (1986)	Sweden[b]	NR	Current smokers Former smokers 1–5 6–10 >10	Males 9.5 7.5 3.0 2.0		Age

NOTE: NR=not reported.
[a] Factors adjusted for in analysis by yr of smoking abstinence.
[b] Estimated from figure 4 of reference.

Graham and Levin 1971; Pathak et al. 1986), Canada (Wigle, Mao, Grace 1980), Europe (Lubin et al. 1984a; Damber and Larsson 1986), Asia (US DHHS 1982; Gao et al. 1988), and Latin America (Joly, Lubin, Caraballoso 1983). Although only a few studies had information on female former smokers, the pattern of risk reduction was similar to that observed for males. Decrease in risk after smoking cessation also has been reported for each of the major histologic types of lung cancer (Wynder and Stellman 1977; Lubin and Blot 1984; Benhamou et al. 1985; Higgins and Wynder 1988) (Table 5 and Figure 1). Higgins and Wynder (1988) found that the decline in risk after cessation was more consistent for Kreyberg I tumors (primarily squamous cell, small cell, and large cell cancers) than for Kreyberg II tumors (primarily adenocarcinomas and bronchiolo-alveolar carcinomas) (Figure 1). Smokers of filter and nonfilter cigarettes (Wynder and Stellman 1979; Lubin et al. 1984b) and of other tobacco products (Joly, Lubin, Caraballoso 1983; Lubin et al. 1984b; Damber and Larsson 1986; Higgins, Mahan, Wynder 1988) have reduced lung cancer risk following cessation (Table 6). Although the findings of the reviewed studies uniformly indicate lower risk among former smokers, the magnitude and rapidity of the risk reduction with smoking cessation varies among the studies. This variation has several potential explanations.

First, years of abstinence among those who stopped smoking for the longest time interval varied from 5 to 25 years or more. Second, although former smokers have a risk of lung cancer between those of continuing smokers and never smokers, the pattern of declining risk as duration of abstinence lengthens has not been fully characterized. The small number of former smokers in some studies limits the precision with which the decline in risk can be described, particularly for the longer durations of abstinence. Third, aspects of the active smoking history, including cumulative smoking exposure up to the time of quitting, age at initiation, years of smoking, number of cigarettes smoked per day, inhalation practices, types of cigarettes and other tobacco products smoked, age at smoking cessation, and the reason for stopping, may modify the risk of lung cancer after cessation (Chapter 4, see section on Effect of Antecedent Smoking History). The varying extent to which these factors have been considered in analyzing the effect of cessation may partially explain the differences in risk observed in former smokers among the studies. As discussed below, failure to adjust for previous smoking history may exaggerate the benefit of smoking cessation, but adjustment for cumulative smoking history also may result in overadjustment of the risk estimate (Chapter 2). Fourth, the studies vary in the definition of former or ex-smokers and in the analytic treatment of former smokers who have recently stopped smoking. In the case–control studies, former smokers have been defined as individuals who were abstinent at the time of interview, at the time of cancer diagnosis, or at some other reference point (e.g., 1 year before diagnosis of lung cancer and a comparable time for controls).

To reduce the bias introduced by quitting because of illness, former smokers who stopped smoking after developing symptoms or disease may be excluded from analysis. Information on the reason for cessation was collected only in some studies, and persons with symptoms at cessation have not been handled uniformly in the published literature. Finally, results of the relevant studies are not totally comparable because the risks of former smokers were compared with those of never smokers in some studies and with continuing smokers in others.

TABLE 5.—Relative risks of lung cancer among never, current, and former smokers, by number of years since stopping smoking and histologic type

Reference	Population	Smoking status and yr since stopped	Histologic type				
			Males		Females	
			Kreyberg type		Kreyberg type	
			I	II	I	II
Wynder and Stellman (1979)	6 US cities	Never smokers	1.0	1.0	1.0	1.0
		Current smokers	32.3	10.7	10.5	4.4
		Former smokers				
		1–3	53.8	14.2	13.6	6.7
		4–6	24.9	5.9	6.2	3.6
		7–10	17.2	6.6	5.1	4.1
		11–15	13.7	5.4	8.8	5.6
		≥16	5.0	1.2	—	0.9
			Males			
			Kreyberg type			
			I	II		
Benhamou et al. (1985)	French males, European case–control study	Never smokers	1.0	1.0		
		Former smokers				
		1–3	34.6	6.7		
		4–6	12.2	2.1		
		7–10	10.9	—		
		11–19	6.3	1.0		
		≥20	4.2	—		
			Males		Females	
			SQ	ADENO	SQ	ADENO
Lubin and Blot (1984)	European case–control study	Current smokers	1.0	1.0	1.0	1.0
		Former smokers				
		1–4	1.1	1.0	1.1	0.7
		5–9	0.7	0.8	0.9	1.0
		10–14	0.6	0.6	0.4	0.4
		15–19	0.4	0.6	0.4	1.2
		≥20	0.4	0.5	0.3	0.3

NOTE: SQ=squamous cell carcinoma of the lung; ADENO=adenocarcinoma of the lung.

TABLE 6.—Relative risks of lung cancer among never, former, and current smokers by types of tobacco products smoked

Reference	Population	Tobacco product	Smoking status		
			Never smokers	Former smokers	Current smokers
Higgins, Mahan, Wynder (1988)	6 US cities	Cigarettes only	1.0	6.9	16.0
		Cigars only	1.0	2.5	3.1
		Pipes only	1.0	0.7	1.9
		Cigars and pipes	1.0	2.4	2.5
		Mixed smokers	1.0	5.1	10.5
Lubin, Richter, Blot (1984)	European case–control study			Yr since stopped	
				1–4 ≥5	
		Cigars only		0.6 0.7	1.0
		Mixed cigars and cigarettes		4.4 0.9	1.0
		Pipes only		2.0 0.9	1.0
		Mixed pipes and cigarettes		1.2 0.8	1.0
Damber and Larsson (1986)	Sweden			Yr since stopped	
				1–10 >10	
		Cigarettes only[a]		5.0 1.2	9.5
		Pipes only		5.0 4.5	8.0

[a] Estimated from figure 5 of reference; reference group is never smokers.

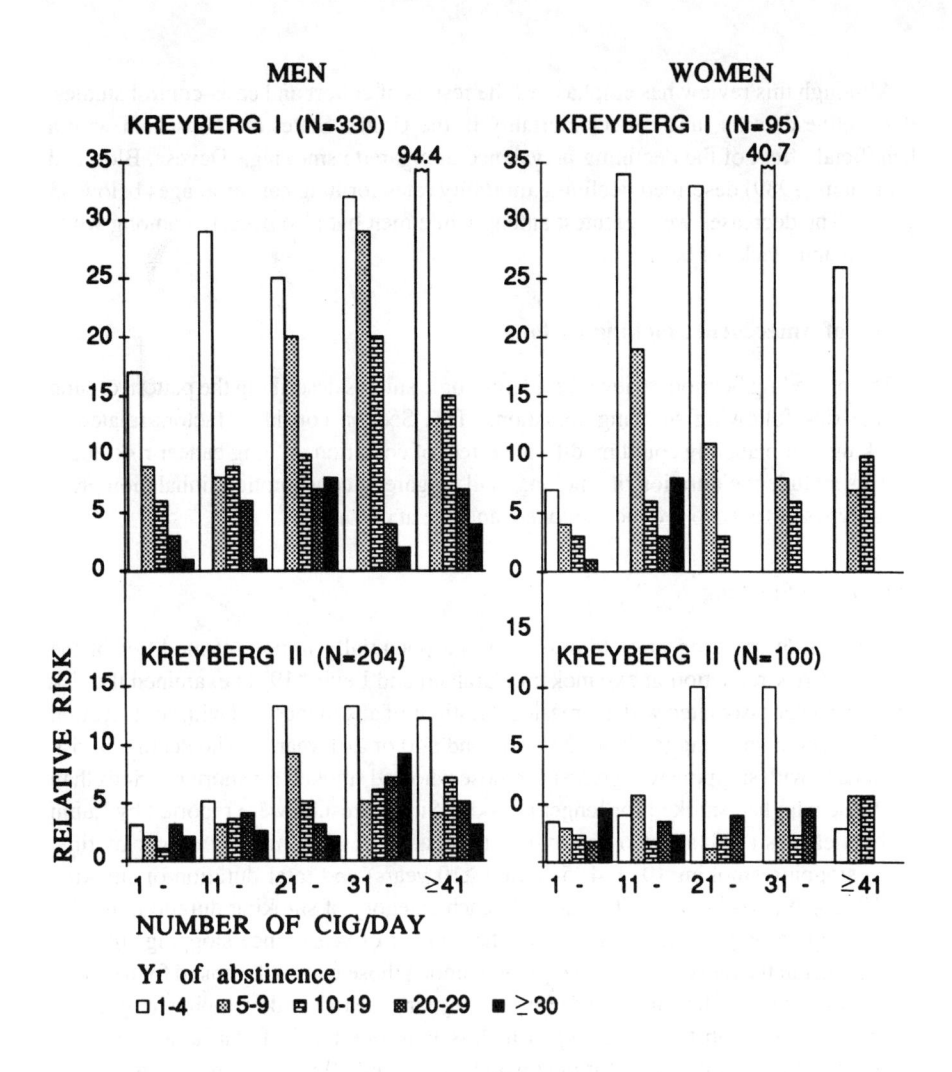

FIGURE 1.—Risk of lung cancer by number of cigarettes smoked per day before quitting, number of years of abstinence, sex, and histologic types

SOURCE: Higgins and Wynder (1988).

Although this review has emphasized the results of cohort and case–control studies, descriptive data on lung cancer mortality in the United States are consistent with a beneficial effect of the declining prevalence of cigarette smoking. Devesa, Blot, and Fraumeni (1989) described declining mortality rates for lung cancer at ages below 45 years. The decreases were greatest among white men but also occurred among white women and blacks of both sexes.

Effect of Antecedent Smoking History

The preceding Section reviewed epidemiologic studies describing the pattern of lung cancer risk following smoking cessation. This Section considers factors related to smoking that plausibly could modify the effect of cessation on lung cancer risk; these factors include the duration of smoking, daily cigarette consumption, inhalation practices, types of tobacco products smoked, and age at cessation.

Duration of Smoking

Duration of smoking prior to cessation is a potentially important modifier of the pattern of risk reduction in ex-smokers. Graham and Levin (1971) examined the risk of lung cancer associated with increasing durations of abstinence and with stratification by duration of smoking (≤ 30 or ≥ 31 years and ≤ 40 or ≥ 41 years). The decline in risk associated with stopping was greater for those who had smoked for shorter periods than for those who had smoked for longer periods. Similar results were reported by Lubin and colleagues (1984a), who determined the risk of developing lung cancer by time since stopping smoking (0, 1–4, 5–9, and ≥ 10 years) and total duration of smoking (1–19, 20–39, 40–49, and ≥ 50 years). In each category of smoking duration, the risk of developing lung cancer decreased as the number of years since stopping smoking increased, but the rate of decline was greater among those who had smoked for a shorter time. Among men who had smoked for 1 to 19 years, the risk of developing lung cancer after 10 years of abstinence dropped to less than one-third of that among current smokers. On the other hand, for men who had smoked 50 years or more and stopped for at least 10 years, the risk was still 90 percent of that for men who continued to smoke. This analysis, which matched for age and controlled for both duration of smoking and length of abstinence, introduces too many variables for the temporal dimensions of cigarette use (Chapter 2). By simultaneously considering attained age, duration of smoking, and length of abstinence, the analytic model incorrectly forces former smokers to have a younger age of starting to smoke than current smokers. In a case–control study in Sweden, Damber and Larsson (1986) also found higher relative risks among former smokers of pipes and cigarettes who had smoked longer.

Brown and Chu (1987) suggested that failure to adjust for previous duration of smoking may result in risk estimates for former smokers that are too low and thus exaggerate the benefits of smoking cessation. Based on reanalysis of data from the large European case–control study, Brown and Chu (1987) reported that the correlation between duration of smoking and time since stopping smoking for ex-smokers was -0.6, indicating that men who had stopped smoking for many years had also smoked for less

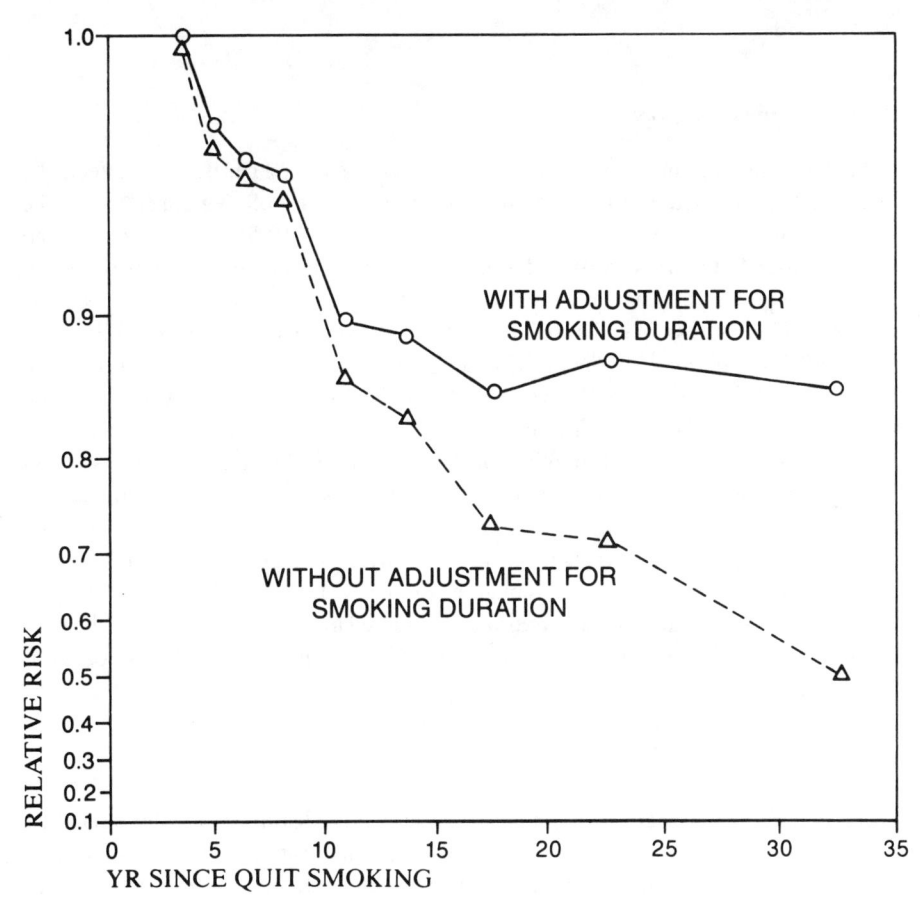

FIGURE 2.—Relative risk of lung cancer among ex-smokers compared with continuing smokers as a function of time since stopped smoking, estimated from logistic regression model, pattern adjusted for smoking duration compared with pattern unadjusted for duration

SOURCE: Brown and Chu (1987).

time than men who had stopped for a shorter time. The relative risk of lung cancer continued to decrease sharply with increasing years of abstinence without adjusting for smoking duration, whereas the decreasing relative risk plateaued when adjusted for duration of smoking (Figure 2). The difference in this pattern was most noticeable for increasing years of smoking abstinence. For those who had stopped smoking for 27 years or more, the relative risk compared with continuing smokers was 0.40 when adjusted for duration, but 0.17 when no adjustment was made. However, control for previous duration of smoking (or cumulative previous smoking history) in determining the risk of lung cancer among former smokers may constitute overadjustment if age and duration of cessation also are included in the model (Chapter 2).

In summary, only limited analyses address the effect of duration of previous smoking on the decline in risk following cessation. The data point to less decline of relative risk following cessation, comparing longer term with shorter term studies, but additional investigation is needed.

Daily Cigarette Consumption

Previous smoking intensity or number of cigarettes smoked per day also affects the pattern of risk reduction after smoking cessation. In the U.S. Veterans Study, the mortality ratios for lung cancer were 1.41, 3.47, 8.34, and 10.05 for ex-smokers who smoked 1 to 9, 10 to 20, 21 to 39, and 40 cigarettes or more per day, respectively (Kahn 1966). The pattern of lung cancer risk reduction by years of smoking abstinence and number of cigarettes smoked has been reported for several studies. In ACS CPS-I and ACS CPS-II (Hammond 1966; Garfinkel and Stellman 1988), the decline in risk with stopping smoking showed a comparable proportional reduction in risk among those who had smoked less (Table 3). In the European case–control study (Lubin et al. 1984a), men who had stopped smoking for 10 years or more, but had previously smoked 30 cigarettes or more per day, had a 40-percent risk of developing lung cancer compared with corresponding current smokers, whereas men who had smoked 1 to 9 cigarettes per day had a 67-percent risk compared with corresponding current smokers. Similar results were observed for female ex-smokers (Lubin et al. 1984a). As previously discussed, duration of smoking was considered in these analyses. Thus, heavier smokers have less reduction of lung cancer risk following cessation than smokers of fewer cigarettes per day.

Inhalation Practices

The pattern of lung cancer risk by years of smoking abstinence and by inhalation practices (i.e., frequency and depth of inhalation) was examined by Lubin and colleagues (1984a). Their analysis indicated a somewhat greater reduction in risk for those ex-smokers who had inhaled less often or less deeply. Among men who had stopped smoking for 10 years or more, relative risk by reported frequency of inhalation compared with current smokers was lowest for those who had rarely or never inhaled (relative risk (RR)=0.39) and for those whose depth of inhalation was reported as only slight or not at all (RR=0.37). In comparison, the relative risk after 10 years or more of abstinence was highest for those who had inhaled all the time (RR=0.50) and for those who had inhaled deeply (RR=0.47). The same pattern was observed among women.

Different Tobacco Products

Differences in the reduction in risk following cessation also have been investigated by types of cigarettes smoked. A lower risk of lung cancer has been observed for smokers of filter cigarettes compared with smokers of nonfilter cigarettes (US DHHS 1982, 1989; Wynder and Kabat 1988), a pattern suggesting that the reduction in risk among former smokers may be more apparent for filter cigarette smokers. However, no significant differences in the trend of risk reduction by years of smoking abstinence (0, 1–4, 5–9, and ≥10) and by type of cigarettes smoked (filter, mixed, nonfilter) were observed by Lubin and coworkers (1984b) in the European case–control study. Among men, the relative risk for former smokers after stopping smoking for 10 years or more was 0.4 for filter cigarette smokers, 0.3 for nonfilter cigarette smokers, and 0.5 for mixed filter and nonfilter cigarette smokers. These data were collected in five western European countries from 1976 to 1980; the tar yields of the products smoked were relatively high in comparison with cigarettes currently smoked in the United States (Lubin et al. 1984b).

In most studies, cigar and pipe smokers have lower lung cancer risks compared with cigarette smokers (US DHHS 1982). Former smokers of only pipes or cigars also showed an intermediate risk of lung cancer compared with current smokers and never smokers of these tobacco products (Table 6). In the U.S. Veterans Study, the lung cancer mortality ratio, compared with never smokers, was 1.67 among current smokers who used only pipes or cigars and 1.50 among former smokers (Kahn 1966). In a case–control study of smoking-related cancers conducted in the United States, Higgins, Mahan, and Wynder (1988) reported that ex-smokers of cigars only showed a relative risk of 2.5 compared with 3.1 among current smokers of cigars only. The relative risk was 0.7 among ex-smokers of pipes only compared with 1.9 among current pipe smokers only. Analysis of the pattern of risk among ex-smokers of cigars and pipes only by considering the amount and duration smoked prior to smoking cessation revealed similar patterns of risk reduction among light and heavy smokers.

Lubin, Richter, and Blot (1984) also examined the pattern of risk reduction by years of smoking abstinence (0, 1–4, ≥5 years) and types of tobacco smoked (cigars only, mixed cigar and cigarette smokers, pipes only, and mixed pipe and cigarette smokers). No apparent differences were observed in the estimated risks, when analyzed by tobacco products, among those who had stopped smoking for at least 5 years, but the numbers of cases who smoked cigars only and pipes only were quite small. On the other hand, Damber and Larsson (1986) reported that the decrease in relative risk among ex-smokers was less pronounced in smokers of pipes compared with cigarette smokers only in a case–control study conducted in Sweden. However, in this population, the risk of lung cancer for pipe smokers (RR=6.9) was similar to that of cigarette smokers (RR=7.0).

In summary, these analyses, limited by the sample sizes within strata of types of products smoked, do not characterize precisely the changing lung cancer risk following cessation for smokers of various tobacco products.

Effect of Age at Cessation

Several researchers have suggested that the reduction in risk after smoking cessation may differ by age at cessation. Wynder and Stellman (1979) reported that the reduction in risk after cessation was appreciably greater for people aged 50 to 69 than for those 70 or older. However, only data for those aged 50 to 69 were presented in this publication. Pathak and associates (1986) also reported a strong interaction between age and duration of cigarette smoking. Risk of lung cancer among ex-smokers was compared with that of current smokers with adjustment for the amount smoked. For ex-smokers less than 65 years of age, the estimated relative risks compared with current smokers declined to 0.49, 0.24, and 0.06 for 5, 10, and 20 years of smoking abstinence, respectively. For those aged 65 or older, the corresponding estimated relative risks were 0.73, 0.54, and 0.29, respectively. These two studies suggest that the risk of lung cancer may decline less steeply with increasing abstinence for older ex-smokers.

Multistage Modeling

Multistage models provide a conceptual framework for facilitating understanding of the relationship of lung cancer incidence with amount smoked, duration of smoking, and time since cessation. These models, proposing theoretical constructs of fundamental biologic mechanisms, have been useful for evaluating epidemiologic data in a biologic framework and thereby furthering the understanding of tobacco carcinogenesis. However, fitting these models to epidemiologic data cannot establish the veracity of the underlying biologic theory. Multistage modeling approaches have been used to describe respiratory carcinogenesis and to assess smoking cessation and lung cancer risk. Although a number of different mathematic models of carcinogenesis have been proposed (e.g., two-stage, multicell, multistage), this discussion primarily addresses the Armitage and Doll (1954, 1957) multistage model, which has been used most extensively in studies of lung cancer.

Based on a series of studies examining age-specific mortality rates for various cancers, Armitage and Doll (1954, 1957) proposed a multistage theory of carcinogenesis. Their model assumes that a single cell can generate a malignant tumor only after undergoing a certain number of genetic changes. Animal studies also support the multistage model. Multistage theories also predict the age pattern of occurrence of many tumors induced in experimental animals by continuous exposure to chemical carcinogens. Experimental regimens involving initiation and promotion provide direct evidence of the effect of early- and late-stage events in the carcinogenic process (Stenback, Peto, Shubik 1981a,b,c).

Using data from the British Physicians Study, Doll (1971) showed that when the incidence of lung cancer in cigarette smokers was plotted against duration of smoking, incidence increased approximately in proportion to the fourth power of duration, similar to the slope of the regression line when incidence in never smokers is plotted against age (Figure 3). Thus, a first-stage effect was implicated because the excess lung cancer risk among smokers increased with the same power of duration of smoking as the risk with age among never smokers. Moreover, the lung cancer mortality rates among ex-smokers decreased somewhat initially and then increased slowly in keeping with the increase in risk among never smokers with age (Doll 1971). Armitage (1971) noted that the stabilization of excess lung cancer risk at the level when smoking stopped suggested that smoking also affected a late stage, namely, the penultimate stage in the carcinogenic process.

Day and Brown (1980) conducted a detailed analysis of the pattern of change in cancer risk after cessation of an exposure. The results supported the Armitage–Doll model. In addition, Day and Brown proposed that the stage affected by the agent and the relative magnitude of the effect of the agent on early and late stages of the carcinogenic process are critical in the determination of risk subsequent to cessation of an exposure. To quantify the magnitude of smoking effects on the two stages, Brown

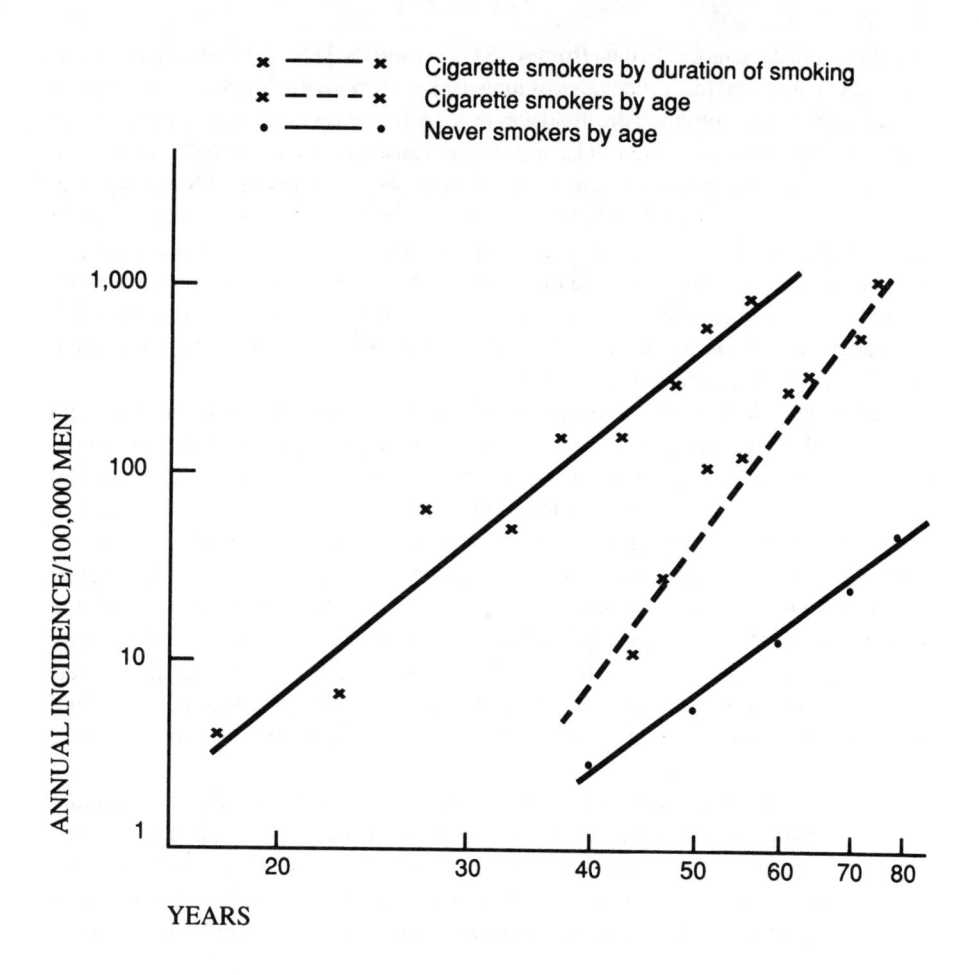

FIGURE 3.—Incidence of bronchial carcinoma among continuing cigarette smokers in relation to age and duration of smoking and among never smokers in relation to age, double logarithmic scale

SOURCE: Doll (1971), with correction of printing error in the original figure.

and Chu (1987) reexamined data on ex-smokers from the European case–control study of lung cancer (Lubin et al. 1984a) and concluded that smoking had an almost double relative effect on late-stage events compared with first-stage events. Using data from a case–control study in New Mexico, Whittemore (1988) developed a predictive model for lung cancer that showed a twofold stronger effect on late-stage than on early-stage events; the model overpredicted cases among ex-smokers and underpredicted cases among current smokers. Therefore, Whittemore suggested that smoking may have an even stronger effect on late-stage events than was assumed in the model.

Alternative models and interpretation of data on former smokers and lung cancer have also been suggested in several recent studies. Freedman and Navidi (1989) tested the fit of the multistage model to data from ACS CPS-I and the U.S. Veterans Study. These researchers observed that crude rates of lung cancer decreased with increasing years of smoking abstinence although the trend was less steep when average amount of smoking and ages when smoking started and stopped were considered in the analysis. Moreover, the observed lung cancer rates among ex-smokers were compared with the expected rates, which were computed in three ways—risk at the time of quitting, risk at current age with excess risk frozen at the time of quitting, and never smokers of the same age. For each comparison approach, the ratio of observed to expected rates decreased with increasing years of smoking abstinence. Freedman and Navidi (1989) concluded that this pattern was incompatible with the multistage model, which predicts stabilization of excess risk when an individual stops smoking.

Gaffney and Altshuler (1988) reexamined data from the British Physicians Study and found that the best-fitting model among current smokers predicted an increase in the excess incidence among ex-smokers, which was inconsistent with the observed decreased rates. These researchers found that a two-stage model fit the incidence of lung cancer in both current smokers and ex-smokers. Gaffney and Altshuler (1988) then proposed a two-stage model with clonal growth in which cigarette smoke induced the initial transition and promoted clonal growth in these cells initiated by cigarette smoke. Moolgavkar, Dewanji, and Luebeck (1989) questioned the biologic plausibility of the proposal by Gaffney and Altshuler (1988) and noted that their model only fit part of the British physicians data set, did not consider each age–smoking level, and discounted the possibility that smoking affected two transition rates in the carcinogenic process.

Moolgavkar, Dewanji, and Luebeck (1989) reanalyzed the British Physicians Study within the framework of the two-mutation, recessive oncogenesis model. Based on this model, the second-mutation rate would be affected by smoking, and a sudden decline in risk after cessation of smoking would be predicted. However, this model implies that smoking affects the last stage in a multistage process, contrary to current considerations.

In summary, multistage models have been used to describe the interrelationships among number of cigarettes smoked daily, duration, time since exposure ended, and lung cancer incidence. Several investigators have interpreted the data on risk among former smokers in different ways. The epidemiologic data clearly indicate that the risk among former smokers is between that of continuing smokers and never smokers. Various models can be fit to the different data sets. The expected pattern of risk among former smokers is sensitive to the model selected and dependent on the relative magnitude of the effect of smoking on early versus late stages of the process of carcinogenesis. Using multistage models, the data on former smokers are insufficient to allow precise quantification of the relative effects of smoking on the early and late stages of the carcinogenic process, which smoking is assumed to affect. Nevertheless, data indicate that smoking has an effect on the late stages of the carcinogenic process and that cessation reduces lung cancer occurrence.

Cessation After Developing Disease

Individuals who stopped smoking are not a randomly selected group in most studies (Chapter 2). Often, smokers quit as a result of developing symptoms of a life-threatening disease or immediately after diagnosis of cancer. This phenomenon is evidenced by the increase in risk of lung cancer in the immediate period after cessation. Some studies have grouped these former smokers with the continuing smokers or have excluded them from the analysis.

A few epidemiologic studies have assessed the risk of lung cancer among those who quit for health reasons and for non-health-related reasons. In the U.S. Veterans Study, about 10 percent of the smokers quit because of a doctor's orders; these smokers were presumably ill. The lung cancer mortality ratio relative to never smokers for ex-smokers who stopped because of non-health-related reasons was 4.43 compared with 5.83 among ex-smokers who stopped on a doctor's orders and 8.98 among continuing smokers (Kahn 1966). In the European case–control study, Brown and Chu (1987) reported that the relative risk of lung cancer for those who stopped smoking because of health reasons compared with those who stopped for reasons other than health was 1.3 ($p<0.001$). Moreover, the percentage who stopped for health reasons decreased with increasing years of abstinence. Among those who had stopped for 1 year or less, 95.8 percent stopped because of health reasons compared with 65.7 percent of longer term ex-smokers. In ACS CPS-II, men and women who did not have a history of heart disease, stroke, or cancer at the time of interview showed a decreased risk of lung cancer in the first 2 years after smoking cessation when compared with continuing smokers. In contrast, the risks for all subjects combined (i.e., those with and without a history of previous chronic disease) were increased during the first 2 years after smoking cessation when compared with continuing smokers. The lower risks among the group with no history of previous disease compared with the total group persisted for subsequent periods of smoking abstinence (Table 7).

Cessation After Diagnosis of Lung Cancer

Two studies examined the relationship between smoking status and treatment outcome of patients with small cell lung cancer. In the study by Johnston-Early and associates (1980), survival was prolonged in patients who were ex-smokers or who had stopped smoking at diagnosis, whereas no difference in survival by smoking status was detected in the study by Bergman and Sorenson (1988).

The study by Johnston-Early and colleagues (1980) involved 112 patients with small cell lung cancer; 20 had stopped smoking before diagnosis; 35 had stopped at diagnosis; and 57 continued smoking. Therapies included chemotherapy with radiation therapy, with or without thymosin fraction V. The three patient groups were similar in disease extent, pretreatment performance status, pack-years smoked, and age and sex distribution. The patients who had stopped smoking prior to diagnosis had the best survival, followed by those who had stopped at diagnosis, and finally by those who continued smoking; the median survival for the three groups was 70, 52, and 47 weeks, respectively. Overall survival differences remained after individually adjusting for disease

TABLE 7.—Standard mortality ratios of lung cancer among former smokers in ACS-CPS II (relative to never smokers) by years of smoking abstinence, daily cigarette consumption at time of cessation, and history of chronic disease

	No history of chronic disease[a]		All respondents	
	1–20 cig/day	≥21 cig/day	1–20 cig/day	≥21 cig/day
Males				
Current smokers	23.5	31.5	18.8	26.9
Former smokers (yr since stopped)				
<1	16.8	23.4	26.7	50.7
1–2	16.7	25.3	22.4	33.2
3–5	19.7	20.5	16.5	20.9
6–10	8.6	14.2	8.7	15.0
11–15	6.3	13.6	6.0	12.6
≥16	3.3	5.3	3.1	5.5

	No history of chronic disease[a]		All respondents	
	1–19 cig/day	≥20 cig/day	1–19 cig/day	≥20 cig/day
Females				
Current smokers	10.5	24.1	7.3	16.3
Former smokers (yr since stopped)				
<1	3.4	21.1	7.9	34.3
1–2	9.0	18.2	9.1	19.5
3–5	2.5	13.2	2.9	14.6
6–10	1.1	12.0	1.0	9.1
11–15	1.1	2.9	1.5	5.9
≥16	1.6	2.4	1.4	2.6

[a] No history of cancer, heart disease, or stroke.
SOURCE: Unpublished tabulations, American Cancer Society.

extent, performance status, and type of protocol treatment. Similarly, statistical significance was maintained after simultaneous adjustment for both thymosin and radiation therapy.

The study by Bergman and Sorenson (1988) involved 154 small cell lung cancer patients who received combination chemotherapy. Thirty-two had stopped smoking at least 6 months before the initiation of treatment or had never smoked, 51 patients stopped smoking less than 6 months prior to the start of treatment, and 71 patients continued to smoke during the treatment period; the median survival was 39, 42, and 40 weeks, respectively. Reasons for differences in results between the two studies are not clear. Overall, patients in the study by Bergman and Sorenson (1988) had smoked fewer pack-years, but the median survival and performance status of each of the three smoking status groups were poorer than for the comparable smoking status groups in the study by Johnston-Early and associates (1980).

LARYNGEAL CANCER

Pathophysiologic Framework

Smoking has been firmly established as a cause of laryngeal cancer (US DHHS 1982, 1989) based on numerous epidemiologic studies. These studies have employed diverse methodologies and have been performed in different countries and covered various time periods. Tobacco smoke exposure has been measured by number of cigarettes smoked per day, number of years of smoking, age when started to smoke, type of cigarettes smoked, and depth of inhalation (US DHHS 1982).

In the larynx, as in the bronchus, a sequence of histologic changes occurs with continued smoking. These changes progress from cells with atypical nuclei, to carcinoma in situ, to invasive carcinoma. Autopsy studies show that recovery of the laryngeal epithelium can follow smoking cessation. Auerbach, Hammond, and Garfinkel (1970) studied postmortem specimens of laryngeal epithelium from 942 men (644 current cigarette smokers, 94 cigar and/or pipe smokers, 116 ex-cigarette smokers, and 88 never smokers). Ex-smokers in this study had stopped smoking for at least 5 years. Compared with current smokers, ex-smokers showed fewer histologic changes; 75 percent of ex-smokers and never smokers showed no cells with atypical nuclei, whereas almost all current smokers showed some cells with atypical nuclei.

Similar findings were reported by Muller and Krohn (1980), who obtained laryngeal epithelial specimens from autopsy. Of the 148 cases in the study, 24 were never smokers and 24 were ex-smokers who had stopped smoking for at least 5 years. Table 8 shows the relative distribution of selected histologic features by smoking status. Occurrence of all histologic changes was lowest among never smokers, intermediate among ex-smokers, and highest among current smokers. However, the histologic findings of ex-smokers in this study were more similar to those of light current smokers (<10 cig/day) than to those of never smokers.

Smoking Cessation and Laryngeal Cancer Risk

A few studies provide data on the relationship between smoking cessation and risk of laryngeal cancer (Table 8). Former smokers are at less risk than current smokers, but have about six times the risk of never smokers. The relative risk of laryngeal cancer is higher immediately after smoking cessation (i.e., 1–3 years after quitting) compared with continuing smokers. However, after approximately 3 to 4 years of smoking abstinence, former smokers show lower relative risks with increasing years of smoking abstinence (Table 8). Based on a case–control study of laryngeal and hypopharyngeal cancer conducted in Europe, Tuyns and colleagues (1988) suggested that the benefit of smoking cessation seemed to appear sooner after cessation for cancer of the hypopharynx/epilarynx than for the larynx.

TABLE 8.—Histologic changes in laryngeal epithelium by smoking status

Smoking status	Normal squamous epithelium	Keratinizing squamous epithelium	Hyperplastic squamous epithelium	Squamous metaplasia
Never smokers	83	4	8	21
Ex-smokers	54	33	29	33
Current smokers				
Light	56	25	12	58
Moderate	46	36	26	46
Heavy	31	44	33	52

Histologic change (% relative frequencies)

SOURCE: Abstracted from text and figures 2–5 in Muller and Krohn (1980).

Risk reduction pattern by years of smoking abstinence and number of cigarettes smoked daily was examined in a few studies (Table 9). In the U.S. Veterans Study, the risk of death from laryngeal cancer was lower among ex-smokers who smoked 10 to 20 or 21 to 39 cigarettes per day than among current smokers, but it was not lower among those smoking 1 to 9 or 40 cigarettes or more per day. However, there were very few laryngeal cancer deaths in the lowest and highest consumption levels (two and one, respectively) (Kahn 1966). In ACS CPS-II, ex-smokers who smoked less than 21 cigarettes per day showed a greater reduction in laryngeal cancer mortality for all durations of smoking abstinence compared with ex-smokers who smoked 21 cigarettes or more per day relative to current smokers. In a case–control study conducted in the Texas Gulf Coast region (Falk et al. 1989), there was no consistent pattern of greater proportion of reduction in risk among those who had smoked fewer cigarettes per day prior to smoking abstinence. Moreover, there was still a threefold increased risk among those who had smoked more than 30 cigarettes daily after 10 years of smoking abstinence (Table 9).

The effect of smoking duration prior to smoking cessation was not considered in the studies mentioned above. There is some indication that the average age at which the ex-smoker developed clinical laryngeal cancer was about 10 years older (68.7) than that of the current smoker (Wynder et al. 1976).

Alcohol has been shown to have an independent effect on risk of laryngeal cancer, but the relationship is weaker than the one between smoking and laryngeal cancer. The relative risks for joint exposure to alcohol and tobacco are consistent with a multiplicative interaction of the two agents (Flanders and Rothman 1982; Elwood et al. 1984; Olsen, Sabroe, Fasting 1985). In this review of the literature, no studies were found that accounted for the effects of alcohol intake in examining risk of laryngeal cancer after smoking cessation.

TABLE 9.—Relative risks of laryngeal cancer by smoking status

Reference	Population	Smoking status	Relative risks				
Kahn (1966)	US veterans	Never smokers Current smokers Former smokers	1.0 9.5 7.2				
Wigle, Mao, Grace (1980)	Alberta, Canada, cancer patients	Never smokers Current smokers Former smokers	1.0 7.8 6.3				
ACS (unpublished tabulations)	ACS CPS-II	Never smokers Current smokers Former smokers	Males 1.0 12.8 6.7	Females 1.0 9.5 6.5			
Falk et al. (1989)	Texas	Never smokers Current smokers Former smokers					
				Cig/day			
			1–10	11–20	21–30	31–40	>40
		(yr since stopped)[a] 3–9 ≥10	3.0 2.8	3.6 1.2	4.0 1.0	7.2 3.1	0.9 3.5

TABLE 9.—Continued

Reference	Population	Smoking status	Relative risks	
			Males	Females
Wynder and Stellman (1977)	6 US cities	Former smokers (yr since stopped)		
		1–3	17.9	6.9
		4–6	8.5	2.6
		7–10	4.0	—
		11–15	3.4	8.8
		≥16	2.5	—
		Current smokers	14.3	11.6
		Never smokers	1.0	1.0
			Males	
			Endolarynx	Hypopharynx
Tuyns et al. (1988)	European countries	Former smokers (yr since stopped)		
		1–4	1.51	1.09
		5–9	0.52	0.28
		≥10	0.28	0.32
		Current smokers	1.0	1.0

NOTE: ACS CPS-II=American Cancer Society Cancer Prevention Study II.
[a] Reference category is never smokers.

CONCLUSIONS

1. Smoking cessation reduces the risk of lung cancer compared with continued smoking. For example, after 10 years of abstinence, the risk of lung cancer is about 30 to 50 percent of the risk for continuing smokers; with further abstinence, the risk continues to decline.

2. The reduced risk of lung cancer among former smokers is observed in males and females, in smokers of filter and nonfilter cigarettes, and for all histologic types of lung cancer.

3. Smoking cessation lowers the risk of laryngeal cancer compared with continued smoking.

4. Smoking cessation reduces the severity and extent of premalignant histologic changes in the epithelium of the larynx and lung.

References

ALDERSON, M.R., LEE, P.N., WANG, R. Risks of lung cancer, chronic bronchitis, ischaemic heart disease, and stroke in relation to type of cigarette smoked. *Journal of Epidemiology and Community Health* 39(4):286–293, December 1985.

AMERICAN CANCER SOCIETY. Unpublished tabulations.

ARMITAGE, P. Discussion on paper by R. Doll. *Journal of the Royal Statistical Society* A134:155–156, 1971.

ARMITAGE, P., DOLL, R. The age distribution of cancer and a multi-stage theory of carcinogenesis. *British Journal of Cancer* 8:1–11, 1954.

ARMITAGE, P., DOLL, R. A two-stage theory of carcinogenesis in relation to the age distribution of human cancer. *British Journal of Cancer* 11:161–169, 1957.

AUERBACH, O., GARFINKEL, L., HAMMOND, E.C. Relation of smoking and age to findings in lung parenchyma: A microscopic study. *Chest* 65(1):29–35, January 1974.

AUERBACH, O., GERE, J.B., FORMAN, J.B., PETRICK, T.G., SMOLIN, H.J., MUEHSAM, G.E., KASSOUNY, D.Y., STOUT, A.P. Changes in the bronchial epithelium in relation to smoking and cancer of the lung. A report of progress. *New England Journal of Medicine* 256(3):97–104, January 17, 1957.

AUERBACH, O., HAMMOND, E.C., GARFINKEL, L. Histologic changes in the larynx in relation to smoking habits. *Cancer* 25(1):92–104, January 1970.

AUERBACH, O., HAMMOND, E.C., GARFINKEL, L., BENANTE, C. Relation of smoking and age to emphysema. Whole-lung section study. *New England Journal of Medicine* 286(16):853–857, April 20, 1972.

AUERBACH, O., STOUT, A.P., HAMMOND, E.C., GARFINKEL, L. Changes in bronchial epithelium in relation to sex, age, residence, smoking and pneumonia. *New England Journal of Medicine* 267(3):111–125, July 19, 1962a.

AUERBACH, O., STOUT, A.P., HAMMOND, E.C., GARFINKEL, L. Bronchial epithelium in former smokers. *New England Journal of Medicine* 267(3):119–125, July 19, 1962b.

AUERBACH, O., STOUT, A.P., HAMMOND, E.C., GARFINKEL, L. Smoking habits and age in relation to pulmonary changes. Rupture of alveolar septums, fibrosis and thickening of walls of small arteries and arterioles. *New England Journal of Medicine* 269(20):1045–1054, November 14, 1963.

AUERBACH, O., STOUT, A.P., HAMMOND, E.C., GARFINKEL, L. Interrelationships among various histologic changes in bronchial tubes and in lung parenchyma. *American Review of Respiratory Disease* 90(6):867–876, December 1964.

BENHAMOU, S., BENHAMOU, E., TIRMARCHE, M., FLAMANT, R. Lung cancer and use of cigarettes: A French case–control study. *Journal of the National Cancer Institute* 74(6):1169–1175, June 1985.

BERGMAN, S., SORENSON, S. Smoking and effect of chemotherapy in small cell lung cancer. *European Respiratory Journal* 1:932–937, 1988.

BIRRER, M.J., MINNA, J.D. Molecular genetics of lung cancer. *Seminars in Oncology* 15(3):226–235, June 1988.

BROWN, C.C., CHU, K.C. Use of multistage models to infer stage affected by carcinogenic exposure: Example of lung cancer and cigarette smoking. *Journal of Chronic Diseases* 40 (Supplement 2):171S–179S, 1987.

CANADIAN DEPARTMENT OF NATIONAL HEALTH AND WELFARE. *A Canadian Study of Smoking and Health.* Department of National Health and Welfare, Epidemiology Division, Health Services Branch, Biostatistics Division, Research and Statistics Directorate, 1966, 137 pp.

CARSTENSEN, J.M., PERSHAGEN, G., EKLUND, G. Mortality in relation to cigarette and pipe smoking: 16 years' observation of 25,000 Swedish men. *Journal of Epidemiology and Community Health* 41:166–172, 1987.

CEDERLOF, R., FRIBERG, L., HRUBEC, Z., LORICH, U. *The Relationship of Smoking and Some Social Covariables to Mortality and Cancer Morbidity. A Ten Year Follow-Up in a Probability Sample of 55,000 Swedish Subjects Age 18–69*, Part 1/2. Stockholm, Sweden: The Karolinska Institute, Department of Environmental Hygiene, 1975.

CORREA, P., PICKLE, L.W., FONTHAM, E., DALAGER, N., LIN, Y., HAENSZEL, W., JOHNSON, W.D. The causes of lung cancer in Louisiana. In: Mizell, M., Correa, P. (eds.) *Lung Cancer: Causes and Prevention. Proceedings of the International Lung Cancer Update Conference.* New Orleans: Verlag Chemie International, Inc., 1984, p. 73.

DAMBER, L.A., LARSSON, L.G. Smoking and lung cancer with special regard to type of smoking and type of cancer. A case–control study in north Sweden. *British Journal of Cancer* 53(5):673–681, May 1986.

DAY, N.E. Epidemiological data and multistage carcinogenesis. In: Börzsönyi, M., Lapis, K., Day, N.E., Yamasaki, H. (eds.) *Models, Mechanisms and Etiology of Tumor Promotion.* Lyon: IARC, 1984, pp. 339–357.

DAY, N.E., BROWN, C.C. Multistage models and primary prevention of cancer. *Journal of the National Cancer Institute* 64(4):977–989, April 1980.

DEVESA, S.S., BLOT, W.J., FRAUMENI, J.F. JR. Declining lung cancer rates among young men and women in the United States: A cohort analysis. *Journal of the National Cancer Institute* 81:1568–1571, 1989.

DOLL, R. The age distribution of cancer: Implications for models of carcinogenesis. *Journal of the Royal Statistical Society* A134:133–166, 1971.

DOLL, R., GRAY, R., HAFNER, B., PETO, R. Mortality in relation to smoking: 22 years' observations on female British doctors. *British Medical Journal* 280(6219):967–971, April 5, 1980.

DOLL, R., HILL, A.B. Mortality in relation to smoking: Ten years' observations of British doctors. *British Medical Journal* 1:1399–1410, May 30, 1964.

DOLL, R., PETO, R. Mortality in relation to smoking: 20 years' observations on male British doctors. *British Medical Journal* 2:1525–1536, December 25, 1976.

DOLL, R., PETO, R. Cigarette smoking and bronchial carcinoma: Dose and time relationships among regular smokers and lifelong non-smokers. *Journal of Epidemiology and Community Health* 32(4):303–313, December 1978.

ELWOOD, J.M., PEARSON, J.C.G., SKIPPEN, D.H., JACKSON, S.M. Alcohol, smoking, social and occupational factors in the aetiology of cancer of the oral cavity, pharynx and larynx. *International Journal of Cancer* 34:603–612, 1984.

FALK, R.T., PICKLE, L.W., BROWN, L.M., MASON, T.J., BUFFLER, P.A., FRAUMENI, J.F. JR. Effect of smoking and alcohol consumption on laryngeal cancer risk in coastal Texas. *Cancer Research* 49(14):4024–4029, July 15, 1989.

FARBER, E. The multistep nature of cancer development. *Cancer Research* 44:4217–4223, October 1984.

FLANDERS, W.D., ROTHMAN, K.J. Interaction of alcohol and tobacco in laryngeal cancer. *American Journal of Epidemiology* 115(3):371–379, March 1982.

FREEDMAN, D.A., NAVIDI, W.C. Multistage models for carcinogenesis. *Environmental Health Perspectives* 81:169–188, May 1989.

GAFFNEY, M., ALTSHULER, B. Examination of the role of cigarette smoke in lung carcinogenesis using multistage models. *Journal of the National Cancer Institute* 80(12):925–931, August 17, 1988.

GAO, Y.T., BLOT, W.J., ZHENG, W., FRAUMENI, J.F., HSU, C.W. Lung cancer and smoking in Shanghai. *International Journal of Epidemiology* 17(2):277–280, June 1988.

GARFINKEL, L., STELLMAN, S.D. Smoking and lung cancer in women: Findings in a prospective study. *Cancer Research* 48(23):6951–6955, December 1, 1988.

GRAHAM, S., LEVIN, M.L. Smoking withdrawal in the reduction of risk of lung cancer. *Cancer* 27(4):865–871, April 1971.

HAENSZEL, W., LOVELAND, D.B., SIRKEN, M.G. Lung-cancer mortality as related to residence and smoking histories. I. White males. *Journal of the National Cancer Institute* 28:947–1001, April 1962.

HAMMOND, E.C. Smoking in relation to the death rates of one million men and women. In: Haenszel, W. (ed.) *Epidemiological Approaches to the Study of Cancer and Other Chronic Diseases*. NCI Monograph 19. U.S. Department of Health, Education, and Welfare, Public Health Service, National Cancer Institute, January 1966, pp. 127–204.

HIGGINS, I.T., WYNDER, E.L. Reduction in risk of lung cancer among ex-smokers with particular reference to histologic type. *Cancer* 62(11):2397–2401, December 1, 1988.

HIGGINS, I.T.T., MAHAN, C.M., WYNDER, E.L. Lung cancer among cigar and pipe smokers. *Preventive Medicine* 17(1):116–128, January 1988.

JOHNSTON-EARLY, A., COHEN, M.H., MINNA, J.D., PAXTON, L.M., FOSSIECK, B.E. JR., IHDE, D.C., BUNN, P.A. JR., MATTHEWS, M.J., MAKUCH, R. Smoking abstinence and small cell lung cancer survival. *Journal of the American Medical Association* 244(19):2175–2179, November 14, 1980.

JOLY, O.G., LUBIN, J.H., CARABALLOSO, M. Dark tobacco and lung cancer in Cuba. *Journal of the National Cancer Institute* 70(6):1033–1039, June 1983.

KAHN, H.A. The Dorn study of smoking and mortality among U.S. veterans: Report on eight and one-half years of observation. In: Haenszel, W. (ed.) *Epidemiological Approaches to the Study of Cancer and Other Chronic Diseases*. NCI Monograph 19. U.S. Department of Health, Education, and Welfare, Public Health Service, National Cancer Institute. January 1966, pp. 1–125.

LUBIN, J.H., BLOT, W.J. Assessment of lung cancer risk factors by histologic category. *Journal of the National Cancer Institute* 73(2):383–389, August 1984.

LUBIN, J.H., BLOT, W.J., BERRINO, F., FLAMANT, R., GILLIS, C.R., KUNZE, M., SCHMAHL, D., VISCO, G. Modifying risk of developing lung cancer by changing habits of cigarette smoking. *British Medical Journal* 288(6435):1953–1956, June 30, 1984a.

LUBIN, J.H., BLOT, W.J., BERRINO, F., FLAMANT, R., GILLIS, C.R., KUNZE, M., SCHMAHL, D., VISCO, G. Patterns of lung cancer risk according to type of cigarette smoked. *International Journal of Cancer* 3:569–576, 1984b.

LUBIN, J.H., RICHTER, B.S., BLOT, W.J. Lung cancer risk with cigar and pipe use. *Journal of the National Cancer Institute* 73(2):377–381, August 1984.

MCDOWELL, E.M., HARRIS, C.C., TRUMP, B.F. Histogenesis and morphogenesis of bronchial neoplasm. In: Shimosato, Y., Melamed, M., Nettesheim, P. (eds.) *Morphogenesis of Lung Cancer*, Volume I. Boca Raton, Florida: CRC Press, 1982, pp. 1–36.

MOOLGAVKAR, S.H., DEWANJI, A., LUEBECK, G. Cigarette smoking and lung cancer: Reanalysis of the British doctors' data. *Journal of the National Cancer Institute* 81(6):415–420, March 15, 1989.

MULLER, K.M., KROHN, B.R. Smoking habits and their relationship to precancerous lesions of the larynx. *Journal of Cancer Research and Clinical Oncology* 96(2):211–217, 1980.

OLSEN, J., SABROE, S., FASTING, U. Interaction of alcohol and tobacco as risk factors in cancer of the laryngeal region. *Journal of Epidemiology and Community Health* 39(2):165–168, June 1985.

PATHAK, D.R., SAMET, J.M., HUMBLE, C.G., SKIPPER, B.J. Determinants of lung cancer risk in cigarette smokers in New Mexico. *Journal of the National Cancer Institute* 76(4):597–604, April 1986.

PETO, J. Early- and late-stage carcinogenesis in mouse skin and in man. In: Börzsönyi, M., Lapis, K., Day, N.E., Yamasaki, H. (eds.) *Models, Mechanisms and Etiology of Tumour Promotion.* Lyon: IARC, 1984, pp. 359–370.

PHILLIPS, D.H., HEWER, A., MARTIN, C.N., GARNER, R.C., KING, M.M. Correlation of DNA adduct levels in human lung with cigarette smoking. *Nature* 336(6201):790–792, December 22–29, 1988.

RANDERATH, E., MILLER, R.H., MITTAL, D., AVITTS, T.A., DUNSFORD, H.A., RANDERATH, K. Covalent DNA damage in tissues of cigarette smokers as determined by ^{32}P-postlabeling assay. *Journal of the National Cancer Institute* 81(5):341–347, March 1, 1989.

ROGOT, E., MURRAY, J.L. Smoking and causes of death among U.S. veterans: 16 years of observation. *Public Health Reports* 95(3):213–222, May–June 1980.

SACCOMANNO, G., ARCHER, V.E., AUERBACH, O., SAUNDERS, R.P., BRENNAN, L.M. Development of carcinoma of the lung as reflected in exfoliated cells. *Cancer* 31(1):256–270, January 1974.

STENBACK, F., PETO, R., SHUBIK, P. Initiation and promotion at different ages and doses in 2200 mice. I. Methods, and the apparent persistence of initiated cells. *British Journal of Cancer* 44(1):1–14, July 1981a.

STENBACK, F., PETO, R., SHUBIK, P. Initiation and promotion at different ages and doses in 2200 mice. II. Decrease in promotion by TPA with ageing. *British Journal of Cancer* 44(1):15–23, July 1981b.

STENBACK, F., PETO, R., SHUBIK, P. Initiation and promotion at different ages and doses in 2200 mice. III. Linear extrapolation from high doses may underestimate low-dose tumour risks. *British Journal of Cancer* 44(1):24–34, July 1981c.

TUYNS, A.J., ESTEVE, J., RAYMOND, L., BERRINO, F., BENHAMOU, E., BLANCHET, F., BOFFETTA, P., CROSIGNANI, P., DEL MORAL, A., LEHMANN, W., ET AL. Cancer of the larynx/hypopharynx, tobacco and alcohol: IARC International Case–Control Study in Turin and Varese (Italy), Zaragoza and Navarra (Spain), Geneva (Switzerland) and Calvados (France). *International Journal of Cancer* 41(4):483–491, April 15, 1988.

U.S. DEPARTMENT OF HEALTH AND HUMAN SERVICES. *The Health Consequences of Smoking: Cancer. A Report of the Surgeon General.* U.S. Department of Health and Human Services, Public Heath Service, Office on Smoking and Health. DHHS Publication No. (PHS) 82-50179, 1982.

U.S. DEPARTMENT OF HEALTH AND HUMAN SERVICES. *The Health Consequences of Smoking: Chronic Obstructive Lung Disease. A Report of the Surgeon General.* U.S. Department of Health and Human Services, Public Health Service, Office on Smoking and Health. DHHS Publication No. (PHS) 84-50205, 1984.

U.S. DEPARTMENT OF HEALTH AND HUMAN SERVICES. *The Health Consequences of Involuntary Smoking. A Report of the Surgeon General.* U.S. Department of Health and Human Services, Public Health Service, Centers for Disease Control. DHHS Publication No. (CDC) 87-8398, 1986.

U.S. DEPARTMENT OF HEALTH AND HUMAN SERVICES. *Reducing the Health Consequences of Smoking: 25 Years of Progress. A Report of the Surgeon General.* U.S. Department of Health and Human Services, Public Health Service, Centers for Disease Control, Center for Chronic Disease Prevention and Health Promotion, Office on Smoking and Health. DHHS Publication No. (CDC) 89-8411, 1989.

U.S. DEPARTMENT OF HEALTH, EDUCATION, AND WELFARE. *Smoking and Health. A Report of the Surgeon General.* U.S. Department of Health, Education, and Welfare, Public Health Service, Office of the Assistant Secretary for Health, Office on Smoking and Health. DHEW Publication No. (PHS) 79-50066, 1979.

U.S. PUBLIC HEALTH SERVICE. *Smoking and Health. Report of the Advisory Committee to the Surgeon General of the Public Health Service.* U.S. Department of Health, Education, and Welfare, Public Health Service, Center for Disease Control. PHS Publication No. 1103, 1964.

WHITTEMORE, A.S. Effect of cigarette smoking in epidemiological studies of lung cancer. *Statistics in Medicine* 7(1–2):223–238, January–February 1988.

WIGLE, D.T., MAO, Y., GRACE, M. Relative importance of smoking as a risk factor for selected cancers. *Canadian Journal of Public Health* 71(4):269–275, July/August 1980.

WU, A.H., HENDERSON, B.E., PIKE, M.C., YU, M.C. Smoking and other risk factors for lung cancer in women. *Journal of the National Cancer Institute* 74(4):747–751, April 1985.

WYNDER, E.L., COVEY, L.S., MABUCHI, K., MUSHINSKI, M. Environmental factors in cancer of the larynx. A second look. *Cancer* 38(4):1591–1601, October 1976.

WYNDER, E.L., KABAT, G.C. The effect of low-yield cigarette smoking on lung cancer risk. *Cancer* 62(6):1223–1230, September 15, 1988.

WYNDER, E.L., STELLMAN, S.D. Comparative epidemiology of tobacco-related cancers. *Cancer Research* 37(12):4608–4622, December 1977.

WYNDER, E.L., STELLMAN, S.D. Impact of long-term filter cigarette usage on lung and larynx cancer risk: A case–control study. *Journal of the National Cancer Institute* 62(3):471–477, March 1979.

CHAPTER 5
SMOKING CESSATION AND NONRESPIRATORY CANCERS

CONTENTS

Introduction 147
Review of Specific Sites 147
    Oral Cancer 147
    Esophageal Cancer 152
    Pancreatic Cancer 155
    Bladder Cancer 159
    Cervical Cancer 165
    Breast Cancer 169
    Endometrial Cancer 169
    Other Cancer Sites 172
Multiple Primary Cancers 176
Summary 177
Conclusions 178
References 179

INTRODUCTION

Lung cancer, the first neoplasm causally linked to cigarette smoking, has been the cancer most thoroughly studied with respect to exposure–response relationships and benefits of cessation (US DHHS 1982). Subsequently, cigarette smoking has been established as a cause of cancer at diverse other sites. For some sites (e.g., oral cavity), the target cells are exposed directly to the various constituents of tobacco smoke. For other sites (e.g., urinary bladder), absorption, transport, and metabolic activation of carcinogens in tobacco smoke result in exposure of target tissues. This Chapter reviews the evidence on smoking cessation and cancer risk at various nonrespiratory sites. The sites selected for review are those for which cigarette smoking has been determined to be a cause of cancer, or contributing cause, or those for which evidence indicates a possible association.

Methodologic issues encountered in inferring causality on the effects of smoking cessation have been discussed in Chapter 2 and will not be reviewed in detail in this Chapter. Potential confounding by differences in prior tobacco exposure at the time of quitting, and by differences between former smokers and continuing smokers in other cancer-related risk factors may pose a greater obstacle to causal inference for the nonrespiratory cancers than for cancers of the lung or larynx; the smoking effects are generally smaller for nonrespiratory cancers, and the potential confounding factors are more numerous.

REVIEW OF SPECIFIC SITES

Oral Cancer

Tobacco use is a major cause of oral cancer (US PHS 1964; US DHHS 1982, 1989). An exposure–response relationship has been identified between the amount of tobacco consumed and the risk of cancer of the oral cavity after considering the effects of alcohol consumption. The proportion of 1985 oral cancer deaths attributable to cigarette smoking in the United States has been estimated to be 92 percent for men and 61 percent for women (US DHHS 1989). The oral cavity, like the lung, receives direct exposure to cigarette smoke. Presumably, the causal association of cigarette smoking with cancer of the oral cavity reflects this contact and the same initiating and promoting agents that are considered to determine the development of lung cancer.

Table 1 summarizes studies that have examined the relationship between smoking cessation and oral cancer risk. In these studies, the risk of oral cancer among current smokers ranges from 2.0 to 18.1 times (median of approximately 4) the risk among never smokers. Oral cancer risks for women who are currently smoking seem lower than those for men in studies conducted prior to the mid-1970s, but little difference by gender has been noted in more recent research. This gender pattern may be because of the initiation of smoking at an older age among earlier birth cohorts of women (US DHHS 1989) born during this century and the resultant low cumulative lifetime exposure of such women.

TABLE 1.—Studies of oral cancer and smoking cessation

Reference	Population (yr of data collection)	Design (number of subjects)	Gender	Current smokers	Former smokers	Yr since quitting	Comments
Kahn (1966)	US veterans (1954–62)	Prospective (248,195)	Male	3.8	1.9	NP	Excludes "doctor's orders" quitters; Cancer mortality
Cederlof et al. (1975)	Sweden (1963–72)	Prospective (27,300) (27,700)	Male Female	2.7 2.0	0.8 0	NP NP	Cancer incidence
Wynder and Stellman (1977)	6 US cities (1969–75)	Case:control (497:6,534)	Male	8.9	9.0 3.5 3.2 3.4 1.6	1–3 4–6 7–10 11–15 ≥16	
		(270:6,522)	Female	4.4	3.8 2.2 1.4 0.6 0.8	1–3 4–6 7–10 11–15 ≥16	
Rogot and Murray (1980)	US veterans (1954–69)	Prospective (293,958)	Male	4.2	1.7	NP	Excludes "doctor's orders" quitters; Cancer mortality; Extension of US Veterans Study

TABLE 1.—Continued

Reference	Population (yr of data collection)	Design (number of subjects)	Gender	Risk relative to never smokers — Current smokers	Risk relative to never smokers — Former smokers	Yr since quitting	Comments
Wigle, Mao, Grace (1980)	Alberta, Canada (1971–73)	Case:control (84:1,002) (41:674)	Male Female	8.7 4.3	3.5 0.8	NP NP	
Spitz et al. (1988)	Houston, TX (1985–87)	Case:control (121:127)	Male	4.5[a]	6.1 2.2 1.0	<5 5–14 ≥15	
		(50:49)	Female	5.5[a]	9.8 4.5 1.5	<5 5–14 ≥15	
Blot et al. (1988)	4 areas in United States (1984–85)	Case:control (762:837)	Male	3.4	1.1 1.1 0.7	1–9 10–19 ≥20	Adjusted for alcohol consumption
		(352:431)	Female	4.7	1.8 0.8 0.4	1–9 10–19 ≥20	
Franco et al. (1989)	Brazil (1986–88)	Case:control (232:464)	Male and female	9.3	2.9 0.6	<10 ≥10	Data for commercially produced cigarettes only

TABLE 1.—Continued

Reference	Population (yr of data collection)	Design (number of subjects)	Gender	Risk relative to never smokers — Current smokers	Risk relative to never smokers — Former smokers	Yr since quitting	Comments
Kabat and Wynder (1989)	18 US cities (1976–83)	Case:control (511:1,057) (226:453)	Male Female	5.5[a] 4.1[a]	2.1 1.5	≥1 ≥1	Adjusted for alcohol
Kabat, Hebert, Wynder (1989)	7 US cities (1983–87)	Case:control (125:107)	Female	2.0	1.0	NP	Adjusted for alcohol and previous number of cig/day
ACS CPS-II (unpublished tabulations)	United States (1982–86)	Prospective (421,623) (605,758)	Male Female	18.1 5.8	6.4 2.5	NP	Cancer mortality

NOTE: NP=not provided; ACS CPS-II=American Cancer Society Cancer Prevention Study II.

[a] Computed as a weighted average from cigarette dose-specific relative risks presented in the paper. Weights are the number of controls within each stratum of smoking.

In each study summarized in Table 1, the risk of oral cancer was lower among former smokers after the first few years of abstinence than for current smokers. After 3 to 5 years of smoking abstinence, oral cancer risk decreased by 50 percent. In a study in Argentina (Iscovich et al. 1987) and in the large multicenter study conducted by the U.S. National Cancer Institute (NCI) (Blot et al. 1988), the risk of oral cancer among former smokers after 10 years of abstinence was comparable with that among never smokers. This observation has been interpreted as an indication that the greatest effect of smoking on oral cancer risk may be in the later (postinitiation) stages of carcinogenesis (Blot et al. 1988).

Although it is well known that smokeless tobacco (ST) increases the risk of oral cancer (Winn et al. 1981; US DHHS 1986) and that stopping the use of ST reduces the prevalence of premalignant tissue changes in the mouth (Gupta et al. 1986), there is little information on the risk of oral cancer in former users of ST.

Compared with current smokers, former smokers may have different alcohol drinking habits before and after smoking cessation, and thus comparisons of risk between current and former smokers may be confounded by alcohol consumption (Chapter 11). In three investigations, the effect of smoking cessation was examined and past alcohol consumption was controlled by multiple logistic regression (Blot et al. 1988; Kabat and Wynder 1989; Kabat, Hebert, Wynder 1989). In the three studies, estimates of relative risks for both current and former smokers were similar to those observed in studies in which alcohol was not included as an adjustment factor. The stability of the relative risk estimates for smoking with adjustment for alcohol intake suggests that alcohol does not substantially confound the relationship between oral cancer risk and cigarette smoking status and that the lower risk of former smokers cannot be explained by lower levels of alcohol consumption (Chapter 11). One study was sufficiently large to permit detailed stratified analysis of the modification of the smoking effect by alcohol consumption (Blot et al. 1988). In this study, former smokers were observed to have a lower risk than current smokers for both men and women at each of five levels of alcohol consumption.

The U.S. Veterans Study (Kahn 1966) demonstrated that at each of three levels of past cigarette smoking exposure, former smokers had lower risk of oral cancer than did current smokers. Kabat, Hebert, and Wynder (1989) controlled for past cigarette exposure by multiple logistic regression and found that relative risk estimates, which were adjusted for past alcohol and cigarette consumption, did not differ from the crude estimates for former smokers (1.0 vs. 1.0 relative to never smokers).

Second primary cancers of the mouth and pharynx occur commonly in persons with an initial primary cancer in the mouth, pharynx, or larynx. Several studies have addressed the incidence of second primaries of the mouth, pharynx, or larynx in relation to smoking status after diagnosis and treatment of the first primary. The findings of these studies are inconclusive, with some indicating reduced risk of a second primary after cessation (Moore 1965; Moore 1971; Wynder et al. 1969; Silverman, Gorsky, Greenspan 1983) and others showing no clear benefit of cessation (Castigliano 1968; Schottenfeld, Gantt, Wynder 1974; Chapter 5, see section on Multiple Primary Cancers).

The results of two studies indicated that continued smoking after diagnosis of oral cancer may reduce survival, particularly in combination with alcohol consumption (Johnston and Ballantyne 1977; Stevens et al. 1983). These analyses, however, did not adjust for the more advanced stage of cancer among users of alcohol and tobacco at presentation (Johnston and Ballantyne 1977).

The results of studies of oral cancer and cigarette smoking cessation indicate that former smokers experience a lower risk of oral cancer than current smokers and that this lower risk does not appear to be a result of confounding by alcohol or level of cigarette consumption prior to cessation. The risk of oral cancer has been shown to drop substantially within 3 to 5 years of cessation.

Esophageal Cancer

Smoking is a major cause of esophageal cancer (US DHHS 1982, 1989). In the United States, the proportion of esophageal cancer deaths attributable to tobacco has been estimated to be 78 percent for men and 75 percent for women (US DHHS 1989). As for cancer of the oral cavity, cigarette smoking is an independent risk factor for esophageal cancer but can also act in conjunction with alcohol to increase cancer risk.

Table 2 summarizes the studies that have examined the relationship between smoking cessation and esophageal cancer risk. In these studies, the risk of esophageal cancer for current smokers ranges from 1.7 to 6.4 times the risk among never smokers (median of approximately 5). These findings are similar to those for oral cancer as shown in Table 1. The risks for smoking and esophageal cancer were similar among males and females.

Three years after cessation, former smokers showed lower risks than current smokers in each study summarized in Table 2, with the exception of the Swedish prospective study (Cederlof et al. 1975) in which smoking-associated risks were considerably lower than in any other study. However, in followup of this cohort, more dramatic elevations in male mortality from esophageal cancer were observed in current smokers relative to never smokers: standardized mortality ratios were 1.1 for 1 to 7 g tobacco per day, 4.5 for 8 to 15 g tobacco per day, and 5.4 for more than 15 g of tobacco per day (Carstensen, Pershagen, Eklund 1987). For former smokers, the standardized mortality ratio was 1.3. Approximately 3 to 5 years after cessation, risk of esophageal cancer was reduced by approximately 50 percent in the two studies providing information by duration of abstinence (Table 2). Data are very scant about the effects of cessation on the risk of esophageal cancer over long periods of abstinence. The U.S. Veterans Study showed that the risk among former smokers was lower at each of four levels of past numbers of cigarettes smoked per day.

A multivariate analysis in which lifetime alcohol consumption was included as an adjustment factor (La Vecchia, Liati et al. 1986) produced relative risks for current and former smokers that were similar to those observed in other studies. In this study, the crude relative risk for ex-smokers was nearly identical to one that was adjusted for alcohol consumption (2.7 vs. 3.0), suggesting that alcohol was not a confounder in the estimates of the benefits of cessation. A study that was limited to nondrinkers (La Vecchia and Negri 1989) also produced risk estimates for smoking that were very

TABLE 2.—Studies of esophageal cancer that have examined the effect of smoking cessation

Reference	Population (yr of data collection)	Design (number of subjects)	Gender	Current smokers	Former smokers	Yr since quitting	Comments
Kahn (1966)	US veterans (1954–62)	Prospective (248,195)	Male	5.3	1.6	NP	Excludes "doctor's orders" quitters; Cancer mortality
Cederlof et al. (1975)	Sweden (1963–72)	Prospective (27,300)	Male	1.7	1.7	NP	Cancer incidence
Wynder and Stellman (1977)	6 US cities (1969–75)	Case:control (159:6,534)	Male	3.6	4.8 1.5 1.4 1.3 1.0	1–3 4–6 7–10 11–15 ≥16	
		(76:6,522)	Female	5.3	3.0 3.1 0 2.2 1.8	1–3 4–6 7–10 11–15 ≥16	
Wigle, Mao, Grace (1980)	Alberta, Canada (1971–73)	Case:control (45:1,002)	Male	5.1	1.1	NP	
Rogot and Murray (1980)	US veterans (1954–69)	Prospective (293,958)	Male	6.4	2.4	NP	Excludes "doctor's orders" quitters; Cancer mortality; Extension of US Veterans Study

TABLE 2.—Continued

Reference	Population (yr of data collection)	Design (number of subjects)	Gender	Risk relative to never smokers — Current smokers	Risk relative to never smokers — Former smokers	Yr since quitting	Comments
La Vecchia, Liati et al. (1986)	Northern Italy (1984–85)	Case:control (129:426)	Male and female	4.3	3.4 2.5	<5 ≥5	Adjusted for SES, diet, and alcohol
La Vecchia and Negri (1989)	Northern Italy (1984–88)	Case:control (30:189)	Male and female	3.6[a]	1.1	NP	Analysis limited to only nondrinkers

NOTE: NP=not provided; SES=socioeconomic status.
[a] Computed as a weighted average from cigarette dose-specific relative risks presented in the paper. Weights are the number of controls within each stratum of smoking.

similar to those derived from other studies, supporting an earlier observation of elevated risk for esophageal cancer in nondrinking smokers (Tuyns 1983).

This review of past research on esophageal cancer and cigarette smoking cessation indicates that former smokers experience a lower risk of esophageal cancer than do current smokers, and that this lower risk is not because of confounding by lower alcohol intake among former smokers.

Pancreatic Cancer

The association, noted for many years, between smoking and cancer of the pancreas is considerably weaker than that between smoking and oral or esophageal cancer (US DHHS 1982). Although the causal mechanisms underlying this association are unclear, smoking has nonetheless been regarded as a contributing factor in cancer of the pancreas (US DHHS 1982, 1989). In the United States in 1985, the proportion of pancreatic cancer deaths attributable to smoking has been estimated to be 29 percent in men and 34 percent in women (US DHHS 1989).

Table 3 summarizes studies of the relationship between pancreatic cancer and smoking cessation. In these studies, current smokers had risks ranging from 1.0 to 5.4 times (median of approximately 2) the risk among never smokers. Risks for pancreatic cancer associated with smoking were similar for males and females.

Former smokers generally had lower risk than current smokers for pancreatic cancer, but the available data do not characterize adequately the change in risk with duration of abstinence. The large case–control study conducted in Los Angeles, CA, (Mack et al. 1986) would suggest that risk is not substantially reduced until after 10 years of abstinence, whereas the smaller English study (Cuzick and Babiker 1989) suggests that substantial risk reduction is more immediate among women than among men; risk reduction may take as long as 20 years among men. This difference in the time course of risk after cessation according to gender has no clear biologic explanation and may be only a chance finding.

The question of potential confounding by differences in cigarette smoking exposure prior to quitting was addressed in the analysis of the U.S. Veterans Study (Kahn 1966). In each of four levels of past cigarette consumption, the risk among former smokers was found to be lower than that among current smokers. In the study conducted by Falk and colleagues (1988), former smokers had a lower risk of pancreatic cancer than current smokers at each of three levels of numbers of cigarettes consumed per day and also at each of four levels of numbers of years smoked.

Because alcohol can cause insult to the pancreas and has been thought to be a possible pancreatic carcinogen (Cubilla and Fitzgerald 1979), two investigators adjusted for lifetime alcohol consumption in multiple logistic regression analyses (Falk et al. 1988; Clavel et al. 1989). These analyses produced relative risk estimates similar to those derived from other studies that did not adjust for alcohol and thus suggested that alcohol consumption is not a confounding factor in the smoking–pancreatic cancer association.

The results of epidemiologic investigations on pancreatic cancer and cigarette smoking cessation indicate that there is a weak, but consistently observed, association between smoking and pancreatic cancer and that former smokers experience a lower

TABLE 3.—Studies of cancer of the pancreas and smoking cessation

Reference	Population (yr of data collection)	Design (number of subjects)	Gender	Current smokers	Former smokers	Yr since quitting	Comments
Kahn (1966)	US veterans (1954–62)	Prospective (248,195)	Male	1.6	1.2	NP	Excludes "doctor's orders" quitters; Cancer mortality
Cederlof et al. (1975)	Sweden (1963–72)	Prospective (27,300) (27,700)	Male Female	2.5 1.0	1.7 3.5	NP NP	Cancer incidence
Rogot and Murray (1980)	US veterans (1954–69)	Prospective (293,958)	Male	1.8	1.2	NP	Excludes "doctor's orders" quitters; Cancer mortality; Extension of US Veterans Study
MacMahon et al. (1981)	Boston, MA (1974–79)	Case:control (218:306) (149:337)	Male Female	1.3[a] 1.6[a]	1.4 1.3	NP NP	
Wynder, Hall, Polanski (1983)	6 US cities (1977–81)	Case:control (153:5,464) (121:2,525)	Male Female	2.2[a] 1.7[a]	1.7 1.4	≥1 ≥1	
Gold et al. (1985)	Baltimore, MD (1978–80)	Case:control (201:201)	Male and female	1.8	1.0	NP	

TABLE 3.—Continued

Reference	Population (yr of data collection)	Design (number of subjects)	Gender	Current smokers	Former smokers	Yr since quitting	Comments
Mack et al. (1986)	Los Angeles, CA (1976–81)	Case:control (490:490)	Male and female	2.3[a]	3.3 2.3 1.0[a]	<5 5–9 ≥10	
Norell et al. (1986)	Sweden (1982–84)	Case:control (98:134)	Male and female	1.6[a]	1.1	NP	Data for population controls
La Vecchia et al. (1987)	Northern Italy (1983–86)	Case:control (99:471) (51:134)	Male Female	1.6 1.1	1.4 0.9	NP NP	Crude relative risk computed from data presented
Mills et al. (1988)	California (1976–83)	Prospective (34,000)	Male and female	5.4	1.5	NP	Cancer mortality study
Falk et al. (1988)	Louisiana (1979–83)	Case:control (363:1234)	Male and female	1.8[a]	1.1[a]	≥3	Adjusted for diet and alcohol
Clavel et al. (1989)	Paris, France (1982–85)	Case:control (98:161) (63:107)	Male Female	1.6[a] 1.5[a]	1.0 0.9	NP NP	Adjusted for alcohol and coffee

TABLE 3.—Continued

Reference	Population (yr of data collection)	Design (number of subjects)	Gender	Current smokers	Former smokers	Yr since quitting	Comments
Cuzick and Babiker (1989)	England (1983–86)	Case:control (123:150)	Male	2.1[a]	3.6 3.6 1.3	<10 10–20 >20	
		(93:129)	Female	1.3[a]	0.8 1.0 1.1	<10 10–20 >20	
Olsen et al. (1989)	Minneapolis–St. Paul, MN (1980–83)	Case:control (212:220)	Male	2.5[a]	0.8	NP	
ACS CPS-II (unpublished tabulations)	United States (1982–86)	Prospective (421,663) (605,758)	Male Female	2.0 2.7	1.2 1.6	NP	Cancer mortality
Farrow and Davis (in press)	Seattle, WA (1982–86)	Case:control (148:188)	Male	3.2	1.0[a]	NP	Adjusted for age, race, and education

NOTE: NP=not provided; ACS CPS-II=American Cancer Society Cancer Prevention Study II.
[a]Computed as a weighted average from cigarette dose-specific relative risks presented in the paper. Weights are the number of controls within each stratum of smoking.

risk of pancreatic cancer than current smokers. This diminution of risk with abstinence serves to strengthen the hypothesis that smoking is a contributing cause of pancreatic cancer. Although alcohol does not appear to be a confounder in the assessment of the benefits of smoking cessation, the possibility of confounding by other factors, such as diet or amount of prior cigarette consumption, has not been adequately studied.

Bladder Cancer

As with pancreatic cancer, the relationship between bladder cancer risk and smoking has been noted for many years. However, because relative risks have not been greatly elevated and because of uncertainty about the effects of unidentified confounding factors in this disease, the causality of this association has been considered less certain compared with other diseases in earlier reports of the Surgeon General (US DHHS 1982). Smoking has nonetheless been regarded as a contributing factor in bladder cancer; in 1985, it was estimated that in the United States 47 percent of bladder cancer deaths in males and 37 percent in females are attributable to smoking (US DHHS 1989). A particular problem with causal inference in smoking and bladder cancer arises because of the inconsistent finding of clear exposure–response relationships in all studies, as has been observed between cigarette smoking and respiratory cancers. However, the usual measures of exposure to tobacco smoke may not accurately index the bladder's dose of tobacco-related carcinogens. The International Agency for Research on Cancer (IARC) concluded, based on evidence available through 1985, that smoking of different forms of tobacco is causally related to cancers of the bladder and renal pelvis (IARC 1986).

In addition to the studies reviewed in the 1982 Surgeon General's Report (US DHHS 1982) and in the 1986 report of IARC (1986), more recent data document a consistent association between cigarette smoking and bladder cancer. In an extended followup of a cohort of 25,000 Swedish males, mortality rates for bladder cancer were increased fourfold among ever smokers compared with never smokers (Carstensen, Pershagen, Eklund 1987). In current smokers, the risk of death from bladder cancer was approximately three times greater at all levels of consumption. The excess mortality from bladder cancer among current smokers was comparable in the American Cancer Society (ACS) Cancer Prevention Study II (CPS-II) (Table 4).

An extension of a large hospital-based case–control study, originally reported in 1977 (Wynder and Goldsmith 1977), showed similar increases in risk among male and female smokers (Augustine et al. 1988). The study included 1,316 male and 505 female cases and 3,940 male and 1,504 female controls interviewed in 9 U.S. cities between 1969 and 1984. For current smokers, odds ratios increased to approximately 3.5 for male and female smokers of 21 to 30 cigarettes per day. Odds ratios were lower among former smokers, although the risk did not decline as the duration of abstinence lengthened (Table 4).

The findings of a recent population-based case–control study documented similar levels of bladder cancer risk associated with cigarette smoking (Slattery et al. 1988). Slattery and coworkers (1988) assessed cigarette smoking and bladder cancer in 332 white male cases and 686 controls in Utah. The overall crude odds ratio for current

TABLE 4.—Studies of bladder cancer and smoking cessation

				Risk relative to never smokers			
Reference	Population (yr of data collection)	Design (number of subjects)	Gender	Current smokers	Former smokers	Yr since quitting	Comments
Kahn (1966)	US veterans (1954–62)	Prospective (248,195)	Male	1.9	1.5	NP	Excludes "doctor's orders" quitters; Cancer mortality
Cederlof et al. (1975)	Sweden (1963–72)	Prospective (27,300) (27,700)	Male Female	1.8 1.0	2.1 0	NP NP	Cancer incidence
Wynder and Stellman (1977)	6 US cities (1969–75)	Case:control (541:6,534)	Male	2.7	2.9 1.9 1.4 1.6 1.1	1–3 4–6 7–10 11–15 ≥16	
		(150:6,522)	Female	2.4	3.1 1.5 0 1.5 2.4	1–3 4–6 7–10 11–15 ≥16	
Wigle, Mao, Grace (1980)	Alberta, Canada (1971–73)	Case:control (204:1,002) (51:674)	Male Female	2.8 3.5	2.1 3.1	NP NP	Adjusted for cumulative past dose
Rogot and Murray (1980)	US veterans (1954–69)	Prospective (293,958)	Male	2.2	1.4	NP	Excludes "doctor's order" quitters; Cancer mortality; Extension of US Veterans Study

TABLE 4.—Continued

Reference	Population (yr of data collection)	Design (number of subjects)	Gender	Risk relative to never smokers — Current smokers	Risk relative to never smokers — Former smokers	Yr since quitting	Comments
Wynder and Goldsmith (1977)	6 US cities (1969–74)	Case:control (574:568)	Male	2.2	2.6	1–3	Cases are from the same series as reported by Wynder and Stellman (1977)
					2.9	4–6	
					1.5	7–9	
					1.6	10–12	
					1.2	13–15	
					1.1	≥16	
		(155:154)	Female	2.2	2.5	1–6	
					1.2	≥7	
Vineis et al. (1983)	Italy (1978–81)	Case:control (355:276)	Male	6.0	3.7	3–9	
					3.6	10–14	
					2.1	≥15	
Cartwright et al. (1983)	England (1978–81)	Case:control (932:1,402)	Male	1.6	1.0	6–15	
					1.1	16–25	
					0.9	≥26	
		(327:579)	Female	1.4	0.5	6–15	
					0.5	≥16	
Morrison et al. (1984)	Boston, MA (1976–77)	Case:control (427:391)	Male	3.1[a]	1.5	≥1	
		(165:142)	Female	5.6[a]	3.4	≥1	
	Manchester, UK (1976–78)	(398:490)	Male	2.6[a]	1.8	≥1	
		(155:241)	Female	2.1[a]	0.7	≥1	
	Nagoya, Japan (1976–78)	(224:442)	Male	2.0[a]	1.0	≥1	
		(66:146)	Female	4.3[a]	NP	NP	

TABLE 4.—Continued

Reference	Population (yr of data collection)	Design (number of subjects)	Gender	Risk relative to never smokers — Current smokers	Risk relative to never smokers — Former smokers	Yr since quitting	Comments
Vineis, Esteve, Terracini (1984)	Italy (1978–83)	Case:control (512:596)	Male	8.0[a,b]	3.1[a] 2.0[a] 2.3[a]	3–9 10–14 ≥15	Adjusted for number of cig/day
Vineis et al. (1985)	Italy (1981–83)	Case:control (55:202)	Female	2.3	1.0	≥3	
Jensen et al. (1987)	Copenhagen, Denmark (1979–81)	Case:control (388:787)	Male and female	3.4	2.0	NP	
Brownson, Chang, Davis (1987)	Missouri (1984–86)	Case:control (823:2,469)	Male	1.9	1.2	NP	Adjusted for alcohol
Hartge et al. (1987)	United States (1977–78)	Case:control (2,982:5,782)	Male and female	2.9	2.2 1.6 1.7 1.4[a]	1–9 10–19 20–29 ≥30	
Iscovich et al. (1987)	Argentina (1983–85)	Case:control (117:234)	Male and female	7.2	4.5 1.8 1.6 1.1	2–4 5–9 10–19 ≥20	
Augustine et al. (1988)	9 US cities (1969–84)	Case:control (1,316:3,940)	Male	2.2[a]	2.4[c] 2.2[c] 2.1[c]	≤6 7–12 ≥13	
		(505:1,504)	Female	0.9[a]	1.7[c] 1.2[c] 1.2[c]	≤6 7–12 ≤13	

TABLE 4.—Continued

Reference	Population (yr of data collection)	Design (number of subjects)	Gender	Risk relative to never smokers — Current smokers	Risk relative to never smokers — Former smokers	Yr since quitting	Comments
Slattery et al. (1988)	Utah (1977–83)	Case:control (332:686)	Male	3.7	3.7 2.7 1.9 1.8	0.5–7 8–15 16–29 ≥30	Adjusted for number of cig/day
Claude, Frenzel-Beyme, Kunze (1988)	Germany (1977–84)	Case:control (531:531)	Male	3.5	1.8	NP	
ACS CPS-II (unpublished tabulations)	United States (1982–86)	Prospective (421,663) (605,758)	Male Female	2.9 2.8	2.0 2.0	NP NP	Cancer mortality
Burch et al. (1989)	Canada (1979–82)	Case:control (627:602) (199:190)	Male Female	2.7 2.6	1.7 1.2	NP NP	

NOTE: NP=not provided; ACS CPS-II=American Cancer Society Cancer Prevention Study II.

[a] Computed as a weighted average from cigarette dose-specific relative risks presented in the paper. Weights are the number of controls within each stratum of smoking.

[b] Includes current and former smokers who quit in the past 2 yr.

[c] Crude (unadjusted) odds ratio calculated from tables presented in the paper.

smoking, compared with never smoking, was 3.69 (95-percent confidence interval (CI), 2.58–5.26). However, an exposure–response relationship was not evident with reported average number of cigarettes smoked daily. The odds ratios for former smokers declined only after 8 years or more of abstinence.

Table 4 summarizes findings from studies that have examined the relationship between cigarette smoking cessation and risk of bladder cancer. Of all the nonrespiratory cancer sites, the relationship between bladder cancer risk and cigarette smoking cessation has been most extensively studied. In these studies, the risk among current smokers ranges from 1.0 to 7.2 times the risk among never smokers (median of approximately 3); risks are similar among males and females. More recent studies conducted since the mid-1970s tend to show higher risks for current smokers than do the earlier studies. The higher risks in more recent studies may reflect the earlier age of starting to smoke of more recent cohorts of smokers (US DHHS 1989) or the presence of a long latency period for the smoking effect to become fully manifest after initiation in susceptible persons.

Beyond the first few years of abstinence, former smokers generally have lower risks than current smokers. The study conducted in six U.S. cities (Wynder and Stellman 1977; Wynder and Goldsmith 1977) indicated an approximate 50-percent reduction in risk after 6 years of abstinence, with risk returning to that of nonsmokers among men after 15 years. A similar return to nonsmoker risk was also observed after 6 years of abstinence in an English study (Cartwright et al. 1983) and in an Argentine study after 20 years (Iscovich et al. 1987). However, results from other studies (Howe et al. 1980; Vineis, Esteve, Terracini 1984; Hartge et al. 1987; Burch et al. 1989) indicated that the reduction in risk in the first few years after cessation is followed by little subsequent additional reduction, even beyond 10 or 15 years of abstinence. These observations are in contrast to those for the other cancer sites reviewed in this Chapter.

In some studies, the analyses controlled for the possible confounding effects of lower cigarette consumption among former smokers prior to cessation. The U.S. Veterans Study (Kahn 1966) showed no reduction in risk for former smokers, compared with current smokers, at levels of past cigarette consumption of 1 pack or less per day. There was an approximate 50-percent reduction in risk, however, for those former smokers who had previously smoked more than 1 pack per day. Most studies that included past cigarette smoking exposure as a covariate in multiple logistic regression analyses (Wigle, Mao, Grace 1980; Howe et al. 1980; Vineis, Esteve, Terracini 1984; Claude, Frentzel-Beyme, Kunze 1988; Slattery et al. 1988; Burch et al. 1989) showed relative risks that were similar to those observed in studies in which no such adjustment was made.

A large multicenter study conducted by NCI (Hartge et al. 1987) contained sufficient numbers of subjects for detailed subgroup analyses. Table 5 displays the findings of this study when both average cigarette dose per day and duration of smoking are cross-classified for current and former smokers. In each of these nine categories, bladder cancer risk was lower among former smokers than among current smokers.

As reviewed above, the amount of evidence supporting cigarette smoking as a cause of bladder cancer has become increasingly compelling since the 1982 Report of the Surgeon General (US DHHS 1982), which focused on cancer. Multiple studies of

TABLE 5.—Bladder cancer risk according to smoking dose, duration of smoking, and smoking status

Smoking dose (cig/day)	Duration of smoking (yr)	Risk relative to never smokers - Current smokers	Risk relative to never smokers - Former smokers
<20	<20	1.7	1.3
	20–39	1.6	1.5
	≥40	2.7	1.9
20–39	<20	2.2	1.4
	20–39	3.8	1.8
	≥40	3.1	2.5
≥40	<20	2.4	1.0
	20–39	4.0	2.1
	≥40	3.8	2.8

SOURCE: Hartge et al. (1987).

varying design conducted throughout the world have shown statistically significant increases in risk of bladder cancer among smokers. Cigarette smoking, determined to be a contributory factor in bladder cancer in past reports of the Surgeon General (US DHHS 1982, 1989), can now be identified as causally associated with bladder cancer. The evidence adequately meets the criteria for causality established in the 1964 Report (US PHS 1964). The decline in risk of bladder cancer with cessation further supports the conclusion that cigarette smoking causes bladder cancer. This diminution in risk cannot be explained by confounding from lower cumulative consumption among former smokers compared with continuing smokers.

Cervical Cancer

Recently, an association has been noted between cancer of the uterine cervix and cigarette smoking (Williams and Horm 1977; Stellman, Austin, Wynder 1980; Lyon et al. 1983; Hellberg, Valentin, Nilsson 1983; Berggren and Sjostedt 1983; Peters et al. 1986; Brock et al. 1988; Nischan, Ebeling, Schindler 1988). However, because of the possibility of confounding by unidentified factors (in particular, a sexually transmitted etiologic agent), this association has not been identified as causal (US DHHS 1982, 1989; IARC 1986). Components of tobacco smoke can be identified in the cervical mucus of smokers (Sasson et al. 1985; Schiffman et al. 1987). These compounds have been found not only to display mutagenic activity in this environment (Holly et al. 1986), but also to have the ability to impair local immunity by reducing the populations of Langerhans' cells within the cervical epithelium (Barton et al. 1988). The reduction in circulating levels of β-carotene caused by cigarette smoking is yet another mechanism whereby cigarettes may increase the risk of cervical cancer (Harris et al. 1986; Brock et al. 1988; Stryker et al. 1988). Thus, the association of cigarette smoking with cervical cancer is biologically plausible.

Table 6 summarizes findings from studies that have examined the relationship between cervical cancer risk and cigarette smoking cessation. In these studies, the risk among current smokers ranges from 1.0 to 5.0 times the risk among never smokers (median of approximately 2). Smoking-associated risks for invasive cancer and for carcinoma in situ are generally similar.

After the first year of abstinence, former smokers have lower cervical cancer risk than current smokers in most studies. Exceptions include the study conducted in Milan (La Vecchia, Franceschi et al. 1986), which showed risk reduction for invasive cancer but not for carcinoma in situ among former smokers, and the study conducted in Central America (Herrero et al. 1989) in which no association with smoking was observed at all, even for current smokers. The effect of time since stopping has not yet been well studied for cervical cancer, but observations from a large multicenter study conducted by NCI (Brinton, Schairer, Haenszel et al. 1986) suggested that risk reduction may occur fairly rapidly after cessation. One study found that smokers tended to have a poorer prognosis for survival after radiation treatment for invasive cervical cancer, but no data were presented regarding smoking cessation (Kucera et al. 1987).

A major concern in studies of smoking and cervical cancer has been the potential for confounding by factors that would predispose a woman to become infected with a sexually transmitted agent that might be causally related to the disease, such as human papilloma virus (Stellman, Austin, Wynder 1980; Winkelstein et al. 1984; IARC 1986). Therefore, it is important to note that those studies that controlled for risk factors for sexually transmitted disease (Trevathan et al. 1983; Greenberg et al. 1985; Herrero et al. 1989; Slattery et al. 1989) produced relative risk estimates for current and former smokers that were quite similar to those from studies that made no such adjustments. The association of smoking and cervical cancer has been considered by some to be a result of residual confounding by inadequately measured indicators of exposure to a sexually transmitted agent. Although factors such as the number of past sexual partners are only surrogates for a hypothetical etiologic infectious agent, they are the very same social correlates of tobacco smoking that would suggest this type of confounding. Therefore, even though such factors as age at first intercourse and the number of sexual partners are imperfect indicators of infection by a possible etiologic agent, their inclusion as covariates in multivariate analyses may be sufficient to control confounding to some extent in the analysis of the effects of smoking on cervical cancer risk.

This review of the evidence on cervical cancer and cigarette smoking cessation indicates that there is a consistently observed association between cervical cancer risk and cigarette smoking and that former smokers experience a lower risk of cervical cancer than current smokers, even after adjusting for the social correlates of smoking and risk of sexually acquired infections. This observed diminution of risk after cessation lends support to the hypothesis that smoking is a contributing cause of cervical cancer. Based on a recent comprehensive review of epidemiologic studies providing data on smoking and cervical cancer, Winkelstein (1990) concluded that smoking is causally associated with cervical cancer.

TABLE 6.—Studies of cervical cancer and smoking cessation

Reference	Location (yr of data collection)	Design (number of subjects)	Current smokers	Former smokers	Yr since quitting	Comments
Cederlof et al. (1975)	Sweden (1963–72)	Prospective (27,700)	5.0	3.0	NR	Cancer incidence
Clarke, Morgan, Newman (1982)	Toronto, Ontario (1973–76)	Case:control (178:855)	2.3	1.7	NR	Invasive cancer
Marshall et al. (1983)	Buffalo, NY (1957–65)	Case:control (513:490)	1.6	0.8	NR	
Trevathan et al. (1983)	Atlanta, GA (1980–81)	Case:control (99:288)	4.2	2.1	NR	Carcinoma in situ. Adjusted for sexual partners, birth control pills, SES
Greenberg et al. (1985)	England (1968–83)	Prospective (17,032)	3.0[a]	0.7	NR	Invasive cancer incidence. Adjusted for age at marriage, birth control pills, SES
Brinton, Schairer, Haenszel et al. (1986)	5 US cities (1982–84)	Case:control (480:797)	1.5	3.2 1.1 1.0 1.1	1 2–4 5–9 ≥10	Adjusted for sexual partners, age at first intercourse, SES
La Vecchia, Franceschi et al. (1986)	Milan, Italy (1981–84)	Case:control (183:183) (230:230)	1.4[b] 1.7	2.5 0.8	NR NR	Carcinoma in situ Invasive cancer

TABLE 6.—Continued

Reference	Location (yr of data collection)	Design (number of subjects)	Risk relative to never smokers — Current smokers	Risk relative to never smokers — Former smokers	Yr since quitting	Comments
Brisson et al. (1988)	Quebec (1982–85)	Case:control (247:137)	3.5	1.9	NR	Carcinoma in situ
Herrero et al. (1989)	4 Central American cities (1986–87)	Case:control (666:1,427)	1.0	1.0	NR	Adjusted for sexual partners
Slattery et al. (1989)	Utah (1984–87)	Case:control (266:408)	3.4	1.4	NR	Adjusted for sexual partners and education
ACS CPS-II (unpublished tabulations)	United States (1982–86)	Prospective (605,758)	2.1	1.9	NR	Cancer mortality

NOTE: NR=not reported; SES=socioeconomic status; ACS CPS-II=American Cancer Society Cancer Prevention Study II.
[a] Computed as a weighted average from cigarette dose-specific relative risks presented in the paper. Weights are the number of incident cases within each stratum of smoking.
[b] Computed as a weighted average from cigarette dose-specific relative risks presented in the paper. Weights are the number of controls within each stratum of smoking.

Breast Cancer

In general, prior research has shown little relation between cigarette smoking and the risk of breast cancer (Baron 1984; Rosenberg et al. 1984; Baron et al. 1986); however, in recent years, several reports have raised the possibility that there might be a weak positive association (Table 7). Because there has been considerable discussion about the possible role of smoking in breast cancer in recent literature, the relationships among cigarette smoking, smoking cessation, and breast cancer risk are reviewed. Cigarette smoking creates a set of physiologic conditions that result in various antiestrogenic effects (Baron 1984; Jensen, Christiansen, Rodbrø 1985; Michnovicz et al. 1986), as well as affecting body mass (Carney and Goldberg 1984; Hofstetter et al. 1986; Chapters 9, 10, 11). The relationship between cigarette smoking and body mass is a particularly important consideration in studies of breast cancer, because body mass has a complex age-dependent association with breast cancer risk, with obesity being protective in premenopausal ages but slightly risk-enhancing later in life (Willett et al. 1985).

Table 7 summarizes findings from studies that have examined the relationship between breast cancer risk and the cessation of cigarette smoking. The risk of breast cancer among current smokers ranges from less than 1.0 to 4.6 times greater than among never smokers (median approximately 1). The relative risks of smoking do not consistently differ in premenopausal and postmenopausal age groups. In addition, there is little consistency regarding the change in risk observed after smoking cessation. Former smokers have lower risks in some studies, but higher risks in others. Adjustment for other breast cancer risk factors does not appear to completely remove the weak association observed in some studies (Schechter, Miller, Howe 1985; Rohan and Baron 1989).

In one study it was found that smokers tended to have a greater prevalence of tumor-positive axillary lymph nodes at the time of diagnosis than did never smokers and former smokers, a finding that could not be explained by patient delay (Daniell 1988). This association was not confirmed, however, in a recent report based on 10-year followup of the Nurses Health Study cohort that included 1,373 cases with information on extent of disease at diagnosis (London et al. 1989).

This review of breast cancer and cigarette smoking suggests that cigarette smoking is not associated with breast cancer. Consistent changes in risk are not observed with smoking cessation.

Endometrial Cancer

The relationship between cigarette smoking and cancer of the endometrium is unique among the associations of smoking with cancers at various sites; of the sites for which smoking has been associated with a change in risk, endometrial cancer is the only cancer for which there is fairly consistent evidence of an inverse (protective) relationship (Baron 1984; Lesko et al. 1985; Stockwell and Lyman 1987), an effect that may be limited to postmenopausal women (Smith, Sowers, Burns 1984; Koumantaki et al. 1989). The reasons for the lower risk among women who smoke are not well under-

TABLE 7.—Studies of breast cancer and smoking cessation

Reference	Location (yr of data collection)	Design (number of subjects)	Menopausal status	Current smokers	Former smokers	Yr since quitting	Comments
Cederlof et al. (1975)	Sweden (1963–72)	Prospective (27,700)	Pre and post	0.6	0.4	NR	Cancer incidence
Schechter, Miller, Howe (1985)	Canada (1980–82)	Case:control (49:134) (71:219)	Pre Post	4.6 1.1	1.8 0.8	≥1 ≥1	Adjusted for several breast cancer risk factors
Hiatt and Fireman (1986)	Northern California (1964–80)	Prospective (84,172)	Pre Post	1.2 1.1	1.2 1.3	NR NR	Cancer incidence
Brinton, Schairer, Stanford et al. (1986)	United States (1973–75)	Case:control (447:503) (614:818)	Pre Post	1.1 1.1	1.4 1.0	NR NR	
Stockwell and Lyman (1987)	Florida (1981)	Case:control (4,011:2,952)	Pre Post	1.3[a] 1.2[a]	0.9 0.9	NR NR	
Brownson et al. (1988)	Missouri (1979–86)	Case:control (114:208) (206:872)	Pre Post	2.3 1.2	1.2 0.7	NR NR	
Adami et al. (1988)	Sweden and Norway (1984–85)	Case:control (422:527)	Pre and post	1.0	0.8		Relative risk calculated from crude data
Rohan and Baron (1989)	Australia (1982–84)	Case:control (146:132) (280:288)	Pre Post	1.3 1.5	2.4 0.9	≥1 ≥1	Adjusted for several breast cancer risk factors

TABLE 7.—Continued

Reference	Location (yr of data collection)	Design (number of subjects)	Menopausal status	Risk relative to never smokers			Comments
				Current smokers	Former smokers	Yr since quitting	
London et al. (1989)	United States (1976–80)	Prospective (117,557)	Pre Post	1.0[a] 1.1[a]	1.1 1.1	NR NR	

NOTE: NR=not reported.

[a]Computed as a weighted average from cigarette dose-specific relative risks presented in the paper. Weights are the number of controls within each stratum of smoking.

stood, but may be due to smoking effects on estrogen production and metabolism, including increased 2-hydroxylation of estradiol in smokers (Michnovicz et al. 1986), an earlier age at menopause in smokers (Baron 1984), and indirect effects of the body weight differences between smokers and nonsmokers, such as the production of estrogens from precursors within adipose tissue (MacDonald et al. 1978; Chapters 8 and 10).

Table 8 includes a summary of findings from studies of endometrial cancer that have examined cigarette smoking cessation. Although the risk of endometrial cancer among current smokers in these studies is approximately 30 percent lower than that among never smokers, the risk among ex-smokers is similar to, or slightly greater than, that among current smokers.

This review of past research on endometrial cancer risk and cigarette smoking cessation suggests that current smokers are at lower risk of endometrial cancer than never smokers, but it is not clear whether this protective effect of smoking on endometrial cancer risk might be reversed soon after cessation of cigarette smoking. Although further investigation of the mechanisms for the protective effect of smoking on endometrial cancer is of scientific interest to better understand the effects of smoking on hormones and of hormones on endometrial cancer risk, this inverse association with smoking has no public health relevance, as the well-substantiated risks to other organ systems from continued smoking far outweigh any potential benefits to the endometrium.

Other Cancer Sites

The metabolic products of tobacco smoke can be found in ovarian follicular fluid (Hellberg and Nilsson 1988). However, there is little evidence that smoking is associated with cancer of the ovary (Byers et al. 1983; Baron 1984; Baron et al. 1986; Stockwell and Lyman 1987; Whittemore et al. 1988; Mori et al. 1988). The risk of ovarian cancer differs little for either current or former smokers, as indicated in the only two studies that have examined the effect of cigarette smoking cessation on ovarian cancer risk (Table 8).

Tobacco has been regarded as a contributing factor for cancer of the kidney (US DHHS 1982, 1989). The U.S. Veterans Study (Kahn 1966; Rogot and Murray 1980) and ACS CPS-II (ACS, unpublished tabulations) suggest only small differences in mortality from renal cancer between current and former smokers (Table 8). A study of renal pelvis and ureteral cancers in Copenhagen (Jensen et al. 1988), however, showed a pattern of risk diminution with abstinence similar to that observed in bladder cancer, a site with the same histologic type of transitional-cell tumors.

Cancers of the anus and penis are considered possibly to result from infection by a sexually transmitted agent in a way analogous to cancer of the uterine cervix (Daniell 1985; Daling et al. 1987; Hellberg et al. 1987). Smokers have been found to be at increased risk both for cancer of the penis (Hellberg et al. 1987) and anus (Daling et al. 1987; Holmes et al. 1988) in recent studies. Only one study has examined the effect of cessation on the risk of these cancers (Hellberg et al. 1987). This study found that

TABLE 8.—Studies of cancer at selected sites that have examined the effect of smoking cessation

Reference	Population (yr of data collection)	Design (number of subjects)	Cancer site	Current smokers	Former smokers	Yr since quitting	Comments
Cederlof et al. (1975)	Sweden (1963–72)	Prospective (27,700)	Endometrium	0.5	1.6	NP	Cancer incidence
Lesko et al. (1985)	8 North American cities (1976–83)	Case:control (508:706)	Endometrium	0.8[a]	0.9	≥1	Adjusted for obesity and exogenous estrogens
Stockwell and Lyman (1987)	Florida (1981)	Case:control (990:2,952)	Endometrium	0.8[a]	0.6	NP	
Cederlof et al. (1975)	Sweden (1963–72)	Prospective (27,700)	Ovary	0.5	1.6	NP	Cancer incidence
Stockwell and Lyman (1987)	Florida (1981)	Case:control (696:2,952)	Ovary	1.1[a]	0.9	NP	
Franks et al. (1987)	United States (1980–82)	Case:control	Ovary	1.1	0.9	≥1	Adjusted for age, parity, and use of oral contraceptives
Kahn (1966)	US veterans (1954–62)	Prospective (248,195)	Kidney	1.4	1.5	NP	Excludes "doctor's orders" quitters Cancer mortality
Rogot and Murray (1980)	US veterans (1954–69)	Prospective (293,958)	Kidney	1.4	1.2	NP	Extension of US Veterans Study
Jensen et al. (1988)	Copenhagen (1979–82)	Case:control (96:288)	Renal pelvis and ureter	3.7	1.9	NP	Crude relative risks computed from data presented

TABLE 8.—Continued

Reference	Population (yr of data collection)	Design (number of subjects)	Cancer site	Current smokers	Former smokers	Yr since quitting	Comments
Hellberg et al. (1987)	Sweden (NP)	Case:control (244:232)	Penis	1.6	1.7	NP	
Cederlof et al. (1975)	Sweden (1963–72)	Prospective (27,300)	Liver	2.4	1.0	NP	Cancer incidence in males
Rogot and Murray (1980)	US veterans (1954–69)	Prospective (248,000)	Liver	2.3	1.8	NP	Cancer mortality
Yu et al. (1983)	Los Angeles, CA (1975–79)	Case:control (76:76)	Liver	1.8[a]	1.1	NP	Abstainers for ≥10 yr were considered never smokers
Kahn (1966)	United States (1954–62)	Prospective (248,195)	Stomach	1.4	1.1	NP	Excludes "doctor's orders" quitters Cancer mortality
Cederlof et al. (1975)	Sweden (1963–72)	Prospective (27,300)	Stomach	1.3	0.7	NP	Cancer incidence in males
Rogot and Murray (1980)	US veterans (1954–69)	Prospective (293,958)	Stomach	1.5	1.1	NP	Extension of US Veterans Study
Nomura et al. (1990)	Japanese men in Hawaii (1965–68)	Prospective (7,990)	Stomach	2.7	1.0	NP	Cohort identified 1965-68 and followed through October 1986
Kahn (1966)	US veterans (1954–62)	Prospective (248,195)	Leukemia	1.4	1.5	NP	Excludes "doctor's orders" quitters Cancer mortality

TABLE 8.—Continued

Reference	Population (yr of data collection)	Design (number of subjects)	Cancer site	Risk relative to never smokers - Current smokers	Risk relative to never smokers - Former smokers	Yr since quitting	Comments
Cederlof et al. (1975)	Sweden (1963–72)	Prospective (27,300) (27,700)	Leukemia (Males) (Females)	1.1 0.4	0.8 1.0	NP NP	Cancer incidence
Rogot and Murray (1980)	US veterans (1954–69)	Prospective (248,000)	Leukemia	1.6	1.5	NP	Extension of US Veterans Study
Trichopoulos et al. (1987)	Greece (1976–84)	Case:control (104:454) (89:454)	Liver HB_sAg^- HB_sAg^+	3.3[a] 1.6[a]	2.8 1.3	NP NP	
ACS CPS-II (unpublished tabulations)	United States (1982–86)	Prospective (421,623) (605,758)	Kidney (Males) (Females)	2.7 1.5	2.1 1.1	NP NP	Cancer mortality

NOTE: NP=not provided; HB_sAg=hepatitis B surface antigen; ACS CPS-II=American Cancer Society Cancer Prevention Study II.
[a]Computed as a weighted average from cigarette dose-specific relative risks presented in the paper. Weights are the number of controls within each stratum of smoking.

current smokers had a penile cancer risk 1.6 times that of never smokers, but the risk among former smokers was similar to that among current smokers (Table 8).

Primary hepatocellular cancer has been associated with smoking in a number of recent studies (Trichopoulous et al. 1980; Lam et al. 1982; Yu et al. 1983; Oshima et al. 1984; Trichopoulos et al. 1987; Hirayama 1989). This association is of potentially great public health importance because of the high incidence of primary liver cancer and the epidemic of cigarette smoking worldwide, which is increasingly involving countries in which liver cancer is the leading cause of cancer mortality. The mechanism whereby smoking might affect liver cancer risk is unknown. Although potential confounding by alcohol consumption is of concern in interpreting this association, the association of smoking with hepatocellular cancer has remained significant in several studies after controlling for alcohol intake (Trichopoulos et al. 1980; Yu et al. 1983; Oshima et al. 1984; Trichopoulos et al. 1987). One case–control study (Yu et al. 1983) and two cohort studies (Cederlof et al. 1975; Carstensen, Pershagen, Eklund 1987; Rogot and Murray 1980) have examined the effects of smoking cessation on liver cancer risk. In all three studies, current smokers were found to have higher risks than either never smokers or former smokers. In the case–control study, potential confounding by different alcohol consumption of current and former smokers was controlled (Yu et al. 1983). Many of the earlier studies (including the prospective studies reviewed in this Chapter) did not exclude the possibility that cancer of the liver may have been primary in another (smoking-related) organ. The possible role of hepatitis B as a modifier of the effect of smoking on the risk of liver cancer is not clear (IARC 1986).

Tobacco has been associated with stomach cancer, but whether this association is causal remains unclear (IARC 1986; US DHHS 1982, 1989). Few studies have considered the effect of cessation on the risk of stomach cancer. The U.S. Veterans Study (Kahn 1966; Rogot and Murray 1980) and the Swedish study (Cederlof et al. 1975) indicate a reduction in stomach cancer risk after cessation, although the relative risks among current smokers were small in these studies (Table 8).

Leukemia has recently been implicated as a smoking-related disease (Austin and Cole 1986; Severson 1987; Kinlen and Rogot 1988), but this observation has not been consistent (for review, see Kinlen and Rogot 1988). The U.S. Veterans Study showed only a slight dose–response relationship for myelogenous leukemias, but there was little difference in risk between current and former smokers (Kahn 1966; Rogot and Murray 1980; Kinlen and Rogot 1988). In the earlier presentation of these data, there was no difference in risk among ex-smokers, compared with current smokers, at any of four levels of prior cigarette smoking (Kahn 1966). The most recent analysis of these data indicated there was little difference in risk among former smokers compared with current smokers for any of the subtypes of leukemia. One study demonstrated a poorer prognosis for patients with myelogenous leukemia who were cigarette smokers (Archimbaud et al. 1989).

MULTIPLE PRIMARY CANCERS

The occurrence of multiple primary cancers may reflect the effects of the same risk factors in the pathogenesis of the multiple cancers, the effects of agents used in treating the initial malignancy, or simply the consequence of chance (Schottenfeld 1982). Thus, multiple primary cancers have been investigated with the goals of examining environmental and host factors increasing cancer risk and of identifying adverse consequences of cancer treatment. Tobacco use, including cigarette smoking, has been examined as a risk factor for the development of a second primary cancer, after diagnosis of a first malignancy at cigarette-associated and non-cigarette-associated sites; the effect of smoking cessation on the occurrence of second cancers has also been addressed in several investigations.

Descriptive studies have shown that an initial malignancy at a smoking-associated site is followed by an increased risk for cancer at the same or another cigarette-associated site (Wynder et al. 1969; Schottenfeld 1982). In an early study of multiple primary cancers, Berg, Schottenfeld, and Ritter (1970) examined the risks of second primary cancers in persons evaluated at Memorial Hospital for squamous cell cancers of the respiratory or upper digestive tract or other histologic types of lung cancer. In comparison with expected numbers of cases based on incidence rates for New York State, significant excesses were observed for cancers of the lip, oral cavity or pharynx, esophagus, larynx, and lung.

Only limited evidence is available on the effects of smoking cessation on the occurrence of multiple primary cancers. Moore reported two studies (1965, 1971) of second primary cancers in persons with an index malignancy of the mouth, pharynx, or larynx; both showed reduced risk for a second primary cancer in persons who stopped smoking after diagnosis of the first cancer. For 1 to 15 years, Silverman, Gorsky, and Greenspan (1983) observed 117 smokers who had a primary cancer of the head and neck region. Thirty percent of continuing smokers developed a second oral primary cancer compared with 15 percent of those reducing smoking and 13 percent of those completely stopping.

In contrast, an effect of cessation was not found in two other studies (Castigliano 1968; Schottenfeld, Gantt, Wynder 1974). Castigliano's 1968 study included 88 subjects with mouth or throat cancer who survived for at least 3 years without evidence of recurrence. During a minimum followup period of 3 years, the occurrence of a second primary cancer was not related to smoking status. Schottenfeld, Gantt, and Wynder (1974) examined multiple primary cancers in 733 patients admitted to Memorial Sloan-Kettering Cancer Center with a primary epidermoid carcinoma of the oral cavity, pharynx, or larynx. During the 5-year followup period, the smoking status of those developing and not developing a second primary did not differ significantly.

Interpretation of these studies is limited by the small numbers of subjects and the limited duration of followup. Furthermore, the interactions of tobacco smoking with other risk factors of cancers of the head and neck, particularly alcohol consumption, complicate interpretation of these data.

SUMMARY

This review of the relationship between cigarette smoking cessation and the risk of nonrespiratory cancers has shown that former smokers tend to have lower risk than current smokers for cancers of the oral cavity, esophagus, pancreas, bladder, and uterine cervix. This lower risk appears to be neither an artifact of a lower exposure to cigarettes in former smokers prior to quitting nor a result of confounding by other known risk factors for these cancers. This observation of a diminution in risk further supports the hypothesis that cigarette smoking is a causal factor for cancers of many sites other than the respiratory system. Although smoking is not as strong a risk factor for nonrespiratory cancers as it is for cancers of the lung and larynx, substantial numbers of cases of many nonrespiratory cancers can be attributed to tobacco use (US DHHS 1989). The patterns of diminution in risk with increasing duration of abstinence indicate that smoking cessation provides a substantial reduction in the risk of nonrespiratory cancer.

CONCLUSIONS

1. Smoking cessation halves the risks for cancers of the oral cavity and esophagus, compared with continued smoking, as soon as 5 years after cessation, with further reduction over a longer period of abstinence.

2. Smoking cessation reduces the risk of pancreatic cancer, compared with continued smoking, although this reduction in risk may only be measurable after 10 years of abstinence.

3. Smoking is a cause of bladder cancer; cessation reduces risk by about 50 percent after only a few years, in comparison with continued smoking.

4. The risk of cervical cancer is substantially lower among former smokers in comparison with continuing smokers, even in the first few years after cessation. This finding supports the hypothesis that cigarette smoking is a contributing cause of cervical cancer.

5. Neither smoking nor smoking cessation are associated with the risk of cancer of the breast.

References

ADAMI, H.O., LUND, E., BERGSTROM, R., MEIRIK, O. Cigarette smoking, alcohol consumption and risk of breast cancer in young women. *British Journal of Cancer* 58(6):832–837, December 1988.

AMERICAN CANCER SOCIETY. Unpublished tabulations provided by L. Garfinkel from the Cancer Prevention Study II. August 1989.

ARCHIMBAUD, E., MAUPAS, J., LECLUZE-PALAZZOLO, C., FIERE, D., VIALA, J.J. Influence of cigarette smoking on the presentation and course of chronic myelogenous leukemia. *Cancer* 63(10):2060–2065, May 15, 1989.

AUGUSTINE, A., HEBERT, J.R., KABAT, G.C., WYNDER, E.L. Bladder cancer in relation to cigarette smoking. *Cancer Research* 48:4405–4408, August 1, 1988.

AUSTIN, H., COLE, P. Cigarette smoking and leukemia. *Journal of Chronic Diseases* 39(6):417–421, 1986.

BARON, J.A. Smoking and estrogen-related disease. *American Journal of Epidemiology* 119(1):9–22, January 1984.

BARON, J.A., BYERS, T., GREENBERG, E.R., CUMMINGS, K.M., SWANSON, M. Cigarette smoking in women with cancers of the breast and reproductive organs. *Journal of the National Cancer Institute* 77(3):677–680, September 1986.

BARTON, S.E., MADDOX, P.H., JENKINS, D., EDWARDS, R., CUZICK, J., SINGER, A. Effect of cigarette smoking on cervical epithelial immunity: A mechanism for neoplastic change? *Lancet* 2(8612):652–654, September 17, 1988.

BERG, J.W., SCHOTTENFELD, D., RITTER, F. Incidence of multiple primary cancers. III. Cancers of the respiratory and upper digestive system as multiple primary cancers. *Journal of the National Cancer Institute* 44:263–274, 1970.

BERGGREN, G., SJOSTEDT, S. Preinvasive carcinoma of the cervix uteri and smoking. *Acta Obstetricia et Gynecologica Scandinavica* 62(6):593–598, 1983.

BLOT, W.J., MCLAUGHLIN, J.K., WINN, D.M., AUSTIN, D.F., GREENBERG, R.S., PRESTON-MARTIN, S., BERNSTEIN, L., SCHOENBERG, J.B., STEMHAGEN, A., FRAUMENI, J.F. JR. Smoking and drinking in relation to oral pharyngeal cancer. *Cancer Research* 48:3282–3287, June 1, 1988.

BRINTON, L.A., SCHAIRER, C., HAENSZEL, W., STOLLEY, P., LEHMAN, H.F., LEVINE, R., SAVITZ, D.A. Cigarette smoking and invasive cervical cancer. *Journal of the American Medical Association* 255(23):3265–3269, 1986.

BRINTON, L.A., SCHAIRER, C., STANFORD, J.L., HOOVER, R.N. Cigarette smoking and breast cancer. *American Journal of Epidemiology* 123(4):614–622, April 1986.

BRISSON, J., ROY, M., FORTIER, M., BOUCHARD, C., MEISELS, A. Condyloma and intraepithelial neoplasia of the uterine cervix: A case–control study. *American Journal of Epidemiology* 128(2):337–342, August 1988.

BROCK, K.E., BERRY, G., MOCK, P.A., MACLENNAN, R., TRUSWELL, A.S., BRINTON, L.A. Nutrients in diet and plasma and risk of in situ cervical cancer. *Journal of the National Cancer Institute* 80(8):580–585, June 15, 1988.

BROWNSON, R.C., BLACKWELL, C.W., PEARSON, D.K., REYNOLDS, R.D., RICHENS, J.W., PAPERMASTER, B.W. Risk of breast cancer in relation to cigarette smoking. *Archives of Internal Medicine* 148(1):140–144, January 1988.

BROWNSON, R.C., CHANG, J.C., DAVIS, J.R. Occupation, smoking, and alcohol in the epidemiology of bladder cancer. *American Journal of Public Health* 77(10):1298–1300, October 1987.

BURCH, J.D., ROHAN, T.E., HOWE, G.R., RISCH, H.A., HILL, G.B., STEELE, R., MILLER, A.B. Risk of bladder cancer by source and type of tobacco exposure: A case–control study. *International Journal of Cancer* 44:622–628, 1989.

BYERS, T., MARSHALL, J., GRAHAM, S., METTLIN, C., SWANSON, M. A case–control study of dietary and nondietary factors in ovarian cancer. *Journal of the National Cancer Institute* 71(4):681–686, October 1983.

CARNEY, R.M., GOLDBERG, A.P. Weight gain after cessation of cigarette smoking. A possible role for adipose-tissue lipoprotein lipase. *New England Journal of Medicine* 310(10):614–616, March 8, 1984.

CARSTENSEN, J.M., PERSHAGEN, G., EKLUND, G. Mortality in relation to cigarette and pipe smoking: 16 years' observation of 25,000 Swedish men. *Journal of Epidemiology and Community Health* 41:166–172, 1987.

CARTWRIGHT, R.A., ADIB, R., APPLEYARD, I., GLASHAN, R.W., GRAY, B., HAMILTON-STEWART, P.A., ROBINSON, M., BARHAM-HALL, D. Cigarette smoking and bladder cancer: An epidemiologic inquiry in West Yorkshire. *Journal of Epidemiology and Community Health* 37(4):256–263, December 1983.

CASTIGLIANO, S.G. Influence of continued smoking on the incidence of second primary cancers involving mouth, pharynx, and larynx. *Journal of the American Dental Association* 77:580–585, 1968.

CEDERLOF, R., FRIBERG, L., HRUBEC, Z., LORICH, U. *The Relationship of Smoking and Some Social Covariables to Mortality and Cancer Morbidity. A Ten Year Follow-up in a Probability Sample of 55,000 Swedish Subjects Age 18–69. Part 1/2*. Stockholm, Sweden: Karolinska Institute, Department of Environmental Hygiene, 1975.

CLARKE, E.A., MORGAN, R.W., NEWMAN, A.M. Smoking as a risk factor in cancer of the cervix: Additional evidence from a case–control study. *American Journal of Epidemiology* 115(1):59–66, January 1982.

CLAUDE, J.C., FRENTZEL-BEYME, R.R., KUNZE, E. Occupation and risk of cancer of the lower urinary tract among men. A case–control study. *International Journal of Cancer* 41(3):371–379, March 15, 1988.

CLAVEL, F., BENHAMOU, E., AUQUIER, A., TARAYRE, M., FLAMANT, R. Coffee, alcohol, smoking and cancer of the pancreas: A case–control study. *International Journal of Cancer* 43(1):17–21, January 15, 1989.

CUBILLA, A.L., FITZGERALD, P.J. Classification of pancreatic cancers (nonendocrine). *Mayo Clinic Proceedings* 54:449–458, 1979.

CUZICK, J., BABIKER, A.G. Pancreatic cancer, alcohol, diabetes mellitus, and gall-bladder disease. *International Journal of Cancer* 43(3):415–421, March 15, 1989.

DALING, J.R., WEISS, N.S., HISLOP, T.G., MADEN, C., COATES, R.J., SHERMAN, K.J., ASHLEY, R.L., BEAGRIE, M., RYAN, J.A., COREY, L. Sexual practices, sexually transmitted diseases, and the incidence of anal cancer. *New England Journal of Medicine* 317(16):973–977, October 15, 1987.

DANIELL, H.W. Re: Causes of anal carcinoma. (Letter.) *Journal of the American Medical Association* 254(3):358, July 19, 1985.

DANIELL, H.W. Increased lymph node metastases at mastectomy for breast cancer associated with host obesity, cigarette smoking, age, and large tumor size. *Cancer* 62(2):429–435, July 15, 1988.

FALK, R.T., PICKLE, L.W., FONTHAM, E.T., CORREA, P., FRAUMENI, J.F. JR. Life-style risk factors for pancreatic cancer in Louisiana: A case–control study. *American Journal of Epidemiology* 128(2):324–336, August 1988.

FARROW, D.C., DAVIS, S. Risk of pancreatic cancer in relation to medical history and the use of tobacco, alcohol and coffee. *International Journal of Cancer*, in press.

FRANCO, E.L., KOWALSKI, L.P., OLIVEIRA, B.V., CURADO, M.P., PEREIRA, R.N., SILVA, M.E., FAVA, A.S., TORLONI, H. Risk factors for oral cancer in Brazil: A case–control study. *International Journal of Cancer* 43(6):992–1000, June 15, 1989.

FRANKS, A.L., LEE, N.C., KENDRICK, J.S., RUBIN, G.L., LAYDE, P.M., THE CANCER AND STEROID HORMONE STUDY GROUP. Cigarette smoking and the risk of epithelial ovarian cancer. *American Journal of Epidemiology* 126(1):112–117, 1987.

GOLD, E.B., GORDIS, L., DIENER, M.D., SELTSER, R., BOITNOTT, J.K., BYNUM, T.E., HUTCHEON, D.F. Diet and other risk factors for cancer of the pancreas. *Cancer* 55(2):460–467, January 15, 1985.

GREENBERG, E.R., VESSEY, M., MCPHERSON, K., YEATES, D. Cigarette smoking and cancer of the uterine cervix. *British Journal of Cancer* 51:139–141, January 1985.

GUPTA, P.C., PINDBORG, J.J., BHONSLE, R.B., MURTI, P.R., MEHTA, F.S., AGHI, M.B., DAFTARY, D.K., SHAH, H.T., SINOR, P.N. Intervention study for primary prevention of oral cancer among 36,000 Indian tobacco users. *Lancet* 1(8492):1235–1239, May 31, 1986.

HARRIS, R.W., FORMAN, D., DOLL, R., VESSEY, M.P., WALD, N.J. Cancer of the cervix uteri and vitamin A. *British Journal of Cancer* 53(5):653–659, May 1986.

HARTGE, P., SILVERMAN, D., HOOVER, R., SCHAIRER, C., ALTMAN, R., AUSTIN, D., CANTOR, K., CHILD, M., KEY, C., MARRETT, L.D., MASON, T.J., MEIGS, J.W., MYERS, M.H., NARAYANA, A., SULLIVAN, J.W., SWANSON, G.M., THOMAS, D., WEST, D. Changing cigarette habits and bladder cancer risk: A case–control study. *Journal of the National Cancer Institute* 78(6):1119–1125, June 1987.

HELLBERG, D., NILSSON, S. Smoking and cancer of the ovary. (Letter.) *New England Journal of Medicine* 318(12):782–783, March 24, 1988.

HELLBERG, D., VALENTIN, J., EKLUND, T., STAFFAN, N. Penile cancer: Is there an epidemiological role for smoking and sexual behaviour? *British Medical Journal* 295(6609):1306–1308, November 21, 1987.

HELLBERG, D., VALENTIN, J., NILSSON, S. Smoking as a risk factor for cervical neoplasia. (Letter.) *Lancet* 2(8365/8366):1497, December 24–31, 1983.

HERRERO, R., BRINTON, L.A., REEVES, W.C., BRENES, M.M., TENORIO, F., DEBRITTON, R.C., GAITAN, E., GARCIA, M., RAWLS, W.E. Invasive cervical cancer and smoking in Latin America. *Journal of the National Cancer Institute* 81(3):205–211, February 1, 1989.

HIATT, R.A., FIREMAN, B.H. Smoking, menopause, and breast cancer. *Journal of the National Cancer Institute* 76:833–838, 1986.

HIRAYAMA, T. A large-scale cohort study on risk factors for primary liver cancer, with special reference to the role of cigarette smoking. *Cancer Chemotherapy and Pharmacology* 23(Supplement):S114–S117, 1989.

HOFSTETTER, A., SCHUTZ, Y., JEQUIER, E., WAHREN, J. Increased 24-hour energy expenditure in cigarette smokers. (Letter.) *New England Journal of Medicine* 314(25):1641, June 19, 1986.

HOLLY, E.A., PETRAKIS, N.L., FRIEND, N.F., SARLES, D.L., LEE, R.E., FLANDER, L.B. Mutagenic mucus in the cervix of smokers. *Journal of the National Cancer Institute* 76(6):983–986, June 1986.

HOLMES, F., BOREK, D., OWEN-KUMMER, M., HASSANEIN, R., FISHBACK, J., BEHBEHANI, A., BAKER, A., HOLMES, G. Anal cancer in women. *Gastroenterology* 95(1):107–111, July 1988.

HOWE, G.R., BURCH, J.D., MILLER, A.B., COOK, G.M., ESTEVE, J., MORRISON, B., GORDON, P., CHAMBERS, L.W., FODOR, G., WINSOR, G.M. Tobacco use, occupation, coffee, various nutrients, and bladder cancer. *Journal of the National Cancer Institute* 64(4):701–713, April 1980.

INTERNATIONAL AGENCY FOR RESEARCH ON CANCER. *Tobacco Smoking*, IARC Monographs on the Evaluation of the Carcinogenic Risk of Chemicals to Humans, Volume 38. Lyon: International Agency for Research on Cancer, 1986.

ISCOVICH, J., CASTELLETTO, R., ESTEVE, J., MUNOZ, N., COLANZI, R., CORONEL, A., DEAMEZOLA, I., TASSI, V., ARSLAN, A. Tobacco smoking, occupational exposure and bladder cancer in Argentina. *International Journal of Cancer* 40(6):734–740, December 15, 1987.

JENSEN, J., CHRISTIANSEN, C., RODBRØ, P. Cigarette smoking, serum estrogens, and bone loss during hormone-replacement therapy early after menopause. *New England Journal of Medicine* 313:973–975, 1985.

JENSEN, O.M., KNUDSEN, J.B., MCLAUGHLIN, J.K., SORENSON, B.L. The Copenhagen case–control study of renal pelvis and ureter cancer: Role of smoking and occupational exposures. *International Journal of Cancer* 41(4):557–561, April 15, 1988.

JENSEN, O.M., WAHRENDORF, J., BLETTNER, M., KNUDSEN, J.B., SORENSEN, B.L. The Copenhagen case–control study of bladder cancer: Role of smoking in invasive and non-invasive bladder tumours. *Journal of Epidemiology and Community Health* 41(1):30–36, March 1987.

JOHNSTON, W.D., BALLANTYNE, A.J. Prognostic effect of tobacco and alcohol use in patients with oral tongue cancer. *American Journal of Surgery* 134:444–447, 1977.

KABAT, G.C., HEBERT, J.R., WYNDER, E.L. Risk factors for oral cancer in women. *Cancer Research* 49(10):2803–2806, May 15, 1989.

KABAT, G.C., WYNDER, E.L. Type of alcoholic beverage and oral cancer. *International Journal of Cancer* 43(2):190–194, February 15, 1989.

KAHN, H.A. The Dorn study of smoking and mortality among US veterans: Report on eight and one-half years of observation. In: Haenzel, W. (ed.) *Epidemiological Approaches to the Study of Cancer and Other Chronic Diseases.* NCI Monograph 19. U.S. Department of Health, Education, and Welfare, U.S. Public Health Service, National Cancer Institute, January 1966, pp. 1–125.

KINLEN, L.J., ROGOT, E. Leukemia and smoking habits among United States veterans. *British Medical Journal* 297(6649):657–659, September 10, 1988.

KOUMANTAKI, Y., TZONOU, A., KOUMANTAKIS, E., KAKLAMANI, E., ARAVANTINOS, D., TRICHOPOULOS, D. A case–control study of cancer of the endometrium in Athens. *International Journal of Cancer* 43(5):795–799, May 15, 1989.

KUCERA, H., ENZELSBERGER, H., EPPEL, W., WEGHAUPT, K. The influence of nicotine abuse and diabetes mellitus on the results of primary irradiation in the treatment of carcinoma of the cervix. *Cancer* 60(1):1–4, July 1, 1987.

LA VECCHIA, C., FRANCESCHI, S., DECARLI, A., FASOLI, M., GENTILE, A., TOGNONI, G. Cigarette smoking and the risk of cervical neoplasia. *American Journal of Epidemiology* 123(1):22–29, January 1986.

LA VECCHIA, C., LIATI, P., DECARLI, A., NEGRELLO, I., FRANCESCHI, S. Tar yields of cigarettes and the risk of oesophageal cancer. *International Journal of Cancer* 38:381–385, 1986.

LA VECCHIA, C., LIATI, P., DECARLI, A., NEGRI, E., FRANCESCHI, S. Coffee consumption and risk of pancreatic cancer. *International Journal of Cancer* 40:309–313, September 15, 1987.

LA VECCHIA, C., NEGRI, E. The role of alcohol in oesophageal cancer in non-smokers, and the role of tobacco in non-drinkers. *International Journal of Cancer* 43(5):784–785, May 15, 1989.

LAM, K.C., YU, M.C., LEUNG, J.W.C., HENDERSON, B.E. Hepatitis B virus and cigarette smoking: Risk factors for hepatocellular carcinoma in Hong Kong. *Cancer Research* 42(12):5246–5248, December 1982.

LESKO, S.M., ROSENBERG, L., KAUFMAN, D.W., HELMRICH, S.P., MILLER, D.R., STROM, B., SCHOTTENFELD, D., ROSENSHEIN, N.B., KNAPP, R.C., LEWIS, J., SHAPIRO, S. Cigarette smoking and the risk of endometrial cancer. *New England Journal of Medicine* 313(10):593–596, 1985.

LONDON, S.J., COLDITZ, G.A., STAMPFER, M.J., WILLETT, W.C., ROSNER, B.A., SPEIZER, F.E. Prospective study of smoking and the risk of breast cancer. *Journal of the National Cancer Institute* 81(21):1625–1631, November 1, 1989.

LYON, J.L., GARDNER, J.W., WEST, D.W., STANISH, W.M., HEBERTSON, R.M. Smoking and carcinoma in situ of the uterine cervix. *American Journal of Public Health* 73(5):558–562, May 1983.

MACDONALD, P.C., EDMAN, C.D., HEMSELL, D.L., PORTER, J.C., SIITERI, P.K. Effect of obesity on conversion of plasma androstenedione to estrone in postmenopausal women with and without endometrial cancer. *American Journal of Obstetrics and Gynecology* 130:448–455, 1978.

MACK, T.M., YU, M.C., HANISCH, R., HENDERSON, B.E. Pancreas cancer and smoking, beverage consumption, and past medical history. *Journal of the National Cancer Institute* 76(1):49–60, January 1986.

MACMAHON, B., YEN, S., TRICHOPOULOS, D., WARREN, K., NARDI, G. Coffee and cancer of the pancreas. *New England Journal of Medicine* 304(11):630–633, March 12, 1981.

MARSHALL, J.R., GRAHAM, S., BYERS, T., SWANSON, M., BRASURE, J. Diet and smoking in the epidemiology of cancer of the cervix. *Journal of the National Cancer Institute* 70(5):847–851, May 1983.

MICHNOVICZ, J.J., HERSHCOPF, R.J., NAGANUMA, H., BRADLOW, H.L., FISHMAN, J. Increased 2-hydroxylation of estradiol as a possible mechanism for the anti-estrogenic effect of cigarette smoking. *New England Journal of Medicine* 315(21):1305–1309, November 1986.

MILLS, P.K., BEESON, W.L., ABBEY, D.E., FRASER, G.E., PHILLIPS, R.L. Dietary habits and past medical history as related to fatal pancreas cancer risk among Adventists. *Cancer* 61(12):2578–2585, June 15, 1988.

MOORE, C. Smoking and cancer of the mouth, pharynx, and larynx. *Journal of the American Medical Association* 191(4):107–110, January 25, 1965.

MOORE, C. Cigarette smoking and cancer of the mouth, pharynx, and larynx. A continuing study. *Journal of the American Medical Association* 218(4):553–558, October 25, 1971.

MORI, M., HARABUCHI, I., MIYAKE, H., CASAGRANDE, J.T., HENDERSON, B.E., ROSS, R.K. Reproductive, genetic, and dietary risk factors for ovarian cancer. *American Journal of Epidemiology* 128(4):771–777, October 1988.

MORRISON, A.S., BURING, J.E., VERHOEK, W.G., AOKI, K., LECK, I., OHNO, Y., OBATA, K. An international study of smoking and bladder cancer. *Journal of Urology* 131(4):650–654, April 1984.

NISCHAN, P., EBELING, K., SCHINDLER, C. Smoking and invasive cervical cancer risk. Results from a case–control study. *American Journal of Epidemiology* 128(1):74–77, July 1988.

NOMURA, A., GROVE, J.S., STEMMERMANN, G.N., SEVERSON, R.K. A prospective study of stomach cancer and its relation to diet, cigarettes, and alcohol consumption. *Cancer Research* 50:627–631, February 1, 1990.

NORELL, S.E., AHLBOM, A., ERWALD, R., JACOBSON, G., LINDBERG-NAVIER, I., OLIN, R., TORNBERG, B., WIECHEL, K.L. Diet and pancreatic cancer: A case–control study. *American Journal of Epidemiology* 124(6):894–902, December 1986.

OLSEN, G.W., MANDEL, J.S., GIBSON, R.W., WATTENBERG, L.W., SCHUMAN, L.M. A case–control study of pancreatic cancer and cigarettes, alcohol, coffee, and diet. *American Journal of Public Health* 79(8):1016–1019, 1989.

OSHIMA, A., TSUKUMA, H., HIYAMA, T., FUJIMOTO, I., YAMANO, H., TANAKA, M. Follow-up study of HBs Ag-positive blood donors with special reference to effect of drinking and smoking on development of liver cancer. *International Journal of Cancer* 34:775–779, 1984.

PETERS, R.K., THOMAS, D., HAGAN, D.G., MACK, T.M., HENDERSON, B.E. Risk factors for invasive cervical cancer among Latinas and non-Latinas in Los Angeles County. *Journal of the National Cancer Institute* 77(5):1063–1077, November 1986.

ROGOT, E., MURRAY, J.L. Smoking and causes of death among U.S. veterans: 16 years' of observation. *Public Health Reports* 95(3):213–222, May/June 1980.

ROHAN, T.E., BARON, J.A. Cigarette smoking and breast cancer. *American Journal of Epidemiology* 129(1):36–42, January 1989.

ROSENBERG, L., SCHWINGL, P.J., KAUFMAN, D.W., MILLER, D.R., HELMRICH, S.P., STOLLEY, P.D., SCHOTTENFELD, D., SHAPIRO, S. Breast cancer and cigarette smoking. *New England Journal of Medicine* 310(2):92–94, January 12, 1984.

SASSON, I.M., HALEY, N.J., HOFFMANN, D., WYNDER, E.L., HELLBERG, D., NILSSON, S. Cigarette smoking and neoplasia of the uterine cervix: Smoke constituents in cervical mucus. *New England Journal of Medicine* 312(5):315–316, January 31, 1985.

SCHECHTER, M.T., MILLER, A.B., HOWE, G.R. Cigarette smoking and breast cancer: A case–control study of screening participants. *American Journal of Epidemiology* 121(4):479–487, April 1985.

SCHIFFMAN, M.H., HALEY, N.J., FELTON, J.S., ANDREWS, A.W., KASLOW, R.A., LANCASTER, W.D., KURMAN, R.J., BRINTON, L.A., LANNOM, L.B., HOFFMANN, D. Biochemical epidemiology of cervical neoplasia: Measuring cigarette smoke constituents in the cervix. *Cancer Research* 47(14):3886–3888, July 15, 1987.

SCHOTTENFELD, D. Multiple primary cancers. In: Schottenfeld, D., Fraumeni, J.F. Jr. (eds.) *Cancer Epidemiology and Prevention*. Philadelphia: W.B. Saunders, Co., 1982, p. 1025.

SCHOTTENFELD, D., GANTT, R.C., WYNDER, E.L. The role of alcohol and tobacco in multiple primary cancers of the upper digestive system, larynx and lung: A prospective study. *Preventive Medicine* 3(2):277–293, June 1974.

SEVERSON, R.K. Cigarette smoking and leukemia. *Cancer* 60(2):141–144, July 15, 1987.

SILVERMAN, S. JR., GORSKY, M., GREENSPAN, D. Tobacco usage in patients with head and neck carcinomas: A follow-up study on habit changes and second primary oral/oropharyngeal cancers. *Journal of the American Dental Association* 106(1):33–35, January 1983.

SLATTERY, M.L., ROBISON, L.M., SCHUMAN, K.L., FRENCH, T.K., ABBOTT, T.M., OVERALL, J.C. JR., GARDNER, J.W. Cigarette smoking and exposure to passive smoke are risk factors for cervical cancer. *Journal of the American Medical Association* 261(11):1593–1598, March 17, 1989.

SLATTERY, M.L., SCHUMACHER, M.C., WEST, D.W., ROBISON, L.M. Smoking and bladder cancer. The modifying effect of cigarettes on other factors. *Cancer* 61(2):402–408, January 15, 1988.

SMITH, E.M., SOWERS, M.F., BURNS, T.L. Effects of smoking on the development of female reproductive cancers. *Journal of the National Cancer Institute* 73(2):371–376, August 1984.

SPITZ, M.R., FUEGER, J.J., GOEPFERT, H., HONG, W.K., NEWELL, G.R. Squamous cell carcinoma of the upper aerodigestive tract. A case comparison analysis. *Cancer* 61:203–208, 1988.

STELLMAN, S.D., AUSTIN, H., WYNDER, E.L. Cervix cancer and cigarette smoking: A case–control study. *American Journal of Epidemiology* 111(4):383–388, April 1980.

STEVENS, M.H., GARDNER, J.W., PARKIN, J.L., JOHNSON, L.P. Head and neck cancer survival and life-style change. *Archives of Otolaryngology* 109(11):746–749, November 1983.

STOCKWELL, H.G., LYMAN, G.H. Cigarette smoking and the risk of female reproductive cancer. *American Journal of Obstetrics and Gynecology* 157(1):35–40, July 1987.

STRYKER, W.S., KAPLAN, L.A., STEIN, E.A., STAMPFER, M.J., SOBER, A., WILLETT, W.C. The relation of diet, cigarette smoking, and alcohol consumption to plasma beta-carotene and alpha-tocopherol levels. *American Journal of Epidemiology* 127(2):283–296, 1988.

TREVATHAN, E., LAYDE, P., WEBSTER, L.A., ADAMS, J.B., BENIGNO, B.B., ORY, H. Cigarette smoking and dysplasia and carcinoma in situ of the uterine cervix. *Journal of the American Medical Association* 250(4):499–502, July 22–29, 1983.

TRICHOPOULOS, D., DAY, N.E., KAKLAMANI, E., TZONOU, A., MUÑOZ, N., ZAVITSANOS, X., KOUMANTAKI, Y., TRICHOPOULOU, A. Hepatitis B virus, tobacco smoking and ethanol consumption in the etiology of hepatocellular carcinoma. *International Journal of Cancer* 39(1):45–49, January 1987.

TRICHOPOULOS, D., MACMAHON, B., SPARROS, L., MERIKAS, G. Smoking and hepatitis B-negative primary hepatocellular carcinoma. *Journal of the National Cancer Institute* 65(1):111–114, July 1980.

TUYNS, A.J. Oesophageal cancer in non-smoking drinkers and non-drinking smokers. *International Journal of Cancer* 32(4):443–444, October 15, 1983.

U.S. DEPARTMENT OF HEALTH AND HUMAN SERVICES. *The Health Consequences of Smoking: Cancer. A Report of the Surgeon General.* U.S. Department of Health and Human Services, Public Health Service, Office on Smoking and Health. DHHS Publication No. (PHS) 82-50179, 1982.

U.S. DEPARTMENT OF HEALTH AND HUMAN SERVICES. *The Health Consequences of Using Smokeless Tobacco. A Report of the Advisory Committee to the Surgeon General.* U.S. Department of Health and Human Services, Public Health Service, National Institutes of Health. NIH Publication No. 86-2874, April 1986.

U.S. DEPARTMENT OF HEALTH AND HUMAN SERVICES. *Reducing the Health Consequences of Smoking: 25 Years of Progress. A Report of the Surgeon General.* U.S. Department of Health and Human Services, Public Health Service, Centers for Disease Control, Center for Chronic Disease Prevention and Health Promotion, Office on Smoking and Health. DHHS Publication No. (CDC) 89-8411, 1989.

U.S. PUBLIC HEALTH SERVICE. *Smoking and Health. Report of the Advisory Committee to the Surgeon General of the Public Health Service.* U.S. Department of Health, Education, and Welfare, Public Health Service, Center for Disease Control. PHS Publication No. 1103, 1964.

VINEIS, P., CICCONE, G., GHISETTI, V., TERRACINI, B. Cigarette smoking and bladder cancer in females. *Cancer Letters* 26(1):61–66, February 1985.

VINEIS, P., ESTEVE, J., TERRACINI, B. Bladder cancer and smoking in males: Types of cigarettes, age at start, effect of stopping and interaction with occupation. *International Journal of Cancer* 34(2):165–170, August 15, 1984.

VINEIS, P., FREA, B., UBERTI, E., GHISETTI, V., TERRACINI, B. Bladder cancer and cigarette smoking in males: A case–control study. *Tumori* 69(1):17–22, February 28, 1983.

WHITTEMORE, A.S., WU, M.L., PAFFENBARGER, R.S. JR., SARLES, D.L., KAMPERT, J.B., GROSSER, S., JUNG, D.L., BALLON, S., HENDRICKSON, M. Personal and environmental characteristics related to epithelial ovarian cancer. II. Exposures to talcum powder, tobacco, alcohol, and coffee. *American Journal of Epidemiology* 128(6):1228–1240, December 1988.

WIGLE, D.T., MAO, Y., GRACE, M. Relative importance of smoking as a risk factor for selected cancers. *Canadian Journal of Public Health* 71(4):269–275, July–August 1980.

WILLETT, W.C., BROWNE, M.L., BAIN, C., LIPNICK, R.J., STAMPFER, M.J., ROSNER, B., COLDITZ, G.A., HENNEKENS, C.H., SPEIZER, F.E. Relative weight and risk of breast cancer among premenopausal women. *American Journal of Epidemiology* 122:731–740, 1985.

WILLIAMS, R.R., HORM, J.W. Association of cancer sites with tobacco and alcohol consumption and socioeconomic status of patients: Interview study from the Third National Cancer Survey. *Journal of the National Cancer Institute* 58(3):525–547, March 1977.

WINKELSTEIN, W. JR. Smoking and cervical cancer—Current status: A review. *American Journal of Epidemiology* 131(6): 945–957, June 1990.

WINKELSTEIN, W. JR., SHILLITOE, E.J., BRAND, R., JOHNSON, K.K. Further comments on cancer of the uterine cervix, smoking, and herpesvirus infection. *American Journal of Epidemiology* 119(1):1–8, January 1984.

WINN, D.M., BLOT, W.J., SHY, C.M., PICKLE, L.W., TOLEDO, A., FRAUMENI, J.F. Snuff dipping and oral cancer among women in the southern United States. *New England Journal of Medicine* 304(13):745–749, March 26, 1981.

WYNDER, E.L., DODO, H., BLOCH, D.A., GANTT, R.C., MOORE, O.S. Epidemiologic investigation of multiple primary cancer of the upper alimentary and respiratory tracts. I. A retrospective study. *Cancer* 24:730–739, 1969.

WYNDER, E.L., GOLDSMITH, R. The epidemiology of bladder cancer. A second look. *Cancer* 40(3):1246–1268, September 1977.

WYNDER, E.L., HALL, N.E.L, POLANSKY, M. Epidemiology of coffee and pancreatic cancer. *Cancer Research* 43(8):3900–3906, August 1983.

WYNDER, E.L., STELLMAN, S.D. Comparative epidemiology of tobacco related cancers. *Cancer Research* 37(12):4608–4622, December 1977.

YU, M.C., MACK, T., HANISCH, R., PETERS, R.L., HENDERSON, B.E., PIKE, M.C. Hepatitis, alcohol consumption, cigarette smoking, and hepatocellular carcinoma in Los Angeles. *Cancer Research* 43(12, Part 1):6077–6079, December 1983.

CHAPTER 6
SMOKING CESSATION AND CARDIOVASCULAR DISEASE

CONTENTS

Introduction	191
Pathophysiologic Framework	191
Smoking and Development of CHD	191
Atherosclerosis	191
Thrombosis	193
Spasm	195
Arrhythmias	195
Reduced Blood Oxygen Delivery	195
Smoking and Development of Peripheral Arterial Disease	196
Smoking and Development of Cerebrovascular Disease	196
Anticipated Effects of Smoking Cessation on Risk of Cardiovascular Diseases Based on Knowledge of Mechanisms	197
Smoking Cessation and CHD	197
Cross-Sectional Studies	199
Studies of Smoking Cessation and Risk of MI Among Healthy Persons	200
Case–Control Studies	200
Cohort Studies	205
Intervention Trials	224
Smoking Cessation and CHD Risk Among Persons With Diagnosed CHD	229
Summary of Smoking Cessation and CHD Risk	239
Smoking Cessation and Aortic Aneurysm	241
Studies of Smoking Cessation and Risk of Aortic Aneurysm	241
Smoking Cessation and Peripheral Arterial Occlusive Disease	241
Smoking Cessation and Development of Peripheral Artery Disease	243
Smoking Cessation and Prognosis of Peripheral Artery Disease	243
Summary	244
Smoking Cessation and Cerebrovascular Disease	245
Studies of Smoking Cessation and Risk of Cerebrovascular Disease	246
Cross-Sectional Studies	246
Case–Control Studies	246
Prospective Cohort Studies	249
Summary of Observational Studies	251
Intervention Studies	251
Influence of Prior Levels of Smoking	251
Effect of Duration of Abstinence	252
Oral Contraceptives and Smoking Cessation	258
Effect of Smoking Cessation After Stroke	260
Summary	260
Conclusions	260
References	261

INTRODUCTION

Cigarette smoking is firmly established as an important cause of coronary heart disease (CHD), arteriosclerotic peripheral vascular disease, and stroke (US DHHS 1983, 1989). Eliminating smoking presents an opportunity for bringing about a major reduction in the occurrence of CHD, the leading cause of death in the United States. Before examining the epidemiologic evidence relating smoking cessation and risk of CHD and other forms of cardiovascular disease (CVD), the mechanisms by which smoking leads to these diseases are briefly reviewed. The objectives in considering these mechanisms are to address the plausibility that smoking cessation reduces risk of CVD, to estimate the expected magnitude in risk reduction, and to assess the rapidity with which any risk reduction might occur. Whether these mechanisms are immediately reversible, irreversible, or slowly reversible is of particular relevance to the rapidity with which smoking cessation will reduce risk. The role of smoking in the pathogenesis of CHD is discussed at length. The etiologies of peripheral vascular disease and stroke share several common features with CHD; thus, discussion focuses on distinguishing features.

PATHOPHYSIOLOGIC FRAMEWORK

Smoking and Development of CHD

Pathogenesis of CHD, which includes the clinical manifestations of myocardial infarction (MI), angina pectoris, and sudden death, is extremely complex and mediated by multiple mechanisms and etiologic factors (Munro and Cotran 1988). At least five interrelated processes are likely to contribute to the clinical manifestations of MI—atherosclerosis, thrombosis, coronary artery spasm, cardiac arrhythmia, and reduced capacity of the blood to deliver oxygen. Smoking appears to influence many steps in the development of CHD. Although not all of these effects are proven fully, the evidence for an influence on several mechanisms is convincing. The exact components of cigarette smoke that are responsible are not known in each instance, but experimental data have implicated nicotine and carbon monoxide (CO) in several processes. Other products of cigarette smoking, such as cadmium, nitric oxide, hydrogen cyanide, and carbon disulfide, have been hypothesized to play a role, but their quantitative contributions remain unknown (US DHHS 1983).

Atherosclerosis

Atherosclerosis is the mechanical narrowing of medium-sized arteries by the proliferation of smooth muscle cells, lipid accumulation, and ultimately, plaque formation and calcification (Munro and Cotran 1988). These lesions develop over decades and are not immediately reversible; whether they are substantially reversible at all in humans is a matter of current interest. Reversibility has been demonstrated in nonhuman primates (Clarkson et al. 1984; Malinow and Blaton 1984) and suggested in studies of humans using repeated arteriography (Blankenhorn et al. 1987). Smoking is clearly associated with the presence of atherosclerosis of the coronary arteries, small arteries of the myocardium, the aorta, and other vessels as demonstrated in many autopsy and angiographic studies (US DHHS 1983). The development of atherosclerosis is complex, and several processes are likely to be important.

Endothelial damage is thought to play a primary role in the development of atherosclerosis by exposing the arterial intima to blood lipids and white cells and by stimulating platelet adhesion. The endothelial damage can be an actual physical denudation, but toxic functional damage may have similar consequences. In animal studies, serum nicotine at levels similar to those of human smokers caused endothelial damage (Krupski et al. 1987; Zimmerman and McGeachie 1987). Evidence that smoking has a direct toxic effect on human endothelium is provided by the observation that smoking 2 tobacco cigarettes approximately doubled the number of nuclear-damaged endothelial cells in circulating blood (Davis et al. 1985, 1986); smoking non-tobacco cigarettes had little effect. In addition, Asmussen and Kjeldsen (1975) found pronounced degenerative changes of the umbilical artery endothelium at the time of delivery among mothers who smoked; these changes were not present in the arteries of nonsmoking mothers.

Smooth muscle cell proliferation is a primary feature of atherosclerotic lesions and may result from several stimuli; the most clearly demonstrated is platelet-derived growth factor from adherent platelets. Smoking appears to increase the adherence of platelets to arterial endothelium; blood drawn from persons after smoking 2 cigarettes results in a more-than-hundredfold adhesion of platelets to rabbit endothelium than does blood drawn from persons before smoking or from never smokers (Pittilo et al. 1984). Platelets from chronic smokers have a greater tendency to aggregate on an artificial surface than do those from nonsmokers (Rival, Riddle, Stein 1987). In minipigs, both cigarette smoke and CO increase the adhesion of platelets to arterial endothelium (Marshall 1986). The influence of smoking on platelet activity is discussed further in the following section.

Lipid infiltration of the arterial intima, largely cholesterol, is another primary feature of atherosclerosis and is directly related to higher blood levels of low-density lipoprotein cholesterol (LDL-C) and reduced blood levels of high-density lipoprotein cholesterol (HDL-C). Smoking reduces the level of HDL-C. A strong inverse association between daily cigarette consumption and HDL-C has been observed in many cross-sectional studies in the United States (Freedman et al. 1987; Gordon and Doyle 1986; Reichley, Mueller, Hanis et al. 1987; Willett et al. 1983) and in other countries (Assmann, Schulte, Schriewer 1984; Goldbourt et al. 1986; Gomo 1986; Jacobsen and Thelle 1987; Pelletier and Baker 1987; Robinson et al. 1987; Tuomilehto et al. 1986). In a longitudinal, community-based study, HDL-C decreased among persons starting to smoke and increased among those who stopped smoking (Fortmann, Haskell, Williams 1986). In other prospective studies, smoking abstinence has been associated with substantial increases in HDL-C levels in both men and women (Hulley, Cohen, Widdowson 1977; Hubert et al. 1987; Rabkin 1984). In a study among young adults in Louisiana, those who began smoking experienced substantial reductions in HDL-C compared with those who did not start (Freedman et al. 1986). HDL-C increased among 13 adult women who successfully stopped smoking for 48 days, but decreased to its previous levels among those who returned to smoking (Stamford et al. 1986). Thus, data indicate that smoking reduces the level of HDL-C, a potent protective factor against CHD.

In a number of studies, smokers have been found to have higher levels of triglycerides (Freedman et al. 1986; Jacobsen and Thelle 1987; Gomo 1986; Willett et al. 1983); however, the independent relation of triglyceride level with risk of CHD is not clear. Smoking appears to have little, if any, relation with LDL-C level. However, smokers have approximately twice the level of serum malondialdehyde of nonsmokers (Nadiger, Mathew, Sadasivudu 1987); malondialdehyde can alter LDL-C and may promote its incorporation into arterial wall macrophages (Steinberg et al. 1989). In a metabolic study among young men, smokers had a decreased cholesterol net transport from cell membranes into plasma, which could partially explain the accumulation of cholesterol in arterial walls (de Parscau and Fielding 1986).

Thrombosis

Coronary artery thrombosis, resulting from platelet-fibrin thrombi, is a key element in most cases of MI. Thrombi are visualized in a high percentage of coronary arteries studied angiographically within hours of the onset of infarction (DeWood et al. 1980), and agents that lyse thrombi are effective treatments for MI (Stampfer et al. 1982; Loscalzo and Braunwald 1988). The efficacy of aspirin, an antiplatelet agent, in preventing MI further supports the role of thrombus formation (Steering Committee of the Physicians' Health Study Research Group 1989). The finding that smoking is associated with history of MI even after controlling for atherosclerosis (Hartz et al. 1981) emphasizes the importance of mechanisms in addition to those that promote atherosclerosis.

Platelets play a central role in thrombus formation in addition to releasing growth factors that stimulate the proliferation of smooth muscle cells in arterial intima (Packham and Mustard 1986). Platelets can form microthrombi that become incorporated into the arterial wall, thus contributing to plaque formation and participating in generation of larger platelet-fibrin thrombi that may acutely occlude a coronary artery. Smoking cigarettes acutely increases spontaneous platelet aggregation in humans (Davis et al. 1985) and in dogs with coronary artery stenosis (Folts and Bonebrake 1982). Madsen and Dyerberg (1984) observed that smoking 2 high-nicotine cigarettes substantially reduced bleeding time among healthy young men, although ex vivo tests of platelet aggregability were only minimally inhibited. In this study, smoking low-nicotine cigarettes and inhalation of CO had little effect on bleeding time. Shortened platelet survival, an indirect indicator of activation, was observed in smokers and reverted to normal after 4 weeks of smoking abstinence (Fuster et al. 1981).

Studies of smoking and platelet aggregation ex vivo in response to the typical stimuli used in the laboratory, such as adenosine diphosphate (ADP) or thrombin, are inconsistent. Increased aggregation has been seen with platelets from chronic smokers (Belch et al. 1984) and in blood drawn 10 minutes after smoking 1 cigarette (Renaud et al. 1985; Renaud et al. 1984); in the latter study, aggregation was associated with blood nicotine levels but not with carboxyhemoglobin (COHb) levels. However, in other studies, ex vivo platelet aggregation was not related to cigarette smoking (Pittilo et al. 1984; Dotevall et al. 1987; de Lorgeril et al. 1985; Madsen and Dyerberg 1984). In one large study, aggregation in response to ADP stimulation was actually somewhat greater in nonsmokers (Meade et al. 1985). Studies of the effect of smoking on platelet production of thromboxane, which mediates the aggregatory effect, have also been inconsistent. In some studies, smoking was found to acutely increase thromboxane blood levels, which reflect the capacity to produce thromboxane in response to stimulation, and urinary metabolites, which reflect the normal steady-state production (Toivanen, Ylikorkala, Viinikka 1986; Marasini et al. 1986; Fischer et al. 1986). However, serum thromboxane B_2 levels were found to be similar among chronic smokers compared with nonsmokers in another study (Dotevall et al. 1987). The serious limitations of ex vivo aggregability measurements in the evaluation of in vivo platelet activity have been noted (Fitzgerald, Oates, Nowak 1988). These researchers measured urinary excretion of a thromboxane metabolite and found elevated levels in chronic smokers that were reduced to the level of nonsmokers after aspirin administration, suggesting a platelet origin of the excess excretion (Nowak et al. 1987).

The lack of a consistent relation between smoking and ex vivo tests of platelet aggregability despite the demonstration that platelets of smokers adhere more readily to endothelium has led to the suggestion that smoking inhibits the production in arterial walls of prostacyclin, an inhibitor of platelet aggregation (Madsen and Dyerberg 1984). Reinders and coworkers (1986) demonstrated that the production of prostacyclin by cultured human endothelial cells is impaired by incubation with cigarette smoke condensate. Pittilo and colleagues (1982) also found that smoking reduces endothelial cell synthesis of prostacyclin in rats. Thus, in vivo smoking-related effects on platelet function may be mediated in part by an interaction with endothelium.

Fibrinogen levels have been found to be elevated among smokers in numerous cross-sectional studies (Meade et al. 1986; Kannel, D'Agostino, Belanger 1987; Wilhelmsen et al. 1984; Dotevall et al. 1987; Belch et al. 1984; Balleisen et al. 1985). Fibrinogen levels, in turn, are strongly related to risk of CHD and stroke (Meade et al. 1986; Kannel, D'Agostino, Belanger 1987; Wilhelmsen et al. 1984). Smoking cessation resulted in a decrease in fibrinogen levels after 4 weeks among 9 female smokers (Harenberg et al. 1985) and after 8 weeks among 14 male smokers (Ernst and Matrai 1987). In the latter study, the levels after 8 weeks were similar to those among never smokers. When fibrinogen was remeasured after 5 years, values had decreased to the levels of never smokers among men who had stopped smoking and had increased among those who started or resumed smoking (Meade, Imeson, Stirling 1987). In multivariate analyses of data from the Framingham Study (Kannel, D'Agostino, Belanger 1987) and Northwick Park Study (Meade et al. 1986) that both included cigarette smoking as well as fibrinogen levels, fibrinogen retained a clear independent association with risk of CHD, whereas the effect of smoking was substantially reduced after the inclusion of fibrinogen in the model. This analysis suggests that elevated fibrinogen levels may mediate a quantitatively important part of the effect of smoking on CHD risk.

Other clotting abnormalities, such as increased plasma viscosity and reduced red cell deformability, that tend to promote thrombus formation have also been observed in smokers (Belch et al. 1984). In addition, levels of plasminogen, which promotes lysis of thrombi, are lower in smokers (Wilhelmsen et al. 1984; Belch et al. 1984), but the levels increase after smoking cessation (Harenberg et al. 1985).

Spasm

Coronary artery spasm can cause acute ischemia manifested as angina pectoris and may promote thrombus formation at the site of repeated arterial constriction (Folts and Bonebrake 1982). Both chronic and acute cigarette smoking have a demonstrable vasoconstrictor effect on the coronary vasculature (Klein 1984). Compared with never smokers, current smokers have an approximately twentyfold risk of vasospastic angina pectoris (Scholl et al. 1986). Coronary artery spasm has also been identified by angiography after smoking a single cigarette (Maouad et al. 1984). Smoking-induced vasoconstriction has been demonstrated in patients with atherosclerotic coronary artery disease (Martin et al. 1984) that is mediated by an α-adrenergic increase in coronary artery tone (Winniford et al. 1986). In addition, smoking acutely increases platelet and plasma vasopressin (Nussey et al. 1986) as well as the carrier protein of vasopressin and oxytocin (de Lorgeril et al. 1985). In addition to causing acute arterial spasm, cigarette smoking appears to be associated with a reduction in long-term coronary artery diameter independent of atherosclerotic plaque (Fried, Moore, Pearson 1986), although the mechanism for this relationship is unclear.

Arrhythmias

In some instances, arrhythmias can precipitate MI by reducing cardiac output or increasing myocardial demand. More importantly, arrhythmias are a major complication of infarction. Thus, reducing the threshold for serious arrhythmias tends to increase the case-fatality rate of MI. Cigarette smoking was found to lower the threshold for ventricular fibrillation in a study of animals (Downey et al. 1977) and was found to be associated with a 21-percent increased prevalence of ventricular premature beats on two-minute electrocardiographic rhythm strips obtained from 10,119 men (Hennekens et al. 1980). Smoking-related ventricular arrhythmias may contribute to the occurrence of sudden death and to increased case-fatality ratios during the course of MI.

Reduced Blood Oxygen Delivery

Cigarette smoking acutely increases myocardial oxygen demand by raising peripheral resistance, blood pressure, and heart rate (Martin et al. 1984; Klein 1984). Concurrently, the capacity of the blood to deliver oxygen is reduced by increased COHb, greater viscosity (Galea and Davidson 1985), and higher coronary vascular resistance. Imbalance between oxygen requirement and delivery as a result of these factors is not likely to be a cause of MI but may contribute to infarction in the presence of significant atherosclerotic narrowing of vessels. Consistent with these mechanisms, low levels of COHb exacerbate myocardial ischemia during graded exercise (Allred et al. 1989), and smoking is associated with more frequent and longer ischemic episodes detected by ambulatory electrocardiographic monitoring among patients with chronic stable CHD (Barry et al. 1989). Blood and plasma viscosities among former smokers are lower than those among current smokers and similar to those among never smokers (Ernst and Matrai 1987). In the same study, both blood and plasma viscosity decreased after smoking cessation and were similar to levels of never smokers after 8 weeks. Reduced oxygen delivery to the myocardium may play a role in lowering the threshold for ventricular arrhythmias.

In addition to influencing the development of CHD, smoking has been hypothesized to have direct toxic effects on the myocardium. Hartz and coworkers (1984) found a nearly threefold increased prevalence of diffuse ventricular hypokinesis among heavy smokers compared with never smokers within a population of patients undergoing diagnostic coronary angiography and ventriculography.

Smoking and Development of Peripheral Arterial Disease

The extremely strong association between smoking and peripheral artery disease is likely to be mediated largely through the mechanisms that promote atherosclerosis (Criqui et al. 1989). The peripheral vasoconstrictive effects of smoking, mediated by nicotine-stimulated release of catecholamines (US DHHS 1983), are likely to play a further important role (Lusby et al. 1981).

Smoking and Development of Cerebrovascular Disease

Cerebrovascular disease represents a heterogeneous group of pathologic processes that include infarction due to stenosis and thrombosis (referred to here as ischemic stroke), embolism from the heart, and hemorrhage from medium-sized vessels in the subarachnoid space (subarachnoid hemorrhage) and from microaneurysms of small penetrating vessels (intracerebral hemorrhage). The association of smoking with ischemic stroke is likely to be mediated largely through the mechanisms that promote atherosclerosis and thrombus formation. Associations between smoking and extent of cerebral artery atherosclerosis have been observed at autopsy among persons who have died of causes unrelated to CVD (Reed et al. 1988) and among volunteers in a cross-sectional study evaluated by a noninvasive method (Rogers et al. 1983). Smoking was also a strong predictor of the extent and severity of cerebral vessel atherosclerosis in an Italian multicenter study of reversible cerebral ischemic attacks (Passero et al. 1987) and in an investigation of 28 pairs of Finnish twins (Haapanen et al. 1989).

The mechanistic basis is unknown for the strong relation between smoking and subarachnoid hemorrhage (US DHHS 1989; Shinton and Beevers 1989), which is thought to result most commonly from the rupture of a saccular aneurysm. Although hypertension is associated with this occurrence, chronic smoking is unrelated to sustained elevation in blood pressure. A weak and clinically unimportant inverse relation with hypertension has been seen in several studies (Schoenenberger 1982; US DHHS 1983), although the association between cigarette smoking and risk of hypertension was observed in a large prospective investigation (Witteman et al. 1990).

Anticipated Effects of Smoking Cessation on Risk of Cardiovascular Diseases Based on Knowledge of Mechanisms

The possible effects of smoking cessation on the risk of CHD are illustrated in Figure 1. The incidence of CHD increases sharply with age among both smokers and never smokers; similar patterns are seen with other smoking-related cardiovascular diseases. At each age, the rates are higher for smokers, and the increase with age is more rapid among smokers (US DHHS 1983; ACS, unpublished tabulations), probably because of the ongoing, cumulative damage caused by smoking. Thus, the absolute excess incidence or mortality (attributable risk) of CHD due to smoking, represented by the vertical difference between the lines for smokers and never smokers in Figure 1, increases with age. However, the relative risk, represented by the ratio of incidence or mortality rates, tends to decrease with age.

Theoretically possible outcomes of smoking cessation are depicted by lines A, B, and C (Figure 1). Line A represents an immediate and complete reversal of the effect of smoking, so that the quitter almost instantly assumes the rate of the never smoker. Line B represents the worst-case scenario; although the stimulus for progressive damage is removed, no reversibility exists so that the former smoker assumes a constant absolute excess risk above that of the never smoker. In this case, it is apparent that quitting would still provide a substantial benefit compared with not quitting and that the relative risk for a former smoker compared with a never smoker would decline over time. An intermediate effect of smoking cessation is depicted by line C; the effects of smoking are slowly reversed, and the rate for the quitter gradually approaches that of the never smoker.

The effects of smoking on CHD are probably mediated by multiple mechanisms, several of which are well established. Some of the effects of smoking appear to be reversible within days or weeks, including the increase in platelet activation, clotting factors, COHb, coronary artery spasm, and increased susceptibility to ventricular arrhythmias. Other effects may be irreversible or only slowly reversible, such as the development of atherosclerosis as a result of smooth muscle proliferation and lipid deposition in the arterial intima resulting from lower HDL-C levels. Thus, persons who stop smoking are likely to experience a component of rapid decline in risk compared with those who continue to smoke and another component that more slowly approaches the risk of never smokers. Because the effects of smoking are multiple and complex, the rapidity and magnitude of risk reduction achieved by smoking cessation can best be estimated by empirical data based on epidemiologic studies in humans. Available data are examined in detail in the remaining sections of this Chapter.

SMOKING CESSATION AND CHD

Epidemiologic evidence on smoking and CHD has been reviewed in detail in previous reports of the U.S. Surgeon General (US PHS 1964; US DHEW 1971, 1979; US DHHS 1983, 1989). After an exhaustive review of the data, the 1983 Report of the Surgeon General concluded that "cigarette smoking is a major cause of CHD in the United States for both men and women" and "should be considered the most important of the known

CHD Mortality
(per 100,000 person-years)

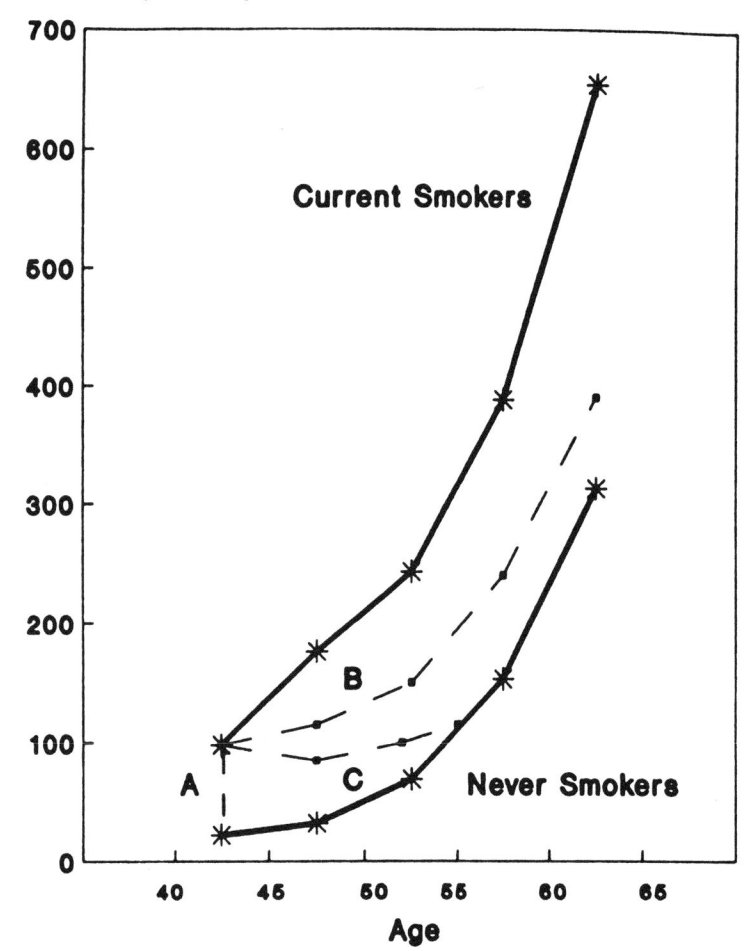

FIGURE 1.—Hypothetical effects of smoking cessation on risk of CHD if mechanisms are predominantly rapidly reversible (A), irreversible (B), or slowly reversible (C). (CHD mortality rates shown in solid lines are for men in ACS CPS-II, 1982–86.)

NOTE: CHD=coronary heart disease; ACS CPS-II=American Cancer Society Cancer Prevention Study II.

SOURCE: Unpublished tabulations, American Cancer Society.

modifiable risk factors for CHD" (US DHHS 1983, p.6). Overall, the Report noted that smokers have about a 70-percent excess death rate from CHD, and heavier smokers have an even greater excess risk.

Since 1983, additional evidence has accumulated to further support these conclusions. Some of these data were presented or summarized in the 1989 Report of the Surgeon General (US DHHS 1989). For 1985, cigarette smoking was estimated to be responsible for 21 percent of all CHD deaths in the United States among men aged 65 years or older and for 45 percent of CHD deaths among younger men. Twelve percent of the CHD deaths among women aged 65 or older and 41 percent of those in younger women were attributed to cigarette smoking. In 1985, 115,000 deaths from CHD were attributed to cigarette smoking.

A large amount of data supports the view that active cigarette smoking substantially increases risk of CHD. Data also indicate that former smokers have a lower risk of CHD than do current smokers. Despite methodologic and geographic differences, the studies are remarkably consistent in demonstrating a reduced risk of CHD among former smokers. Much of this literature has been reviewed in earlier reports of the Surgeon General (US DHEW 1979; US DHHS 1983) as well as by Kuller and colleagues (1982).

This Section reviews the epidemiologic evidence of the effects of cigarette smoking cessation on CHD risk, specifically MI and CHD death. The relevant studies may be divided into those that examine the effect among apparently healthy individuals (primary prevention) and the effect among individuals already diagnosed with CHD for risk of recurrence or CHD death (secondary prevention). Cross-sectional studies of the extent of coronary atherosclerosis also provide relevant information.

Cross-Sectional Studies

In a detailed study of coronary atherosclerosis, Auerbach and coworkers (1976) examined 1,056 autopsied hearts from patients at the East Orange Veterans Administration Hospital and found that smokers had more severe disease than never smokers, with past smokers having intermediate levels. Those who died from CHD or diabetes or those who had hearts weighing more than 500 g were excluded. After adjustment for age, current cigarette smokers had a prevalence of advanced CHD that ranged from 11.7 to 23.4 percent, depending on the number of cigarettes smoked per day. The prevalence among never smokers was 5.3 percent compared with 11.0 percent among former smokers. The prevalence odds ratio of advanced versus no disease or minimal disease was 2.4, when former smokers were compared with never smokers. In contrast, among current smokers of 1 to 2 packs per day, the ratio was 6.7. A similar pattern was observed for different pathologic manifestations of CHD. The effect of duration of abstinence among former smokers was not analyzed.

Ramsdale and coworkers (1985) used arteriography to assess the extent of coronary atherosclerosis before surgery for valve replacement among 387 patients. All patients provided a smoking history, including age at initiation of smoking and cessation of smoking and average number of cigarettes smoked per week. Among never smokers, 87 percent had no stenosis greater than 50 percent; only 60 percent of past smokers and 60 percent of current smokers were without this degree of stenosis. Of never smokers, only 2.6 percent had three or more arteries affected compared with 10.6 percent of former smokers and 12.2 percent of current smokers. Both current and past smokers had more severe coronary artery disease. The median score among never smokers and current smokers was 0.2 and 2.8, respectively. For past smokers, the data were presented by duration since quitting. There was no evidence for a trend of decreased effect by increasing time since cessation. The median score for those quitting within the previous 5 years was 5.0; for 5 to 10 years, 5.0; and for 10 years or more, 7.5. Coronary atherosclerosis was positively correlated with lifetime number of cigarettes smoked among both current or past smokers. In this study, past smokers had a slightly worse coronary risk profile than other groups. No information was provided about past or concurrent illness that may have motivated the former smokers to quit. Nonetheless, this study supports the view that cigarette smoking is a risk factor for atherosclerosis and that a substantial duration of abstinence may be necessary to appreciably reduce its extent.

Weintraub and coworkers (1985) evaluated smoking history in 1,349 coronary arteriography patients. Of these patients, 984 had significant coronary disease (75 percent or more obstruction). Amount of current smoking was not a significant predictor of serious obstruction after total pack-years were considered. On average, the risk for such obstruction increased by about 1 percent per pack-year.

Cross-sectional studies of arteriographic findings can be difficult to interpret because patients undergoing angiography are clearly not representative of the general population. Nonetheless, these studies support the view that smoking causes an increase in atherosclerosis and that very recent quitting has little impact on coronary stenosis.

Fried, Moore, and Pearson (1986) studied the effects of smoking by assessing the coronary diameter in 31 men who had normal coronary arteriograms. Men with any detectable stenosis in the main coronary arteries or more than 25 percent in any coronary branch were excluded to assess the effects of smoking on the caliber of coronary arteries in the absence of atherosclerosis. These researchers found that after adjustment for alcohol intake (which is associated with wider arteries), current and former smokers had 40 to 50 percent narrower arteries than did never smokers. The past smokers had somewhat narrower arteries than current smokers although this was not statistically significant. Of the 11 ex-smokers, 6 had quit in the previous year. This study suggests the possibility of another persisting effect of smoking, apart from promoting atherosclerosis, not rapidly reversed by cessation.

Studies of Smoking Cessation and Risk of MI Among Healthy Persons

Case–Control Studies

Table 1 summarizes data from case–control studies (Willett et al. 1981; Rosenberg, Kaufman, Helmrich, Miller et al. 1985; LaVecchia et al. 1987; Rosenberg, Palmer, Shapiro 1990), of men and women from the United States and abroad. Prospective studies of CHD are generally considered less prone to bias than case–control studies, although case–control studies are probably less susceptible to misclassification resulting from resumption of smoking among former smokers. For example, an individual diagnosed with a recent MI can probably recall his or her smoking status just before the infarction with considerable accuracy (Chapter 2). Thus, case–control studies may

TABLE 1.—Case–control studies of CHD risk among former smokers

Reference	Population	Number of cases	Number of controls	Source of controls	Number of cases among former smokers	Former smokers[a]	Current smokers[a]
Willett et al. (1981)	Nurses Health Study: women aged 30–55	263	5,260	Nested in cohort	29	Overall 1.0 (0.7–1.6) Quit 1–4 yr 1.5 (0.7–3.1) Quit 5–9 yr 1.5 (0.8–3.0) Quit ≥10 yr 0.6 (0.3–1.3)	3.0 (2.3–4.0)
Rosenberg, Kaufman, Helmrich, Shapiro (1985)	Eastern US men aged <55	1,873	2,775	Hospital-based	348	1.1 (0.9–1.4)	2.9 (2.4–3.4)
Rosenberg, Kaufman, Helmrich, Miller et al. (1985)	Eastern US women aged <50	555	1,864	Hospital-based	35	1.0 (0.7–1.6)	1.4–7.0 depending on cig/day
LaVecchia et al. (1987)	Italian women aged <55	168	251	Hospital-based	3	0.8 (0.2–3.8)	3.6–13.1 depending on cig/day

[a] Relative risk as compared with never smokers

TABLE 1.—Continued

Reference	Population	Number of cases	Number of controls	Source of controls	Number of cases among former smokers	Relative risk as compared with never smokers[a] Former smokers	Relative risk as compared with never smokers[a] Current smokers
Rosenberg, Palmer, Shapiro (1990)	Eastern US women aged <65	910	2,375	Hospital-based	149	Overall 1.2 (1.0–1.7) Quit <24 mo 2.6 (1.8–3.8) Quit 24–35 mo 1.3 Quit ≥36 mo 0.8–1.1	3.6 (3.0–4.4)

NOTE: CHD=coronary heart disease.
[a] 95% confidence interval shown in parentheses when available.

be quite valuable in assessing the time course for the decline in risk. However, the lack of detailed data on fatal cases is a potential limitation of the case–control approach.

In a case–control study of women in the Nurses Health Study cohort, Willett and coworkers (1981) identified 263 women who reported a nonfatal MI on the baseline Nurses Health Study questionnaire in 1976 when they were 30 to 55 years of age. Their smoking histories were compared with randomly selected controls corresponding in age with a case–control ratio of 1:20. Women who were former smokers did not experience increased risk of MI, with a relative risk compared with never smokers of 1.0 (95-percent confidence interval (CI), 0.7–1.6). In contrast, current smokers had a significantly elevated threefold higher risk of MI. When duration of abstinence was assessed, it appeared that those who quit either 1 to 4 or 5 to 9 years earlier had a nonsignificantly elevated risk of 1.5, and those who quit 10 years or more earlier had a relative risk of 0.6. Because there were only 29 cases among former smokers, the estimates for risk by duration of abstinence are not precise.

Rosenberg, Kaufman, Helmrich, and Shapiro (1985) specifically analyzed the impact of smoking cessation on risk of first MI among 4,648 men less than 55 years of age, using a hospital-based case–control design. Men with known preexisting heart disease were excluded. The 2,775 controls were mostly persons with fracture or sprain, disk disorders, and gastrointestinal disorders thought not to be related to cigarette smoking. There were 1,873 cases and 2,775 controls. For current smokers (smoked within the past year), the age-adjusted relative risk was 2.9 (95-percent CI, 2.4–3.4) and for past smokers overall, it was 1.1 (95-percent CI, 0.9–1.4). The relative risk for those who had not smoked for 12 to 23 months was 2.0 (95-percent CI, 1.1–3.8). For those with longer durations of abstinence, the relative risk was 1.1 (95-percent CI, 0.9–1.4) (Figure 2). The risk was increased for those smoking more cigarettes per day among current smokers as well as recent quitters. For longer durations of abstinence, the amount previously smoked appeared to have little impact. These investigators also examined the effect of quitting within categories of other risk factors; in general, there were no marked differences other than for diabetics among whom the benefits of cessation appeared to be greater. The same group of investigators (Rosenberg, Kaufman, Helmrich, Shapiro 1985) addressed the possibility that continuing smokers and former smokers may differ in their underlying risk of heart disease. They found that those who quit had a slightly higher risk profile. Hence, the benefit of cessation in this study cannot be attributed to overall better health among those who quit.

Rosenberg and associates (1985) also conducted a hospital-based case–control study of first nonfatal MI among women less than 50 years of age (Rosenberg, Kaufman, Helmrich, Miller et al. 1985). Women who smoked in the year before admission were classified as current smokers. Participants consisted of 555 cases and 1,864 controls who were hospitalized for trauma, orthopedic disorders, and other conditions thought to be unrelated to smoking. Current smokers had relative risks increasing from 1.4 to 7.0, depending on the number of cigarettes smoked per day. In contrast, former smokers (at least 1 year of abstinence) had the same risk as never smokers, with a relative risk of 1.0 (95-percent CI, 0.7–1.6).

In a recent report, Rosenberg, Palmer, and Shapiro (1990) further examined the decline in risk of MI among women who stopped smoking. Cases included 910 women

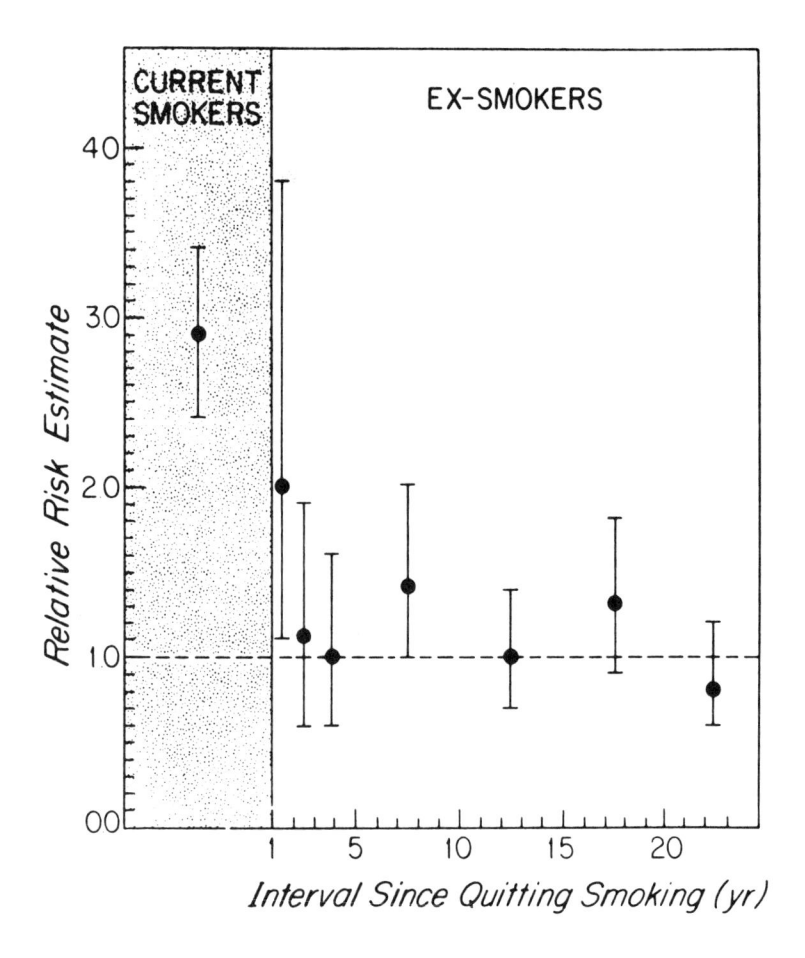

FIGURE 2.—Estimated relative risk of MI after quitting smoking among men
under age 55, adjusted for age; 95% CIs are indicated by
vertical line; relative risk for men who never smoked is 1.0

NOTE: MI=myocardial infarction; CI=confidence interval.
SOURCE: Rosenberg, Kaufman, Helmrich, Shapiro (1985).

with first infarction; their smoking histories were compared with those of 2,375 hospitalized controls. Among former smokers overall, the relative risk of MI was 1.2 (95-percent CI) compared with never smokers; for current smokers the relative risk was 3.6. When former smokers were subdivided according to duration of abstinence, women who had stopped smoking within the previous 24 months had a relative risk of 2.6 (95-percent CI, 1.8–3.8). The relative risk was 1.3 for those who stopped smoking 24 to 35 months earlier. After 3 years of abstinence, relative risks ranged from 0.8 to 1.1 and were indistinguishable from that of women who had never smoked.

Cohort Studies

Data from prospective cohort studies are summarized in Table 2. The British Physicians Study of Doll and Hill (1954, 1956) was one of the important early studies that established the link between smoking and risk of CHD and the health benefits of cessation. The study is based on a survey of 40,637 British physicians who responded to a 1951 questionnaire inquiring about smoking behavior. A second questionnaire was mailed to men in 1957–58 and to women in 1960–61; the response rate was 98 percent. The 10-year followup (Doll and Hill 1964) used the updated data to assess risk among former smokers. Additional questionnaires were distributed in 1966 and 1972, with response rates of 96 and 98 percent, respectively. The 20-year followup of 34,440 men (Doll and Peto 1976) showed a reduction in CHD mortality among former smokers. The benefits were more apparent in the younger age group, and the excess risk declined with increasing duration of abstinence. In men aged 30 to 54 years, the relative risk among former smokers of 1 to 4 years' duration was 1.9 compared with never smokers; relative risk further declined to 1.4 to 1.3 with a maximum of 20 years' duration of abstinence. In contrast, persistent smokers had a relative risk of 3.5. In this study, those who quit had smoked about 10 percent fewer cigarettes per day before quitting than did persistent smokers.

The British Physicians Study also included 6,194 women, for whom the data were reported separately (Doll et al. 1980). These women completed questionnaires in 1951, 1961, and 1973. In contrast to most studies among adults, a substantial minority of nonsmoking women in this cohort initiated cigarette smoking between 1951 and 1961. Thus, the rates of smoking-related diseases among those classified as never smokers are likely to be overestimated because never smokers, defined according to the 1951 data, included a proportion of subsequent current smokers. Overall, the relative risk of CHD mortality among former smokers was 0.9 compared with 1.0 to 2.2 among current smokers, depending on the amount smoked. Because there were only 26 cases among former smokers, a detailed analysis was not performed.

The first large-scale American Cancer Society (ACS) cohort was assembled in 1952 when 187,783 men aged 50 to 69, living in 9 States, completed a questionnaire related primarily to smoking (Hammond and Horn 1958a,b). The men were enrolled by over 22,000 ACS volunteers each of whom was asked to enroll 10 individuals, excluding those who were seriously ill. There was no further update of cigarette use. These men were studied for fatal outcomes for an average of 44 months, for a total of 667,753 person-years. Cause of death for 11,870 individuals was determined by death certificate. Compared with never smokers, the relative risk of death due to CHD among current smokers of less than 1 pack per day was 1.75. Among former smokers of less than 1 pack per day, those quitting within the previous year had a relative risk of 2.09, those quitting 1 to 10 years earlier had a risk of 1.54, and those quitting for more than 10 years had a relative risk of 1.09. A similar pattern was observed among smokers of 1 pack or more per day: among current smokers, the relative risk was 2.2; among quitters within the past year, 3.00; among quitters of 1 to 10 years, 2.06; and among quitters of more than 10 years, 1.60 (Figure 3). The authors speculated that the elevated

TABLE 2.—Cohort studies of CHD risk among former smokers

Reference	Population	Followup	Number of cases among former smokers	Former smokers	Current smokers	Comments
Doll and Hill (1964)	British physicians: 34,445 men	10 yr for CHD deaths	28 61 59 40	Quit 1–4 yr 1.05 5–9 yr 1.25 10–14 yr 1.16 ≥15 yr 1.12	1.41	Smoking ascertained 1951, updated 1958
Doll and Peto (1976)	British physicians: 34,440 men	20 yr for CHD deaths		Aged 30–54	3.5	Smoking data assessed at baseline and after 7 yr
			7 10 10 7	Quit 1–4 yr 1.9 5–9 yr 1.3 10–14 yr 1.4 ≥15 yr 1.3		
				Aged 55–64	1.7	
			19 34 38 45	Quit 1–4 yr 1.9 5–9 yr 1.4 10–14 yr 1.7 ≥15 yr 1.3		
				Aged ≥65	1.3	
			24 76 62 148	Quit 1–4 yr 1.0 5–9 yr 1.3 10–14 yr 1.2 ≥15 yr 1.1		

Relative risks compared with never smokers[a]

TABLE 2.—Continued

Reference	Population	Followup	Number of cases among former smokers	Former smokers	Current smokers	Comments
				Relative risks compared with never smokers[a]		
Doll et al. (1980)	British physicians: 6,194 women	22 yr for CHD deaths	26	0.91	1.0–2.2 depending on amount smoked	Smoking assessed at baseline and after 9 yr
Hammond and Horn (1958a,b)	187,783 men aged 50–60	44 mo for CHD deaths		Previously <1 ppd	1.75 (143 cases)	
			23	Quit <1 yr 2.09		
			80	1–10 yr 1.54		
			40	>10 yr 1.09		
				Previously ≥1 ppd	2.20 (122 cases)	
			18	Quit <1 yr 3.00		
			64	1–10 yr 2.06		
			40	>10 yr 1.60		
Hammond and Garfinkel (1969)	ACS CPS-I: 358,534 men free of diagnosed CHD	6 yr for CHD mortality		Previously 1–19 cig/day	1.90 (1,063 cases)	
			29	Quit <1 yr 1.62		
			57	1–4 yr 1.22		
			55	5–9 yr 1.26		
			52	10–14 yr 0.96		
			70	≥20 yr 1.08		

TABLE 2.—Continued

Reference	Population	Followup	Number of cases among former smokers	Relative risks compared with never smokers[a]		Comments
				Former smokers	Current smokers	
Hammond and Garfinkel (1969) (continued)				Previously ≥20 cig/day	2.55 (2,822 cases)	
			62	Quit <1 yr 1.61		
			154	1–4 yr 1.51		
			135	5–9 yr 1.16		
			133	10–14 yr 1.25		
			80	≥15 yr 1.05		
ACS (unpublished tabulations)	ACS CPS-II: 1.2 million men and women	4 yr for CHD deaths		Men <21 cig/day	1.93	Persons with cancer, heart disease, and stroke excluded at baseline
			14	Quit <1 yr 1.43		
			48	1–2 yr 1.61		
			47	3–5 yr 1.49		
			88	6–10 yr 1.28		
			90	11–15 yr 0.99		
			359	≥16 yr 0.88		
				Men ≥21 cig/day	2.02	
			19	Quit <1 yr 2.56		
			33	1–2 yr 1.57		
			36	3–5 yr 1.41		
			67	6–10 yr 1.63		
			71	11–15 yr 1.16		
			182	≥16 yr 1.09		

TABLE 2.—Continued

Reference	Population	Followup	Number of cases among former smokers	Relative risks compared with never smokers[a] Former smokers	Current smokers	Comments
ACS (unpublished tabulations) (continued)				Women <20 cig/day	1.76	
			3	Quit <1 yr 2.13		
			7	1–2 yr 0.87		
			11	3–5 yr 1.31		
			12	6–10 yr 0.74		
			17	11–15 yr 1.20		
			82	≥16 yr 1.17		
				Women ≥20 cig/day	2.27	
			9	Quit <1 yr 1.41		
			10	1–2 yr 1.16		
			16	3–5 yr 0.96		
			24	6–10 yr 1.88		
			12	11–15 yr 1.37		
			32	≥16 yr 1.12		
Dorn (1959); Kahn (1966); Rogot and Murray (1980)[b]	US veterans: 248,046 men	16 yr for cardiovascular deaths	9,027	Stopped (overall) 1.15	1.58	Those who quit on doctor's orders were excluded
				<5 yr 1.40		
				5–9 yr 1.40		
				10–14 yr 1.30		
				15–19 yr 1.20		
				≥20 yr 1.00		

TABLE 2.—Continued

Reference	Population	Followup	Number of cases among former smokers	Relative risks compared with never smokers[a] — Former smokers	Relative risks compared with never smokers[a] — Current smokers	Comments
Dorn (1959); Kahn (1966); Rogot and Murray (1980)[b] (continued)		For CHD deaths		Stopped (overall) 1.16 <5 yr 1.40 5–9 yr 1.40 10–14 yr 1.30 15–19 yr 1.20 ≥20 yr 1.10	1.58	No update of smoking information
Doyle et al. (1962)	Framingham and Albany cohorts 4,120 healthy men aged 30–62	6–8 yr for fatal and nonfatal MI	10	0.9	2.3	Only baseline smoking data used
Doyle et al. (1964)	Framingham and Albany cohorts of 4,120 healthy men aged 30–62	10 yr (Framingham) 8 yr (Albany) MI and CHD deaths	13	1.1 (0.5–2.2)	2.0–3.0 depending on amount smoked	No data on duration
Gordon, Kannel, McGee (1974)	2,336 men in Framingham Heart Study, aged 29–62	18 yr for CHD excluding angina	24	0.7	1.3	Smoking information updated biennially
Rosenman et al. (1975)	3,154 healthy California men aged 39–59	8–9 yr for fatal and nonfatal CHD	16	Aged 39–40 1.9 Aged 50–59 1.1	2.5	Only baseline smoking data used

TABLE 2.—Continued

Reference	Population	Followup	Number of cases among former smokers	Former smokers	Current smokers	Comments
Cederlof et al. (1975)	Sample of 51,911 Swedish men aged 18–69	10 yr	97	Quit 1–9 yr 1.5 total Smoked <20 cig/day 0.9 Smoked ≥20 cig/day 1.6	1.7	Only baseline smoking data used
			86	Quit ≥10 yr 1.0 total Smoked <20 cig/day 0.9 Smoked ≥20 cig/day 1.1		
Fuller et al. (1983)	Whitehall civil servants: 18,403 men aged 40–64	10 yr for CHD deaths	208	171 normo-glycemic 1.3 23 glucose intolerant 0.7 14 diabetics 3.8	2.5 1.5 2.9	Prevalent cases of CHD not excluded
Friedman et al. (1981)	25,917 Kaiser-Permanente subscribers in the San Francisco area, aged 20–79	4 yr for CHD deaths	31	0.9	1.6	Prevalent cases of CHD not omitted; exclusion of those cases increased the apparent benefit of quitting

[a]

TABLE 2.—Continued

Reference	Population	Followup	Number of cases among former smokers	Relative risks compared with never smokers[a] — Former smokers	Relative risks compared with never smokers[a] — Current smokers	Comments
Keys (1980)	7-Countries Study of 12,096 men free of CHD	10 yr for CHD deaths	About 13[c] (Northern Europe)	2.3	2.4–4.5 depending on amount	Relative risk based on only about 5 cases in never smokers, very small numbers
			About 9 (Italy, Greece, Yugoslavia)	0.8	0.7–1.8 depending on amount	
			About 7[c] (US)	0.7	1.6–3.0 depending on amount	Numbers extrapolated from figures
Shapiro et al. (1969)	HIP cohort about 39,000 men aged 35–64	3 yr for MI	NR	1.0	1.8	
Jajich, Ostfeld, Freeman (1984)	2,674 poor persons in Cook County, IL aged 64–75	4.5 yr for CHD deaths	20	1.11	1.94	Stroke excluded but prevalent CHD not excluded at baseline
Willett et al. (1987)	Nurses Health Study: 121,700 US women aged 30–55	6 yr for nonfatal MI and CHD deaths	55	1.5 (1.0–2.1)	2.1–10.8 depending on amount smoked	

TABLE 2.—Continued

Reference	Population	Followup	Number of cases among former smokers	Relative risks compared with never smokers[a] — Former smokers	Relative risks compared with never smokers[a] — Current smokers	Comments
Floderus, Cederlof, Friberg (1988)	10,495 Swedish twins aged 36–75	21 yr for CHD deaths	188 men 10 women	1.0 (0.8–1.1) 0.6 (0.4–1.0)	1.4–1.8 depending on amount smoked	No reassessment of smoking during followup; no data on duration
Lannerstad, Isacsson, Lindell (1979)	703 Malmö men, age 55	5 yr	0	CHD deaths	2.0	No cases among former smokers; only 2 in never smokers
Holme et al. (1980)	14,816 healthy Oslo men, aged 40–49	4.7	NR			Never and ex-smokers had about 40% of the risk of cigarette smokers
Netterstrom and Juel (1988)	2,465 Danish bus drivers	7.75 yr for MI and CHD death	9	3.2 (0.4–25.6)	5.0 (0.7–36.0)	

NOTE: CHD=coronary heart disease; ppd=packs/day; ACS CPS-I and -II=American Cancer Society Cancer Prevention Studies I and II; HIP=health insurance plan; MI=myocardial infarction; NR=not reported.
[a]95% confidence interval shown in parentheses when available.
[b]Breakdowns of relative risk derived from figure presented in paper cited.
[c]Extrapolated from figure presented in paper cited.

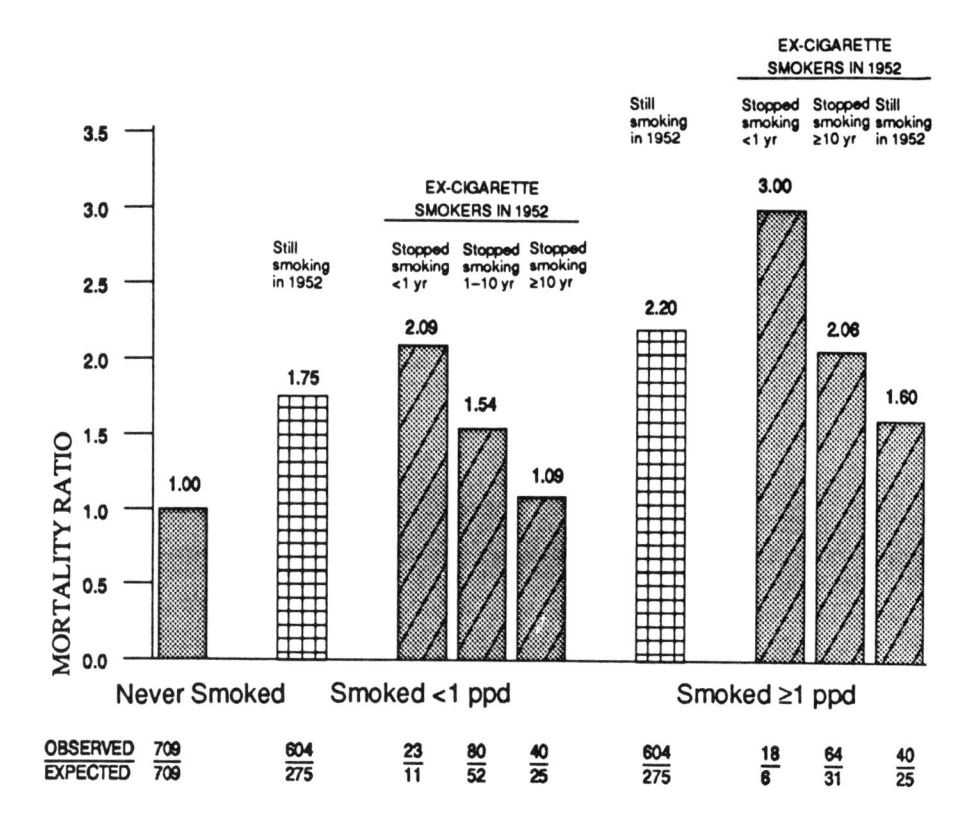

FIGURE 3.—Mortality ratios due to coronary artery diseases; rates for men who have stopped smoking are compared with those for men who never smoked and those for men still smoking in 1952

NOTE: ppd=packs/day.
SOURCE: Hammond and Horn (1958b).

risk among recent quitters reflected the inclusion of men who stopped smoking because of early symptoms of heart disease.

A second cohort study, the ACS Cancer Prevention Study I (CPS-I) (formerly called the ACS 25-State Study), was undertaken between 1959 and 1972. Recruitment was by family, and eligible families had at least one person aged 45 or older. All family members aged 35 or older were asked to participate in the study; more than 1 million persons were enrolled. In a 6-year followup of 358,534 men free of diagnosed serious illness, clear reductions in risk of CHD mortality were observed among former smokers compared with current smokers (Hammond and Garfinkel 1969). Among those smoking less than 1 pack per day, the relative risk among current smokers was 1.90. Among those who stopped in the previous year, the relative risk was 1.62, and among those with 10 years or more of abstinence, the risk was nearly the same as that for never smokers. A similar pattern was observed among those smoking 1 pack or more per day. Current smokers at that level had a relative risk of 2.55. Quitters of less than 1 year had a relative risk of 1.61, and those with between 10 and 20 years of abstinence had only a slightly elevated relative risk of 1.25. Because of the very large number of deaths and the careful followup, the estimates of effect are relatively precise. In this period, cigarette smoking declined substantially, especially in the predominantly white, middle- to upperclass groups represented by the study population. Hence, some misclassification of the current smoking group may have occurred, but the relative risks among former smokers, apart from the most recent quitters (some of whom inevitably resumed smoking), are likely to be accurate.

In 1982, a third ACS cohort, CPS-II, was initiated in 50 States. The methods for recruitment and the population enrolled were similar to CPS-I, but the cohort was larger, with more than 1.2 million participants (Chapter 3). Preliminary data based on 4 years of followup were published in the 1989 Surgeon General's Report (US DHHS 1989). Among men, former smokers aged 35 or younger had relative risks of CHD of 1.41, those aged 36 to 64 had 1.75, and those 65 or older had 1.29; the relative risks among current smokers were 1.94, 2.81, and 1.62, respectively. A generally similar pattern was seen among women.

When the data are examined by amount of previous smoking and time since quitting, the pattern of changing risk is influenced by the presence of disease at enrollment. When those who reported themselves as sick or as having previously diagnosed cancer, heart disease, or stroke at baseline were not excluded from the analysis, men who previously smoked fewer than 21 cigarettes per day and who had quit smoking within the previous 3 years experienced a CHD mortality rate that was about 6 percent higher than that among current smokers. However, with increasing duration of abstinence, the risk among former smokers came very close to that of never smokers; after 16 years or more, the relative risk was 1.01 (US DHHS 1989). It is likely that the early peak in mortality among recent quitters partly reflects the effect of having included those who quit because of smoking-related illness. After excluding those with cancer, heart disease, and stroke at baseline, this early excess mortality is less apparent (Table 2). In all categories, those who quit 1 to 2 years earlier had relative risks substantially lower than those of current smokers. Findings are less consistent for those who quit within the past year, presumably because of a high incidence of smoking resumption in that group and the possible inclusion of persons who stopped smoking as a result of symptoms due to undiagnosed illness. A very similar pattern was observed among men who smoked 21 cigarettes or more per day, except that the relative risks were higher for all but those with the shorter period of abstinence. The absolute rates were lower for women, as expected, and the relative risks are thus statistically unstable. Nevertheless, the overall patterns among female smokers were generally similar to those among male smokers.

To examine the effects of smoking cessation at different ages, CPS-II data on cumulative mortality rates due to CHD were tabulated for 5-year categories of age at cessation. (See Table 3 and Chapter 3 for a description of the methods used to calculate these rates.) The mortality rates used for these calculations were based on subjects not

TABLE 3.— Estimated probability of dying from ischemic heart disease in the next 16.5-year interval (95% CI) for quitting at various ages compared with never smoking and continuing to smoke, by amount smoked and sex

Age at quitting or at start of interval	Never smokers	Continuing smokers <21[a]	Continuing smokers ≥21[a]	Former smokers <21[a]	Former smokers ≥21[a]
MEN					
40–44	0.01 (.01–.01)	0.03 (.02–.03)	0.03 (.03–.04)	0.01 (.00–.02)	0.02 (.01–.02)
45–49	0.02 (.01–.02)	0.04 (.04–.05)	0.04 (.04–.05)	0.02 (.01–.03)	0.02 (.01–.03)
50–54	0.04 (.03–.03)	0.07 (.06–.07)	0.06 (.06–.07)	0.04 (.03–.05)	0.04 (.02–.05)
55–59	0.05 (.05–.06)	0.10 (.08–.11)	0.09 (.07–.10)	0.05 (.04–.07)	0.08 (.06–.10)
60–64	0.10 (.09–.11)	0.14 (.12–.16)	0.16 (.10–.21)	0.12 (.09–.15)	0.10 (.06–.15)
65–69	0.15 (.13–.17)	0.20 (.16–.25)	0.13 (.08–.19)	0.14 (.07–.21)	0.12 (.00–.24)
70–74[b]	0.13 (.11–.14)	0.17 (.13–.22)	0.10 (.05–.16)	0.19 (.10–.29)	0.11 (.02–.20)

sick at interview or giving a history of heart disease, cancer, or stroke. For both women and men, during the next decade-and-a-half cumulative CHD mortality for those who stopped smoking before age 60 was about half that of those who continued to smoke. This same pattern of reduced risk extended to those who stopped smoking between ages 60 and 64. After age 65, few persons stopped smoking, as indicated by wide confidence intervals, so that no clear patterns could be determined.

Because the methods used in CPS-I and CPS-II are similar, it is appropriate to compare the results of the two studies. In CPS-II, the relative risks of CHD for current smoking among men and women are substantially higher at every age than those observed in CPS-I. The higher relative risks for CHD and other smoking-related diseases among women in CPS-II are possibly due to the earlier age of smoking

TABLE 3.—Continued

Age at quitting or at start of interval	Never smokers	Continuing smokers <20[a]	Continuing smokers ≥20[a]	Former smokers <20[a]	Former smokers ≥20[a]
WOMEN					
40–44	0.00 (.00–.00)	0.01 (.00–.01)	0.01 (.01–.01)	0.00 (.00–.01)	0.00 (.00–.01)
45–49	0.00 (.00–.01)	0.01 (.01–.01)	0.01 (.01–.02)	0.00 (.00–.00)	0.01 (.00–.01)
50–54	0.01 (.01–.01)	0.02 (.02–.03)	0.03 (.02–.03)	0.01 (.00–.02)	0.02 (.01–.02)
55–59	0.02 (.02–.02)	0.04 (.03–.05)	0.05 (.04–.06)	0.01 (.00–.02)	0.02 (.01–.04)
60–64	0.04 (.03–.04)	0.06 (.04–.07)	0.08 (.06–.10)	0.02 (.00–.05)	0.04 (.01–.06)
65–69	0.07 (.07–.08)	0.11 (.07–.15)	0.12 (.07–.18)	0.12 (.03–.21)	0.09 (.01–.17)
70–74[b]	0.07 (.06–.07)	0.09 (.05–.13)	0.11 (.05–.16)	0.03 (.00–.08)	0.02 (.00–.05)

NOTE: Based on subjects not sick at enrollment or giving a history of cancer, heart disease, or stroke; 95% confidence interval (CI) shown in parentheses.
[a] Cig/day.
[b] Estimates for quitting at this age are estimates of the probability of dying in the next 12.5-yr interval.
SOURCE: Unpublished tabulations, American Cancer Society.

initiation in the more recent cohort (US DHHS 1989). The higher relative risks among men are more difficult to explain because the age of initiation has not changed substantially among men over time (US DHHS 1989).

The large size and careful methodology of the three ACS cohorts provide considerable evidence for the benefit of quitting in reducing risk of CHD. These studies also provide strong evidence that there is some residual risk of CHD attributable to past smoking that persists for a considerable duration after cessation.

The U.S. Veterans Study (Dorn 1959; Kahn 1966; Rogot 1974; Rogot and Murray 1980) has also provided useful information on the health effects of smoking. The population was drawn from 293,958 U.S. veterans who held Government life insurance policies in December 1953. In 1954, a total of 198,820 individuals returned mailed questionnaires about their smoking behavior, and in 1957, an additional 49,226 responded. Those who stopped smoking on a physician's orders were excluded from the analysis. Mortality in this cohort was monitored, and death certificates were obtained to assess cause of death. Smoking status after the baseline questionnaire was not ascertained. After 16 years of followup, quitters at enrollment when compared with never smokers had relative risks of 1.15 for all cardiovascular mortality and 1.16 for CHD death specifically (Rogot and Murray 1980). In contrast, men who were current smokers at baseline had relative risks of 1.58 for these two categories. Among past smokers, risk of death due to CVD increased with higher previous usual daily cigarette consumption. The relative risks among past smokers, compared with never smokers, ranged from 1.02 for less than 10 cigarettes per day to 1.34 for 40 cigarettes or more per day. This gradient was more pronounced among current smokers (Figure 4).

A gradient was also apparent for decreasing risk with increasing duration of smoking abstinence. For both cardiovascular and coronary mortality, there was a moderate decrease in risk with short duration of abstinence and a smaller, but consistent decline in risk with longer periods of abstinence (Figure 5). After 20 years or more of abstinence, the relative risk of CVD was 1.04, and for coronary death, the risk was 1.05.

The major strength of the U.S. Veterans Study is the large numbers, with 21,413 deaths from CVD among smokers and 9,027 among former smokers. The long followup period without reclassification of smoking status is a limitation, which will tend to lead to an underestimate of the effect of sustained smoking and an underestimate of the benefits of quitting (Chapter 2). This source of potential bias may not have markedly distorted the estimates in this study: in the followup of this cohort (Rogot and Murray 1980), the relative risk for cardiovascular mortality associated with current smoking at enrollment was 1.62 at 8.5 years and 1.58 at 16 years; for coronary disease, the relative risk was 1.61 at 8.5 years and 1.58 at 16 years. Thus, the impact of misclassification of current smokers who quit (and therefore lowered their risk) as persistent smokers appears to be slight. A similar comparison of the relative risks among former smokers is less informative in assessing the impact of misclassification. Most quitters who resume smoking do so within 2 years after cessation. Therefore, misclassification of ex-smokers between 8.5 and 16 years of cessation is likely to be small. For both cardiovascular mortality and coronary mortality, the relative risks among ex-smokers declined slightly from 1.21 at 8.5 years of followup to 1.15 and 1.16 at 16 years of followup. This is consistent with the inverse relation between duration of smoking cessation and mortality ratio.

Among current smokers in the U.S. Veterans Study, the relative risks of coronary disease were slightly higher after 8.5 years of followup (relative risk (RR)=1.95 for >20 cig/day) than after 2.5 years of followup (RR=1.75) (Dorn 1959). As expected, those who stopped smoking on a physician's orders were at higher risk of death regardless of their smoking status.

An early report of combined data from the Framingham and Albany Heart Studies (Doyle et al. 1962) included 4,120 men free from coronary disease at entry into the study. The Framingham Study data were based on 6 years of followup and the Albany Heart Study data on 8 years of followup. Among the 411 former smokers in the combined cohort, the relative risk of MI (age-adjusted) was 0.9 compared with never

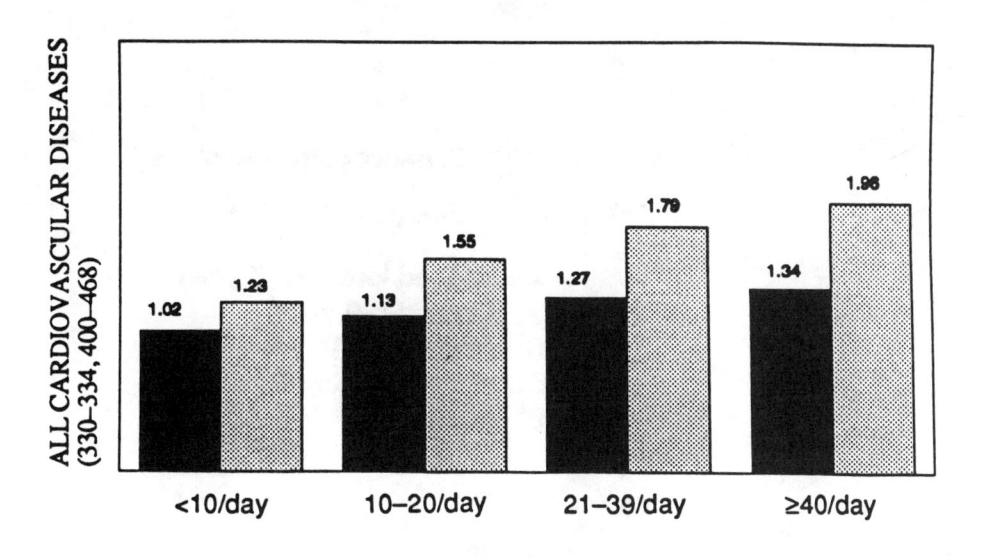

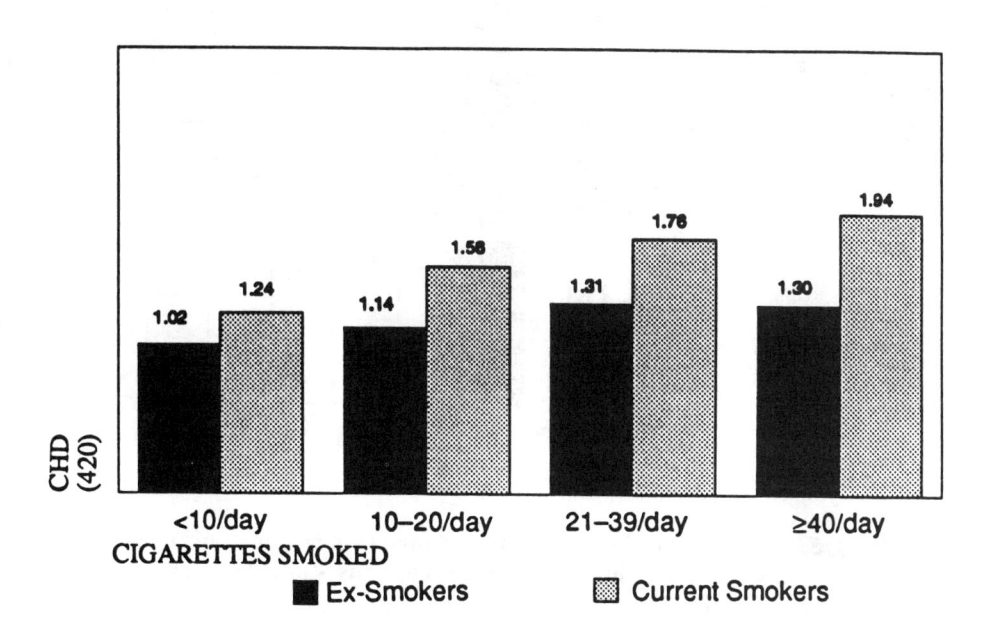

FIGURE 4.—Mortality ratios for all cardiovascular diseases and CHD, by daily cigarette consumption, US Veterans Study, 1954–69

NOTE: Ex-smokers includes only former cigarette smokers who stopped smoking for reasons other than physician's orders.

SOURCE: Rogot and Murray (1980).

Current cigarette smokers

Ex-cigarette smokers

A: stopped less than 5 years
B: stopped 5-9 years
C: stopped 10-14 years
D: stopped 15-19 years
E: stopped 20 or more years

All cardiovascular diseases (330-334, 400-468)

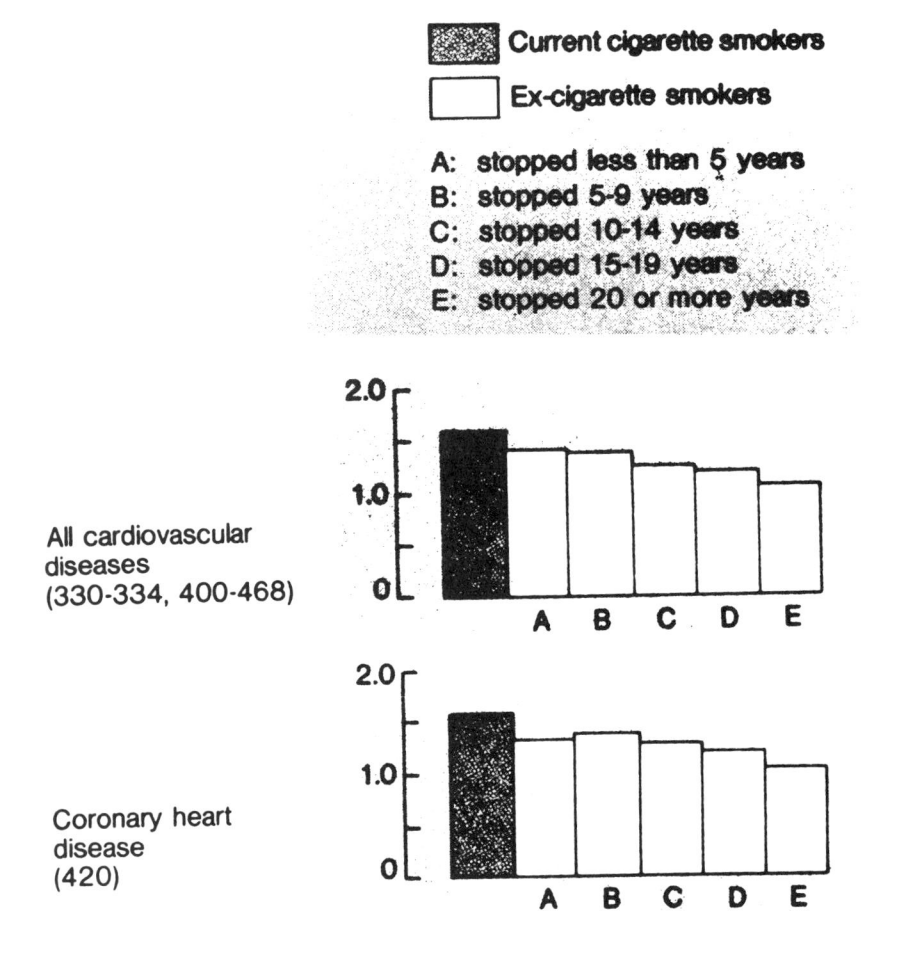

Coronary heart disease (420)

FIGURE 5.—Mortality ratio for current and former cigarette smokers by years of smoking cessation, US Veterans Study, 1954–69

NOTE: Ex-smokers includes only former cigarette smokers who stopped smoking for reasons other than physician's orders.

SOURCE: Rogot and Murray (1980).

smokers, 60 percent lower than among current smokers. A more detailed analysis was not possible because only 10 cases occurred among former smokers.

In a second report using the combined data from the Framingham Study and the Albany cohort (Doyle et al. 1964), the relative risk for former versus never smokers was 1.1 (95-percent CI, 0.5–2.2). Current smokers had significantly elevated relative risks ranging from 2.0 to 3.0, depending on the amount smoked.

In a later report from the Framingham Study based on 18 years of followup biennial examinations, Gordon, Kannel, and McGee (1974) assessed the effects of smoking cessation. In this analysis, anyone who smoked for 1 year or more during the most recent 2-year interval between examinations was considered a current smoker. Approximately 20 percent of men who reported that they had quit smoking at entry into the study resumed smoking; about half of those smoked very little or only intermittently after resumption. Compared with current smokers, former smokers had a 30-percent reduction in fatal and nonfatal CHD (excluding angina); the relative risk among current smokers compared with that among never smokers was 1.3. Other coronary risk factors were examined in detail; there were no significant differences between persistent smokers and those who quit, but those who quit were more likely to be ill. Hence, it would be expected that adjustment for confounding would have revealed even greater benefit from cessation. The benefit of quitting seemed more marked in younger men. However, there were only 24 cases of CHD among the quitters so that a detailed analysis could not be performed.

The Western Collaborative Group Study monitored a cohort of 3,524 men for an average of 8.5 years for CHD incidence (Rosenman et al. 1975). Information collected at baseline among men aged 39 to 49 indicated that former smokers had a relative risk of 1.9 compared with that of never smokers, 20 percent lower than among current smokers. For men aged 50 to 59, former smokers had a relative risk of 1.1 compared with never smokers, 40 percent less than among current smokers. This effect of cessation was slightly greater than that observed after 4.5 years of followup (Jenkins, Rosenman, Zyzanski 1968). The difference between the age groups could be a true effect or may reflect different levels of misclassification; it is possible that a greater proportion of the quitters in the younger group than in the older group resumed smoking.

In 1963, a prospective study of smoking and mortality was conducted in Sweden by sending questionnaires to a probability sample of men aged 18 to 69 (Cederlof et al. 1975). A total of 51,911 respondents provided some information; a subsample of 11,739 were sent followup questionnaires in 1969. In that interval, 12 percent of the former smokers had resumed cigarette smoking, and an additional 8 percent initiated pipe or cigar smoking. The men were monitored for 10 years for mortality and cancer morbidity. Men who quit within the past 9 years had a significantly elevated relative risk (RR=1.5) that was nearly as high as the relative risk for current smokers (RR=1.7). In contrast, those with a longer duration of abstinence had a relative risk of 1.0. Men with diseases at baseline were not excluded, so it is likely that the benefits of recent cessation are obscured by the inclusion of men with disease-induced quitting.

The Whitehall Civil Servants Study (Rose et al. 1977; Fuller et al. 1983) is another important source of data on risk factors for CHD. Between 1967 and 1969, a total of 18,403 male civil servants aged 40 to 64 were examined. In the 19-year followup, the age-adjusted CHD mortality rate among 17,051 persons with normal blood sugar was 50 percent lower for quitters than for current smokers. When compared with never smokers, the relative risk for former smokers among normoglycemics was 1.3. Among the 999 men with glucose intolerance (but not diabetes), the risk for former smokers was 30 percent lower than that for current smokers. Overall, the 224 diabetic men experienced a very high risk of CHD; among this group the risk for former smokers was 30 percent higher than for current smokers (based on 10 cases among the current smokers). These data are generally consistent with other studies in the overall findings, but suggest that smoking cessation may not have the same benefit for diabetics as for the general population; however, this finding is based on small numbers, and the severity of diabetes was not considered in the analysis. This study did not provide any information on the time course of the decline in risk after cessation. It is also likely that during the long followup period, a substantial percentage of current smokers quit smoking.

The effect of differences in coronary risk factors other than smoking was examined in quitters and persistent smokers by Friedman and colleagues (1979). As expected, there were a number of differences between quitters and persistent smokers when they were studied at a time in which individuals in both groups were smoking. A followup analysis of this same population was conducted to assess the impact of quitting on risk of CHD and to evaluate the effect of differences between these groups that might alter CHD risk (Friedman et al. 1981). Smoking was assessed by questionnaire at approximately annual multiphasic health checkups given at the Kaiser-Permanente Medical Centers in San Francisco and Oakland, CA. There were 9,394 persistent smokers, 2,856 persistent quitters (those who denied smoking at 2 sessions after an examination when they were currently smoking), and 12,697 never smokers. The cohort was monitored for an average of 4 years for a total followup of 188,436 person-years. The age-, sex-, and race-adjusted death rates (per thousand person-years) associated with CHD were 2.6 among smokers, 1.4 among quitters, and 1.6 among never smokers. After adjustment for baseline differences, quitters had a risk of fatal CHD that was 55 percent lower (95-percent CI, 74–22) compared with persistent smokers. By excluding individuals with frank coronary disease at baseline, a slightly higher benefit for quitting was demonstrated. Further adjustment for measures of smoking intensity slightly attenuated the reduction in risk to 47 percent, suggesting that only a small part of the apparent benefit of quitting is attributable to the fact that quitters were less intense smokers at initiation of smoking. Only the number of cigarettes smoked had any measurable impact; depth of inhalation and duration of smoking had no effect. Except for women during the first half of this century, most smokers begin to smoke during adolescence; thus, duration is very highly correlated with age in most populations. These findings generally confirmed previous results from the same study (Friedman, Dales, Ury 1979).

The Seven Countries Study (Keys 1980) provided a valuable resource for analysis of risk factors for CHD. A total of 16 cohorts of men, aged 40 to 59, living in 7 countries, were examined and monitored for 10 years for CHD incidence. The cohorts were assembled between 1958 and 1964, and consisted of 12,096 men free from CVD. In each grouping of cohorts, former smokers had a lower risk of CHD than did current smokers. However, only about 28 cases of CHD death among former smokers were reported; therefore, no detailed analysis was possible.

Data on the health effects of smoking cessation are also available from the Health Insurance Plan of Greater New York. The incidence of MI was ascertained over a

3-year interval among 110,000 individuals (Shapiro et al. 1969). A total of 613 cases of MI were reported among men aged 35 to 64 in this group. Compared with current smokers, those who quit in the preceding 5 years had a 50-percent lower risk; compared with never smokers, the relative risk was 1.0. As in other studies, the percent reduction in risk associated with smoking cessation tended to be lower in the older age groups, but a decreased risk associated with quitting was apparent among all ages.

Many studies of smoking cessation have focused on middle-aged men and women. Even as recently as the late 1970s, current smoking was considered to be a minor risk factor for CHD beyond age 65 (US DHEW 1979), and the benefits of cessation among older persons have been questioned (Seltzer 1974, 1975). Jajich, Ostfeld, and Freeman (1984) assessed the effect of quitting among 2,674 recipients of public assistance aged 64 to 75 in Cook County, IL. Of the 2,674 individuals studied, 270 were past smokers, 873 were current smokers, and 1,248 were never smokers. Participants were screened at baseline and monitored for 4 years for CHD mortality. Overall, former smokers had a relative risk of CHD mortality of 1.11 (based on 20 exposed cases), whereas current smokers had a relative risk of 1.94. The number of cases was inadequate for a detailed analysis of the effect of duration of abstinence. Persons with heart problems were not excluded at baseline. Approximately one-third of the CHD deaths were among those with such a history; therefore, it is likely that the apparent benefits of quitting may be understated because of the tendency of such individuals at high risk to quit because of illness. These data provide some evidence that the benefits of cessation extend to older adults.

The British Regional Heart Study (Cook et al. 1986) monitored 7,735 men aged 40 to 59 who were randomly selected from general practice lists in the United Kingdom. The men were screened at baseline and studied for 5 to 7.5 years for incidence of fatal and nonfatal CHD; in this interval, there were 336 CHD outcomes. Those with CHD at baseline were not excluded. Compared with never smokers, quitters had a relative risk of approximately 2.5; compared with current smokers, the relative risk was approximately 30 percent lower. Men who quit smoking within the previous 5 years had a relative risk of approximately 3.3, compared with 3.6 among persistent smokers. Those who had quit more than 5 years earlier had a relative risk of approximately 2.3, but there was no evidence for a trend of decreasing risk with increasing duration since cessation. Even those who had quit 20 or more years earlier had an elevated risk. After adjustment for other risk factors, the relative risk in this group was 1.6 ($p=0.11$).

As expected, the prevalence of CHD at baseline among quitters was significantly higher than for either current or never smokers. Presumably, the diagnosis of disease provided a motivation to quit. When these men were excluded, the relative risks were attenuated. Nonetheless, for those who had quit in the previous 5 years, the relative risk was still elevated at 3.2. The total years of smoking was suggested as the most important variable. It was also suggested that cessation lowered risk primarily by preventing the accumulation of further years of smoking. It is noteworthy that although results of this study are adequate to show an elevated risk among past smkers, the number of cases among former smokers is too small to provide precise estimates of risk at the various durations since quitting. For example, there are only 11 cases in the group that quit 20 or more years earlier.

Many studies of large cohorts examined the effects of smoking primarily among men. However, the Nurses Health Study investigators reported on smoking and CHD in a cohort of 121,700 women monitored through biennial questionnaires from 1976 to 1982 (Willett et al. 1987). Women with previously diagnosed CHD were excluded from the analysis. Compared with never smokers, former smokers had a relative risk of 1.5 (95-percent CI, 1.0–2.1). In contrast, current smokers had a substantially elevated relative risk, ranging from 2.1 for smokers of 5 to 14 cigarettes per day to 10.8 for those who smoked 45 cigarettes or more per day. There was no further analysis for the effect of duration of abstinence. The authors suggested that the slight elevation in risk of ex-smokers was due, in part, to resumption of smoking by some fraction of the former smokers. Adjustment for age; obesity; menopausal status; estrogen use; family history of MI; and personal history of diabetes, hypertension, and high cholesterol in a multivariate analysis led to an identical relative risk of 1.5, demonstrating the absence of confounding by these coronary risk factors in this population.

In another cohort study, Floderus, Cederlof, and Friberg (1988) monitored 10,945 twins born in Sweden between 1886 and 1925. Smoking behavior was ascertained at baseline in 1961, and the cohort was studied for mortality for 21 years using matched-pair analysis. Among the males, former smokers compared with never smokers had a risk of coronary mortality of 1.0 (95-percent CI, 0.8–1.1). In contrast, current smokers had relative risks ranging from 1.4 to 1.8 depending on amount smoked. There were no data on duration of abstinence at baseline, and there may have been changes in smoking prevalence during the long followup that would tend to attenuate the relative risk.

In a unique cohort design, Raichlen and coworkers (1986) examined progression of atherosclerosis among 32 men who underwent coronary angiographies at least 2 years apart. Among current smokers, progression of disease was statistically significant and was correlated with pack-years smoked during the interval. Among past smokers, the degree of progression of atherosclerosis was far less than among current smokers; it was not statistically different from lack of progression.

Several other cohort studies have reported on the relation of smoking cessation with risk of CHD; however, the number of subjects was generally too small to contribute substantially to knowledge in this area (Table 2).

Intervention Trials

In several clinical trials, an attempt has been made to evaluate the effect of altering risk factors for CHD, including smoking (Chapter 3). Most of the trials including smoking cessation have also incorporated interventions for other CHD risk factors making it difficult to assess the independent effect of quitting. Nonetheless, these data have extended the understanding of the effects of smoking cessation on CHD risk. Assessing self-report of smoking cessation or decrease in cigarette consumption is another potential difficulty. There may be a tendency for subjects in a trial to seek approval and avoid negative feedback by reporting less cigarette use than is actually the case (Chapter 2). Such a tendency would have the effect of misclassification and would yield an underestimate of the benefits of cessation (Table 4).

TABLE 4.—Intervention trials of smoking cessation and CHD risk

Reference	Population	Intervention	Outcome	Cases among former smokers	Overall effect of intervention	Effect of smoking cessation (nonrandomized)
Hughes et al. (1981); MRFIT Research Group (1982, 1986); Grimm (1986);	MRFIT: 12,866 healthy US men aged 35–57 at high CHD risk	Diet, reduction in weight, hypertension, and smoking	CHD deaths	15	7% decline in intervention group	44% reduction compared with persistent smokers
Ockene et al. (1990)	MRFIT: 7,663 participant smokers at entry	Diet, reduction in weight, hypertension, and smoking	CHD deaths	33	—	Quitters had 42% reduction (16–60%) comparing quitters at first annual exam to smokers at that time
	MRFIT: 6,943 participant smokers at entry	Diet, reduction in weight, hypertension, and smoking	CHD deaths	12	—	Quitters had 65% reduction (37–80%) comparing 3-yr persistent quitters with persistent smokers
Hjermann et al. (1981)	Oslo study: 1,232 healthy Oslo men aged 40–49 at high CHD risk	Diet and smoking	Fatal and nonfatal MI	16	47% decline in intervention group	Smoking cessation accounted for about 25% of the difference between the groups
Kornitzer et al. (1983)	19,409 male Belgian factory workers, aged 40–59	Antismoking, hypertension control	Fatal and nonfatal MI	169	24.5% reduction in intervention group	No specific analysis conducted for effect of smoking cessation

TABLE 4.—Continued

Reference	Population	Intervention	Outcome	Cases among former smokers	Overall effect of intervention	Effect of smoking cessation (nonrandomized)
Rose, Tunstall-Pedoe, Heller (1983)	12 pairs of factories in UK, 18,210 men aged 40–59	Diet, antismoking, hypertension control	Nonfatal MI and CHD deaths	403	4% net reduction in prevalence of current smoking, virtually no difference in outcome between the two groups	No specific analysis of ex-smokers
Rose et al. (1982)	1,445 healthy British civil servants all smoking at high CHD risk	Antismoking advice	CHD deaths	49	19% reduction in intervention group	19% CHD reduction in group offered antismoking advice, not statistically significant
Wilhelmsen et al. (1986)	10,004 random Göteborg men aged 45–55	Antihypertensive, dietary, antismoking advice	Major CHD	NR	No difference	Intervention achieved only small differences between the groups for smoking and other risk factors

NOTE: CHD=coronary heart disease; MRFIT=Multiple Risk Factor Intervention Trial; MI=myocardial infarction; NR=not reported.

The Multiple Risk Factor Intervention Trial (MRFIT) was designed to test whether reduction of diastolic blood pressure, serum cholesterol, and cigarette smoking decreases the incidence of CHD (Hughes et al. 1981; MRFIT Research Group 1986; Grimm 1986). Men aged 35 to 57 were screened; of those in the upper 15 percent of CHD risk (based on coefficients from the Framingham Study), but without overt CHD, 6,428 were randomized to special intervention, and 6,438 were assigned to usual care. Men in the special intervention group were given intensive instructions concerning diet and smoking cessation and were treated for hypertension. Those in the usual care group were referred to their regular source of medical care. The difference in total cholesterol between the two groups was only half that expected; because of better than anticipated hypertension treatment in the usual care group, the difference in blood pressure was also substantially less than expected. At the outset, 59 percent of the participants were current cigarette smokers. After 12 months, 31 percent of the smokers in the intervention group had quit (verified by thiocyanate (SCN^-) levels) compared with 12 percent of the smokers in the control group. At the end of the 6-year trial, 46 percent of smokers in the intervention group had quit compared with 29 percent in the control group. Mortality resulting from CHD was only 7 percent lower in the special care group, a difference that did not approach statistical significance. The authors suggested that the small decrease in risk was due in part to the smaller than anticipated differences in risk factor levels between the two groups and that some of the benefit in risk factor reduction might possibly have been counterbalanced by an unfavorable response to antihypertensive therapy in some of the hypertensive patients (MRFIT Research Group 1982). Within the intervention group, those who quit in the first year had a multivariate-adjusted relative risk 50 percent lower than that of persistent smokers; in the control group, adjusted relative risk 30 percent lower than that of persistent smokers. In this trial, risk of sudden CHD death was reduced 65 percent among quitters compared with persistent smokers. Because all participants were seen at least annually, the possible misclassification of smoking status was minimized.

The 10.5-year followup data from MRFIT have recently been published (MRFIT Research Group 1990). Deaths due to CHD were 10.6 percent lower in the special intervention group (95-percent CI,–23.7 to 4.9) compared with the usual care group (two-sided p value=0.24). This reduction in risk was largely attributable to a 24.3-percent lower risk of death due to acute MI (2-sided p value=0.04). Total cardiovascular mortality was 7.1 percent lower after 10.5 years in the special intervention group compared with the usual care group (p>0.05). In one analysis not based on randomized groups, CHD mortality rates of smokers who had quit within the first 12 months of the trial and of those who were still smoking at that time were compared (Ockene et al. 1990). Quitters had a 37-percent reduction in mortality. After adjustment for other CHD risk factors, the reduction was 42 percent (95-percent CI, 16–60). The slightly greater benefit observed after adjustment for risk factors indicates that there was little confounding and that it was in the direction that would tend to underestimate the benefit of cessation. This analysis ignored any changes in smoking status after the first annual examination. To the extent that either some of the quitters resumed smoking or some of the current smokers quit, that analysis would yield an underestimate of the benefits of cessation. A second analysis compared quitters who remained abstinent at the first three annual examinations with persistent smokers. In this analysis, which would be affected to a lesser extent by misclassification, former smokers had a 65-percent reduction in risk compared with persistent smokers (95-percent CI, 37–80).

A trial using a somewhat similar design was conducted in Oslo, Norway (Hjermann et al. 1981; Hjermann, Holme, Leren 1986). Males aged 40 to 49 were screened for coronary risk, and normotensive men at high risk of CHD due to elevated serum cholesterol, smoking, and other risk factors were identified. The participants had no clinical CHD at the time of randomization to the intervention or control group (N=604 and N=628, respectively). The intervention consisted of advice and instruction on altering diet and reducing smoking. Participants were examined at least annually during the 5 years of followup. After 5 years, fatal and nonfatal CHD was reduced in the interventiongroup by 47 percent. There was greater success in reducing cholesterol in this trial than in inducing smoking cessation. The mean serum cholesterol was approximately 13 percent lower in the intervention group than among the controls. However, only 25 percent of the smokers in the intervention group and 17 percent in the control group quit entirely, although many reduced the amount smoked. There was an inverse relation between CHD incidence and percentage change in tobacco consumption, but this did not attain statistical significance. The authors calculated that approximately 25 percent of the difference in CHD incidence between the two groups was attributable to differences in smoking.

A second report (Hjermann, Holme, Leren et al. 1986) included followup through 102 months. Statistically significant reductions among the intervention group compared with the control group were seen for fatal coronary events (reduced 59 percent), total coronary events (reduced 44 percent), and total cardiovascular events (reduced 61 percent).

The World Health Organization European Collaborative Trial in the multifactorial prevention of CHD was conducted at several sites in Europe. Pooled results were reported from centers in the United Kingdom, Belgium, Italy, and Poland (WHO European Collaborative Group 1983); separate reports have also been published from centers in the United Kingdom (Rose, Tunstall-Pedoe, Heller 1983) and Belgium (Kornitzer et al. 1983). A total of 66 factories involving 49,781 men were randomized to a multifactorial risk factor reduction program or to the control group. The reduction of levels of risk factors varied considerably among the centers. Overall, the reduction in risk factor levels was modest, and there was no significant decline in CHD endpoints in the intervention group. The effect on CHD was broadly correlated with changes in risk factors. There was no specific analysis on the impact of smoking cessation.

The Belgian center was the largest in the European Collaborative Trial. Fifteen pairs of factories were randomly allocated to the intervention or control groups, which included 19,409 men aged 40 to 59 years. The intervention included advice about smoking cessation and reduction of hypertension and elevated cholesterol. Subjects were screened as part of the trial, but referred to their own physicians for therapy. After 6 years, there was a 24.5-percent reduction in fatal and nonfatal CHD in the intervention group compared with the control group (p=0.03) (Kornitzer et al. 1983). The rates in the intervention and control groups continued to diverge throughout the followup period. No specific analysis was conducted to assess the independent effect of smoking cessation on risk of CHD.

The multifactor primary prevention trial in Göteborg, Sweden focused on reduction of hypertension, elevated serum cholesterol, and smoking (Wilhelmsen et al. 1986). A random sample of 10,004 men aged 45 to 55 years was included in the intervention group, and 2 other random samples of the same size were identified as controls. Of those invited to participate in the intervention group, 7,495 attended the first screening examination. At the outset, within the intervention and control groups combined, 20.6 percent were former smokers. After 4 years, the proportion of former smokers increased to 27.7 percent, and after 10 years to 39.4 percent in the intervention group. In the control group, the percentage of former smokers also increased—to 22.3 percent at 4 years and to 36.1 percent at 10 years. The differences achieved for other risk factors between the intervention and control groups were also quite small. After 10 years, there were virtually no differences in fatal and nonfatal outcomes between the groups.

The center in the United Kingdom was also large (Rose, Tunstall-Pedoe, Heller 1983), with 12 pairs of factories and 18,210 men aged 40 to 59 years. There were only very modest changes in risk factors other than cigarette smoking. The reported number of cigarettes smoked per day in the intervention group decreased by 16 percent, but the proportion of current cigarette smokers decreased by only 4 percent. Rose and Hamilton (1978) stated that whereas self-report of cessation is likely to be reasonably accurate, reported decreases in smoking are probably exaggerated. With such small net changes in risk factors, it is not surprising that there was virtually no difference in the rate of CHD between the two groups.

Only one trial has attempted to assess the effect of advice for smoking cessation without intervening for other risk factors simultaneously. In theory, trials of this design can provide the clearest indication of the effect of such advice in the absence of other effects. Participants were selected from a cohort of 16,016 from the Whitehall Civil Servants Study (Fuller et al. 1983). From this group, 1,445 high-risk male smokers aged 40 to 59 were randomized to a normal care group or the intervention group that received antismoking advice. At year one, 51 percent of the intervention group reported that they were not smoking, and at year three, 36 percent reported the same. In the normal care group, the corresponding percentages were 10 and 14 percent. A third of the quitters reported smoking cigars or a pipe. It is important to note that the questionnaire response rate at 3 years was 64 percent in the intervention group and 70 percent in the normal care group (Rose and Hamilton 1978). The 9-year response rate was 83 percent. At that point, 55 percent of responders in the intervention group reported quitting, as did 41 percent in the normal care group. Despite the similarity of smoking prevalence of the two groups, at 10 years CHD mortality decreased by 18 percent in the intervention group. This difference did not attain statistical significance (95-percent CI, –43 to +18 percent) (Rose et al. 1982).

Smoking Cessation and CHD Risk Among Persons With Diagnosed CHD

Studies examining smoking cessation and CHD risk among persons with diagnosed CHD may be less prone to some of the methodologic pitfalls discussed in Chapter 2.

In many instances, studies are primarily of individuals who were smokers up to the time of the infarction. Such a major health event can be a powerful motivation to quit smoking permanently. Moreover, the timing of quitting often coincides with the infarction and is therefore ascertained quite accurately. Because those with a prior diagnosis of CHD are at such high risk for another event, the estimates of effect can be relatively precise, even with a modest number of individuals under study. One difficulty in interpreting these studies is in the comparison of quitters with never smokers. Never smokers who suffer MI tend to have a worse CHD risk factor profile (apart from smoking) than smokers (Mulcahy 1983). However, most of the other risk factors are less amenable to change than smoking. After smoking is removed as a risk factor among former smokers, the effect is often a better prognosis than that for never smokers. Several of these issues and a review of the literature prior to 1983 are discussed by Mulcahy (1983). This researcher found that studies were quite consistent in showing that quitters had about half the risk of recurrent MI or CHD death compared with persistent smokers (Mulcahy 1983). Nearly all studies of this issue have indicated a benefit of cessation (Table 5).

A cohort of 213 patients who survived for 28 days a first attack of coronary insufficiency or MI was studied for 5 years (Mulcahy et al. 1977). Of these, 190 were smokers at the time of the event. Of the 89 who stopped, the cumulative 5-year death rate was 14.6 percent. Of the 42 who reduced cigarette use, the rate was 14.2 percent. However, among the 59 persistent smokers, 28.8 percent died within 5 years. Nearly all of the deaths were associated with CHD.

This study was extended by further accrual of patients and followup of 551 men less than 60 years of age (Daly et al. 1987). Of the 406 current smokers at the time of the event, 140 had stopped by year two. Those quitters had a 10-percent reduction in risk of sudden death and a 40-percent reduction in risk of total mortality compared with those who continued to smoke.

A 1978 report from the Framingham Study (Sparrow, Dawber, Colton 1978) compared the survival of 56 individuals who quit smoking after a first MI with 139 who continued to smoke after the diagnosis. Within 2 to 3 years after diagnosis, former smokers had a significantly better survival rate than persistent smokers. The 6-year mortality rate (estimated by life table methods) was 18.8 percent among quitters compared with 30.4 percent among persistent smokers. When the risk of recurrent MI was assessed, the authors found that former smokers had a lower risk than persistent smokers, with a 6-year reinfarction rate of 15.5 percent in quitters versus 21.5 percent among smokers. However, with only eight reinfarctions among the quitters, the differences were not statistically significant. The rate of decline in risk could not be assessed because of the small samples.

Framingham Study investigators (Hubert, Holford, Kannel 1982) conducted a long-term followup study of 130 subjects with angina pectoris. They found that smoking status at the examination ascertaining angina was modestly associated with subsequent risk of a later, more serious CHD outcome. Apparently, the change in smoking behavior explained this finding. Of the angina patients who smoked, 14 percent quit between the onset of disease and the biennial examination when the diagnosis was confirmed. Another 29 percent quit during the followup period. In this cohort, the heavier smokers

TABLE 5.—Studies of the effect of smoking cessation on persons with diagnosed CHD

Reference	Population	Followup	Cases among former smokers	Reduction in risk compared with persistent smokers[a]	Comments
Mulcahy et al. (1977)	190 Dublin men aged <60 who smoked at time of first coronary insufficiency or MI	5 yr	13 deaths	50%	Smokers (N=42) who reduced cig/day also had a lower mortality compared with persistent smokers
Daly et al. (1987)	373 men aged <60 who smoked at time of first MI or unstable angina and survived 2 yr	Average 9.4 yr; ≤16 yr	NR	10% for sudden death; 40% for total mortality	No further classification of smoking; some of same patients as in Daly 1983
Sparrow, Dawber, and Colton (1978)	Framingham Heart Study: 195 cohort members who smoked at time of first MI	6 yr	10 deaths	40%	
Hubert, Holford, Kannell (1982)	Framingham Heart Study: subjects with angina	≤26 yr	NR	10-yr followup: <60 yr 90% ≥60 yr 60% 26-yr followup: <60 yr 70% ≥60 yr 10%	Only 25 cases in baseline smokers, so estimates are statistically unstable
Salonen (1980)	North Karelia, Finland: 523 men aged <65 who smoked at first MI	3 yr	26 deaths; 22 CHD deaths	40% (60–10) 40% (60–0)	Followup began 6 mo after MI; apparent benefit more pronounced in first 6 mo of followup (60%)

TABLE 5.—Continued

Reference	Population	Followup	Cases among former smokers	Reduction in risk compared with persistent smokers[a]	Comments
Von der Lippe and Lund-Johansen (1982)	1,330 participants in the Norwegian timolol trial who smoked at time of MI	17 mo	31 deaths in those who stopped smoking before entering the trial	None	Study not designed to examine effects of smoking cessation; no details provided on possible confounding
			37 deaths in those who stopped in the first months of the trial	10%	
Rønnevik, Gunderson, Abrahamsen (1985)	1,330 participants in the Norwegian timolol trial who smoked at time of MI	17 mo	44 recurrent nonfatal MI	33% reduction; 8% in quitters, 12% in persistent smokers	
Shapiro, Howat, Singh (1982)	142 MI survivors aged <45	≤10 yr	NR	80% (former and never smokers vs. persistent smokers)	Former and never smokers considered together, not separately
Aberg et al. (1983)	983 Göteborg male smokers at time of MI	≤10.5 yr	104 recurrent nonfatal MI; 80 CHD deaths	30%; difference between groups increased with time	30% quitters had worse predicted prognosis at baseline; no further assessment of smoking beyond 3 mo after initial MI
Daly et al. (1983)	374 Dublin men, smokers at time of MI diagnosis or angina	Mean 7.4 yr, ≤13 yr	80 deaths	60% overall; 40% first 6 yr; 80% 7–13 yr	Followup began 2 yr after MI, when smoking status was assessed

TABLE 5.—Continued

Reference	Population	Followup	Cases among former smokers	Reduction in risk compared with persistent smokers[a]	Comments
Johansson et al. (1985)	156 Göteborg women aged ≤65, smokers at time of first MI	5 yr	12 deaths	60% (80–20)	Quitters had worse baseline prognosis; differences between groups were apparent early and increased with time
Perkins and Dick (1985)	119 UK patients who smoked at first MI	5 yr	9 deaths	60%	
Vlietstra et al. (1986)	11,605 patients in CASS who smoked at time CHD was diagnosed by angiography	5 yr	By risk quartile: (best) 1: 13 2: 21 3: 44 (worst) 4: 156 overall: 234	Total mortality: 40% 40% 50% 20% 40% (50–20)	Quitters had worse baseline prognosis; exclusion of those with mixed smoking behavior and close followup reduced likelihood of misclassification of exposure; also, hospitalization for MI was substantially reduced in former smokers
Hermanson et al. (1988)	3,045 CASS patients with CHD aged 35–54	5.3 yr for MI or death	35–54 yr: NR	40% (50–30)	Reanalysis of a subset of patients analyzed by Vlietstra (1986)
	1,893 CASS patients with CHD aged ≥55		55–59 yr: 99 60–64 yr: 92 65–69 yr: 48 >70 yr: 29	30% (50–20) 30% (50–10) 30% (60–0) 70% (80–30)	

TABLE 5.—Continued

Reference	Population	Followup	Cases among former smokers	Reduction in risk compared with persistent smokers[a]	Comments
Hallstrom, Cobb, Ray (1986)	310 survivors of out of hospital arrest, smokers at that time	Mean 47.5 mo		35% for fatal recurrent cardiac arrest	Borderline statistical significance
Green (1987)	2,199 men who smoked at time of MI	2 yr	NR	30% for CHD	
Hedback and Perk (1987)	157 smokers at time of MI	5 yr	13 fatal and nonfatal CHD	50%	Trial of rehabilitation including smoking cessation
Galan et al. (1988)	160 patients re-angiographed after angioplasty	Mean 7 mo		31% decreased for restenosis	Groups were similar at baseline
Phillips et al. (1988)	530 male British former smokers with non-MI CHD	Mean 7.5 yr		33% for fatal or nonfatal CHD	No update of smoking data; no assessment of severity of baseline CHD
	175 former smokers with MI, aged 40–59			10%	
Goldberg, Szklo, Chandra (1981)	325 post-MI patients	≤10 yr		Survival Quit at MI Not quit 1 yr 99% 98% 5 yr 97% 84% 10 yr 95% 51%	Independent of multiple risk factors; no update of smoking status

NOTE: CHD=coronary heart disease; MI=myocardial infarction; NR=not reported; CASS=Coronary Artery Surgery Study.
[a] 95% confidence interval shown in parentheses when available.

were more likely to quit than the lighter smokers. Former smokers had a lower rate of subsequent CHD. There was a suggestion that older persons benefited less; however, this finding could not be confirmed because only a small fraction of the 25 older smokers actually quit.

Salonen (1980) monitored a Finnish cohort of men less than 65 years of age whose smoking behavior was assessed 6 months after MI. Of these, 352 were never smokers, 302 were persistent smokers, and 221 quit smoking within 6 months after MI. Three years after MI, quitters had a 40-percent reduction in risk of total mortality (95-percent CI, 10–60 percent) and of CHD death (95-percent CI, 10–60 percent) compared with persistent smokers. The reduction in risk was more pronounced in earlier periods; between 6 months and 1 year, mortality was reduced by 60 percent (95-percent CI, 10–80 percent). It is possible that the apparent decline in benefit may represent misclassification because current smokers continued to quit but were still analyzed as current smokers. The benefits of quitting were strongest among those with the best prognosis after infarction. Of post-MI deaths, 28 percent were estimated to be attributable to continued smoking.

As part of the Norwegian trial of timolol use after MI, mortality of the 1,884 participants was ascertained over an average of 17 months according to smoking status. Virtually no differences were observed (Von der Lippe and Lund-Johansen 1982). Across both the timolol and placebo groups, 8 percent of the nonsmokers died, compared with 8 percent of those who stopped smoking before entry into the trial, 7 percent among those who quit in the first month of the trial, and 8 percent among persistent smokers. However, there was a reduction in reinfarctions, 8 percent among those who quit in the first month of the trial compared with 12 percent among persistent smokers (Rønnevik, Gundersen, Abrahamsen 1985).

Shapiro, Howat, and Singh (1982) monitored 142 patients who survived a first MI that occurred when the patient was younger than age 45. Of these patients, 50 who continued to smoke more than 20 cigarettes per day had substantially higher mortality rates (58-percent 10-year mortality by life table methods) than did the 61 never and former smokers (12-percent mortality). The survival curves began to diverge 1 year after MI. Unfortunately, data were not presented separately for former smokers, and apparently there were only a small number of never smokers.

Aberg and colleagues (1983) studied 983 men aged 67 years or less who were listed in the MI Register of Göteborg between 1968 and 1977. The men were smokers within 3 months of their initial MI, who survived hospitalization. Not all men listed in the Register were included in the study, but the selection process did not introduce bias. Quitting was defined as not smoking 3 months after the infarction. Followup began at that point and continued for 10.5 years. The 542 males who had stopped smoking by 3 months after infarction had a significantly worse prognosis, based on predischarge characteristics, than did the 441 persistent smokers. Those who quit had substantially more left ventricular failure and higher peak enzyme levels during hospitalization. Based on these and other preinfarction and hospitalization variables, those who quit had a predicted 2-year mortality that was 8 to 9 percent higher than that of persistent smokers. However, despite this slightly worse baseline prognosis, quitters had a significantly lower mortality than did persistent smokers. Overall, the 5-year mortality was significantly reduced among quitters, with a cumulative mortality rate 30 percent lower. The effect was somewhat stronger among those aged 50 or older than among younger men, but was significant in both age groups. The cumulative 5-year reduction in recurrence of MI was 30 percent. These estimates almost certainly underrepresent te true effect of cessation for two reasons: quitters at baseline had a distinctly worse prognosis, and smoking cessation was defined only at the point 3 months after infarction. It is likely that some of the smokers quit at a later point; this would tend to dilute the smoking group with ex-smokers who enjoy a lower risk. Thus, the rates of mortality and reinfarction among truly persistent smokers would be underestimated in this study. The two groups began to diverge for both endpoints after as little as 1 year postinfarction, and the differences increased with time. This report confirmed and extended initial findings from that study (Wilhelmsson et al. 1975).

Several studies have monitored patients with angiographically diagnosed coronary disease. Kramer and coworkers (1983) studied 278 men with sequential coronary angiograms. These researchers found that neither cigarette smoking at the initial or followup examination nor smoking cessation was predictive of progression of atherosclerosis.

Daly and colleagues (1983) studied 217 men who stopped smoking after a first diagnosis of unstable angina or MI and 157 persistent smokers. Smoking status was defined 2 years after the first diagnosis. As in the Aberg study (1983), those who quit tended to have a more serious diagnosis than the persistent smokers. However, quitters enjoyed substantial protection compared with persistent smokers. For total mortality, risk was reduced by 60 percent among those who quit smoking compared with continuing smokers; for fatal reinfarction, risk was also reduced by 60 percent. During the first 6 years of followup, the reduction in risk was 40 percent (95-percent CI, 10–60 percent), but in the followup period of 7 to 13 years, the benefits of quitting were more marked, with a reduction in risk of 80 percent (95-percent CI, 50–90 percent). The benefits of quitting were more marked among those with less severe initial disease. In this study, quitters had a lower cumulative mortality than did never smokers with these diagnoses. Those never smokers may have had more coronary risk factors other than smoking which may be less amenable to change than smoking.

In a later study with some of the same patients, Daly and coworkers (1985) found that 1 year after the initial event, 241 quitters had a 40-percent lower prevalence of angina compared with 143 persistent smokers. However, by 6 years of followup, the prevalence of angina was the same in both groups and remained similar throughout the followup period of 17 years. Green (1985) noted that the prevalence of angina 6 months after infarction among 851 ex-smokers was equivalent to that among smokers. However, it is unclear whether the ex-smokers were smoking at the time of the event.

Most studies of the effect of post-MI cessation have been conducted among men. Johansson and colleagues (1985) examined 156 women in Göteberg, younger than 65, who were smokers at the time of their first MI. The definitions and criteria were the same as those in the study by Aberg and coworkers (1983). Three months after infarction, 75 women continued to smoke and 81 had stopped. As in the Göteberg Study of men (Aberg et al. 1983), women who quit had more severe infarctions. Despite the worse prognosis normally associated with the higher enzyme elevations and other indications of severity, the quitters had a significantly better survival. The reduction in risk compared with smokers remained at 60 percent (95-percent CI, 20–80 percent), and after adjustment for prognostic features before and during the infarction, the reduction remained at 60 percent. When compared with never smokers, the relative risk among quitters was 1.1. The reinfarction rate was slightly, though not significantly, higher among persistent smokers.

Similar findings for a rapid benefit were observed in the small study of Perkins and Dick (1985). For 5 years, these researchers monitored 52 patients (including 11 women) who stopped smoking at the time of the infarction and 67 persistent smokers (of whom 18 were women). Men who quit had a 50-percent reduced risk of death; for women it was 60 percent lower.

As part of the Coronary Artery Surgery Study, the effect of smoking cessation on risk of clinical CHD outcomes was assessed in men with documented coronary atherosclerosis by angiography (Vlietstra et al. 1986). The death rates among 1,490 quitters were compared with those of 2,675 persistent smokers and 2,912 never smokers. Men who were quitters at baseline but who subsequently resumed smoking and those who were smokers initially but later stopped were excluded from the analysis. Hence, this study was largely free of misclassification. As in most of the other studies, the quitters had slightly worse prognoses than did the persistent smokers. At every level of risk, however, quitters had a significantly better 5-year survival. Overall, the reduction in risk (from Cox regression) was 40 percent (95-percent CI, 20–50 percent). The benefit was slightly more pronounced among those with the worst baseline prognosis. Overall, the 5-year survival rate among quitters was similar to that of never smokers (85 vs. 87 percent, respectively). Nearly all the benefit was attributable to a decreased rate of CHD death. After adjustment for prognostic score, the rate of hospitalization for MI was substantially higher among persistent smokers than among quitters (11.3 vs. 7.1 percent, respectively). For both fatal and nonfatal endpoints, the rates began to diverge substantially after about 1 year (Figure 6). Because of the careful study design and the unusually large number of cases, the results of this study must be accorded considerable weight.

In an extension of the analysis of survival data from the Coronary Artery Surgery Study, the effects of smoking cessation were examined in a population of individuals aged 55 and older with angiographically documented coronary disease (Hermanson et al. 1988). As in the previous report, persistent smokers were defined as those 1,086 smokers who did not quit throughout the 6-year followup period, and quitters were those 807 who stopped smoking 1 year before the baseline angiogram and who did not resume smoking during followup. The experience of 3,045 younger subjects aged 35 to 54 years was also examined. At every age, quitters had better survival rates than did persistent smokers, and there was no evidence that the benefit was attenuated with increasing age.

Employing a different approach, Hallstrom, Cobb, and Ray (1986) studied a cohort of 310 men who smoked and were discharged from the hospital after an episode of out-of-hospital cardiac arrest. After the arrest, 219 men continued to smoke and 91 men quit. During the average 47.5 months of followup, 67 persistent smokers and 18 former smokers died of a recurrent cardiac arrest. After adjustment across baseline risk

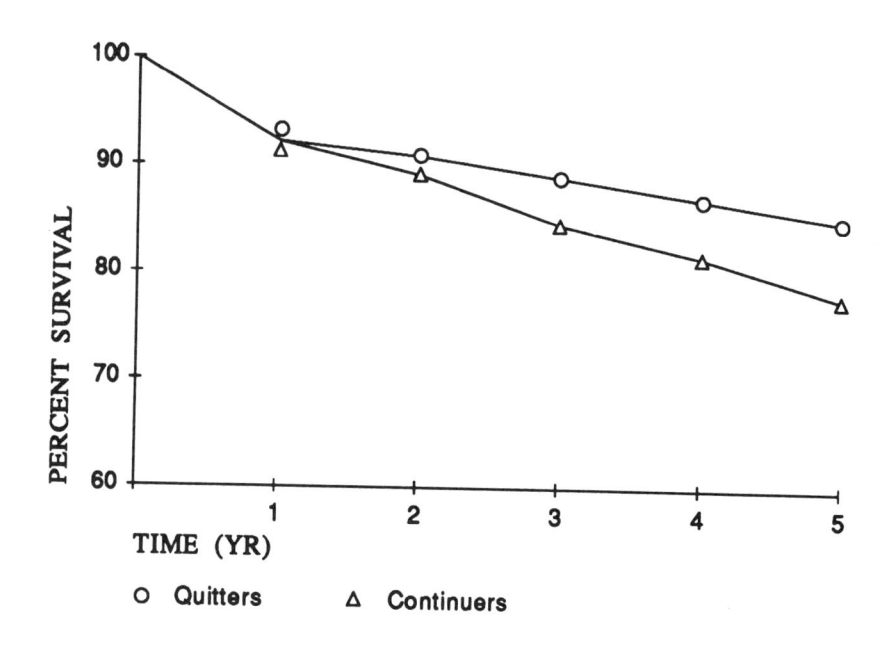

FIGURE 6.—Effect of smoking cessation on survival among men with documented coronary atherosclerosis; pooled survival among quitters (○) (N=1,490) and continuers (△) (N=2,675)

SOURCE: Vlietstra et al. (1986).

strata, this difference was of borderline significance in a life table analysis (p=0.076). After exclusion of crossovers (14 smokers quit ≥6 months after the arrest, and 2 quitters resumed smoking), the benefit of cessation was slightly more pronounced (p=0.048).

Analysis of data from a trial of practolol also provided information on the effects of smoking cessation after MI (Green 1987). There were 855 never smokers, 1,344 persistent smokers, and 851 individuals who quit smoking after the entry MI. Those who stopped smoking had a worse outcome initially than persistent smokers, and the benefit from cessation did not appear until 2 years after the event. When events in the first 6 weeks after the index MI were excluded, the benefits of cessation appeared at about 18 months. By 24 months, those who stopped had a 30-percent CHD risk reduction. As in other studies, former smokers when compared with continuing smokers tended to have more severe MI, with significantly more pulmonary congestion noted when x-rayed and significantly greater occurrence of faster dysrhythmia. This supports the view that those with a worse MI are more likely to quit, and it explains why quitters in the study had a worse initial outcome.

In a trial of rehabilitation after MI, 147 patients in a Swedish hospital were routinely invited to participate in a rehabilitation program; 158 patients in a comparable hospital were not (Hedback and Perk 1987). The cardiovascular experience in the intervention group was favorable, and when the specific effect of smoking cessation was examined among the 82 patients from both groups who quit after MI, approximately 15.9 percent died in the subsequent 5 years compared with 30.6 percent among the persistent smokers and 11.8 percent among the never smokers.

The influence of smoking cessation on frequency of restenosis after coronary angioplasty was assessed by comparing 84 persistent smokers with 76 individuals who stopped at the time of angioplasty (Galan et al. 1988). Patients were reexamined angiographically after an average of 7 months. Restenosis was significantly higher in persistent smokers (55 vs. 38 percent, p=0.03). Several other studies (Fleck et al. 1988; Vandormael et al. 1987) failed to find an association between smoking at angioplasty and subsequent restenosis, but those studies did not consider the impact of cessation at the time of angioplasty. Although the mechanisms of restenosis are not clear, the findings of Galan and coworkers (1988) are consistent with a fairly rapidly acting process for decreased risk after cessation.

As part of the British Regional Heart Study described above, investigators also monitored 1,515 men with evidence of CHD but without MI and 428 men with evidence of prior MI at entry (Phillips et al. 1988). Smoking behavior was assessed at baseline, and the men, aged 40 to 59, were studied for an average of 7.5 years. There was no update of the smoking information. After adjustment for age and other risk factors, for those with non-MI CHD at baseline, the relative risk comparing former with never smokers was 1.4; for current smokers, it was 2.1. For those with a history of MI, the relative risk for former smokers was 1.7; and for current smokers, it was 1.9. The degree of misclassification that may have occurred during the followup period is difficult to assess. No information is available on the duration of abstinence or the degree of severity of CHD as distributed by smoking status.

In a community-based followup of 325 post-MI patients in Baltimore, MD, Goldberg, Szklo, and Chandra (1981) found that after control for several clinical and sociodemographic factors, survival among those who quit at the time of MI was substantially improved. The 1-, 5-, and 10-year survival rates among those who quit were 99, 97, and 95 percent, respectively; in contrast, the rates among persistent smokers were 98, 84, and 51 percent, respectively. Despite the lack of updates on smoking behavior, there was a trend for diverging survival between the two groups.

Summary of Smoking Cessation and CHD Risk

Within the past 40 years, large amounts of data regarding the effect of smoking cessation on CHD risk have been accumulated from numerous studies. However diverse in design and location, these studies consistently find that the risk of CHD is reduced among former smokers compared with those who continued to smoke. The data are compatible with a rapid, partial decline in risk, followed by a more gradual decline reaching levels of never smokers after a prolonged period. The initial decline appears to occur within 1 year of cessation or perhaps even less and constitutes a reduction of about one-half or more of the excess risk associated with current smoking. The remaining decline in excess risk is more gradual, with the risks reaching those of never smokers only after a number of years of smoking abstinence. This pattern of decline in excess risk is compatible with multiple effects of smoking on the process of developing CHD, including both short-term influences on platelets and other factors relating to thrombosis which may be more rapidly reversible and long-term increases in atherosclerosis which are only slowly reversible.

Persistent smokers may differ from those who quit in other ways that could affect the risk of developing CHD. A number of investigators have examined whether such differences would account for some or all of the decline in risk among those who stop smoking. The risk profiles of quitters and persistent smokers vary among studies: In some studies, there are no material differences; however, in other studies, quitters have a healthier profile; the opposite is true for still other studies. In the studies of primary prevention, none of these differences could explain even a minor portion of the decreased risk among quitters. Most studies of cessation after an MI have found that quitters had a higher baseline risk; however, their risk decreased compared with persistent smokers. Thus, both in primary and secondary prevention studies, confounding effects of other risk factors do not explain the apparent benefits of cessation. To the contrary, in many studies, the decrease in risk is even more pronounced after adjustment for baseline characteristics.

Only a few studies have examined the impact of smoking cessation in relation to various other CHD risk factors. No data are available to suggest that the relative risks differ substantially in the presence or absence of other CHD risk factors; that is, the percentage reduction in risk most likely occurs across risk factor categories. However, because individuals at high risk for other reasons such as family history, hypertension, or elevated cholesterol have higher rates of CHD, a given percentage decrease in risk among these individuals is a greater absolute decrease than among those with a lower risk profile. Hence, it is of especially great importance to achieve high rates of cessation among individuals who are otherwise at high risk for CHD.

Most data on the effects of smoking cessation are derived from white males, but sufficient information is available about women to indicate that the findings are similar for both sexes. Less is known about the effects of cessation among minority groups; however, there is no reason to believe that the benefits of cessation would be any different for these groups.

Several studies have examined the effect of smoking cessation after age 60 on subsequent CHD risk. Data are now available that demonstrate that the benefits of cessation extend to older adults as well as to young and middle-aged adults for both primary (Table 3) and secondary prevention (Hermanson et al. 1988). Although the relative risks of CHD among current smokers tend to be lower among older persons than among younger persons, smoking cessation among older persons can have a greater absolute effect because their rates of CHD are so much higher.

Considerable data address the effects of smoking cessation among individuals with diagnosed CHD. A reduction in risk of further CHD-related morbidity and mortality that accompanies smoking cessation has been conclusively demonstrated. Cigarette smoking is considered the leading modifiable CHD risk factor; overwhelming evidence demonstrates that cessation reduces that risk substantially.

SMOKING CESSATION AND AORTIC ANEURYSM

Abdominal aortic aneurysm refers to the dilatation or expansion of the aorta because of degenerative or inflammatory destruction of the components of the arterial wall. Most abdominal aortic aneurysms are a result of atherosclerosis, although other conditions cause abdominal aortic aneurysms. The preponderance of evidence from autopsy studies reviewed in the 1983 Report of the Surgeon General suggests that cigarette smoking aggravates or accelerates aortic atherosclerosis (US DHHS 1983). In addition, epidemiologic studies published up to that time indicated that smokers had elevated death rates from ruptured abdominal aneurysm compared with nonsmokers (Hammond and Garfinkel 1969; Hammond and Horn 1958a,b; Kahn 1966; Weir and Dunn 1970). Mechanisms whereby smoking causes atherosclerosis are reviewed in this Chapter.

Studies of Smoking Cessation and Risk of Aortic Aneurysm

Several of the larger prospective cohort studies reviewed above have reported results for mortality by cause of death. The data on mortality among former smokers from abdominal aortic aneurysms reported in five prospective cohort studies are summarized in Table 6. A consistent pattern is seen among men in these studies, with an excess risk of mortality approximately 50 percent lower among former smokers than among current smokers. However, excess risk among former smokers has remained about two to three times higher than that among never smokers. A similar pattern was also present for women in ACS CPS-II. Although data for women are limited, Doll and associates (1980) reported 11 deaths due to aortic aneurysm occurring during 22 years of followup among 6,194 women. Overall, these data indicate that former smokers have a reduced risk of death from aortic aneurysm compared with current smokers. More detailed analyses by duration of smoking abstinence have not been presented.

SMOKING CESSATION AND PERIPHERAL ARTERIAL OCCLUSIVE DISEASE

The peripheral arteries include those branches of the aorta that supply the upper and lower extremities and the abdominal viscera. Most peripheral arterial occlusive disease results from atherosclerosis, although other conditions may cause obstruction of these arteries. Symptomatic atherosclerosis of peripheral arteries occurs most often in the vessels of the lower extremities. The 1983 Report of the Surgeon General reviewed risk factors and epidemiologic data relating to the etiology of peripheral artery disease (US DHHS 1983). In that Report, an extremely strong association between cigarette smoking and diagnosis of peripheral artery disease was observed (US DHHS 1983). Cigarette smoking was the strongest risk factor for peripheral artery disease in the Framingham Study (Kannel, McGee, Gordon 1976). In this Section, the impact of smoking cessation on risk of developing peripheral artery disease is reviewed. In addition, the influence of cessation on treadmill time, rest pain, progression to amputation, and survival among patients with diagnosed peripheral artery disease is discussed.

TABLE 6.—Studies of smoking cessation and risk of death due to aortic aneurysm

Reference	Population	Followup	Cases among former smokers	Standardized mortality ratios compared with never smokers — Former smokers	Standardized mortality ratios compared with never smokers — Current smokers
Doll and Peto (1976)	British physicians: 34,440 men	20 yr	30	3.2	5.2
Doll et al. (1980)	British physicians: 6,194 women	22 yr	NR	3.0	1–14 cig/day: 1.3 15–24 cig/day: 1.3
Rogot and Murray (1980)	US veterans: 293,958 men	15 yr	253	2.58	5.23
Carstensen, Pershagen, Eklund (1987)	25,129 Swedish men	16 yr	12	1.4	1–7 g/day: 1.7 8–15 g/day: 2.7 >15 g/day: 3.0
US DHHS (1989)	ACS CPS-I (25-State Study)	6 yr	NR	Women 3.67[a] Men 2.40	4.64 4.11

NOTE: NR=not reported; ACS CPS-I=American Cancer Prevention Study I.
[a] Indicates current and former smokers.

Smoking Cessation and Development of Peripheral Artery Disease

Two studies provide sufficient detail to calculate the risk of peripheral vascular disease among former smokers compared with current smokers. Jacobsen and coworkers (1984) compared a consecutive series of 53 patients with intermittent claudication with age-matched controls free from symptoms of claudication. All patients with claudication were either current or former smokers. Among former smokers, the risk of developing peripheral arterial disease was 50 percent lower than that of current smokers.

Hughson, Mann, and Garrod (1978) reported risk factors for intermittent claudication among 54 patients and 108 controls. Smoking was the risk factor most strongly associated with the development of intermittent claudication. Former smokers had an estimated 58-percent lower risk than that of current smokers.

Smoking Cessation and Prognosis of Peripheral Artery Disease

In a study of 91 men with mild intermittent claudication monitored for at least 6 months, patients who stopped or decreased smoking had slightly less progression of symptoms during 2.5 years of followup, but this finding was not statistically significant (Cronenwett et al. 1984). Changes in treadmill exercise tolerance were assessed among 41 patients suffering from intermittent claudication who continued to smoke during the followup period and among 16 patients who stopped smoking after the first test and remained nonsmokers until the end of study (Quick and Cotton 1982). The maximum treadmill walking distance did not change significantly among continuing smokers (23 meter improvement, p=0.17). However, among those who stopped smoking, the improvement in maximum treadmill distance was statistically significant (86.2 meters, p=0.02). The two groups were not compared directly.

During a 6-year period, the risk of developing pain at rest was studied in 224 consecutive nondiabetic patients with intermittent claudication (Jonason and Ringgvist 1985). The cardiovascular risk profiles were almost identical for 30 never smokers and 34 patients who stopped smoking within 1 year after initial examination. These two groups were combined and compared with 160 patients who continued to smoke. The cumulative percentage of patients with pain at rest after 6 years was 8 percent among those who had stopped smoking within 1 year after the initial examination or who were never smokers; among smokers and those who stopped smoking more than 1 year after the initial examination, 21 percent developed pain at rest (p<0.03 after adjustments for difference in presence of multiple stenoses at baseline). These data are difficult to interpret because never and former smokers were combined, but suggest that the rate of development of rest pain is decreased among former and never smokers compared with those who continue to smoke.

In a followup study of 60 patients who underwent operation for intermittent claudication, those who stopped or reduced smoking after referral had a much improved prognosis (Hughson et al. 1978). At baseline, clinical characteristics or the number of cigarettes smoked did not differ between those patients who decreased or stopped smoking and those who continued to smoke during the followup period. The interval between initial and repeat operations was significantly shorter in those who continued to smoke (Mann-Whitney test, p<0.05). Those who stopped or reduced smoking attained a significant improvement in overall survival by 12 months. A second series of 160 patients was studied for 8 years after their first hospital admission. Those who were smoking at the time of referral had a significantly poorer survival pattern than those who had stopped smoking or had reduced smoking. Similar results were observed by Jonason and Bergström (1987) who studied 343 consecutive patients with intermittent claudication and by Faulkner, House, and Castleden (1983) who studied 133 patients.

A retrospective record review was undertaken at Mayo Clinic to identify nondiabetic patients with a clinical diagnosis of arteriosclerosis obliterans, and Juergens, Barker, and Hines (1960) reported the survival and amputation rates among these patients. Of 159 patients who smoked at the time of diagnosis and who survived 5 years, 88 continued to smoke and 71 abstained from smoking after diagnosis. Of the total number of patients who continued to smoke, 11.4 percent required an amputation within the 5-year period. In contrast, none of the abstainers required amputation during this period.

In a recent retrospective 5-year followup study, Ameli and colleagues (1989) reported the rates of amputation and patency of 136 arterial reconstructions performed for lower limb ischemia. Of 121 patients, 103 smoked before the operation, and of the smokers 43 postoperatively discontinued smoking. The 34 patients who continued to smoke more than 15 cigarettes per day had a fivefold increase in risk for amputation at 2 years and a threefold increase in risk for amputation at 5 years compared with the 87 nonsmokers (including never and former smokers) and smokers of 15 cigarettes or less per day (p=0.013). Five years after surgery, 28 percent of patients smoking more than 15 cigarettes per day had undergone amputation compared with 11 percent of the patients who were nonsmokers or smoked 15 cigarettes or less per day.

The effect of smoking on the patency of femoropopliteal vein bypass grafts used for treating peripheral arterial occlusion was studied among 157 patients monitored for 1 year (Wiseman et al. 1989). Patients who continued to smoke, identified by elevated serum SCN^-, had a graft patency of 63 percent after 1 year compared with 84 percent among nonsmokers (p<0.02). However, the analysis did not separate never smokers from those who stopped smoking near or at the time of surgery (p<0.02). Only serum fibrinogen levels were a stronger predictor of graft failure than serum SCN^-.

Summary

Overall, these studies show a lower risk of peripheral artery disease among former smokers compared with current smokers and a consistent reduction in complications of peripheral vascular disease among patients who stop smoking. Those who quit have improved performance and improved overall survival.

SMOKING CESSATION AND CEREBROVASCULAR DISEASE

Stroke is the third leading cause of death in the United States. It is also a major cause of morbidity, with approximately 400,000 Americans suffering strokes each year (Graves 1989). The two major types of stroke are ischemic strokes due to occlusion of a vessel by an embolus or thrombus and hemorrhagic strokes resulting from subarachnoid or parenchymal hemorrhage. The terms cerebrovascular accident and stroke are nonspecific and usually refer to clinical syndromes resulting from cerebral infarction or hemorrhage. A thrombotic or embolic stroke may be caused by atherosclerotic disease of the extra- or intracranial blood vessels. Embolization from the heart or extracranial arteries is also an important cause of stroke. In the Framingham Study, atherothrombotic brain infarction (referred to in this Chapter as ischemic stroke) accounted for 52.9 percent of strokes (Wolf et al. 1988). Improved diagnostic methods have provided a better categorization of the causes of stroke.

The 1964 Report of the Surgeon General (US PHS 1964) noted a moderate increase in the mortality rate from cerebrovascular disease in cigarette smokers compared with nonsmokers in the original ACS 9-State Study (Hammond and Horn 1958a,b) and the U.S. Veterans Study (Dorn 1959). In the 1971 Report, six major prospective epidemiologic studies were reviewed (US DHEW 1971). Cigarette smokers in these studies experienced increased stroke mortality compared with nonsmokers. The 1980 Report noted that women who smoke have an increased risk of subarachnoid hemorrhage (US DHHS 1980). The 1983 Report reviewed the data associating cigarette smoking with stroke and found an increased risk of stroke among smokers that was most evident among younger age groups (US DHHS 1983). It also noted that female cigarette smokers have an increased risk of subarachnoid hemorrhage and that the concurrent use of cigarettes and oral contraceptives greatly increased this risk.

The 1989 Report of the Surgeon General reviewed four additional large cohort studies that addressed the relation between cigarette smoking and risk of stroke and concluded that cigarette smoking is a cause of stroke (US DHHS 1989).

In a recent meta-analysis, Shinton and Beevers (1989) summarized the relation between cigarette smoking and stroke using 32 separate case–control and cohort studies. The overall relative risk of stroke associated with cigarette smoking was 1.5 (95-percent CI, 1.4–1.6). Relatve risks differed considerably for the subsets of stroke: cerebral infarction 1.9, cerebral hemorrhage 0.7, and subarachnoid hemorrhage 2.9. Relative risks decreased with increasing age; for persons less than 55 years of age, the relative risk was 2.9; for those aged 55 to 74 years, the relative risk was 1.8; and for those 75 years and older, the relative risk was 1.1. A dose–response relation was observed between the number of cigarettes smoked and risk of stroke, and women had a slightly greater relative risk than men (RR=1.72 vs. 1.43).

Based on the data from ACS CPS-II, the 1989 Report of the Surgeon General estimated that 51 percent of cerebrovascular disease deaths among men aged less than 65 years were attributable to cigarette smoking, and among women of the same age, 55 percent of cerebrovascular disease deaths were attributable to smoking (US DHHS 1989). For persons 65 years of age or older, 24 percent of cerebrovascular disease among men was attributable to smoking; among women, 6 percent was estimated to be attributable to smoking.

Studies of Smoking Cessation and Risk of Cerebrovascular Disease

In this Section, data from cross-sectional, case–control, prospective cohort, and intervention studies are reviewed. As discussed in Chapter 2, misclassification of former smokers because of recidivism during the followup period is a general concern in prospective studies. However, case–control studies of stroke are limited by the relatively high fatality rate for incident cerebrovascular events, particularly for subarachnoid hemorrhage. This often excludes many incident cases or forces the use of proxy information from next of kin or other relatives. In all epidemiologic studies of past smoking and risk of stroke, careful classification of stroke by pathophysiologic type is important. Details of the relation between past smoking and risk of stroke are presented in Tables 7 and 8 for each type of stroke reported by investigators.

Cross-Sectional Studies

In a cross-sectinal analysis of 1,692 black and white men and women admitted for diagnostic evaluation of the carotid arteries, Tell and coworkers (1989) reported a significant relation between cigarette smoking an the thickness of carotid artery plaque assessed using B-mode ultrasonography. Based on self-report, patients were characterized as either nonsmokers (never smoked or quit more than 10 years earlier), former smokers (quit between 10 years and 1 month earlier), or current smokers. After adjusting for a patient's age, race, sex, and history of diabetes mellitus and hypertension, the mean plaque scores differed significantly among the three smoking groups. The mean difference in plaque thickness compared with that which could be expected was –0.31 mm for nonsmokers, 0.04 mm for former smokers, and 0.32 mm for current smokers. The absolute difference in mean plaque scores between nonsmokers and current smokers was 0.63 mm (95-percent CI, 0.45–0.81 mm), between nonsmokers and former smokers, 0.35 mm (95-percent CI, 0.17–0.54 mm), and between former and current smokers, 0.27 mm (95-percent CI, 0.08–0.47 mm). These data suggest a slower rate of progression of atherosclerosis among persons who have quit smoking compared with those who continue to smoke.

In a cross-sectional study of cerebral blood flow levels in 268 neurologically normal volunteers, Rogers and coworkers (1985) observed that subjects who quit smoking had significantly higher cerebral perfusion levels than subjects who continued to smoke.

Case–Control Studies

Case–control studies addressing the relation between smoking and risk of stroke are summarized in Table 7. In many other published case–control studies, former smokers have not been specifically identified as a distinct exposure group. In those studies that identify former smokers, the number of cases has been very small or unspecified except for the study by Donnan and colleagues (1989). In several studies (Bell and Ambrose

TABLE 7.—Case–control studies of smoking cessation and risk of stroke

Reference	Source and case–control numbers	Outcome	Strokes among former smokers		Former smokers	Current smokers
					Relative risk as compared with never smokers[a]	
Bonita et al. (1986)	New Zealand: 132 cases; 1,586 community controls	Stroke, excluding subarachnoid hemorrhage	NR		1.4 (0.8–2.6)	2.4
Bonita (1986)	New Zealand: 115 cases; 1,586 community controls	Subarachnoid hemorrhage	NR		1.0 (0.5–1.9)	3.8
Bell and Ambrose (1982)	Scotland: 236 cases; general population control; (sample from survey by Tobacco Research Council)	73.3% of consecutive series with smoking data recorded		Men		
			10	Hemorrhage	0.19	0.16
			4	Infarction	0.14	0.88
			1	Hemorrhagic infarction	0.63	1.14
				Women		
			3	Hemorrhage	0.58	0.76
			1	Infarction	0.33	1.99
			0	Hemorrhagic infarction	NR	3.00
Taha, Ball, Illingworth (1982)	England: 178 cases, compared to UK population	Survived subarachnoid hemorrhage	7	Men	2.1[b]	4.7
			12	Women	1.5	2.6

TABLE 7.—Continued

Reference	Source and case–control numbers	Outcome	Strokes among former smokers		Relative risk as compared with never smokers[a]	
					Former smokers	Current smokers
Bell and Symon (1979)	England: 106 men, 1,628 women; general UK population 1965	Subarachnoid hemorrhage	NR	Men Women	1.92 2.52	3.89 3.72
Collaborative Group for the Study of Stroke in Young Women (1975)	US: 430 cases (15–44 yr); 429 hospital controls; 451 neighborhood controls	Thrombosis Hemorrhage	21 26		1.14 1.76	1.18 3.27
Donnan et al. (1989)	422 consecutive cases; 422 community controls	Cerebral ischemia	145	Quit <2 yr 2–5 yr 5–10 yr >10 yr	2.0 (1.3–3.1) 3.2 3.1 2.1 1.7	3.7

NOTE: NR=not reported.
[a]95% confidence interval shown in parentheses when available.
[b]Relative risk calculated from data presented in original paper.

1982; Taha, Ball, Illingworth 1982; Bell and Symon 1979), population smoking rates rather than a true concurrent control group were used for comparison purposes. Despite these limitations, the risk of stroke among former smokers has been consistently lower than that among current smokers. Data for subarachnoid hemorrhage (Bell and Symon 1979; Taha, Ball, Illingworth 1982) show a persistent elevation in risk among former smokers compared with never smokers; however, this risk is lower than among current smokers.

Prospective Cohort Studies

To date, a total of 14 prospective cohort studies have reported sufficient detail to categorize former smokers as a specific subgroup monitored for incidence of stroke. These studies have obtained information on smoking status at baseline through interview or self-administered questionnaire and have observed populations for 2 years (Nomura et al. 1974) to 26 years (Wolf et al. 1988). Other cohort studies have reported the relation between cigarette smoking and stroke but have not included sufficient details to categorize ex-smokers as a unique exposure group.

In each of the studies included in Table 7, the risks among former smokers and among current smokers are reported compared with the risk among never smokers. The earlier prospective studies tended not to show a positive relation between smoking and stroke, and in several studies, the risk among past smokers was higher than that among current smokers. In a multivariate analysis of data from the Whitehall Civil Servants Study (18,403 male British civil servants), the relative risk of stroke was 2.2 among current smokers of 15 cigarettes per day compared with never smokers, whereas the relative risk among former smokers was 1.5 (Fuller et al. 1983). Among British women, current smokers experienced a 3.0 relative risk of subarachnoid hemorrhage, and former smokers experienced a 2.3 relative risk (Vessey, Lawless, Yeates 1984). Lower elevations in risk were found among individuals experiencing ischemic strokes.

No excess risk of stroke was observed among 2,748 current or former smokers, residents of Cook County, IL (Ostfeld et al. 1974), or in 47,423 residents of Washington County, MD (Nomura et al. 1974). Doll and Peto (1976) studied 34,440 male British physicians for 20 years and updated information on cigarette smoking after 6 and 15 years. These researchers used similar methods for studying female British physicians among whom smoking status was updated after 10 years (Doll et al. 1980). Only slight elevations in risks of stroke were seen among male current or former smokers, and no excess risk was found among female current smokers. Similarly, Okada and colleagues (1976) found no significant elevation in risk of stroke among current or former smokers in a Japanese population.

In 14 cohort studies published after 1980, the relative risks among former smokers were lower than those reported for current smokers (Table 7). Rogot and Murray (1980) observed U.S. veterans and defined the population of former smokers as those who had stopped smoking for reasons other than a doctor's orders. These former smokers had a relative risk of 1.02; current smokers had a relative risk of 1.32.

In a study of 7,895 Hawaiian men of Japanese ancestry (Abbott et al. 1986), 658 smokers who quit in the first 6 years of followup were monitored for another 6 years;

their age-adjusted relative risk for total stroke was 1.5 compared with never smokers (95-percent CI, 1.0–2.3). Risks were similar for ischemic and hemorrhagic strokes. Concurrently, current smokers had a relative risk of 3.5 compared with never smokers. Former smokers had a significant reduction in risk of total stroke compared with current smokers (p<0.05). This analysis suggests that after adjusting for other risk factors, former smokers may be at increased risk of stroke. This residual risk may be due to the irreversibility or slow reversibility of the underlying mechanisms of smoking-attributable stroke, or the resumption of smoking among former smokers.

Welin and colleagues (1987) followed 789 men born in 1913 for 18.5 years. Smoking information was updated during a followup examination after 6 years. Investigators then identified a subgroup of former smokers who were monitored for 12 years. Among these former smokers, the relative risk of stroke was 1.18 compared with 1.67 for current smokers.

Wolf and coworkers (1988) studied 4,255 men and women in the Framingham Study and updated cigarette smoking information at 2-year intervals. Among current smokers, the relative risks of overall stroke were 1.42 for men and 1.61 for women. During the 26 years of followup, 50 percent of the normotensive smokers quit smoking compared with 44 percent of the hypertensive smokers (p<0.05). Former smokers had a significantly lower risk compared with current smokers. This relation was observed among men and women in each of the blood pressure categories. Benefits of smoking cessation were observed in the hypertensive and normotensive subjects.

In the Nurses Health Study, current smoking was strongly associated with risk of both subarachnoid hemorrhage and thromboembolic stroke (RR=10.3 and 3.1, respectively, for 25 cigarettes or more per day) (Colditz et al. 1988). The relative risks for former smokers were substantially lower.

As described in the 1989 Report of the Surgeon General, the relative risks of stroke for smokers showed an increase when CPS-II data from 1982 to 1986 were compared with CPS-I data from 1959 to 1965 (US DHHS 1989). These studies, using the same design and methods, showed an increase in the relative risk of death from stroke among current smokers for men aged 35 to 64 years from 1.79 in 1959–65 to 3.67 in 1982–86. For women of the same age, the relative risk increased from 1.92 to 4.80. The number of former smokers among women in CPS-I was too small to report these data separately. However, for males, the relative risk of stroke among former smokers has shown little increase and remained only slightly higher than among never smokers.

The reasons are unclear for the stronger associations between cigarette smoking and risk of stroke noted in more recent studies. However, this tendency for higher relative risks in the more recent studies has been documented for a wide variety of smoking-related diseases (US DHHS 1989). One likely explanation is that the effect of smoking is related to duration of smoking, and the cohorts of persons (especially women) who started smoking before age 20 are only now reaching middle and late adulthood (Garfinkel and Stellman 1988). Control of hypertension has improved in the United States during the last decade, and the incidence of stroke has declined. Thus, smoking may now play a relatively greater role in the etiology of this disease than it did in earlier periods when uncontrolled hypertension was more common.

Summary of Observational Studies

In a meta-analysis of cohort and case–control studies of cigarette smoking and stroke (Shinton and Beevers 1989), the overall relative risk of stroke among former smokers was 1.17 compared with never smokers (95-percent CI, 1.05–1.30). This estimate is based on a summary of 18 relative risks from 13 studies that separately identified former smokers (Kahn 1966; Doll and Peto 1976; Abbott et al. 1986; Colditz et al. 1988; Ostfeld et al. 1974; Kono et al. 1985; Khaw et al. 1984; Vessey, Lawless, Yeates 1984; Bell and Symon 1979; Bell and Ambrose 1982; Bonita et al. 1986; Bonita 1986; Taha, Ball, Illingworth 1982). As observed for the relation between current smoking and stroke, the risk among former smokers was greater when the analysis was repeated using only those studies with stroke occurring before age 75 (RR=1.47, 95-percent CI, 1.15–1.88 compared with never smokers). By comparison, the relative risks for current smokers were 2.9 for those younger than 55 years and 1.8 for persons aged 55 to 74 years. Thus, although a modest elevation in risk persisted among younger former smokers, this relative risk was substantially less than that which was observed among current smokers.

Intervention Studies

Intervention trials described above provide little direct evidence relating to change in risk of stroke after smoking cessation. Only the trial of smoking cessation conducted among 1,445 British men used a single intervention (Rose et al. 1982). During 10 years of followup, five men in the normal care group died because of stroke, and seven men in the intervention group died because of stroke. The small numbers in each group and the small difference in smoking cessation rates between the intervention and control groups limit any conclusion regarding the impact of smoking cessation in this population.

Other intervention studies have included management of hypertension and cholesterol as well as smoking cessation programs. As discussed under randomized trials of smoking cessation and CHD, these multiple interventions make drawing conclusions difficult regarding the relation between smoking cessation and risk of stroke (Steinbach et al. 1984; Wilhelmsen et al. 1986; MRFIT Research Group 1982, 1986; Salonen, Puska, Mustaniemi 1979; Hjermann 1980; Holme 1982).

In a nonrandomized intervention, Rogers and colleagues (1985) measured changes in cerebral artery blood flow among volunteers who were encouraged to abstain from cigarettes. Cerebral perfusion was improved after smoking abstinence.

Influence of Prior Levels of Smoking

Using data from the followup of 248,046 U.S. veterans monitored for 15 years, Rogot and Murray (1980) reported the mortality ratio for stroke among former cigarette smokers who stopped smoking for reasons other than a physician's orders according to the level of prior cigarette smoking. Based on 1,279 strokes among past smokers, the mortality ratio for stroke among former smokers relative to never smokers increased with higher previous daily cigarette consumption from 0.94 for those smoking less than 10 cigarettes per day to 1.34 for those smoking 40 cigarettes or more per day compared with never smokers (Figure 7). Data from ACS CPS-II also address this relationship (Table 8). Within each level of previous smoking, the risk of stroke was clearly lower for former smokers than for continuing smokers, except among men who smoked 21 cigarettes or more per day. Other studies have had too few former smokers to classify them according to previous number of cigarettes smoked.

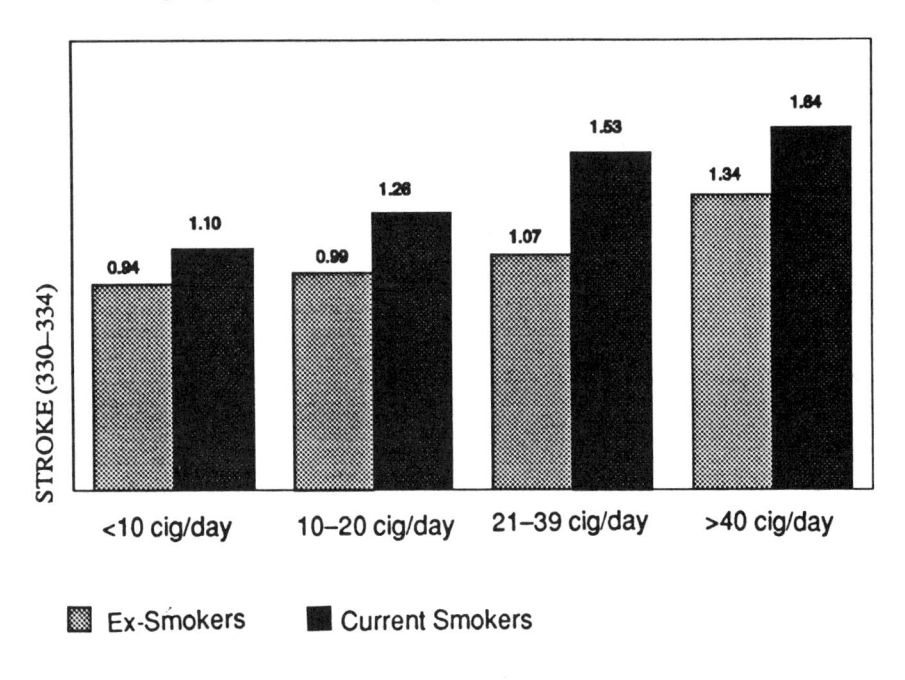

FIGURE 7.—Mortality ratios for stroke for current smokers and ex-smokers compared with never smokers, by daily cigarette consumption, US Veterans Study, 1954–69

SOURCE: Adapted from Rogot and Murray (1980).

Effect of Duration of Abstinence

The relation between duration of abstinence and risk of stroke has been addressed in only a few studies. In a case–control study that included 145 former smokers who suffered stroke, Donnan and coworkers (1989) observed that the relative risk of stroke declined monotonically over the 10 years following quitting; at the end of 10 years, a significant excess risk of stroke was still evident.

Using 5-year intervals, Rogot and Murray (1980) reported the mortality ratios for those who had abstained. Assuming that an individual classified as a former smoker at the beginning of the study would remain a former smoker throughout the 15 years of

TABLE 8.—Prospective cohort studies of smoking cessation and risk of stroke

Reference	Population	Followup	Cases among former smokers	Outcome	Former smokers	Current smokers
Ostfeld et al. (1974)	2,748 Cook County, IL residents receiving old age assistance aged 65–74	3 yr	23	All strokes	0.91[b]	1–9 cig/day: 1.29 10–19 cig/day: 0.85 ≥20 cig/day: 0.81
Nomura et al. (1974)	47,423 Washington County, MD residents	2 yr morbidity	27 (men)	Thrombosis Hemorrhage Undifferentiated Total	1.03[b] 0.79 1.00 0.97	0.79 0.86 1.30 0.90
			8 (women)	Thrombosis Hemorrhage Undifferentiated Total	1.08 2.00 1.14 1.26	1.14 0.91 0.36 0.92
Doll and Peto (1976)	British physicians: 34,440 men	20 yr	NR	Cerebral thrombosis mortality	1.22	1.24
Okada et al. (1976)	4,186 Japanese	6 yr	NR	Cerebrovascular attacks	Relative risk of cerebral hemorrhage in nonsmokers was lower than in smokers or ex-smokers, but the difference was not statistically significant

[a] Relative risk compared with never smokers

TABLE 8.—Continued

Reference	Population	Followup	Cases among former smokers	Outcome	Former smokers	Current smokers
Doll et al. (1980)	British physicians: 6,194 women	22 yr	NR	Death due to cerebral thrombosis	1.18	1–14 cig/day: 0.93 14–24 cig/day: 0.45 ≥25 cig/day: 0.19
Rogot and Murray (1980)	US veterans: 248,046 men	15 yr	1,279	Stroke ICD 330–343 (7th revision)	1.02	1.32
Fuller et al. (1983)	Whitehall civil servants: 18,403 men aged 40–64	10 yr	34	Stroke mortality	1.52	1–9 cig/day: 1.0[c] 10–19 cig/day: 2.0 ≥20 cig/day: 2.3
Vessey, Lawless, Yeates (1984)	17,000 UK women aged 25–39	10–16 yr	2 4	Subarachnoid Nonhemorrhagic	2.3[b] 1.3	3.0 1.4
Abbott et al. (1986)	Honolulu Heart Study: 7,895 men of Japanese origin; 658 smokers who quit in first 6 yr	12 yr; 6 yr	11 3	Thromboembolic Hemorrhagic Total	1.6 (0.7–3.8) 1.8 (0.4–9.0) 1.5 (1.0–2.3)	3.00 6.10 3.50
Welin et al. (1987)	789 men living in Gothenburg, 678 examined	18.5 yr; 11 yr	NR	Excluded subarachnoid hemorrhage	1.18[b]	1.67
Carstensen, Pershagen, Eklund (1987)	25,159 Swedes	16 yr	124	Cerebrovascular mortality ICD 430–438	1.10	1–7 g/day: 0.9 8–15 g/day: 0.9 >15 g/day: 1.1

Relative risk compared with never smokers[a]

TABLE 8.—Continued

Reference	Population	Followup	Cases among former smokers	Outcome	Former smokers	Current smokers
					Relative risk compared with never smokers[a]	
Wolf et al. (1988)	Framingham Study: 4,255 men and women	26 yr	N/A	Stroke and transient ischemic attack	Risk significantly lower than that of current smokers	Men: 1.42 stroke 1.56 brain infarction Women: 1.61 stroke 1.86 brain infarction
Colditz et al. (1988)	Nurses Health Study: 118,539 US women aged 30–55	8 yr	65	Subarachnoid hemorrhage	3.0 (1.3–6.6)	1–14 cig/day: 4.3 15–24 cig/day: 5.1 ≥25 cig/day: 10.3
				Thromboembolic stroke	1.3 (0.7–6.6)	1–14 cig/day: 1.8 15–24 cig/day: 3.2 ≥25 cig/day: 3.1
				Total stroke	1.5 (1.1–2.2)	1–14 cig/day: 2.5 15–24 cig/day: 2.9 ≥25 cig/day: 3.8
US DHHS (1989)	ACS CPS-I (25-State Study)	6 yr (1959–65)	NR		Men[d] 35–64 yr: 1.02 (0.83–1.25)[a] ≥65 yr: 0.93 (0.80–1.08)[a]	1.79 (1.55–2.08)[a] 1.15 (1.02–1.30)[a]

TABLE 8.—Continued

Reference	Population	Followup	Cases among former smokers	Outcome	Relative risk compared with never smokers[a]		
						Former smokers	Current smokers
ACS (unpublished tabulations)	ACS CPS-II (50-State Study)[e]	4 yr (1982-86)	NR	Mortality due to cerebrovascular disease	Men <21 cig/day		
					Quit <1 yr	3.94	2.43
					1–2 yr	1.11	
					3–5 yr	1.55	
					6–10 yr	1.64	
					11–15 yr	0.62	
					≥16 yr	0.72	
					Men ≥21 cig/day		
					Quit <1 yr	0.37	2.07
					1–2 yr	1.43	
					3–5 yr	1.39	
					6–10 yr	2.27	
					11–15 yr	2.34	
					≥16 yr	1.92	
					Women <20 cig/day		
					Quit <1 yr	NR	1.77
					1–2 yr	1.92	
					3–5 yr	0.79	
					6–10 yr	0.59	
					11–15 yr	1.23	
					≥16 yr	0.93	

TABLE 8.—Continued

Reference	Population	Followup	Cases among former smokers	Outcome	Relative risk compared with never smokers[a]		
						Former smokers	Current smokers
ACS (unpublished tabulations) (continued)					Women ≥20 cig/day		2.33
					Quit <1 yr	0.29	
					1–2 yr	0.51	
					3–5 yr	0.71	
					6–10 yr	0.84	
					11–15 yr	0.23	
					≥16 yr	0.73	

NOTE: N/A=not applicable; ACS CPS-I and -II=American Cancer Society Cancer Prevention Studies I and II; NR=not reported; ICD=International Classification of Disease.
[a]95% confidence interval shown in parentheses when available.
[b]Relative risk calculated from data presented in original paper.
[c]Relative risk reported by Shinton and Beevers (1989)
[d]Data for women former smokers not presented separately.
[e]Excluding those with a history of cancer, heart disease, or stroke at enrollment.

followup, these investigators reported mortality ratios close to 1.0 for all durations except for 5 to 9 years after quitting.

Based on 26 years of studying 4,255 men and women in the Framingham Study (Wolf et al. 1988), the risk of stroke among persons who stopped was significantly lower than that among persons who continued to smoke cigarettes. Furthermore, persons who quit smoking developed stroke at the rate of never smokers soon after discontinuing cigarette smoking (Figure 8). Wolf and coworkers (1988) estimated that the risk of stroke among smokers had decreased significantly 2 years after quitting and reverted to the level of never smokers within 5 years. These results persisted after controlling for age, blood pressure, serum cholestrol level, relative weight, left ventricular hypertrophy on electrocardiogram, and blood glucose level. Thus, the reduction in risk after smoking cessation is not attributable to differences in other risk factors for stroke between those who quit and those who continue to smoke.

In the Nurses Health Study (Colditz et al. 1988), a lower risk of stroke was observed with increasing time from cessation. Compared with the risk among never smokers, the relative risk was 2.6 among women who had stopped for less than 2 years (95-percent CI, 1.4–4.7). However, among women who had stopped for 2 years or more, the relative risk was reduced to 1.4 (95-percent CI, 1.0–2.0). Women currently smoking 15 to 24 cigarettes per day had a relative risk of 2.9 compared with never smokers. Again, the elevation of the relative risk during the first 2 years after cessation is consistent with high recidivism among these women.

Prospective data from ACS CPS-II showed that among men who quit smoking, the risk of stroke returned to that of never smokers after 11 years or more of smoking abstinence for those originally smoking fewer than 21 cigarettes per day. However, for men who previously smoked 21 cigarettes or more per day, the risk among former smokers did not return to the level of never smokers, even after 16 years or more of cessation. Among women who quit, the rate of decrease was much more rapid; by 3 to 5 years after cessation, the risk of stroke was similar to that of never smokers (Table 8).

Oral Contraceptives and Smoking Cessation

In two studies the risk of subarachnoid hemorrhage was augmented among cigarette smokers who also take oral contraceptives (Petitti and Wingerd 1978; Collaborative Group for the Study of Stroke in Young Women 1975). In the Collaborative Group Study of stroke among young women (1975), the category of former smokers was not clearly defined; rather, a group of "once regular smokers" was compared with "never regular smokers." In this study there was no association between current smoking or former smoking and risk of thrombotic stroke. Overall, the relative risk for hemorrhagic stroke was 1.8 among once regular smokers and 3.3 among current smokers. Within the group of once regular smokers, women currently using oral contraceptives had approximately twice the risk compared with women not using oral contraceptives. The Royal College of General Practitoners study of oral contraceptives did not separate former smokers from never smokers (Layde, Beral, Kay 1981). Hence, data to address the relationship among oral contraceptives, smoking cessation, and risk of subarachnoid

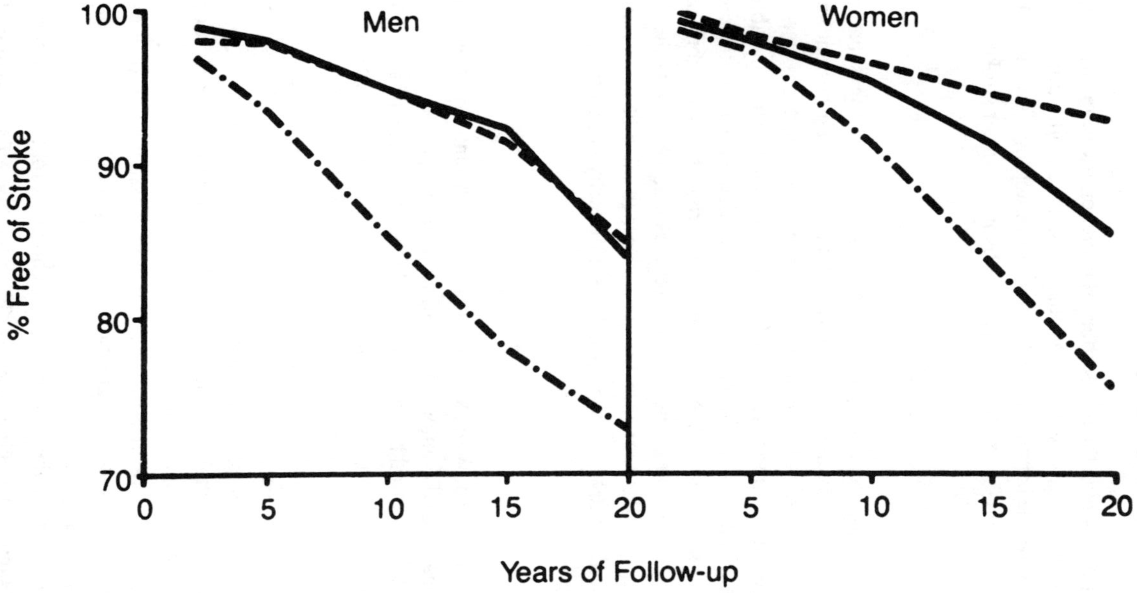

FIGURE 8.—Survival free of stroke in cigarette smokers (dotted line), never smokers (solid line), and former smokers (dashed line), aged 60, using Cox proportional hazard regression model, among men and women

SOURCE: Wolf et al. (1988).

hemorrhage are not available from that study. Because oral contraceptive preparations used today provide substantially lower doses, the risk of cardiovascular disease associated with their use and their interaction with cigarette smoking may be different than observed for the early high-dose preparations.

Effect of Smoking Cessation After Stroke

In contrast with CHD, in which the focus after MI is prevention of recurrent disease, the center of attention after a major cerebrovascular event is rehabilitation. For CHD, substantial evidence shows the benefits of abstaining from smoking after onset of CHD. Comparable data are not available on the benefits of abstinence after stroke.

Summary

Risk of stroke resulting from occlusion of the cerebral arteries and from subarachnoid hemorrhage is increased approximately twofold to fourfold among current smokers compared with never smokers. After cessation, the excess risk decreases steadily. In some studies, the risk of stroke among former smokers becomes indistinguishable from that of never smokers within 5 years; in other studies, this decrease did not occur until after 10 years or more of smoking abstinence. The reduced risk of stroke among persons who stop smoking is independent of the amount previously smoked and other known risk factors for stroke. Similar reductions in risk of stroke after cessation are seen among men and women, but few data are available for minority populations.

CONCLUSIONS

1. Compared with continued smoking, smoking cessation substantially reduces risk of coronary heart disease (CHD) among men and women of all ages.
2. The excess risk of CHD caused by smoking is reduced by about half after 1 year of smoking abstinence and then declines gradually. After 15 years of abstinence, the risk of CHD is similar to that of persons who have never smoked.
3. Among persons with diagnosed CHD, smoking cessation markedly reduces the risk of recurrent infarction and cardiovascular death. In many studies, this reduction in risk of recurrence or premature death has been 50 percent or more.
4. Smoking cessation substantially reduces the risk of peripheral artery occlusive disease compared with continued smoking.
5. Among patients with peripheral artery disease, smoking cessation improves exercise tolerance, reduces the risk of amputation after peripheral artery surgery, and increases overall survival.
6. Smoking cessation reduces the risk of both ischemic stroke and subarachnoid hemorrhage compared with continued smoking. After smoking cessation, the risk of stroke returns to the level of never smokers; in some studies this has occurred within 5 years, but in others as long as 15 years of abstinence were required.

References

ABBOTT, R.D., YIN, Y., REED, D.M., YANO, K. Risk of stroke in male cigarette smokers. *New England Journal of Medicine* 315(12):717–720, September 18, 1986.

ABERG, A., BERGSTRAND, R., JOHANSSON, S., ULVENSTAM, G., VEDIN, A., WEDEL, H., WILHELMSSON, C., WILHELMSEN, L. Cessation of smoking after myocardial infarction. Effects on mortality after 10 years. *British Heart Journal* 49(5):416–422, May 1983.

ALLRED, E.N., BLEECKER, E.R., CHAITMAN, B.R., DAHMS, T.E., GOTTLIEB, S.O., HACKNEY, J.D., PAGANO, M., SELVESTER, R.H., WALDEN, S.M., WARREN, J. Short-term effects of carbon monoxide exposure on the exercise performance of subjects with coronary artery disease. *New England Journal of Medicine* 321(21):1426–1432, November 23, 1989.

AMELI, F.M., STEIN, M., PROVAN, J.L., PROSSER, R. The effect of postoperative smoking on femoropopliteal bypass grafts. *Annals of Vascular Surgery* 3(1):20–25, January 1989.

AMERICAN CANCER SOCIETY. Cancer Prevention Study II. Unpublished tabulations.

ASMUSSEN, I., KJELDSEN, K. Intimal ultrastructure of human umbilical arteries. Observations on arteries from newborn children of smoking and nonsmoking mothers. *Circulation Research* 36(5):579–589, May 1975.

ASSMANN, G., SCHULTE, H., SCHRIEWER, H. The effects of cigarette smoking on serum levels of HDL cholesterol and HDL apolipoprotein A-I. *Journal of Clinical Chemistry and Clinical Biochemistry* 22(6):397–402, June 1984.

AUERBACH, O., CARTER, H.W., GARFINKEL, L., HAMMOND, E.C. Cigarette smoking and coronary artery disease. A macroscopic and microscopic study. *Chest* 70(6):697–705, December 1976.

BALLEISEN, J., BAILEY, J., EPPING, P.H., SCHULTE, H., VAN DE LOO, J. Epidemiological study on Factor VII, Factor VIII and fibrinogen in an industrial population: I. Baseline data on the relation to age, gender, body-weight, smoking, alcohol, pill-using, and menopause. *Thrombosis and Haemostasis* 54(2):475–479, August 1985.

BARRY, J., MEAD, K., NABEL, E.G., ROCCO, M.B., CAMPBELL, S., FENTON, T., MUDGE, G.H. JR., SELWYN, A.P. Effect of smoking on the activity of ischemic heart disease. *Journal of the American Medical Association* 261(3):398–402, January 20, 1989.

BELCH, J.J.F., MCARDLE, B.M., BURNS, P., LOWE, G.D.O., FORBES, C.D. The effects of acute smoking on platelet behaviour, fibrinolysis and haemorheology in habitual smokers. *Thrombosis and Haemostasis* 51(1):6–8, February 28, 1984.

BELL, B.A., AMBROSE, J. Smoking and the risk of a stroke. *Acta Neurochirurgica* 64(1–2):1–7, 1982.

BELL, B.A., SYMON, L. Smoking and subarachnoid haemorrhage. *British Medical Journal* 1(6163):577–578, March 3, 1979.

BLANKENHORN, D.H., NESSIM, S.A., JOHNSON, R.L., SANMARCO, M.E., AZEN, S.P., CASHILL-HEMPHILL, L. Beneficial effects of combined colestipol-niacin therapy on coronary atherosclerosis and coronary venous bypass grafts. *Journal of the American Medical Association* 257(23):3233–3240, June 19, 1987.

BONITA, R. Cigarette smoking, hypertension and the risk of subarachnoid hemorrhage: A population-based case–control study. *Stroke* 17(5): 831–835, September–October 1986.

BONITA, R., SCRAGG, R., STEWART, A., JACKSON, R., BEAGLEHOLE, R. Cigarette smoking and risk of premature stroke in men and women. *British Medical Journal* 293(6538): 6–8, July 1986.

CARSTENSEN, J.M., PERSHAGEN, G., EKLUND, G. Mortality in relation to cigarette and pipe smoking: 16 years' observation of 25,000 Swedish men. *Journal of Epidemiology and Community Health* 41:166–172, 1987.

CEDERLOF, R., FRIBERG, L., HRUBEC, Z., LORICH, U. *The relationship of smoking and some social covariables to mortality and cancer morbidity. A ten year follow-up in a probability sample of 55,000 Swedish subjects age 18–69, Part 1/2.* Stockholm, Sweden: Karolinska Institute, Department of Environmental Hygiene, 1975.

CLARKSON, T.B., BOND, M.G., BULLOCK, B.C., MCLAUGHLIN, K.J., SAWYER, J.K. A study of atherosclerosis regression in Macaca mulatta. V. Changes in abdominal aorta and carotid and coronary arteries from animals with atherosclerosis induced for 38 months and then regressed for 24 to 48 months at plasma cholesterol concentrations of 300 or 200 mg/dL. *Experimental and Molecular Pathology* 41(1):96–118, August 1984.

COLDITZ, G.A., BONITA, R., STAMPFER, M.J., WILLETT, W.C., ROSNER, B., SPEIZER, F.E., HENNEKENS, C.H. Cigarette smoking and risk of stroke in middle-aged women. *New England Journal of Medicine* 318(15):937–941, April 14, 1988.

COLLABORATIVE GROUP FOR THE STUDY OF STROKE IN YOUNG WOMEN. Oral contraceptives and stroke in young women. Associated risk factors. *Journal of the American Medical Association* 231(7):718–722, February 17, 1975.

COOK, D.G., POCOCK, S.J., SHAPER, A.G., KUSSICK, S.J. Giving up smoking and the risk of heart attacks. A report from the British Regional Heart Study. *Lancet* 2(8520):1376–1380, December 13, 1986.

CRIQUI, M.H., BROWNER, D., FRONEK, A., KLAUBER, M.R., COUGHLIN, S.S., BARRETT-CONNOR, E., GABRIEL, S. Peripheral arterial disease in large vessels is epidemiologically distinct from small vessel disease. An analysis of risk factors. *American Journal of Epidemiology* 129(6):1110–1119, June 1989.

CRONENWETT, J.L., WARNER, K.G., ZELENOCK, G.B., WHITEHOUSE, W.M. JR., GRAHAM, L.M., LINDENAUER, S.M., STANLEY, J.C. Intermittent claudication: Current results of nonoperative management. *Archives of Surgery* 119(4):430–436, April 1984.

DALY, L.E., GRAHAM, I.M., HICKEY, N., MULCAHY, R. Does stopping smoking delay onset of angina after infarction? *British Medical Journal* 291(6500):935–937, October 5, 1985.

DALY, L.E., HICKEY, N., GRAHAM, I.M., MULCAHY, R. Predictors of sudden death up to 18 years after a first attack of unstable angina or myocardial infarction. *British Heart Journal* 58(6):567–571, December 1987.

DALY, L.E., MULCAHY, R., GRAHAM, I.M., HICKEY, N. Long term effect on mortality of stopping smoking after unstable angina and myocardial infarction. *British Medical Journal* 287(6388):324–326, July 30, 1983.

DAVIS, J.W., SHELTON, L., EIGENBERG, D.A., HIGNITE, C.E., WATANABE, I.S.. Effects of tobacco and non-tobacco cigarette smoking on endothelium and platelets. *Clinical Pharmacology and Therapeutics* 37(5):529–533, May 1985.

DAVIS, J.W., SHELTON, L., HARTMAN, C.R., ET AL. Smoking-induced changes in endothelium and platelets are not affected by hydroxyethylrutosides. *British Journal of Experimental Pathology* 67(5):765–771, October 1986.

DE LORGERIL, M., REINHARZ, A., BUSSLINGER, B., REBER, G., RIGHETTI, A. Acute influence of cigarette smoke in platelets, catecholamines and neurophysins in the normal conditions of daily life. *European Heart Journal* 6(12):1063–1068, December 1985.

DE PARSCAU, L., FIELDING, C. Abnormal plasma cholesterol metabolism in cigarette smokers. *Metabolism* 35(11):1070–1073, November 1986.

DEWOOD, M.A., SPORES, J., NOTSKE, R., MOUSER, L.T., BURROUGHS, R., GOLDEN, M.S., LANG, H.T. Prevalence of total coronary occlusion during the early hours of transmural myocardial infarction. *New England Journal of Medicine* 303(16):897–902, October 16, 1980.

DOLL, R., GRAY, R., HAFNER, B., PETO, R. Mortality in relation to smoking: 22 years' observations on female British doctors. *British Medical Journal* 280(6219):967–971, April 5, 1980.

DOLL, R., HILL, A.B. The mortality of doctors in relation to their smoking habits. A preliminary report. *British Medical Journal* 1(4877):1451–1455, June 26, 1954.

DOLL, R., HILL, A.B. Lung cancer and other causes of death in relation to smoking. A second report on the mortality of British doctors. *British Medical Journal* 2:1071–1081, November 10, 1956.

DOLL, R., HILL, A.B. Mortality in relation to smoking: Ten years' observations of British doctors. *British Medical Journal* 1:1460–1467, June 6, 1964.

DOLL, R., PETO, R. Mortality in relation to smoking: 20 years' observations on male British doctors. *British Medical Journal* 2:1525–1536, December 25, 1976.

DONNAN, G.A., ADENA, M.A., O'MALLEY, H.M., MCNEIL, J.S., DOYLE, A.E., NEILL, G.C. Smoking as a risk factor for cerebral ischaemia. *Lancet* 2(8664):643–647, September 16, 1989.

DORN, H.F. Tobacco consumption and mortality from cancer and other diseases. *Public Health Reports* 74(7):581–593, July 1959.

DOTEVALL, A., KUTTI, J., TEGER-NILSSON, A.C., WADENVIK, H., WILHELMSEN, L. Platelet reactivity, fibrinogen and smoking. *European Journal of Haematology* 38(1):55–59, January 1987.

DOWNEY, H.F., BASHOUR, C.A., BOUTROS, I.S., BASHOUR, F.A., PARKER, P.E. Regional myocardial blood flow during nicotine infusion: Effects of beta adrenergic blockade and acute coronary artery occlusion. *Journal of Pharmacology and Experimental Therapeutics* 202(1):55–68, July 1977.

DOYLE, J.T., DAWBER, T.R., KANNEL, W.B., HESLIN, A.S., KAHN, H.A. Cigarette smoking and coronary heart disease. Combined experience of the Albany and Framingham studies. *New England Journal of Medicine* 266(16):796–801, April 19, 1962.

DOYLE, J.T., DAWBER, T.R., KANNEL, W.B., KINCH, S.H., KAHN, H.A. The relationship of cigarette smoking to coronary heart disease. *Journal of the American Medical Association* 190(10):108–112, December 7, 1964.

ERNST, E., MATRAI, A. Abstention from chronic cigarette smoking normalizes blood rheology. *Atherosclerosis* 64(1):75–77, March 1987.

FAULKNER, K.W., HOUSE, A.K., CASTLEDEN, W.M. The effect of cessation of smoking on the accumulative survival rates of patients with symptomatic peripheral vascular disease. *Medical Journal of Australia* 1(5):217–219, March 5, 1983.

FISCHER, S., BERNUTZ, C., MEIER, H., WEBER, P.C. Formation of prostacyclin and thromboxane in man as measured by the main urinary metabolites. *Biochimica et Biophysica Acta* 876(2):194–199, April 15, 1986.

FITZGERALD, G.A., OATES, J.A., NOWAK, J. Cigarette smoking and hemostatic function. *American Heart Journal* 115:267–271, 1988.

FLECK, E., REGITZ, V., LEHNERT, A., DACIAN, S., DIRSCHINGER, J., RUDOLPH, W. Restenosis after balloon dilatation of coronary stenosis, multivariate analysis of potential risk factors. *European Heart Journal* 9(Supplement C):15–18, March 1988.

FLODERUS, B., CEDERLOF, R., FRIBERG, L. Smoking and mortality: A 21-year follow-up based on the Swedish Twin Registry. *International Journal of Epidemiology* 17(2):332–340, June 1988.

FOLTS, J.D., BONEBRAKE, F.C. The effects of cigarette smoke and nicotine on platelet thrombus formation in stenosed dog coronary arteries: Inhibition with phentolamine. *Circulation* 65(3):465–470, March 1982.

FORTMANN, S.P., HASKELL, W.L., WILLIAMS, P.T. Changes in plasma high density lipoprotein cholesterol after changes in cigarette use. *American Journal of Epidemiology* 124(4):706–710, October 1986.

FREEDMAN, D.S., SRINIVASAN, S.R., SHEAR, C.L., HUNTER, S.M., CROFT, J.B., WEBBER, L.S., BERENSON, G.S. Cigarette smoking initiation and longitudinal changes in serum lipids and lipoproteins in early adulthood: The Bogalusa Heart Study. *American Journal of Epidemiology* 124(2):207–219, August 1986.

FREEDMAN, D.S., SRINIVASAN, S.R., SHEAR, C.L., WEBBER, L.S., CHIANG, Y.K., BERENSON, G.S. Correlates of high density lipoprotein cholesterol and apolipoprotein A-I levels in children. The Bogalusa Heart Study. *Arteriosclerosis* 7(4):354–360, July–August 1987.

FRIED, L.P., MOORE, R.D., PEARSON, T.A. Long-term effects of cigarette smoking and moderate alcohol consumption on coronary artery diameter. Mechanisms of coronary artery disease independent of atherosclerosis or thrombosis? *American Journal of Medicine* 80(1):37–44, January 1986.

FRIEDMAN, G.D., DALES, L.G., URY, H.K. Mortality in middle-aged smokers and nonsmokers. *New England Journal of Medicine* 300(5):213–217, February 1, 1979.

FRIEDMAN, G.D., PETITTI, D.B., BAWOL, R.D., SIEGELAUB, A.B. Mortality in cigarette smokers and quitters. Effect of base-line differences. *New England Journal of Medicine* 304(23):1407–1410, June 4, 1981.

FRIEDMAN, G.D., SIEGELAUB, A.B., DALES, L.G., SELTZER, C.C. Characteristics predictive of coronary heart disease in ex-smokers before they stopped smoking: Comparison with persistent smokers and nonsmokers. *Journal of Chronic Diseases* 32:175–190, 1979.

FULLER, J.H., SHIPLEY, M.J., ROSE, G., JARRETT, R.J., KEEN, H. Mortality from coronary heart disease and stroke in relation to degree of glycaemia: The Whitehall Study. *British Medical Journal* 287(6396):867–870, September 24, 1983.

FUSTER, V., CHESEBRO, J.H., FRYE, R.L., ELVEBACK, L.R. Platelet survival and the development of coronary artery disease in the young adult: Effects of cigarette smoking, strong family history and medical therapy. *Circulation* 63(3):546–551, March 1981.

GALAN, K.M., DELIGONUL, U., KERN, M.J., CHAITMAN, B.R., VANDORMAEL, M.G. Increased frequency of restenosis in patients continuing to smoke cigarettes after percutaneous transluminal coronary angioplasty. *American Journal of Cardiology* 61:260–263, 1988.

GALEA, G., DAVIDSON, R.J.L. Haematological and haemorheological changes associated with cigarette smoking. *Journal of Clinical Pathology* 38(9):978–984, September 1985.

GARFINKEL, L., STELLMAN, S.D. Smoking and lung cancer in women: Findings in a prospective study. *Cancer Research* 48(23):6951–6955, December 1, 1988.

GOLDBERG, R., SZKLO, M., CHANDRA, V. The effect of cigarette smoking on the long-term prognosis of myocardial infarction. *American Journal of Epidemiology* 114(3):431, September 1981.

GOLDBOURT, U., YAARI, S., COHEN-MANDELZWEIG, L., NEUFELD, H.N. High-density lipoprotein cholesterol: Correlation with biochemical, anthropometric, behavioral, and clinical parameters in 6,500 Israeli men. *Preventive Medicine* 15(6):569–581, November 1986.

GOMO, Z.A.R. The effect of age, sex, alcohol consumption and cigarette smoking on serum concentrations of lipids and apolipoproteins in Zimbabwean blacks. *Atherosclerosis* 61(2):149–154, August 1986.

GORDON, T., DOYLE, J.T. Alcohol consumption and its relationship to smoking, weight, blood pressure, and blood lipids. The Albany Study. *Archives of Internal Medicine* 146(2):262–265, February 1986.

GORDON, T., KANNEL, W.B., MCGEE, D. Death and coronary attacks in men after giving up cigarette smoking. *Lancet* 2(7893):1345–1348, December 7, 1974.

GRAVES, E.J. National Hospital Discharge Survey. *Vital and Health Statistics* Series 13(99):1–60, April 1989.

GREEN, K.G. Does stopping smoking delay onset of angina after infarction? (Letter.) *British Medical Journal* 291(6504):1281, November 2, 1985.

GREEN, K.G. Falsely favourable early prognosis for continuing smokers following recovery from acute myocardial infarction. Information from the multi-centre practolol trial. *British Journal of Clinical Practice* 41(6):785–788, June 1987.

GRIMM, R.H. JR. The drug treatment of mild hypertension in the Multiple Risk Factor Intervention Trial. A review. *Drugs* 31(Supplement 1):13–21, 1986.

HAAPANEN, A., KOSKENVUO, M., KAPRIO, J., KESANIEMI, Y.A., HEIKKILA, K. Carotid arteriosclerosis in identical twins discordant for cigarette smoking. *Circulation* 80(1):10–16, July 1989.

HALLSTROM, A.P., COBB, L.A., RAY, R. Smoking as a risk factor for recurrence of sudden cardiac arrest. *New England Journal of Medicine* 314(5):271–275, 1986.

HAMMOND, E.C., GARFINKEL, L. Coronary heart disease, stroke, and aortic aneurysm. Factors in etiology. *Archives of Environmental Health* 19:167–182, August 1969.

HAMMOND, E.C., HORN, D. Smoking and death rates—Report on forty-four months of follow-up of 187,783 men. I. Total mortality. *Journal of the American Medical Association* 166(10):1159–1172, March 8, 1958a.

HAMMOND, E.C., HORN, D. Smoking and death rates—Report on forty-four months of follow-up of 187,783 men. II. Death rates by cause. *Journal of the American Medical Association* 166(11):1294–1308, March 15, 1958b.

HARENBERG, J., STAIGER, C., DE VRIES, J.X., WEBER, E., ZIMMERMAN, R., SCHETTLER, G. The effects of a combination of cigarette smoking and oral contraception on coagulation and fibrinolysis in human females. *Klinische Wochenschrift* 63(5):221–224, March 1, 1985.

HARTZ, A.J., ANDERSON, A.J., BROOKS, H.L., MANLEY, J.C., PARENT, G.T., BARBORIAK, J.J. The association of smoking with cardiomyopathy. *New England Journal of Medicine* 311(19):1201–1206, November 8, 1984.

HARTZ, A.J., BARBORIAK, P.N., ANDERSON, A.J., HOFFMANN, R.G., BARBORIAK, J.J. Smoking, coronary artery occlusion, and nonfatal myocardial infarction. *Journal of the American Medical Association* 246(8):851–853, August 21, 1981.

HEDBACK, B., PERK, J. 5-year results of a comprehensive rehabilitation programme after myocardial infarction. *European Heart Journal* 8(3):234–242, March 1987.

HENNEKENS, C.H., LOWN, B., ROSNER, B., GRUFFERMAN, S., DALEN, J. Ventricular premature beats and coronary risk factors. *American Journal of Epidemiology* 112(1):93–99, July 1980.

HERMANSON, B., OMENN, G.S., KRONMAL, R.A., GERSH, B.J. Beneficial six-year outcome of smoking cessation in older men and women with coronary artery disease: Results from the CASS Registry. *New England Journal of Medicine* 319(21):1365–1369, November 24, 1988.

HJERMANN, I. Smoking and diet intervention in healthy coronary high risk men. Methods and 5-year follow-up of risk factors in a randomized trial. The Oslo Study. *Journal of the Oslo City Hospitals* 30(1):3–17, January 1980.

HJERMANN, I., HOLME, I., LEREN, P. Oslo study diet and antismoking trial: Results after 102 months. *American Journal of Medicine* 80(Supplement 2A):7–12, February 14, 1986.

HJERMANN, I., HOLME, I., VELVE BYRE, K., LEREN, P. Effect of diet and smoking intervention on the incidence of coronary heart disease. *Lancet* 2(8259):1303–1310, December 12, 1981.

HOLME, I. On the separation of the intervention effects of diet and antismoking advice on the incidence of major coronary events in coronary high risk men. The Oslo Study. *Journal of the Oslo City Hospitals* 32(3/4):31–54, March–April 1982.

HOLME, I., HELGELAND, A., HJERMANN, I., LEREN, P., LUND-LARSEN, P.G. Four and two-thirds years incidence of coronary heart disease in middle-aged men: The Oslo Study. *American Journal of Epidemiology* 112(1):149–160, July 1980.

HUBERT, H.B., EAKER, E.D., GARRISON, R.J., CASTELLI, W.P. Life-style correlates of risk factor change in young adults: An eight-year study of coronary heart disease risk factors in the Framingham offspring. *American Journal of Epidemiology* 125(5):812–831, May 1987.

HUBERT, H.B., HOLFORD, T.R., KANNEL, W.B. Clinical characteristics and cigarette smoking in relation to prognosis of angina pectoris in Framingham. *American Journal of Epidemiology* 115(2):231–242, February 1982.

HUGHES, G.H., HYMOWITZ, N., OCKENE, J.K., SIMON, N., VOGT, T.M. The Multiple Risk Factor Intervention Trial (MRFIT). V. Intervention on smoking. *Preventive Medicine* 10(4):476–500, July 1981.

HUGHSON, W.G., MANN, J.I., GARROD, A. Intermittent claudication: Prevalence and risk factors. *British Medical Journal* 1(6124):1379–1381, May 27, 1978.

HUGHSON, W.G., MANN, J.I., TIBBS, D.J., WOODS, H.F., WALTON, I. Intermittent claudication: Factors determining outcome. *British Medical Journal* 1(6124):1377–1379, May 27, 1978.

HULLEY, S.B., COHEN, R., WIDDOWSON, G. Plasma high-density lipoprotein cholesterol level. Influence of risk factor intervention. *Journal of the American Medical Association* 238(21):2269–2271, November 21, 1977.

JACOBSEN, B.K., THELLE, D.S. The Tromso Heart Study: Food habits, serum total cholesterol, HDL cholesterol, and triglycerides. *American Journal of Epidemiology* 125(4):622–630, April 1987.

JAJICH, C.L., OSTFELD, A.M., FREEMAN, D.H. JR. Smoking and coronary heart disease mortality in the elderly. *Journal of the American Medical Association* 252(20):2831–2834, November 23–30, 1984.

JENKINS, C.D., ROSENMAN, R.H., ZYZANSKI, S.J. Cigarette smoking: Its relationship to coronary heart disease and related risk factors in the Western Collaborative Group Study. *Circulation* 38(6):1140–1155, December 1968.

JOHANSSON, S.., BERGSTRAND, R., PENNERT, K., ULVENSTAM, G., VEDIN, A., WEDEL, H., WILHELMSSON, C., WILHELMSEN, L., ABERG, A. Cessation of smoking after myocardial infarction in women. Effects on mortality and reinfarctions. *American Journal of Epidemiology* 121(6):823–831, June 1985.

JONASON, T., BERGSTRÖM, R. Cessation of smoking in patients with intermittent claudication: Effects on the risk of peripheral vascular complications, myocardial infarction and mortality. *Acta Medica Scandinavica* 221:253–260, 1987.

JONASON, T., RINGGVIST, I. Factors of prognostic importance for subsequent rest pain in patients with intermittent claudication. *Acta Medica Scandinavica* 218(1):27–33, 1985.

JUERGENS, J.L., BARKER, N.W., HINES, E.A. JR. Arteriosclerosis obliterans: Review of 520 cases with special reference to pathogenic and prognostic factors. *Circulation* 21(2):188–195, February 1960.

KAHN, H.A. The Dorn study of smoking and mortality among U.S. veterans: Report on eight and one-half years of observation. In: Haenszel, W. (ed.) *Epidemiological Approaches to the Study of Cancer and Other Chronic Diseases.* NCI Monograph No. 19. U.S. Department of Health, Education, and Welfare, U.S. Public Health Service, National Cancer Institute. January 1966, pp. 1–125.

KANNEL, W.B., D'AGOSTINO, R.B., BELANGER, A.J. Fibrinogen, cigarette smoking, and risk of cardiovascular disease: Insights from the Framingham Study. *American Heart Journal* 113(4):1006–1010, April 1987.

KANNEL, W.B., MCGEE, D., GORDON, T. A general cardiovascular risk profile: The Framingham Study. *American Journal of Cardiology* 38(1):46–51, July 1976.

KEYS, A. Smoking habits. In: Keys, A. (ed.) *Seven Countries: A Multivariate Analysis of Death and Coronary Heart Disease.* Cambridge, Massachusetts: Harvard University Press, 1980, pp. 136–160.

KHAW, K.-T., BARRETT-CONNOR, E., SUAREZ, L., CRIQUI, M.H. Predictors of stroke-associated mortality in the elderly. *Stroke* 15(2):244–248, March–April 1984.

KLEIN, L.W. Cigarette smoking, atherosclerosis and the coronary hemodynamic response: A unifying hypothesis. *Journal of the American College of Cardiology* 4(5):972–974, November 1984.

KONO, S., IKEDA, M., TOKUDOME, S., NISHIZUMI, M., KURATSUNE, M. Smoking and mortalities from cancer, coronary heart disease and stroke in male Japanese physicians. *Journal of Cancer Research and Clinical Oncology* 110(2):161–164, 1985.

KORNITZER, M., DE BACKER, G., DRAMAIX, M., KITTEL, F., THILLY, C., GRAFFAR, M., VUYLSTEEK, K. Belgian Heart Disease Prevention Project: Incidence and mortality results. *Lancet* 1(8333):1066–1070, May 14, 1983.

KRAMER, J.R., KITAZUME, H., PROUDFIT, W.L., MATSUDA, Y., WILLIAMS, G.W., SONES, F.M. JR. Progression and regression of coronary atherosclerosis: Relation to risk factors. *American Heart Journal* 105(1):134–144, January 1983.

KRUPSKI, W.C., OLIVE, G.C., WEBER, C.A., RAPP, J.H. Comparative effects of hypertension and nicotine on injury-induced myointimal thickening. *Surgery* 102(2):409–415, August 1987.

KULLER, L., MEILAHN, E., TOWNSEND, M., WEINBERG, G. Control of cigarette smoking from a medical perspective. *Annual Review of Public Health* 3:153–178, 1982.

LAVECCHIA, C., FRANCESCHI, S., DECARLI, A., PAMPALLONA, S., TOGNONI, G. Risk factors for myocardial infarction in young women. *American Journal of Epidemiology* 125(5):832–843, May 1987.

LANNERSTAD, O., ISACSSON, S.-O., LINDELL, S.-E. Risk factors for premature death in men 56–60 years old. A prospective study of men born in 1914, living in Malmo, Sweden. *Scandinavian Journal of Social Medicine* 7(1):41–47, 1979.

LAYDE, P.M., BERAL, J., KAY, C.R. Further analyses of mortality in oral contraceptive users. Royal College of General Practitioners' oral contraceptive study. *Lancet* 1(8219):541–546, March 7, 1981.

LOSCALZO, J., BRAUNWALD, E. Tissue plasminogen activator. *New England Journal of Medicine* 319(14):925–931, October 6, 1988.

LUSBY, R.J., BAUMINGER, B., WALTERS, G., DAVIES, P.W., SKIDMORE, R., BAIRD, R.N. Cigarette smoking induced vasoconstriction in habitual smokers with and without arterial occlusive disease. In: Greenhalgh, R.M. (ed.) *Smoking and Arterial Disease.* Woodstock, New York: Beekman Publications, Inc., August 1981, pp. 218–225.

MADSEN, H., DYERBERG, J. Cigarette smoking and its effects on the platelet-vessel wall interaction. *Scandinavian Journal of Clinical Laboratory Investigation* 44(3):203–206, May 1984.

MALINOW, M.R., BLATON, V. Regression of atherosclerotic lesions. *Arteriosclerosis* 4(3):292–295, May–June 1984.

MAOUAD, J., FERNANDEZ, F., BARRILLON, A., GERBAUX, A., GAY, J. Diffuse or segmental narrowing (spasm) of the coronary arteries during smoking demonstrated on angiography. *American Journal of Cardiology* 53(2):354–355, January 15, 1984.

MARASINI, B., BIONDI, M.L., BARBESTI, S., ZATTA, G., AGOSTONI, A. Cigarette smoking and platelet function. *Thrombosis Research* 44(1):85–94, October 1, 1986.

MARSHALL, M. Ultrastructural findings on platelet depositions in initial atherogenesis. *Wiener Klinische Wochenschrift* 98(7):212–214, April 4, 1986.

MARTIN, J.L., WILSON, J.R., FERRARO, N., LASKEY, W.K., KLEAVELAND, J.P., HIRSHFELD, J.W. JR. Acute coronary vasoconstrictive effects of cigarette smoking in coronary heart disease. *American Journal of Cardiology* 54(1):56–60, July 1, 1984.

MEADE, T.W., IMESON, J., STIRLING, Y. Effects of changes in smoking and other characteristics on clotting factors and the risk of ischaemic heart disease. *Lancet* 2(8566):986–988, October 31, 1987.

MEADE, T.W., MELLOWS, S., BROZOVIC, M., MILLER, G.J., CHAKRABARTI, R.R., NORTH, W.R., HAINES, A.P., STIRLING, Y., IMESON, J.D., THOMPSON, S.G. Haemostatic function and ischaemic heart disease: Principal results of the Northwick Park Heart Study. *Lancet* 2(8506):533–537, September 6, 1986.

MEADE, T.W., VICKERS, M.V., THOMPSON, S.G., STIRLING, Y., HAINES, A.P., MILLER, G.J. Epidemiological characteristics of platelet aggregability. *British Medical Journal* 290:428–432, February 9, 1985.

MULCAHY, R. Influence of cigarette smoking on morbidity and mortality after myocardial infarction. *British Heart Journal* 49(5):410–415, May 1983.

MULCAHY, R., HICKEY, N., GRAHAM, I.M., MACAIRT, J. Factors affecting the 5 year survival rate of men following acute coronary heart disease. *American Heart Journal* 93(5):556–559, May 1977.

MULTIPLE RISK FACTOR INTERVENTION TRIAL RESEARCH GROUP. Multiple Risk Factor Intervention Trial. Risk factor changes and mortality results. *Journal of the American Medical Association* 248(12):1465–1477, September 24, 1982.

MULTIPLE RISK FACTOR INTERVENTION TRIAL RESEARCH GROUP. Coronary heart disease death, nonfatal acute myocardial infarction and other clinical outcomes in the Multiple Risk Factor Intervention Trial. *American Journal of Cardiology* 58(1):1–13, July 1, 1986.

MULTIPLE RISK FACTOR INTERVENTION TRIAL RESEARCH GROUP. Mortality rates after 10.5 years for participants in the Multiple Risk Factor Intervention Trial. *Journal of the American Medical Association* 263(13):1795–1801, April 4, 1990.

MUNRO, J.M., COTRAN, R.S. The pathogenesis of antherosclerosis: Atherogenesis and inflammation. *Laboratory Investigation* 58(3):249–261, March 1988.

NADIGER, H.A., MATHEW, C.A., SADASIVUDU, B. Serum malanodialdehyde (TBA reactive substance) levels in cigarette smokers. *Atherosclerosis* 64(1):71–73, March 1987.

NETTERSTROM, B., JUEL, K. Impact of work-related and psychosocial factors on the development of ischemic heart disease among urban bus drivers in Denmark. *Scandinavian Journal of Work and Environmental Health* 14(4):231–238, August 1988.

NOMURA, A., COMSTOCK, G.W., KULLER, L., TONASCIA, J.A. Cigarette smoking and strokes. *Stroke* 5(4):483–486, July–August 1974.

NOWAK, J., MURRAY, J.J., OATES, J.A., FITZGERALD, G.A. Biochemical evidence of a chronic abnormality in platelet and vascular function in healthy individuals who smoke cigarettes. *Circulation* 76(1):6–14, July 1987.

NUSSEY, S.S., ANG, V.T., BEVAN, D.H., JENKINS, J.S. Human platelet arginine vasopressin. *Clinical Endocrinology* 24(4):427–433, April 1986.

OCKENE, J.K., KULLER, L.H., SVENDSEN, K.H., MEILAHN, E. The relationship of smoking cessation to coronary heart disease and lung cancer in the Multiple Risk Factor Intervention Trial (MRFIT). *American Journal of Public Health* 80(8):954–958, August 1990.

OKADA, H., HORIBE, H., YOSHIYUKI, O., HAYAKAWA, N., AOKI, N. A prospective study of cerebrovascular disease in Japanese rural communities, Akabane and Asahi. Part I: Evaluation of risk factors in the occurrence of cerebral hemorrhage and thrombosis. *Stroke* 7(6):599–607, November–December 1976.

OSTFELD, A.M., SHEKELLE, R.B., KLAWANS, H., TUFO, H.M. Epidemiology of stroke in an elderly welfare population. *American Journal of Public Health* 64(5):450–458, May 1974.

PACKHAM, M.S., MUSTARD, J.F. The role of platelets in the development and complications of atherosclerosis. *Seminars in Hematology* 23(1):8–26, January 1986.

PASSERO, S., ROSSI, G., NARDINI, M., BONELLI, G., D'ETTORRE, M., MARTINI, A., BATTISTINI, N., ALBANESE, V., BONO, G., BRAMBILLA, G.L., ET AL. Italian multicenter study of reversible cerebral ischemic attacks. Part 5. Risk factors and cerebral atherosclerosis. *Atherosclerosis* 63(2–3):211–224, February 1987.

PELLETIER, D.L., BAKER, P.T. Physical activity and plasma total- and HDL-cholesterol levels in western Samoan men. *American Journal of Clinical Nutrition* 46(4):577–585, October 1987.

PERKINS, J., DICK, T.B. Smoking and myocardial infarction: Secondary prevention. *Postgraduate Medical Journal* 61(714):295–300, April 1985.

PETITTI, D.A., WINGERD, J. Use of oral contraceptives, cigarette smoking, and risk of subarachnoid haemorrhage. *Lancet* 2(8083):234–236, July 29, 1978.

PHILLIPS, A.N., SHAPER, A.G., POCOCK, S.J., WALKER, M., MACFARLANE, P.W. The role of risk factors in heart attacks occurring in men with pre-existing ischaemic heart disease. *British Heart Journal* 60(5):404–410, November 1988.

PITTILO, R.M., CLARKE, J.M., HARRIS, D., MACKIE, I.J., ROWLES, P.M., MACHIN, S.J., WOOLF, N. Cigarette smoking and platelet adhesion. *British Journal of Haematology* 58(4):627–632, December 1984.

PITTILO, R.M., MACKIE, I.J., ROWLES, P.M., MACHIN, S.J., WOOLFF, N. Effects of cigarette smoking on the ultrastructure of rat thoracic aorta and its ability to produce prostacyclin. *Thrombosis and Haemostasis* 48:173–176, October 29, 1982.

QUICK, C.R.G., COTTON, L.T. Measured effect of stopping smoking on intermittent claudication. *British Journal of Surgery* 69(Supplement):S24–S26, June 1982.

RABKIN, S.W. Effect of cigarette smoking cessation on risk factors for coronary atherosclerosis: A control clinical trial. *Atherosclerosis* 52:173–184, November 1984.

RAICHLEN, J.S., HEALY, B., ACHUFF, S.C., PEARSON, T.A. Importance of risk factors in the angiographic progression of coronary artery disease. *American Journal of Cardiology* 57(1):66–70, January 1, 1986.

RAMSDALE, D.R., FARAGHER, E.B., BRAY, C.L., BENNETT, D.H., WARD, C., BETON, D.C. Smoking and coronary artery disease assessed by routine coronary arteriography. *British Medical Journal* 290(6463):197–200, January 19, 1985.

REED, D.M., STRONG, J.P., HAYASHI, T., NEWMAN, W.P. III, TRACY, R.E., GUZMAN, M.A., STEMMERMANN, G.N. Comparison of two measures of atherosclerosis in a prospective epidemiology study. *Arteriosclerosis* 8(6):782–787, November–December 1988.

REICHLEY, K.B., MUELLER, W.H., HANIS, C.L. Centralized obesity and cardiovascular disease risk in Mexican Americans. *American Journal of Epidemiology* 125(3):373–386, March 1987.

REINDERS, J.H., BRINKMAN, H.J.M., VAN MOURIK, J.A., DE GROOT, P.G. Cigarette smoke impairs endothelial cell prostacyclin production. *Arteriosclerosis* 6(1):15–23, January–February 1986.

RENAUD, S., BLACHE, D., DUMONT, E., THEVENON, C., WISSENDANGER, T. Platelet function after cigarette smoking in relation to nicotine and carbon monoxide. *Clinical Pharmacology and Therapeutics* 36(3):389–395, September 1984.

RENAUD, S., DUMONT, E., BAUDIER, F., ORTCHANIAN, E., SYMINGTON, I.S. Effect of smoking and dietary saturated fats on platelet functions in Scottish farmers. *Cardiovascular Research* 19(3):155-159, March 1985.

RIVAL, J., RIDDLE, J.M., STEIN, P.D. Effects of chronic smoking on platelet function. *Thrombosis Research* 45(1):75-85, January 1, 1987.

ROBINSON, D., FERNS, G.A., BEVAN, E.A., STOCKS, J., WILLIAMS, P.T., GALTON, D.J. High density lipoprotein subfractions and coronary risk factors in normal men. *Arteriosclerosis* 7(4):341-346, July-August 1987.

ROGERS, R.L., MEYER, J.S., JUDD, B.W., MORTEL, K.F. Abstention from cigarette smoking improves cerebral perfusion among elderly chronic smokers. *Journal of the American Medical Association* 253(20):2970-2974, May 24-31, 1985.

ROGERS, R.L., MEYER, J.S., SHAW, T.G., MORTEL, K.F., HARDENBERG, J.P., ZAID, R.R. Cigarette smoking decreases cerebral blood flow suggesting increased risk for stroke. *Journal of the American Medical Association* 250(20):2796-2800, November 25, 1983.

ROGOT, E. *Smoking and General Mortality Among U.S. Veterans, 1954-1969.* National Heart and Lung Institute, Publication No. (NIH) 74-544, 1974, p. 65.

ROGOT, E., MURRAY, J.L. Smoking and causes of death among U.S. veterans: 16 years of observation. *Public Health Reports* 95(3):213-222, May-June 1980.

RØNNEVIK, P.K., GUNDERSEN, T., ABRAHAMSEN, A.M. Effect of smoking habits and timolol treatment on mortality and reinfarction in patients surviving acute myocardial infarction. *British Heart Journal* 54(2):134-139, August 1985.

ROSE, G., HAMILTON, P.J.S. A randomized controlled trial of the effect on middle-aged men of advice to stop smoking. *Journal of Epidemiology and Community Health* 32(4):275-281, December 1978.

ROSE, G., HAMILTON, P.J.S., COLWELL, L., SHIPLEY, M.J. A randomised controlled trial of anti-smoking advice: 10-year results. *Journal of Epidemiology and Community Health* 36(2):102-108, June 1982.

ROSE, G., HAMILTON, P.J.S., KEEN, H., REID, D.D., MCCARTNEY, P., JARRETT, R.J. Myocardial ischaemia, risk factors and death from coronary heart-disease. *Lancet* 1(8003):105-109, January 15, 1977.

ROSE, G., TUNSTALL-PEDOE, H.D., HELLER, R.F. UK Heart Disease Prevention Project: Incidence and mortality results. *Lancet* 1(8333):1062-1065, May 14, 1983.

ROSENBERG, L., KAUFMAN, D.W., HELMRICH, S.P., MILLER, D.R., STOLLEY, P.D., SHAPIRO, S. Myocardial infarction and cigarette smoking in women younger than 50 years of age. *Journal of the American Medical Association* 253(20):2965-2969, May 24-31, 1985.

ROSENBERG, L., KAUFMAN, D.W., HELMRICH, S.P., SHAPIRO, S. The risk of myocardial infarction after quitting smoking in men under 55 years of age. *New England Journal of Medicine* 313(24):1511-1514, December 12, 1985.

ROSENBERG, L., PALMER, J.R., SHAPIRO, S. Decline in the risk of myocardial infarction among women who stop smoking. *New England Journal of Medicine* 322(4):213-217, January 25, 1990.

ROSENMAN, R.H., BRAND, R.J., JENKINS, C.D., FRIEDMAN, M., STRAUS, R., WURM, M. Coronary heart disease in the Western Collaborative Group Study. Final follow-up experience of 8.5 years. *Journal of the American Medical Association* 233(8):872-877, August 25, 1975.

SALONEN, J.T. Stopping smoking and long-term mortality after acute myocardial infarction. *British Heart Journal* 43(4):463-469, April 1980.

SALONEN, J.T., PUSKA, P., MUSTANIEMI, H. Changes in morbidity and mortality during comprehensive community programme to control cardiovascular diseases during 1972-7 in North Karelia. *British Medical Journal* 2(6199):1178-1183, November 10, 1979.

SCHOENENBERGER, J.C. Smoking change in relation to changes in blood pressure, weight, and cholesterol. *Preventive Medicine* 11:441–453, 1982.

SCHOLL, J.M., BENACERRAF, A., DUCIMETIERE, P., CHABAS, D., BRAU, J., CHAPELLE, J., THERY, J.L. Comparison of risk factors in vasospastic angina without significant fixed coronary narrowing to significant fixed coronary narrowing and no vasospastic angina. *American Journal of Cardiology* 57:199–202, February 1, 1986.

SELTZER, C.C. Cigarette smoking and longevity in the elderly. *Medical Counterpoint* 6(2):29–33, February 1974.

SELTZER, C.C. Smoking and coronary heart disease in the elderly. *American Journal of the Medical Sciences* 269(3):309–315, May–June 1975.

SHAPIRO, L.M., HOWAT, A.P., SINGH, S.P. The mortality and morbidity of young survivors of myocardial infarction. *Quarterly Journal of Medicine* 51(203):366–371, Summer 1982.

SHAPIRO, S., WEINBLATT, E., FRANK, C.W., SAGER, R.V. Incidence of coronary heart disease in a population insured for medical care (HIP): Myocardial infarction, angina pectoris, and possible myocardial infarction. *American Journal of Public Health* 59(6)(Supplement 2):1–101, June 1969.

SHINTON, R., BEEVERS, G. Meta-analysis of relation between cigarette smoking and stroke. *British Medical Journal* 298(6676):789–794, March 25, 1989.

SPARROW, D., DAWBER, T.R., COLTON, T. The influence of cigarette smoking on prognosis after a first myocardial infarction. A report from The Framingham Study. *Journal of Chronic Diseases* 31(6/7):425–432, 1978.

STAMFORD, B.A., MATTER, S., FELL, R.D., PAPANEK, P. Effects of smoking cessation on weight gain, metabolic rate, caloric consumption, and blood lipids. *American Journal of Clinical Nutrition* 43(4):486–494, April 1986.

STAMPFER, M.J., GOLDHABER, S.Z., YUSUF, S., PETO, R., HENNEKENS, C.H. Effect of intravenous streptokinase on acute myocardial infarction: Pooled results from randomized trials. *New England Journal of Medicine* 307(19):1180–1182, November 4, 1982.

STEERING COMMITTEE OF THE PHYSICIANS' HEALTH STUDY RESEARCH GROUP. Final report on the aspirin component of the ongoing Physicians' Health Study. *New England Journal of Medicine* 321(3):129–135, July 20, 1989.

STEINBACH, M., CONSTANTINEANU, M., GEORGESCU, M., HARNAGEA, P., THEODORINI, S., GALFI, L., DAMSA, T., SCHIOIU, L., MITU, S., POPESCU, A., ET AL. The Bucharest Multifactorial Prevention Trial of Coronary Heart Disease—Ten year follow-up: 1971–1982. *Revue Roumaine de Medecine Interne* 22(2):99–106, April–June 1984.

STEINBERG, D., PARTHASARATHY, S., CAREW, T.E., KHOO, J.C., WITZTUM, J.L. Beyond Cholesterol: Modifications of low-density lipoprotein that increase its atherogenicity. *New England Journal of Medicine* 320(14):915–924, April 6, 1989.

TAHA, A., BALL, K.P., ILLINGWORTH, R.D. Smoking and subarachnoid haemorrhage. *Journal of the Royal Society of Medicine* 75(5):332–335, May 1982.

TELL, G.S., HOWARD, G., MCKINNEY, W.M., TOOLE, J.F. Cigarette smoking cessation and extracranial carotid atherosclerosis. *Journal of the American Medical Association* 261(8):1178–1180, February 24, 1989.

TOIVANEN, J., YLIKORKALA, O., VIINIKKA, L. Effects of smoking and nicotine on human prostacyclin and thromboxane production in vivo and in vitro. *Toxicology and Applied Pharmacology* 82(2):301–306, February 1986.

TUOMILEHTO, J., TANSKANEN, A., SALONEN, J.T., NISSINEN, A., KOSKELA, K. Effects of smoking and stopping smoking on serum high-density lipoprotein cholesterol levels in a representative population sample. *Preventive Medicine* 15(1):35–45, January 1986.

U.S. DEPARTMENT OF HEALTH AND HUMAN SERVICES. *The Health Consequences of Smoking for Women. A Report of the Surgeon General.* U.S. Department of Health and Human Services, Public Health Service, Office of the Assistant Secretary for Health, Office on Smoking and Health, 1980.

U.S. DEPARTMENT OF HEALTH AND HUMAN SERVICES. *The Health Consequences of Smoking: Cardiovascular Disease. A Report of the Surgeon General.* U.S. Department of Health and Human Services, Public Health Service, Office on Smoking and Health. DHHS Publication No. (PHS) 84-50204, 1983.

U.S. DEPARTMENT OF HEALTH AND HUMAN SERVICES. *Reducing the Health Consequences of Smoking: 25 Years of Progress. A Report of the Surgeon General.* U.S. Department of Health and Human Services, Public Health Service, Centers for Disease Control, Center for Chronic Disease Prevention and Health Promotion, Office on Smoking and Health. DHHS Publication No. (CDC) 89-8411, 1989.

U.S DEPARTMENT OF HEALTH, EDUCATION, AND WELFARE. *The Health Consequences of Smoking. A Report to the Surgeon General: 1971.* U.S. Department of Health, Education, and Welfare, Public Health Service, Health Services and Mental Health Administration. DHEW Publication No. (HSM) 71-7513, 1971.

U.S DEPARTMENT OF HEALTH, EDUCATION, AND WELFARE. *Smoking and Health. A Report of the Surgeon General.* U.S. Department of Health, Education, and Welfare, Public Health Service, Office of the Assistant Secretary for Health, Office on Smoking and Health. DHEW Publication No. (PHS) 79-50066, 1979.

U.S. PUBLIC HEALTH SERVICE. *Smoking and Health. Report of the Advisory Committee to the Surgeon General of the Public Health Service.* U.S. Department of Health, Education, and Welfare, Public Health Service, Center for Disease Control. PHS Publication No. 1103, 1964.

VANDORMAEL, M.G., DELIGONUL, U., KERN, M.J., HARPER, M., PRESANT, S., GIBSON, P., GALAN, K., CHAITMAN, B.R. Multilesion coronary angioplasty: Clinical and angiographic follow-up. *Journal of the American College of Cardiology* 10(2):246–252, August 1987.

VESSEY, M.P., LAWLESS, M., YEATES, D. Oral contraceptives and stroke: Findings in a large prospective study. *British Medical Journal* 289(6444):530–531, September 1, 1984.

VLIETSTRA, R.E., KRONMAL, R.A., OBERMAN, A., FRYE, R.L., KILLIP, T. III. Effect of cigarette smoking on survival of patients with angiographically documented coronary artery disease: Report from the CASS Registry. *Journal of the American Medical Association* 255(8):1023–1027, February 28, 1986.

VON DER LIPPE, G., LUND-JOHANSEN, P. Reduction of sudden deaths after myocardial infarction by treatment with beta-blocking drugs. In: Zanchetti, A. (ed.) *Advances in Beta-Blocker Therapy II. Proceedings of the Second International Bayer Beta-Blocker Symposium, October 16–17, 1981.* Venice, 1982, pp. 100–105.

WEINTRAUB, W.S., KLEIN, L.W., SEELAUS, P.A., AGARWAL, J.B., HELFANT, R.H. Importance of total life consumption of cigarettes as a risk factor for coronary artery disease. *American Journal of Cardiology* 55(6):669–672, March 1, 1985.

WEIR, J.M., DUNN, J.E. JR. Smoking and mortality: A prospective study. *Cancer* 25(1):105–112, January 1970.

WELIN, L., SVARDSUDD, K., WILHELMSEN, L., LARSSON, B., TIBBLIN, G. Analysis of risk factors for stroke in a cohort of men born in 1913. *New England Journal of Medicine* 317(9):521–526, August 27, 1987.

WILHELMSEN, L., BERGLUND, G., ELMFELDT, D., TIBBLIN, G., WEDEL, H., PENNERT, K., VEDIN, A., WILHELMSSON, C., WERKO, L. The Multifactor Primary Prevention Trial in Göteborg, Sweden. *European Heart Journal* 7(4):279–288, April 1986.

WILHELMSEN, L., SVARDSUDD, K., KORSAN-BENGTSEN, K., LARSSON, B., WELIN, L., TIBBLIN, G. Fibrinogen as a risk factor for stroke and myocardial infarction. *New England Journal of Medicine* 311(8):501–505, August 23, 1984.

WILHELMSSON, C., VEDIN, J.A., ELMFELDT, D., TIBBLIN, G., WILHELMSEN, L. Smoking and myocardial infarction. *Lancet* 1(7904):415–420, February 22, 1975.

WILLETT, W., HENNEKENS, C.H., CASTELLI, W.P., ROSNER, B., EVANS, D., TAYLOR, J., KASS, E.H. Effects of cigarette smoking on fasting triglyceride, total cholesterol, and HDL-cholesterol in women. *American Heart Journal* 105(3):417–421, March 1983.

WILLETT, W.C., HENNEKENS, C.H., BAIN, C., ROSNER, B., SPEIZER, F.E. Cigarette smoking and non-fatal myocardial infarction in women. *American Journal of Epidemiology* 113(5):575–582, May 1981.

WILLETT, W.C., GREEN, A., STAMPFER, M.J., SPEIZER, F.E., COLDITZ, G.A., ROSNER, B., MONSON, R.R., STASON, W., HENNEKENS, C.H. Relative and absolute excess risks of coronary heart disease among women who smoke cigarettes. *New England Journal of Medicine* 317(21):1303–1309, November 19, 1987.

WINNIFORD, M.D., WHEELAN, K.R., KREMERS, M.S., UGOLINI, V., VAN DEN BERG, E. JR., NIGGEMANN, E.H., JANSEN, D.E., HILLIS, L.D. Smoking-induced coronary vasoconstriction in patients with atherosclerotic coronary artery disease: Evidence for adrenergically mediated alterations in coronary artery tone. *Circulation* 73(4):662–667, April 1986.

WISEMAN, S., KENCHINGTON, G., DAIN, R., MARSHALL, C.E., MCCOLLUM, C.N., GREENHALGH, R.M., POWELL, J.T. Influence of smoking and plasma factors on patency of femoropopliteal vein grafts. *British Medical Journal* 299:643–646, September 9, 1989.

WITTEMAN, J.C., WILLETT, W.C., STAMPFER, M.J., COLDITZ, G.A., KOK, F.J., SACKS, F.M., SPEIZER, F.E., ROSNER, B., HENNEKENS, C.H. Relation of moderate alcohol consumption and risk of systemic hypertension in women. *American Journal of Cardiology* 65(9):633–637, March 1, 1990.

WOLF, P.A., D'AGOSTINO, R.B., KANNEL, W.B., BONITA, R., BELANGER, A.J. Cigarette smoking as a risk factor for stroke: The Framingham Study. *Journal of the American Medical Association* 259(7):1025–1029, February 19, 1988.

WORLD HEALTH ORGANIZATION EUROPEAN COLLABORATIVE GROUP. Multifactorial trial in the prevention of coronary heart disease. 3. Incidence and mortality results. *European Heart Journal* 4:141–147, 1983.

ZIMMERMAN, M., MCGEACHIE, J. The effect of nicotine on aortic endothelium. A quantitative ultrastructural study. *Atherosclerosis* 63:33–41, 1987.

CHAPTER 7
SMOKING CESSATION AND NONMALIGNANT RESPIRATORY DISEASES

CONTENTS

Introduction 279

Part I. Smoking Cessation and Respiratory Morbidity 285
   Respiratory Symptoms 285
      Clinical Studies 285
      Cross-Sectional Studies of Populations 288
      Occupational Groups 296
      Longitudinal Studies 299
      Clinical Studies of Possible Mechanisms 304
   Respiratory Infections 305
      Smoking Cessation and Respiratory Infection 307

Part II. Pulmonary Function Among Former Smokers 308
   Cross-Sectional Population Studies of FEV_1 308
   Pulmonary Function Studies After Smoking Cessation 316
      Changes in Spirometric Parameters After Cessation 319
      Tests of Small Airways Function 323
      Diffusing Capacity Among Former Smokers 327
      Other Measures 328
   Longitudinal Population-Based Studies 328

Part III. Airway Responsiveness, Cigarette Smoking, and Smoking Cessation 337
   Mechanisms of Heightened Airway Responsiveness in Smokers and Former Smokers 338
   Cross-Sectional Studies 338
   Longitudinal Studies 339
   Clinical Studies 340

Part IV. Effects of Smoking Cessation on COPD Mortality 341

Part V. Former Smokers With Established Chronic Obstructive Pulmonary Disease 345
   Effect of Smoking Cessation on FEV_1 Decline Among COPD Patients 345
   Effect of Smoking Cessation on Mortality Among COPD Patients 347

Conclusions 349

References 351

INTRODUCTION

Obstructive airways diseases constitute a heterogeneous group of disorders that include but are not limited to emphysema, asthma, chronic bronchitis, and chronic obstructive pulmonary disease (COPD). These four clinical conditions are the most prevalent of the obstructive airways diseases and are responsible for substantial morbidity and mortality. Over 18 million Americans suffer from asthma, and about 12 million Americans have COPD, which is the fifth leading cause of death and the most rapidly increasing cause of death among adults older than 65 years (Feinleib et al. 1989). The 1984 Report on the health consequences of smoking reviewed information on chronic obstructive lung diseases (US DHHS 1984). The Report concluded that "cigarette smoking is the major cause of chronic obstructive lung disease in the United States for both men and women. The contribution of cigarette smoking to chronic obstructive lung disease morbidity and mortality far outweighs all other factors" (US DHHS 1984, p. 8). Approximately 84 percent of COPD mortality among men and 79 percent among women is attributable to cigarette smoking (US DHHS 1989). The annual toll of smoking-attributable COPD in the United States is estimated to be 57,000 deaths (US DHHS 1989), which are responsible for more than 500,000 years of potential life lost before the average life expectancy (Davis and Novotny 1989).

The nosology of obstructive airways diseases has been evolving since the CIBA Foundation Guest Symposium in 1959, one of the first attempts to create a standardized classification. For the purposes of this Chapter, emphysema refers to pathologic abnormal permanent enlargement of the airspaces distal to the terminal bronchiole, accompanied by destruction of airspace walls and without obvious fibrosis (American Thoracic Society 1987). Chronic bronchitis refers to chronic cough and/or sputum production for at least 3 months per year for 2 consecutive years. Asthma has been defined as "a disease characterized by increased responsiveness of the airways to various stimuli and manifested by slowing down of forced expiration, which changes in severity either spontaneously or as a result of therapy" (American College of Chest Physicians, American Thoracic Society Joint Statement 1975). The term COPD is used to describe persistent obstructive ventilatory impairment as determined by a test of pulmonary ventilatory function (O'Connor, Sparrow, Weiss 1989).

Overlap of these conditions is extremely common, although discrete cases of each can be identified (Figure 1). It is estimated that 60 to 100 percent of COPD patients also have airways hyperresponsiveness (Klein and Salvaggio 1966; Parker, Bilbo, Reed 1965; Ramsdell, Nachtwey, Moser 1982; Ramsdale et al. 1984; Bahous et al. 1984). Almost one-half of all asthmatics suffer from chronic bronchitis (Burrows et al. 1987), and asthma may be a risk factor for the development of chronic airflow obstruction (Fletcher et al. 1976; Schachter, Doyle, Beck 1984; Buist and Vollmer 1987; Peat, Woolcock, Cullen 1987). Although the extent of emphysema, as documented by postmortem examination of the lungs, correlates significantly with the degree of fixed airflow obstruction, the correlation is modest, suggesting that emphysema alone does not fully explain the functional impairment in most persons with COPD (Cosio et al. 1977).

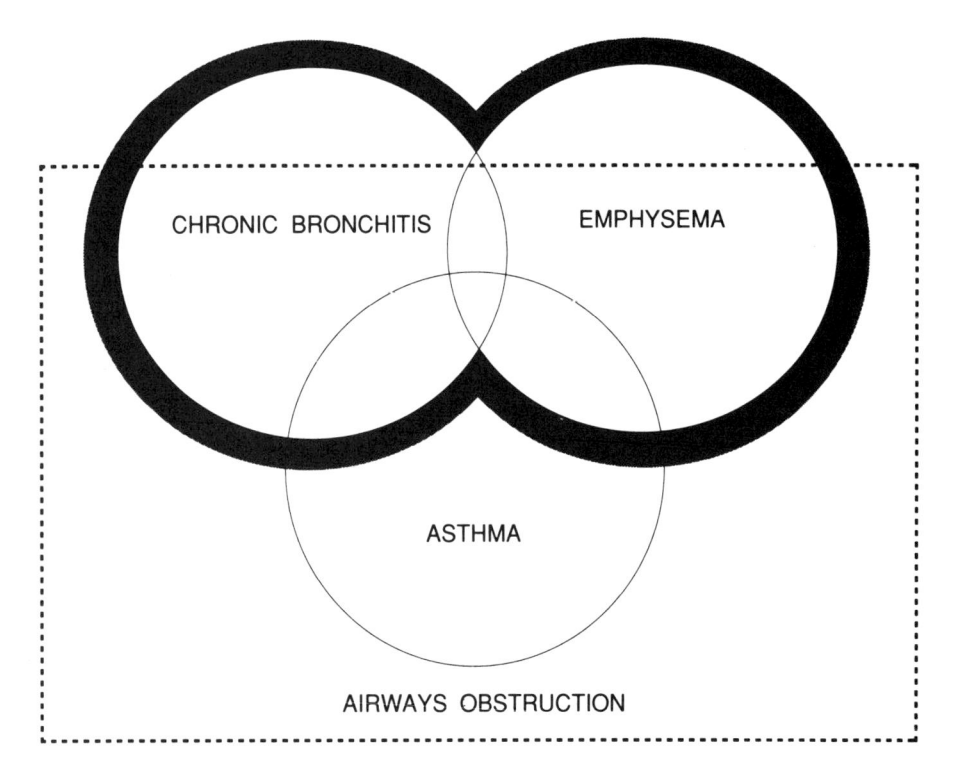

FIGURE 1.—Nonproportional Venn Diagram of the interrelationship among chronic bronchitis, emphysema, asthma, and airways obstruction.
SOURCE: Snider (1988).

Researchers in the United States and the United Kingdom tend to separate asthma from the other obstructive airways diseases and to deemphasize the importance of cigarette smoking in this particular clinical entity. However, the data suggest that cigarette smoking may influence asthma and that allergy and airway hyperresponsiveness, strongly associated with asthma, may play a role in the development of fixed airflow obstruction (O'Connor, Sparrow, Weiss 1989).

The generally accepted model of the pathogenesis of COPD is based on the results of longitudinal investigations of lung function (Fletcher and Peto 1977; Becklake and Permutt 1979; Burrows 1981; Speizer and Tager 1979) (Figure 2). The model suggests that disease development is preceded by a long latent period during which lung function declines at an accelerated rate.

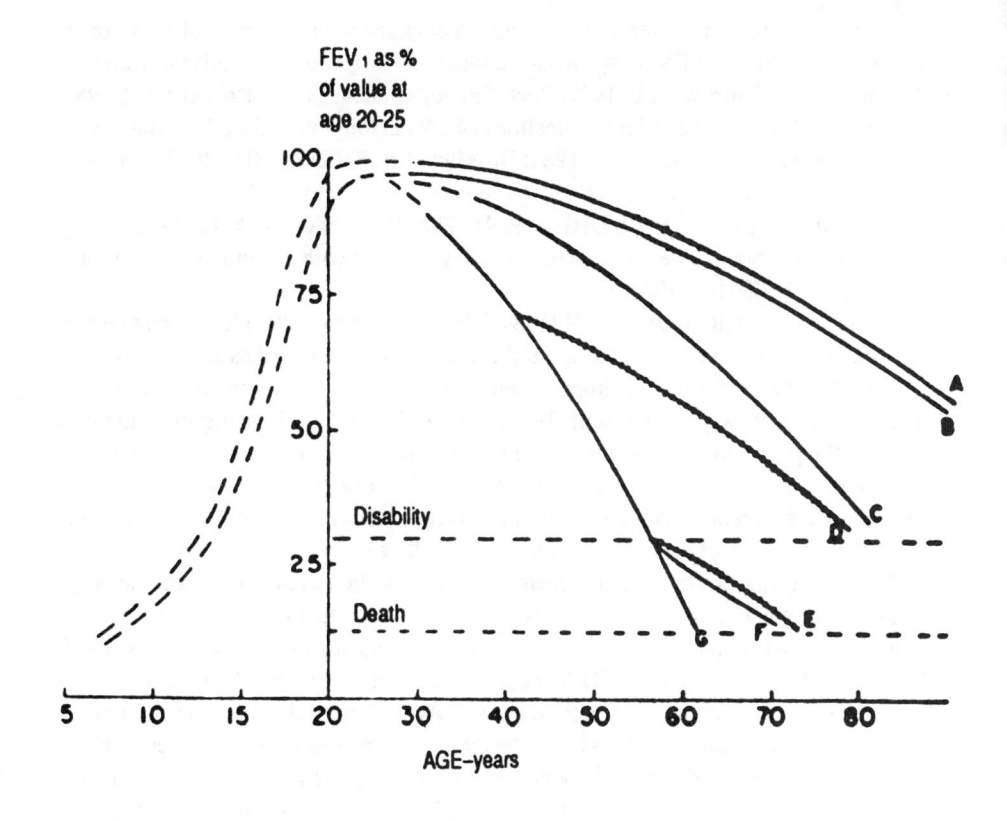

FIGURE 2.—Theoretical curves depicting varying rates of decline of FEV$_1$

NOTE: Curves A and B represent never smokers and smokers, respectively, declining at normal rates. Curve C shows increased decline without development of COPD. Rates of decline for former smokers are represented by curves D and E for those without and with clinical COPD, respectively. Curves F and G show rates of decline with continued smoking after development of COPD.

SOURCE: Speizer and Tager (1979).

Several features of this conceptual model merit emphasis in relation to smoking. First, disease development may occur as a result of factors that accelerate decline in adult life, lead to less than maximal growth, or both. Second, because of the extremely long latent period from the onset of smoking to disease development, factors important in childhood and young adulthood cannot be addressed in longitudinal studies that begin in adulthood. Third, longitudinal studies of children and adults have shown that pulmonary function levels are very stable over time with tracking correlations ranging from 0.70 to 0.90. This high degree of longitudinal correlation, consistent with both environmental and genetic determinants of disease, demonstrates the importance of previous level of function as a major determinant of future disease risk.

Research on risk factors for COPD was reviewed extensively in the 1984 Report of the Surgeon General (US DHHS 1984). The review leads to several general findings with regard to smoking. Cigarette smoking is associated with low levels of 1-sec forced expiratory volume (FEV_1) in cross-sectional investigations (Knudson, Burrows, Lebowitz 1976; Burrows et al. 1977; Beck, Doyle, Schachter 1981; Dockery et al. 1988; US DHHS 1984), with accelerated decline of FEV_1 in longitudinal studies (Burrows et al. 1987; Beck, Doyle, Schachter 1982; Bossé et al. 1981; US DHHS 1984), and with increased mortality from COPD (Best 1966; Doll and Peto 1976; Hammond 1965; Hammond and Horn 1958; US DHHS 1984). The effects of cigarette smoking on lung function level or rate of decline and on mortality increase with the duration and amount of smoking (US DHHS 1984).

Because the development of COPD in adults is associated with a long latent period, the age at which cigarette smoking might have a critical effect has not readily been addressed. Passive smoking impairs lung growth in children and thus, may limit maximal lung growth (Tager et al. 1983; US DHHS 1986). Smoking in adults may shorten the phase when lung function tends to plateau between the ages of 20 and 40 and/or may accelerate the decline in lung function (Tager et al. 1988). Cigarette smoking is the predominant cause of lung function decline at a rate greater than the annual volume loss of 20 to 30 mL associated with aging.

Although cigarette smoking has been clearly established as the major risk factor for COPD, the interactions of the intensity of smoking with factors determining susceptibility have not been fully characterized. For example, Burrows and coworkers (1987) suggested that two subsets of COPD patients can be differentiated by the presence or absence of accompanying asthmatic features. According to this hypothesis, subjects with chronic asthmatic bronchitis have a better long-term prognosis, smaller cumulative exposure to tobacco smoke, and greater prevalence of allergy and airway responsiveness. The second group of patients has emphysema, poorer long-term prognosis, greater cumulative tobacco smoke exposure, and reduced prevalence of allergy and airway hyperresponsiveness (Burrows et al. 1987). Available data do not discriminate the relative contributions of cigarette smoking in these clinical subtypes of patients.

Studies of the mechanisms by which cigarette smoking causes lung injury were reviewed extensively in the 1984 Report of the Surgeon General (US DHHS 1984). That Report and other reviews (Thurlbeck 1976; Snider 1989; Wright 1989) also cover the relationship between the structural changes associated with smoking and the severity of airflow obstruction. Cigarette smoking causes inflammation of both the airways and parenchyma of the lung; the resulting structural damage has functional consequences that can lead to the development of clinically diagnosed COPD if there is sustained smoking. Frank parenchymal damage is preceded by an increase in inflammatory cells in lung parenchyma at the level of the bronchioli (Niewoehner, Kleinerman, Rice 1974). Both neutrophils and alveolar macrophages are important in the development of this inflammatory bronchiolitis. Although neutrophils store and release greater quantities of elastase than alveolar macrophages (Janoff et al. 1979), the macrophage may be an important cell in attracting neutrophils to the lung (Hunninghake and Crystal 1983). Cigarette smoking-induced bronchiolitis is associated with functional abnormalities detectable in the early stages only with sensitive tests of small airway function (Buist et al. 1979; Cosio et al. 1977; McCarthy, Craig, Cherniack 1976; Ingram and Schilder 1967; Ingram and O'Cain 1971). Even before significant emphysema is present, destruction of peribronchiolar alveoli can be found in the lungs of smokers (Saetta et al. 1985; Wright 1989); the loss of alveolar attachments may result in loss of elastic recoil (Wright 1989).

The protease–antiprotease hypothesis proposes that the destruction of lung tissue resulting in emphysema occurs as a consequence of genetic or acquired imbalance of proteolytic and antiproteolytic enzymes in the lung. As noted in the 1984 Surgeon General's Report (US DHHS 1984), this theory derives from two principal observations: (1) α-1-antitrypsin, a major anti-elastolytic enzyme of the lower respiratory tract, is absent in persons genetically deficient in α-1-antitrypsin; these persons often develop emphysema at an early age (Laurell and Eriksson 1963), and (2) administration of proteolytic enzymes in animal models produces emphysema (Gross et al. 1965). Cigarette smoking is associated with increased numbers of neutrophils and activated macrophages in the lungs of smokers, and neutrophil elastase can cause emphysema in animal models (Harris et al. 1975; Galdston et al. 1984). In addition, the α-1-antiprotease of cigarette smokers has reduced functional activity (Gadek, Fells, Crystal 1979; Gadek et al. 1981).

However, although damage to the airways and parenchyma of the lung by cigarette smoke underlies excess lung function loss and COPD in smokers, the factors determining the development of disease in individual smokers have been only partially characterized. A minority of cigarette smokers develop COPD, and cigarette smoking only partially explains the variability in FEV_1 decline (Burrows et al. 1977; US DHHS 1984). Data suggest that cigarette smoking may influence airway as well as parenchymal inflammation. Thus, host factors determining the response of the airways and parenchyma to cigarette smoking, as well as the intensity of smoking, are likely to determine the development of disease.

Cigarette smoking has a variety of effects on the immune system; those effects may be important in determining the risks of COPD and other respiratory diseases. Cigarette smoking is associated with elevated total serum IgE. This total IgE does not exhibit seasonal variability, as seen in atopic individuals, and the antigens responsible for this increase have not been identified. Cigarette smoking may influence the development of an atopic diathesis via effects on T-cell helper and suppressor activity (Ginns et al. 1982; Miller et al. 1982), epithelial permeability (Jones et al. 1980; Simani, Inoue, Hogg 1974), or functional alterations of antigen-presenting cells (Warr and Martin 1977). Cigarette smoking is associated with skin test positivity among children exposed to maternal cigarette smoking (Weiss et al. 1985; Martinez et al. 1988); however, this association is not seen in studies of active adult smokers (Burrows, Lebowitz, Barbee 1976). In adult subjects, skin test positivity is most prevalent among former smokers (Taylor, Gross et al. 1985). These data are consistent with the hypothesis that atopic individuals may not become or remain regular smokers because of airway inflammation secondary to inflammatory effects of cigarette smoking. Thus, cigarette smoking may interact with atopy in a complex manner, inducing atopy in less susceptible or initially nonatopic subjects and discouraging highly atopic subjects from taking up smoking.

Eosinophils are primary effector cells for allergic inflammation (DeMonchy et al. 1985). Increases in eosinophils are associated with the severity and exacerbations of asthma (Horn et al. 1975). Increased eosinophils are also associated with the occurrence of respiratory symptoms and the level of pulmonary function (Burrows et al. 1980; Kauffman et al. 1986). Cigarette smokers exhibit elevations of the peripheral blood eosinophil count (Taylor, Gross et al. 1985), although it is unknown if allergen-induced and cigarette smoking-induced eosinophilia occur by similar or different mechanisms. Eosinophils in peripheral blood are also related to clinical correlates of emphysema (Nagai, West, Thurlbeck 1985).

Cigarette smoking has also been associated with increased levels of airway responsiveness (Woolcock et al. 1987; Sparrow et al. 1987; Burney et al. 1987). Several mechanisms could explain the relationship between cigarette smoking and increased airway responsiveness, including smoking-associated reduction in prechallenge level of lung function, chronic airway inflammation due to smoking, and smoking-induced impairment of epithelial function. The potential central role of cigarette smoking in parenchymal and airways inflammation is depicted in Figure 3.

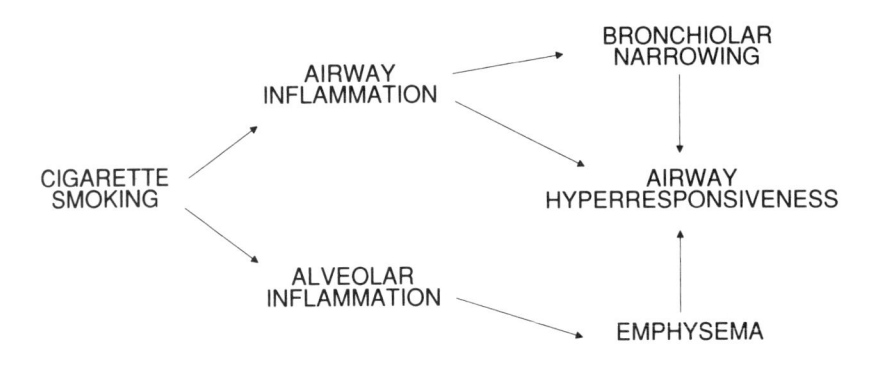

FIGURE 3.—**Hypothesized mechanisms by which airway hyperresponsiveness may be associated with developing or established COPD without necessarily being a preexisting risk factor**

NOTE: COPD=chronic obstructive pulmonary disease.

SOURCE: O'Connor, Sparrow, Weiss (1989).

When considered in this pathophysiologic framework, the potential consequences of smoking cessation on the degree of impairment and future risk of COPD vary with the extent of irreversible changes at cessation and with host characteristics of the quitting smoker. In adults, cigarette smoking cessation is associated with a slowing of FEV_1 decline to the rate of never smokers (Figure 2). To the extent that airway and alveolar inflammation have caused reversible epithelial and parenchymal inflammation, pulmonary function could improve after cessation, particularly if heightened airway responsiveness and bronchiolitis can resolve. To the extent that cigarette smoking has caused permanent damage to lung structure (e.g., emphysema), those changes are unlikely to be reversible. Thus, the amount and duration of smoking, the relative extents of parenchymal and airway inflammation, and the degree of permanent structural damage are probably the key determinants of the level of function after smoking cessation. Even in the setting of established COPD, smoking cessation may potentially reduce the rate of functional loss.

Former smokers may differ from continuing smokers with regard to host characteristics that potentially determine susceptibility to cigarette smoke. Because presmoking levels of atopy and airway responsiveness modify the short-term response to smoke, individuals with atopy or heightened airway responsiveness may be less likely to take up smoking, to reduce smoking, or to quit smoking if respiratory symptoms occur. This potential bias, termed the "healthy smoker effect" by O'Connor, Sparrow, and Weiss (1989), cannot be evaluated in cross-sectional studies.

PART I. SMOKING CESSATION AND RESPIRATORY MORBIDITY

Respiratory Symptoms

Since the 1950s, strong evidence has accumulated documenting increased respiratory symptoms in smokers of all ages compared with nonsmokers (US PHS 1964; US DHEW 1971, 1979; US DHHS 1984). Further, the number of cigarettes smoked per day is the strongest risk factor for the principal chronic respiratory symptoms including chronic cough, phlegm production, wheeze, and dyspnea (Lebowitz and Burrows 1977; Dean et al. 1978; Higgins, Keller, Metzner 1977; Huhti and Ikkala 1980; Higenbottam et al. 1980; Schenker, Samet, Speizer 1982). The widespread effects of chronic smoking on the lung, including decreased tracheal mucous velocity (Lourenço, Klimek, Borowski 1971; Goodman et al. 1978; Thomson and Pavia 1973), increased secretion of mucus on the basis of mucous gland hypertrophy and hyperplasia (Thurlbeck 1976), chronic airway inflammation (Niewoehner, Kleinerman, Rice 1974), increased epithelial permeability (Jones et al. 1980; Minty, Jordon, Jones 1981; Mason et al. 1983), and emphysema (US DHHS 1984), underlie the development of these symptoms. Smoking cessation has been associated with a reduction in respiratory morbidity, presumably through reversal of some of these pathophysiologic abnormalities. Relevant evidence can be found in clinical studies, which involve followup of the symptoms of persons participating in smoking cessation clinics, and epidemiologic studies.

Clinical Studies

Buist and coworkers (1976) found that smoking cessation was associated with a dramatic reduction in respiratory symptoms within 1 month of cessation. These researchers assessed spirometry and respiratory symptoms for over 12 months in 75 cigarette smokers enrolled in a smoking cessation program. Subjects were divided into quitters (those who did not smoke during the entire 12-month period), modifiers (individuals who reduced their cigarette consumption by 25 percent), and nonmodifiers (subjects who continued to smoke at the same level). The three groups were of comparable ages (35 to 39 years) and had a cumulative cigarette consumption of 20 to 26 pack-years. A symptoms ratio was calculated at 1, 3, 6, and 12 months by taking the number of symptoms (e.g., cough, expectoration, shortness of breath, and wheezing) observed and dividing by the total number of possible symptoms for that group. All groups started with ratio values of approximately 0.55. The ratios for quitters declined within 1 month of cessation and continued to decline over the course of the study from 0.52 to 0.08. In contrast, the ratios for modifiers decreased less than quitters, and nonmodifiers had no change in their ratios over 12 months (Figure 4). Data on individual symptoms were not presented, and smoking abstinence was not verified by biologic markers. In a followup study of more than 30 months, Buist, Nagy, and Sexton and colleagues (1979) again showed that among 15 quitters, respiratory symptoms disappeared by the third or fourth month of followup and did not return during the remainder of the study. However, after a small initial decrease in symptoms among 45 continuing smokers, further decreases were not recorded. The small sample sizes and a 41-percent loss to followup must be considered in interpreting the latter findings.

Three studies reported different results for the effect of smoking cessation on respiratory symptoms in asthmatics. Higenbottam, Feyeraband, and Clark (1980) conducted a cross-sectional study of 106 consecutive asthmatic clinic patients and concluded that symptoms decreased after stopping smoking. Age-standardized prevalence rates for chronic cough, chronic cough and phlegm, and wheezing among asthmatics were lower for the 27 former smokers than for the 27 current smokers and the 52 never smokers. Only breathlessness was found more often in former smokers than in the other smoking groups, possibly reflecting irreversible smoking-induced changes. Quantification of smoking history and time since cessation among former smokers was not reported. In contrast, Fennerty and colleagues (1987) as well as Hillerdahl and Rylander (1984) reported increased respiratory symptoms in asthmatics who stopped smoking. Fennerty and coworkers (1987) found that 2 of 14 asthmatics (14.3 percent) who stopped smoking for 24 hours complained that asthmatic symptoms were worsening. Neither of these two subjects showed a decrease in specific airway conductance or peak flow, but one had an increase in airway responsiveness to methacholine. However, four of seven asthmatics who abstained from smoking for 7 days recorded a reduction in symptoms. Hillerdahl and Rylander (1984) studied 59 asthmatics who were recruited from an office practice and who had stopped smoking "permanently or for short periods of time." Using questionnaires, these reseachers found that symptoms worsened in 18 asthmatics (30.5 percent) who had stopped smoking. Three subjects claimed onset of new asthmatic symptoms within months of cessation. Asthmatics younger than 40 years of age were more likely to complain of worsening of their asthma than those subjects older than 40 years of age. Hillerdahl and Rylander (1984) concluded that among asthmatics who smoke, psychological reasons, improved secretion clearance, or both could explain the findings. The uncontrolled nature of these studies, the small numbers of subjects, the potential for selection and information bias, and the noncomparability of treatment regimens among study participants limit the usefulness of these findings.

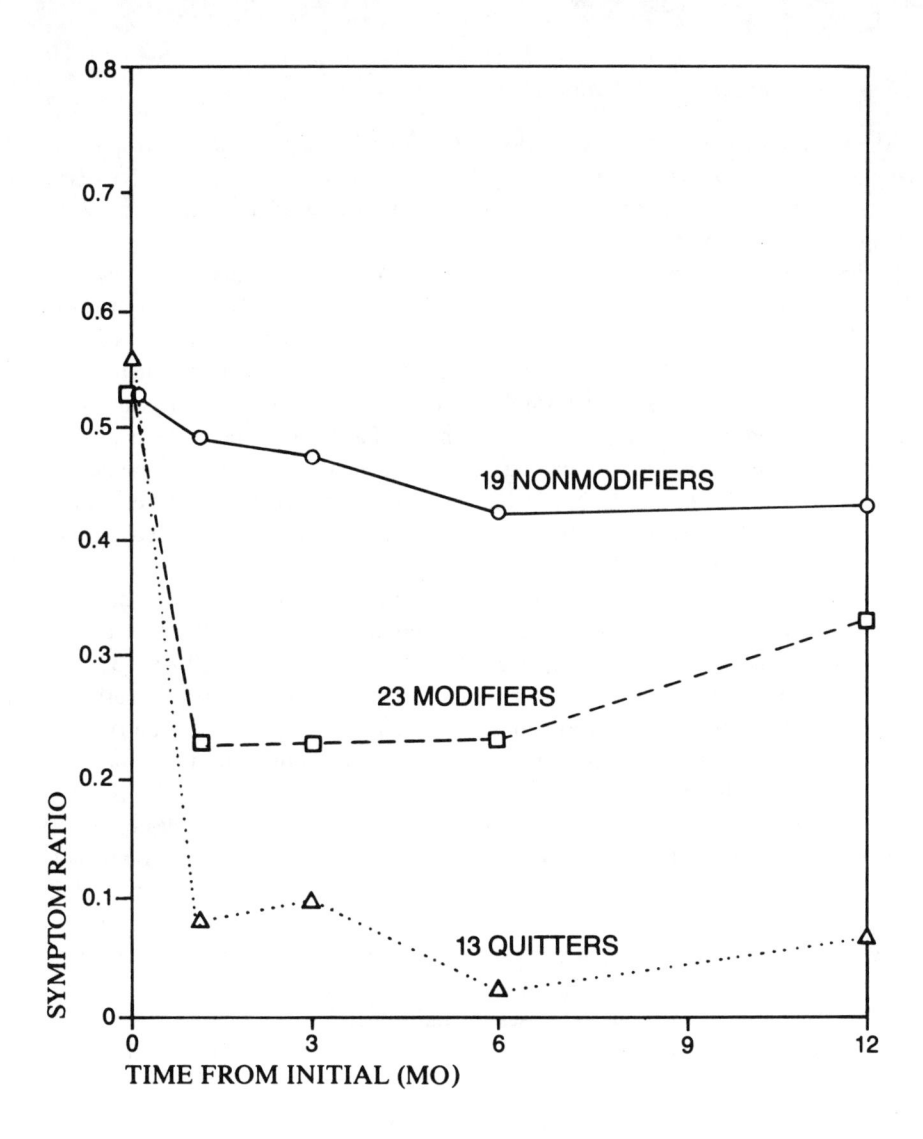

FIGURE 4.—Symptom ratio (number of observed symptoms to number of possible symptoms) in nonmodifiers, modifiers, and quitters at each test period; symptoms are cough, sputum production, wheezing, and shortness of breath

SOURCE: Buist et al. (1976).

In summary, studies of participants of smoking cessation clinics have shown that respiratory symptoms have disappeared rapidly on quitting, even after 20 pack-years of exposure. Limited studies of asthmatics have provided conflicting results.

Cross-Sectional Studies of Populations

The results of community-based studies have shown lower prevalence of respiratory symptoms among former smokers compared with current smokers (Table 1). Two early investigations evaluated symptoms of chronic nonspecific lung disease among smoking groups. Ferris and Anderson (1962) studied a random sample of subjects, aged 25 to 74, from an industrial town in New Hampshire. Using spirometry and interviewer-administered questionnaires, these researchers recorded lung function and symptoms associated with chronic nonspecific respiratory disease in 1,167 individuals. Chronic nonspecific respiratory disease was considered present if (1) phlegm production was reported six or more times per day for 4 days per week for 3 months per year for the past 3 years (chronic bronchitis); (2) if a diagnosis of asthma had been made and was still present; (3) if wheezing or whistling in the chest occurred most days or nights; (4) if shortness of breath occurred while walking at subject's normal pace on level ground; or (5) if an FEV_1 less than 60 percent of forced vital capacity (FVC) was noted (chronic obstructive lung disease). Age-standardized prevalence rates per 100 for chronic nonspecific respiratory disease showed that both male and female ex-smokers had rates of abnormality similar to those of never smokers and lower than those of current smokers (for males, 18.1 vs. 8.4 vs. 50.3, and for females, 17.2 vs. 19.2 vs. 31.0 for never smokers, ex-smokers, and current smokers, respectively). In 1967, a resurvey of the population using a slightly different random sample was performed (Ferris et al. 1971). Again, the age-standardized rates were less for both male and female ex-smokers than for current smokers.

Mueller and colleagues (1971) studied a random sample of one-fifth of the population of Glenwood Springs, CO. Symptoms of chronic nonspecific lung disease, comparable with those defined by Ferris and colleagues (1971), were reported by 20 percent of 55 male former smokers and by 9 percent of 22 female ex-smokers. These percentages were between those of current and never smokers. Age trends were not apparent among males; the small sample size precluded analysis for females.

In the mid-1960s, two surveys assessed the effects of smoking on respiratory symptoms in older men (Table 1). Wilhelmsen and Tibblin (1966) analyzed data from 339 men aged 50 years, born in 1913 and living in Göteborg, an industrial town in Sweden. Of 73 former smokers, the percentages with morning cough for 3 months per year, sputum for 3 months per year, and wheezing other than from colds were lower than those for 182 current smokers of less than or greater than 15 g of tobacco per day and similar to those of 84 never smokers. Dyspnea when walking fast or up a small hill was reported most frequently by current smokers of more than 15 g of tobacco per day; all other groups showed comparable percentages of subjects reporting this symptom.

Weiss and coworkers (1963) studied 350 consecutive men, aged 50 years or older, undergoing routine examination in the Philadelphia Pulmonary Neoplasm Research Project (N=6,137). Fifty-three percent of former cigarette smokers (N=68) reported one or more symptoms of cough, wheeze, or dyspnea compared with 57 percent of current smokers (N=183) and 42 percent of never smokers (N=36). Furthermore, former smokers complained of cough as frequently as never smokers (9 vs. 11 percent) and complained of dyspnea as often as current smokers (46 vs. 44 percent). Only 20

TABLE 1.—Percentages of subjects in cross-sectional studies with respiratory symptoms, by cigarette smoking status and gender

Symptoms[a] Reference	Age (number of subjects)	Current smokers Male (%)	Current smokers Female (%)	Former smokers Male (%)	Former smokers Female (%)	Never smokers Male (%)	Never smokers Female (%)
Cough 3 mo/yr							
Wilhelmsen and Tibblin (1966)	50 (339)	36.2	—	8.2	—	4.8	—
Weiss et al. (1963)	50–69 (287)	41.0	—	9.0	—	11.0	—
Fletcher and Tinker (1961)	40–59 (363)	19.9	—	13.0	—	0.0	—
Mueller et al. (1971)[b]	20–69 (892)	13.0	20.0	5.0	10.0	9.0	5.0
Manfreda, Nelson, Cherniack (1978)							
	25–54 (256)[c]	25.4	20.3	8.1	—	8.3	—
	25–54 (246)[d]	31.5	31.7	2.9	10.0	4.0	4.0
Schenker, Samet, Speizer (1982)[b]	17–74 (5,670)	—	9.1[e] 17.0[f] 31.8[g]	—	7.5	—	5.6
Phlegm 3 mo/yr							
Wilhelmsen and Tibblin (1966)		11.5	—	1.4	—	1.2	—
Fletcher and Tinker (1961)		17.6	—	16.9	—	7.5	—
Mueller et al. (1971)[b]		18.0	10.0	12.0	5.0	4.0	1.0
Manfreda, Nelson, Cherniack (1978)							
	25–54 (256)[c]	16.9	10.2	10.8	—	0.0	0.0
	25–54 (246)[d]	24.7	25.4	5.7	5.0	4.0	4.0
Hawthorne and Fry (1978)	45–64	36.2	23.0	16.1	10.9	10.1	6.7
Miller et al. (1988)[h]	Male (mean): 42.0 (1,169) Female (mean): 42.9 (1,169)	40.8	28.4	14.7	6.9	12.1	0.4

TABLE 1.—Continued

Symptoms[a] Reference	Age (number of subjects)	Current smokers Male (%)	Current smokers Female (%)	Former smokers Male (%)	Former smokers Female (%)	Never smokers Male (%)	Never smokers Female (%)
Schenker, Samet, Speizer (1982)[b]	—	—	7.2[e] 16.7[f] 24.8[g]	—	6.7	—	4.5
Lebowitz and Burrows (1977)	14–96 (2,857)	11.2	11.0	25.9	12.6	45.5	35.8
Dyspnea grade[i]							
Wilhelmsen and Tibblin (1966)[j]		24.7	—	21.9	—	20.2	—
Weiss et al. (1963)[j]		44.0	—	46.0	—	36.0	—
Fletcher et al. (1959) Grades 2 or more	40–59	23.5	29.0	25.0	23.1	10.0	31.4
Fletcher and Tinker (1961) Grade 3 or more		8.7	—	6.5	—	2.5	—
Mueller et al. (1971)[b] Grade 2, Grade 3, or more		29.0 7.0	32.0 13.0	14.0 4.0	41.0 11.0	22.0 6.0	32.0 7.0
Manfreda, Nelson, Cherniack (1978)[k] Grade 2 or more	25–54 (256)[c] 25–54 (246)[d]	5.6 12.3	22.1 17.5	5.4 5.8	6.1 5.0	8.3 4.0	7.0 12.0
Hawthorne and Fry (1978)[j]		13.2	18.6	9.9	20.5	7.0	13.2
Miller et al. (1988)[h] Grade 2 Grade 3		9.3 3.0	15.6 8.9	7.1 3.3	12.7 11.5	3.0 0.4	9.5 2.6
Schenker, Samet, Speizer (1982)[b] Grade 3		—	5.6[e] 6.1[f] 17.6[g]	—	8.2	—	5.9

TABLE 1.—Continued

Symptoms[a] Reference	Age (number of subjects)	Current smokers Male (%)	Current smokers Female (%)	Former smokers Male (%)	Former smokers Female (%)	Never smokers Male (%)	Never smokers Female (%)
Wheeze							
Wilhelmsen and Tibblin (1966)[l]		12.6	—	6.9	—	4.8	—
Weiss et al. (1963)[m]		8.0	—	6.0	—	3.0	—
Fletcher et al (1959)[l]		16.3	12.9	12.5	—	—	2.3
Mueller et al. (1971)[b,l]		18.0	10.0	12.0	5.0	4.0	1.0
Manfreda, Nelson, Cherniack (1978)[n]							
	25–54 (256)[c]	26.8	25.4	10.8	12.1	4.2	3.5
	25–54 (246)[d]	31.5	30.2	14.3	20.0	8.0	8.0
Hawthorne and Fry (1978)[l]		21.8	19.2	9.8	10.6	6.1	6.0
Miller et al. (1988)[h,l]		40.8	28.4	14.7	6.9	12.2	7.4
Schenker, Samet, Speizer (1982)[b,l]		—	14.4[e] 18.5[f] 28.0[g]	—	8.3	—	6.0

[a] Symptoms not mutually exclusive.
[b] Age adjusted.
[c] Urban residents.
[d] Rural residents.
[e] 1–14 cig/day.
[f] 15–24 cig/day.
[g] ≥25 cig/day.
[h] Weighted values to be representative of state as whole.
[i] Grade 2: dyspnea when walking with people of same age on level ground, grade 3: dyspnea when walking at one's own pace on level ground.
[j] Dyspnea not defined.
[k] Shortness of breath compared with persons of same sex and age.
[l] Ever wheeze.
[m] Wheezing not defined.
[n] Wheezing apart from colds.

men reported wheeze, precluding meaningful analysis for this variable. The high symptom rates seen in this study may reflect the older ages of the participants and the selection factors contributing to enrollment in the Philadelphia Pulmonary Neoplasm Research Project.

Three other early investigations confirmed a lower prevalence of specific respiratory symptoms among former smokers (Table 1). Fletcher and coworkers (1959) reported the respiratory symptoms of 244 British post office workers, aged 40 to 59, as part of the study of the relationship between symptoms and tests of lung function. Former smokers of both sexes reported wheezing on most days or nights less often than current smokers, but former smokers also complained of grade 2 dyspnea (i.e., stopping for breath when walking at one's own pace on level ground) as often as current smokers. Fletcher and Tinker (1961) studied respiratory symptoms in 363 London male transport workers. Former smokers had lower prevalence rates for cough, phlegm production, and grade 3 dyspnea (i.e., stopping for breath after walking about 100 yards on level ground) than current smokers of 15 cigarettes or more per day. In a large community-based study in Tecumseh, MI, Payne and Kjelsberg (1964) reported age- and sex-specific prevalence rates for cough and phlegm production that were comparable for former and never smokers (Figure 5). In contrast, sex-specific rates of dyspnea were highest among former smokers and increased with age (Figure 6).

More recent studies have also found lower prevalence of respiratory symptoms among former smokers and documented sex-specific differences among smoking categories (Table 1). Mueller and colleagues (1971) showed that male former smokers had fewer symptoms than current smokers, including cough for 3 months per year, grade 2 dyspnea, and wheezing. Only sputum production for 3 months per year was higher among male former smokers than among never smokers. Female former smokers had lower prevalence rates for cough and phlegm production but higher rates for dyspnea and wheezing than current smokers. Rates for female former smokers were generally higher than those for male former smokers. Manfreda, Nelson, and Cherniack (1978) studied subjects from urban and rural communities in Canada, and found very similar overall and sex-specific prevalence rates for these respiratory symptoms among former smokers. In this study, however, female former smokers had prevalence rates between those of current and never smokers for all symptoms.

In three separate surveys, Hawthorne and Fry (1978) evaluated the association among smoking, respiratory symptoms, and cardiopulmonary mortality in 11,295 men and 7,491 women from southwest Scotland. Former smokers had prevalence rates for phlegm production and wheezing intermediate to those of current and never smokers. Male former smokers reported shortness of breath as often as male never smokers, whereas female former smokers had an increased prevalence of dyspnea compared with current smokers of either sex.

Miller and colleagues (1988) determined sex-specific prevalence rates for a wide range of respiratory symptoms in a stratified random sample from the general population of Michigan. Mean age for the three smoking groups was comparable. Male current and former smokers had similar lifetime cigarette pack consumption (9.09×10^3 vs. 9.93×10^3), whereas female current smokers had almost twice the cigarette consumption of former smokers (8.32×10^3 vs. 4.50×10^3). The prevalence rates of persistent sputum and wheezing were lower among male former smokers compared with current smokers. In contrast, the prevalence of dyspnea was similar for male former and current smokers, and findings were similar among females. Furthermore, female former smokers had higher rates for dyspnea than males but lower rates for all other respiratory variables assessed.

Schenker, Samet, and Speizer (1982) evaluated the effect of smoking status on respiratory symptoms of 5,686 women. Age-adjusted prevalence rates for chronic cough, chronic phlegm, and wheeze most days or nights among former smokers were between those for current and never smokers. Grade 3 dyspnea was reported more often by former smokers than current smokers of 1 to 24 cigarettes per day or by never smokers.

Several reports have addressed the occurrence of symptoms in an epidemiologic study in Tucson, AZ (Lebowitz and Burrows 1977; Paoletti et al. 1985). Cross-sectional analyses, based on the first survey of the population, indicated that former smokers had a higher prevalence of chronic phlegm production than did never smokers

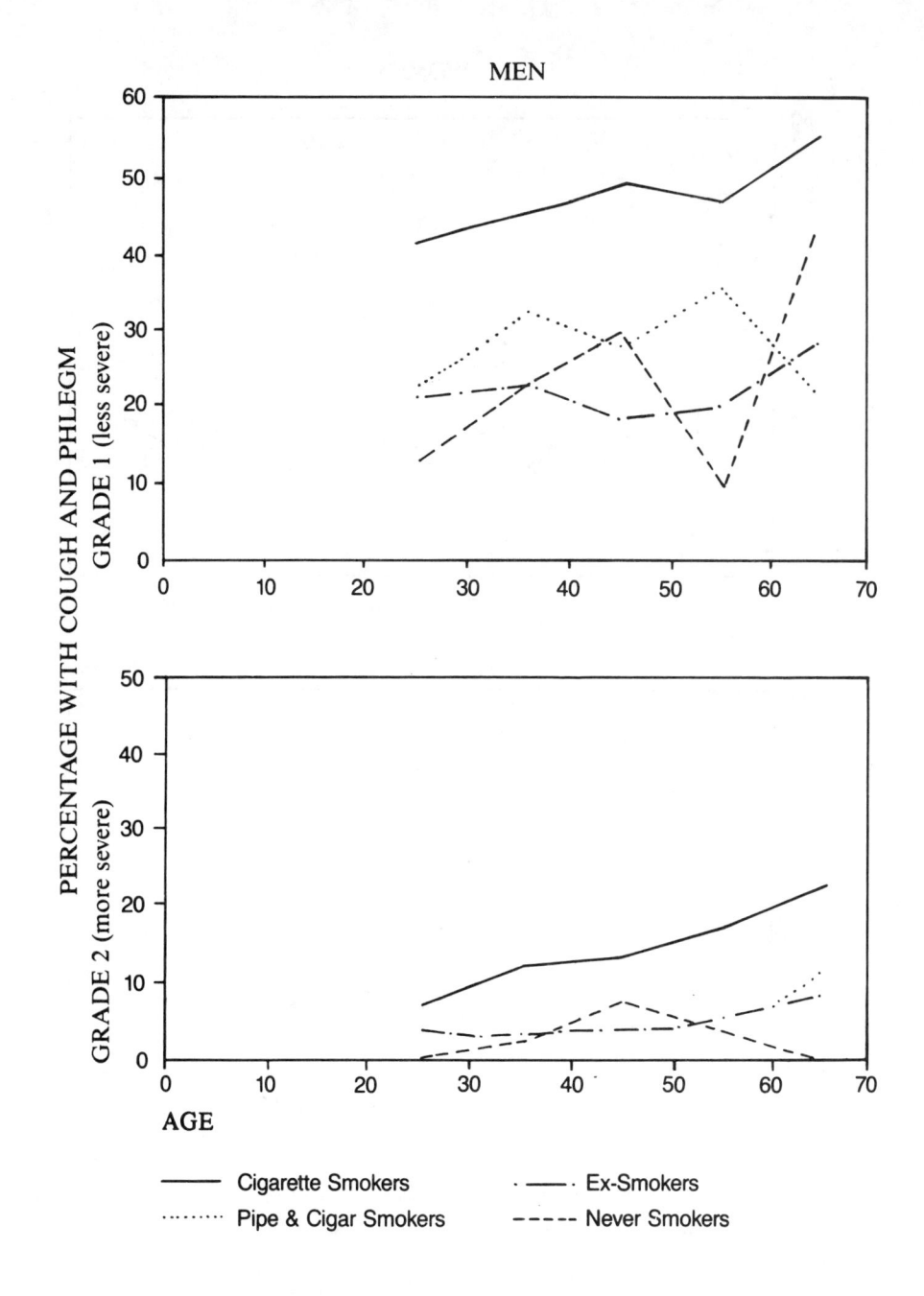

FIGURE 5.—Prevalence of cough and phlegm by smoking group

NOTE: Persons with grade 2 cough and phlegm had both symptoms and at least one symptom for ≥3 mo/yr.

SOURCE: Payne and Kjelsberg (1964).

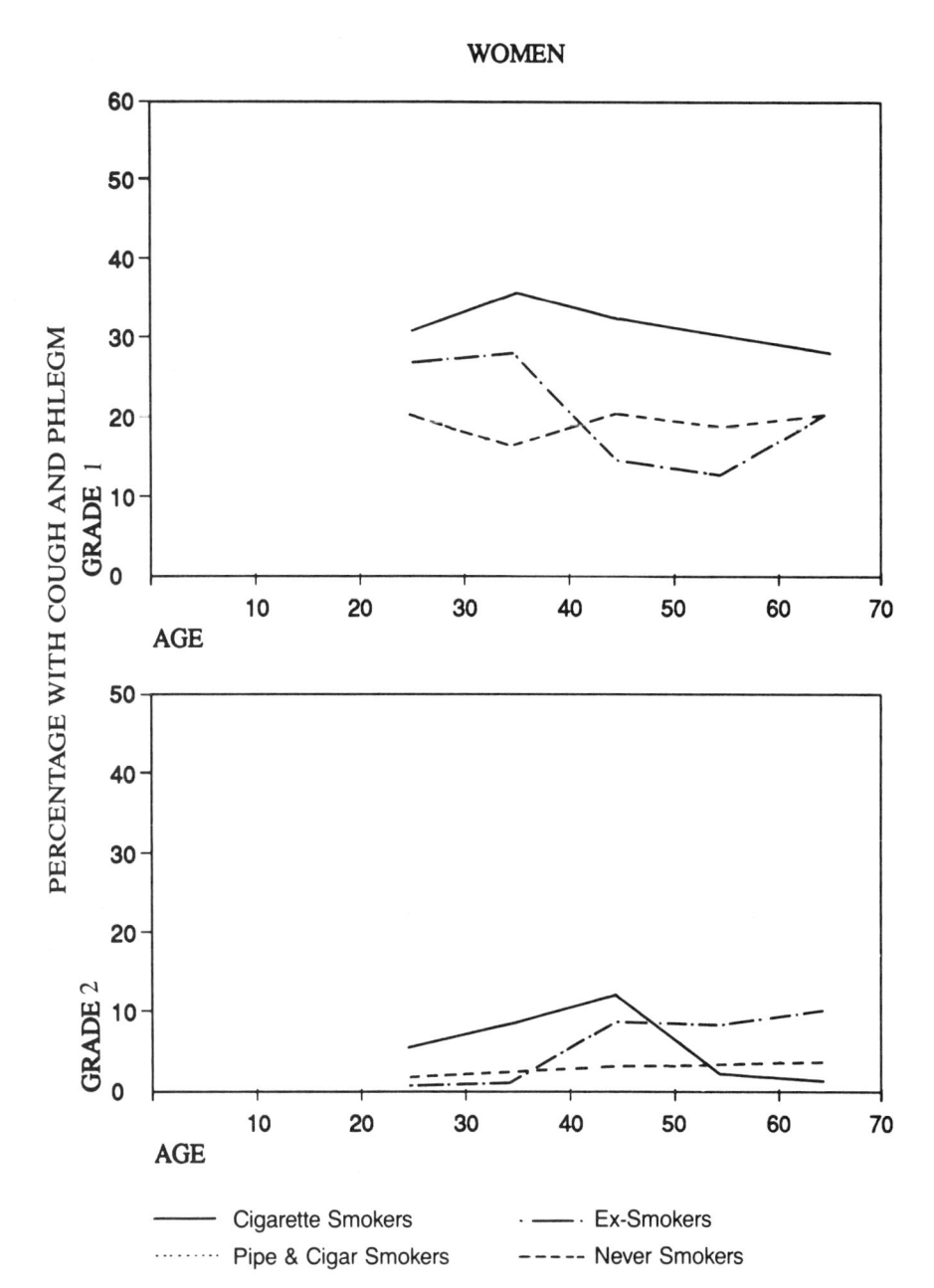

FIGURE 5. (Continued)—Prevalence of cough and phlegm by smoking group

NOTE: Persons with grade 2 cough and phlegm had both symptoms and at least one symptom for ≥3 mo/yr.

SOURCE: Payne and Kjelsberg (1964).

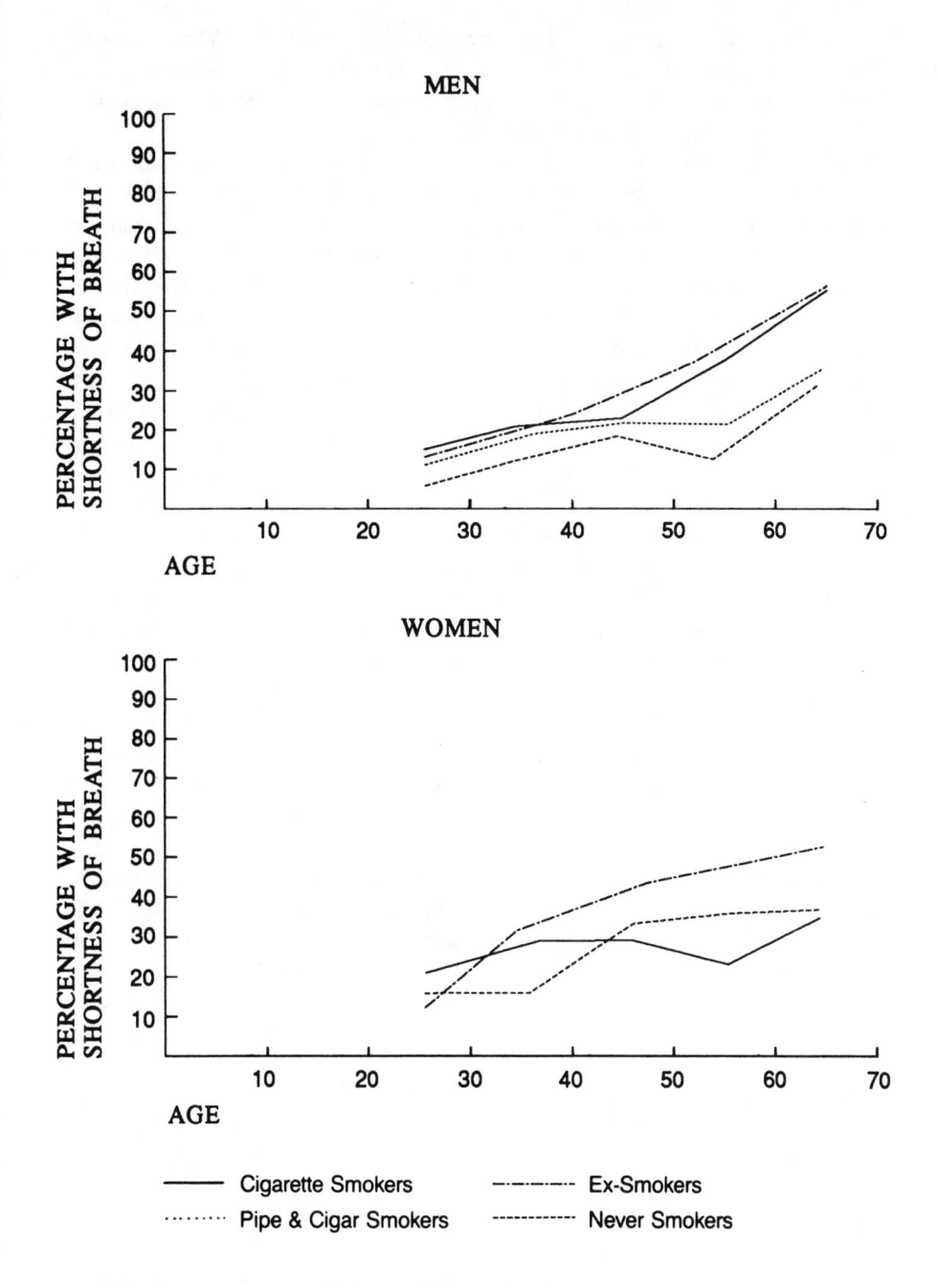

FIGURE 6.—Prevalence of dyspnea by smoking group
SOURCE: Payne and Kjelsberg (1964).

but a lower prevalence compared with current smokers (Table 1). When examined within age groups, the prevalence of chronic phlegm tended to be higher among older male former smokers with substantial past consumption of cigarettes, suggesting that symptoms may not revert quickly to those of never smokers.

To evaluate the effect of cumulative tar consumption on respiratory symptoms and lung function in the Tucson population, Paoletti and coworkers (1985) studied the predictive value of estimated tar exposure and pack-years on respiratory symptoms of 582 current smokers and 621 former smokers. Tar exposure was calculated from the Federal Trade Commission data on tar yield of each type of cigarette smoked and was used to classify retrospectively the smokers' exposures into categories of low and high tar pack-years as well as total tar (kilograms). Only current and former smokers with consistent consumption behavior were analyzed. Ex-smokers had lower prevalence rates of cough, chronic cough, phlegm, and chronic phlegm than did current smokers. Multiple logistic regression analysis was used to determine risk factors for any cough, any wheeze, and dyspnea. Statistical models for former smokers could not be derived using total pack-years, total tar estimates, age, or deep inhalation that significantly predicted respiratory symptoms among former smokers of either sex. The low prevalence rates of symptoms among former smokers may have limited the modeling.

Ballal (1984) analyzed the effect of depth of inhalation on respiratory symptoms in 75 former smokers as part of a larger study of the smoking behavior of 753 Sudanese medical practitioners. The proportion of former smokers complaining of any wheeze increased with degree of inhalation (slightly, moderately, or deeply), but the trend was not statistically significant. Small numbers and subject selection restrict the importance of this finding.

In summary, cross-sectional population-based studies have generally shown that former smokers have reduced prevalence rates for cough, phlegm production, and wheezing compared with current smokers. Dyspnea may not completely reverse after cessation as shown by the comparable prevalence rates for current and ex-smokers in several studies. However, dyspnea may prompt cessation when sustained smoking has caused significant physiologic impairment. Differences in symptom rates by gender have been documented in former smokers; potential explanations include sex-specific differences in reporting, differences in smoking practices, or distinct underlying physiologic responses to cessation by gender. Although the relevant data are limited, reversal of most symptoms reflecting mucous gland hypertrophy and hyperplasia and airways inflammation appears to be rapid and not dependent on cumulative smoking at the time of cessation. Measures of past cigarette consumption have not been associated with current respiratory symptoms among former smokers.

Occupational Groups

Studies of grain elevator workers, dairy farmers, cedar mill workers, and persons exposed to dust, gas, fumes, and asbestos have addressed the influence of occupation and smoking on respiratory symptoms (Table 2). Broder and coworkers (1979) and Dopico and colleagues (1984) compared respiratory symptoms in grain handlers with those of civic outside workers and of city workers, respectively. In both studies, former

TABLE 2.—Percentages of subjects in cross-sectional occupational surveys with respiratory symptoms by smoking and occupational exposure status

Symptoms[a] Reference	Mean age (Total)	Current smokers Occupationally exposed	Control	Former smokers Occupationally exposed	Control	Never smokers Occupationally exposed	Control
Cough 3 mo/yr							
Broder et al. (1979)[b]	Grain elevator workers (A) 39±13 (189)	67.0	—	38.0	—	23.0	—
	Grain elevator workers (B) 41±13 (252)	59.0	—	23.0	—	15.0	—
	Civic outside workers (B) 42±14 (180)	—	56.0	—	15.0	—	5.0
Chan-Yeung et al. (1984)	White cedar mill workers 44.3±14.1 (511)	30.7	—	12.3	—	8.5	—
	Nonwhite cedar mill workers 39.6±9.1 (141)	30.7	—	12.3	—	8.5	—
	White office workers 43.2±11.5 (394)	—	21.8	—	3.0	—	3.5
	Nonwhite office workers 39.0±9.9 (46)	—	21.8	—	3.0	—	3.5
Kilburn, Warshaw, Thornton (1986)	Shipyard workers 58 (288)	55.0	—	33.0	—	33.0	—
	Michigan men 42 (594)	51.0	48.0	30.0	13.0	15.0	3.0
Phlegm 3 mo/yr							
Broder et al. (1979)[c]		45.0	—	17.0	—	15.0	—
Dopico et al. (1984)[d]	Grain handlers 41.0±12.0 (310)	42.0	—	32.0	—	37.0	—
	City workers 41.0±12.0 (239)	—	26.0	—	4.0	—	8.0

TABLE 2.—Continued

Symptoms[a] Reference	Mean age (Total)	Current smokers Occupationally exposed	Control	Former smokers Occupationally exposed	Control	Never smokers Occupationally exposed	Control
Babbott et al. (1980)[e,f]	Dairy farmers (198)	39.0	—	19.0[g]	—	16.0	—
	Industry workers (516)	—	30.0	—	9.0[g]	—	10.0
Chan-Yeung et al. (1984)		26.1	21.8	14.1	8.2	10.0	7.5
Kilburn, Warshaw, Thornton (1986)		55.0	28.0	39.0	15.0	38.0	7.0
Dyspnea > grade 2							
Broder et al. (1979)[h]		23.0	21.0	12.0	11.0	15.0	5.0
		15.0	—	16.0	—	5.0	—
Dopico et al. (1984)[i]		72.0	3.0	58.0	6.0	57.0	2.0
Babbott et al. (1980)[f]		45.0	36.0	51.0[g]	34.0[g]	27.0	19.0
Chan-Yeung et al. (1984)		34.9	21.1	26.4	10.4	18.1	6.4
Kilburn, Warshaw, Thornton (1986)[j]		65.0	7.0	59.0	6.0	54.0	2.0
Wheeze							
Broder et al. (1979)[k]		5.0	4.0	8.0	6.0	4.0	8.0
		3.0	—	7.0	—	3.0	—
Dopico et al. (1984)[l]		22.0	50.0	17.0	41.0	17.0	30.0
Babbott et al. (1980)[f,l]		47.0	45.0	41.0[g]	29.0[g]	31.0	22.0
Chan-Yeung et al. (1984)[m]		23.4	24.8	12.3	7.5	9.2	7.5
Kilburn, Warshaw, Thornton (1986)[l]		68.0	13.0	43.0	8.0	32.0	1.0

[a]Males only; symptoms not mutually exclusive.
[b]Cough for more than a few days/wk.
[c]Phlegm for more than a few days/wk.
[d]Morning expectoration.
[e]Chronic sputum production; sputum most days persisting for at least 3 mo/yr.
[f]Matched on age and cigarette smoking (current, farm: industry 35.59 vs. 35.41; former, 43.20 vs. 43.24; never, 34.01 vs. 33.88).
[g]Matched on years since cessation, farmers 7.95 vs. industry 8.43.
[h]Shortness of breath.
[i]Grade 2 dyspnea.
[j]Dyspnea at two flights of stairs.
[k]Wheeze in attacks.
[l]Ever wheeze.
[m]Persistant wheeze; wheeze with colds or wheeze on most days or nights.

smokers had intermediate prevalence rates for cough, sputum production, wheeze, and shortness of breath compared with current and never smokers. Additionally, former smokers who were grain handlers had more acute and chronic symptoms than ex-smokers who were outside civil or city workers. For grain workers, length of employment had no effect on the prevalence of respiratory symptoms within each smoking group. The results of these two studies differ in that the occupational effect was minimal and less than the smoking effect in the former investigation but significant and greater in the latter. The choice of control subjects may explain this discrepancy.

Babbott and colleagues (1980) assessed the respiratory symptoms of 198 Vermont dairy farmers and 516 nonmineral industrial workers. Former smokers were matched on age (mean 43 years) and years since cessation (mean 8 years). Chronic sputum production, wheezing, and dyspnea were more common among current smokers than among former or never smokers and more frequent among dairy farmers than industrial workers. Similar results were found by Chan-Yeung and coworkers (1984) in a study of 652 cedar mill workers and 440 control office workers. Korn and associates (1987), in a population sample of 8,515 white adults, showed that smoking and exposure to dust, gases, or fumes were independently associated with an increased prevalence of chronic cough, chronic phlegm, persistent wheeze, and breathlessness. Former smokers with gas or fume exposure were more likely to have respiratory symptoms, particularly breathlessness, than exposed current or never smokers. A multiplicative relationship between smoking and occupational exposure was found for breathlessness but not for other symptoms.

Kilburn, Warshaw, and Thornton (1986) conducted an investigation of respiratory symptoms, cardiopulmonary diseases, and asbestosis among 338 male and 81 female shipyard workers and their families. In general, the study group had more symptoms than reported from a similarly stratified random sample of the Michigan population (Miller et al. 1988). The authors suggested that environmental influences in the Los Angeles area may explain the higher rates. Male shipyard workers who were former smokers had more cough, sputum production, and wheezing than shipyard workers who were current smokers, whereas the pattern was reversed for female shipyard workers.

In summary, results from selected occupational groups support the findings from the community-based studies, although work exposures may interact with smoking in determining the occurrence of symptoms among former smokers (US DHHS 1985). The results of these investigations may be affected by misclassification of exposures and by selection or recall bias. As in the community-based studies, limited descriptive information is provided on former smokers.

Longitudinal Studies

Numerous longitudinal population-based studies have found rapid resolution of most respiratory symptoms after smoking cessation (Table 3). A study by Woolf and Zamel (1980) indicated that 302 female former smokers with a mean cigarette consumption of 15 pack-years had dramatic resolution of respiratory symptoms within 5 years. These investigators defined former smokers as women who had not smoked for at least 1 year before entry into the study. Persistent former and never smokers were comparable in

TABLE 3.—Change (%) in presence of respiratory symptoms, longitudinal studies, by cigarette smoking status

Symptoms Reference	Age (mean)		Continuing smokers			Former smokers			Never smokers	
			Lost	No change[a]	Gained	Lost	No change[a]	Gained	Lost	No change[a]	Gained
Cough 3 mo/yr											
Woolf and Zamel (1980)[b]	Smokers Light: 43.2±1.7[c] Moderate: 39.1±1.1 Heavy: 38.6±0.9		18.0	66.0	16.0	2.0	85.0	13.0	5.0	86.0	9.0
Tashkin et al. (1984)[d]	Smokers Male: 45.1 Female: 46.9 Quitters Male: 43.4 Female: 45.6		8.3	77.6	14.1	14.3	82.7	3.0	—	—	—
Comstock et al. (1970)[e]	40–59		Net change: 1.0			Net change: −21.0			Net change: 3.0		
Sharp et al. (1973)[f,g]	43–58		10.7	78.0	11.3	16.7	78.5	4.8	4.5	90.8	4.7
Friedman and Siegelaub (1980)[g]	20–79 White male ≥1 ppd[h] White female ≥1 ppd Black male ≥1 ppd Black female ≥1 ppd		7.6 7.4 5.5 5.0	85.5 85.2 89.2 89.7	6.9 7.4 5.3 5.3	10.1 5.0 1.3 2.9	89.3 92.5 97.4 96.6	0.6 2.5 1.3 1.5	— — — —	— — — —	— — — —
Phlegm 3 mo/yr											
Tashkin et al. (1984)			8.8	77.9	13.3	7.7	86.3	6.0	—	—	—

TABLE 3.—Continued

Symptoms Reference	Age (mean)	Continuing smokers Lost	Continuing smokers No change[a]	Continuing smokers Gained	Former smokers Lost	Former smokers No change[a]	Former smokers Gained	Never smokers Lost	Never smokers No change[a]	Never smokers Gained
Comstock et al. (1970)			Net change: 4.0			Net change: −15.0			Net change: 0.0	
Sharp et al. (1973)		15.4	86.2	6.4	10.2	77.0	12.8	8.0	85.0	7.0
Dyspnea ≥ grade 2										
Woolf and Zamel (1980)[i]		17.0	69.0	13.0	18.0	75.0	8.0	7.0	91.0	2.0
Tashkin et al. (1984)[j]		4.6	89.9	5.5	4.2	89.8	6.0	—	—	—
Comstock et al. (1970)			Net change: 2.0			Net change: 11.0			Net change: 2.0	
Sharp et al. (1973)[k]		11.0	72.8	16.2	14.4	72.8	12.8	10.2	79.8	10.0
Friedman et al. (1973)										
White male ≥1 ppd			Net change: −8.9			Net change: −4.8				
White female ≥1 ppd			Net change: −11.8			Net change: −5.0				
Wheeze										
Woolf and Zamel (1980)[l]		18.0	71.0	11.0	0.0	96.0	5.0	5.0	91.0	4.0
Tashkin et al. (1984)[l]		11.2	77.8	11.0	13.7	82.1	4.2	—	—	—

TABLE 3.—Continued

Symptoms Reference	Age (mean)	Continuing smokers Lost	Continuing smokers No change[a]	Continuing smokers Gained	Former smokers Lost	Former smokers No change[a]	Former smokers Gained	Never smokers Lost	Never smokers No change[a]	Never smokers Gained
Comstock et al. (1970)[m]			Net change: 5.0			Net change: –5.0			Net change: –2.0	
Sharp et al. (1973)[m]		13.4	77.0	9.6	11.1	78.7	10.2	7.3	88.4	4.3

[a] No change indicates that respiratory symptoms were either consistently absent or consistently present.
[b] Only females, cough and/or phlegm, 5-yr study period.
[c] Light=≤70 cig/wk; moderate=71–140 cig/wk; heavy=more than 140 cig/wk.
[d] Former smokers defined as those who stopped between baseline and followup.
[e] Males only, 5–6-yr followup.
[f] Males only, former studies defined as those who stopped between baseline and followup, 7-yr followup.
[g] Former studies defined as those who stopped between baseline and followup, 1.5-yr followup.
[h] ppd=packs/day.
[i] Grade 2 or 3 dyspnea.
[j] Dyspnea not defined.
[k] Dyspnea at ordinary pace.
[l] Wheeze not defined.
[m] Ever wheeze.

age; former smokers had a shorter duration of smoking in years than current smokers of 1/2 to 1 pack per day, but similar cumulative pack-years (11.5 vs. 15.0). More former and never smokers reported consistent absence of cough or sputum, dyspnea, or wheeze compared with current smokers. Thirteen percent of former smokers developed cough or phlegm during the study period compared with 9 percent of never smokers and 16 percent of smokers. At enrollment, smokers had more respiratory symptoms and were more likely to develop symptoms over the 5 years of the study.

Similarly, in a large population study in the Los Angeles area, respiratory symptoms diminished among former smokers after only 5 years of abstinence (Tashkin et al. 1984). In this study, the following 4 smoking groups were defined: 278 persistent smokers; 414 never smokers; 106 quitters, subjects who smoked regularly at baseline but were nonsmokers at the conclusion of the study; and 294 former smokers, individuals who were regular smokers but had quit at least 2 years prior to baseline. The mean age for female quitters (45.6 years) was comparable among the smoking categories; the mean age for male quitters (43.4 years) was similar to the mean ages for current and never smokers; however, it was 6.2 years less than that for former smokers. Quitters and former smokers had smoked similar numbers of cigarettes per day (26.3 vs. 24.6 for males; 19.1 vs. 19.0 for females), but quitters had higher pack-years (38.6 vs. 26.8 for males; 27.4 vs. 16.2 for females). In addition, quitters had pack-years comparable with current smokers (38.6 vs. 40.5 for males; 27.4 vs. 30.9 for females). Over the 5 years of the study, quitters recovered from the symptoms of cough, sputum, and wheeze more frequently than continuing smokers. No difference in shortness of breath was found between the two groups in the 5-year study period. Quitters and former smokers were not compared to determine the relative importance of cumulative exposure versus time since exposure on the observed reduction of symptoms among ex-smokers.

Comstock and coworkers (1970) reported comparable findings in a study of respiratory symptoms in 670 male telephone company employees studied for 5 to 6 years. Symptoms of chronic cough, phlegm production, and wheeze decreased significantly in quitters whose baseline prevalence for these symptoms was similar to persistent smokers but whose followup values were comparable to never smokers. Baseline and followup prevalence rates for breathlessness in quitters were equivalent to those of persistent smokers.

Sharp and colleagues (1973) found similar trends in respiratory symptoms in 1,263 middle-aged males from an industrial population surveyed in 1961 and again in 1968. Former smokers were defined as individuals who stopped smoking after entry into the study; previous smoking histories were not provided. Over the 7 years of the study, 72.3 percent of former smokers with persistent cough and 64.4 percent with persistent phlegm recovered from the symptoms. These rates of recovery were higher than for the other smoking groups with similar symptoms. Additionally, former smokers who originally complained of dyspnea and wheeze tended to lose these symptoms over the study period, but less dramatically (49-percent and 45.5-percent recovery, respectively). New reports of cough and phlegm were made by less than 10 percent of never and former smokers and 16 percent of continuing smokers, whereas new wheeze was found in 13.5 percent of former and 14.1 percent of continuing smokers. In contrast, dyspnea developed in 18.1 percent of former smokers and 22.4 percent of continuing smokers.

In a study of shorter duration, Friedman and Siegelaub (1980) confirmed the findings of Tashkin and coworkers (1984), Comstock and associates (1970), and Sharp and colleagues (1973). Over approximately 1.5 years of observation, 3,825 recent quitters more often reported decreased chronic cough but no exertional dyspnea when compared with 9,392 persistent smokers.

Findings from two Finnish studies and one British study support the results of these North American investigations (Huhti and Ikkala 1980; Poukkula, Huhti, Mäkaräinen 1982; Leeder et al. 1977). In the 10-year study of Huhti and Ikkala (1980), respiratory symptoms increased in all groups of smokers except male quitters, who had lower prevalence of phlegm production and wheezing (Table 4). Similarly, in a 10-year followup of male pulp mill workers, Poukkula, Huhti, and Mäkaräinen (1982) observed a decrease in respiratory symptoms only for quitters and only for cough and phlegm production. No explanation for the increase in symptoms over time for never smokers was provided in either study. During a 6-year period, Leeder and colleagues (1977) evaluated chronic cough and phlegm annually in 3,916 young married adults. Men who gave up smoking had a progressive decline in the reporting of cough and phlegm. Only a small number of female ex-smokers were included.

In summary, the findings from these longitudinal studies agree with those from the cross-sectional surveys and suggest that cough, phlegm production, and wheezing reverse after cessation, regardless of duration or quantity previously smoked. Dyspnea, however, may be less likely to resolve in subjects with longer smoking histories, possibly indicating irreversible damage induced by smoking up to time of cessation.

Clinical Studies of Possible Mechanisms

Few studies have investigated the mechanisms by which respiratory symptoms improve after smoking cessation. Reversal of mucous gland hyperplasia and reduction in airway inflammation have been considered likely mechanisms but have not been documented. Recovery of epithelial integrity has been shown in two small clinical studies of epithelial permeability (Minty, Jordan, Jones 1981; Mason et al. 1983). Improvement in tracheal mucous velocity, another possible mechanism by which respiratory symptoms may decrease after smoking cessation, has also been examined. Goodman and coworkers (1978) reported that five of nine young former smokers had tracheal mucous velocities that were comparable with age-matched never smokers. One subject had a minimally depressed velocity, and three had markedly depressed values. Only one subject was restudied 2 months after baseline and 9 months after cessation, and at that time, tracheal mucous velocity was found still to be reduced. Because subjects were not studied while smoking, the change after cessation could not be determined. Camner, Philipson, and Arvidsson (1973) studied tracheal velocity in subjects before and after smoking cessation. They found that in 11 of 17 male former smokers, tracheal mucous velocity improved 3 months after cessation and that in the remaining 6 former smokers, velocity was slower or similar when compared with baseline values. Improved tracheal mucous velocity may lead to less mucus in the airways and thereby reduce symptoms of cough and wheeze among former smokers.

TABLE 4.—Percentage of subjects with respiratory symptoms by smoking status, 1961 and 1971, in a cohort of middle-aged, rural Finns

	Smoking groups[a]							
	I Never smokers 1961 Never smokers 1971		II Ex-smokers 1961 Ex-smokers 1971		III Smokers 1961 Ex-smokers 1971		IV Smokers 1961 Smokers 1971	
Symptoms	Males (89)	Females (573)	Males (102)	Females (26)	Males (75)	Females (19)	Males (211)	Females (47)
Phlegm all day—winter								
1961	4	2	7	—	9	11	18	4
1971	6	4	7	4	7	—	27	13
Wheezing most days								
1961	—	3	—	—	3	—	4	2
1971	2	6	4	—	1	—	9	11
Weather affects chest								
1961	6	14	10	15	13	11	13	6
1971	19	27	25	23	24	16	39	19
Breathlessness grades 3–4								
1961	4	20	10	12	15	16	11	9
1971	10	24	17	12	16	21	21	6
Chronic bronchitis								
1961	9	5	14	15	29	16	36	21
1971	11	8	15	12	9	5	41	21
Mean age (yr) in 1961	50	51	50	49	50	47	49	46

[a]Figures in parentheses are number of subjects.
SOURCE: Huhti and Ikkala (1980).

Respiratory Infections

Numerous clinical studies have shown alterations in immune and inflammatory function among cigarette smokers compared with never smokers. Studies of peripheral blood have shown that current smokers have as much as 30 percent higher leukocyte counts than never smokers (Corre, Lellouch, Schwartz 1971; Friedman et al. 1973). Increases have been reported in polymorphonuclear leukocytes (Bridges, Wyatt, Rehm 1985), which appear to have normal chemotactic, microbicidal, and secretory functions (Nobel and Penny 1975; Abboud et al. 1983), and monocytes (Nielsen 1985), which may partially lack the ability to kill intracellular *Candida* (Nielsen 1985). Total numbers of T lymphocytes are increased among smokers (Kaszubowski, Wysocki, Machalski 1981; Robertson et al. 1983; Burton et al. 1983; Smart et al. 1986). Light and moderate smokers have increases in OKT3+ (total T cells) and OKT4+ (T-helper cells) (Hughes et al. 1985; Ginns et al. 1982), and heavy smokers have decreases in OKT4+ and increases in OKT8+ (T-suppressor cells) (Ginns et al. 1982; Miller et al. 1982). Additionally, functional changes in T lymphocytes from smokers have been observed (Whitehead et al. 1974; Suciu-Foca et al. 1974; Onari et al. 1980), but these findings remain controversial.

Changes in serum components have also been reported. Smokers have higher levels of C5, C9, C1 inhibitor (Wyatt, Bridges, Halatek 1981), C-reactive protein, and autoantibodies (antinuclear and rheumatoid factors) (Heiskell et al. 1962), but lower levels of specific immunoglobulins (IgG, IgM, and IgA) (Ferson et al. 1979; Vos-Brat and Rumke 1969; Kosmider, Felus, Wysocki 1973; Dales et al. 1974; Wingerd and Sponzilli 1977; Gulsvik and Fagerhol 1979; Gerrard, Heiner et al. 1980; Leitch, Lumb, Kay 1981; Andersen et al. 1982; Bartelik, Ziolo, Bartelik 1984; McSharry, Banham, Boyd 1985). As previously described, IgE is elevated in smokers (Burrows et al. 1981; Zetterström et al. 1981; Hällgren et al. 1982; Warren et al. 1982; Bonini 1982; Stein et al. 1983), and this increase may result from suppression of regulatory T-lymphocyte function (Holt 1987).

Bronchoalveolar lavage has provided evidence on the noncellular and cellular components of the peripheral airways and alveoli among smokers and nonsmokers. Data have indicated that smokers appear to have normal or slightly elevated levels of IgA and IgG (Reynolds and Newball 1974; Warr and Martin 1977; Bell et al. 1981; Velluti et al. 1983; Pre, Bladier, Battesti 1980; Gotoh et al. 1983). Similarly, values for lysozyme (Harris et al. 1975), complement components (Robertson et al. 1976), and fibronectin (Villiger et al. 1981) are elevated in lavage fluid from smokers. The total number of cells retrieved from lavage of smokers is increased with marked elevation in the percentages of activated macrophages and neutrophils (Hunninghake et al. 1979; Harris, Swenson, Johnson 1970). Absolute lymphocyte numbers remain unchanged, although T-cell function may be altered (Daniele et al. 1977; DeShazo et al. 1983). Recovered macrophages have increased chemotactic function (Warr and Martin 1974; Labedzki et al. 1983; Richards et al. 1984) and increased release of damaging products such as superoxide anions (Hoidal et al. 1979; Hoidal et al. 1980; Joseph et al. 1980; Hoidal and Niewoehner 1982; Greening and Lowrie 1983; Razma et al. 1984), but diminished microbicidal activity (Martin and Warr 1977; Fisher et al. 1982; Ando et al. 1984).

Smokers have been shown to have reduced specific immune responses to inhaled antigens in several occupational studies. Farmers who were never smokers had higher levels of serum precipitins to *Micropolyspora faeni* than farmers who smoked (Morgan et al. 1973; Morgan et al. 1975; Gruchow et al. 1981; Cormier and Bélanger 1989; Kusaka et al. 1989), whereas pigeon breeders who had never smoked had higher precipitating antibodies to pigeon 7 globulin compared with their smoking counterparts (McSharry et al. 1984; Andersen and Christensen 1983; Boyd et al. 1977). Similar results have been found in poultry workers (Andersen and Schonheyder 1984) and processing workers (McSharry and Wilkinson 1986) in relation to IgG responses to hen serum antigen and prawn antigen, respectively. Whether smokers have a lower incidence of hypersensitivity pneumonitis has not been adequately studied.

Finally, smokers manifest a blunted immune response to influenza vaccination. Although smokers and nonsmokers have similar postvaccination titers at 3 months (Knowles, Taylor, Turner-Warwick 1981), current smokers have reduced titers at 1 year when compared with nonsmokers (Finklea et al. 1971; Mackenzie, Mackenzie, Holt 1976). In a large clinical trial comparing responses to killed and live attenuated vaccine, smokers had a decreased primary immune response to the killed vaccine (Mackenzie, Mackenzie, Holt 1976).

Although effects of smoking on the immune system have been demonstrated, few studies have investigated the association between smoking and acute respiratory illnesses of presumed infectious etiology. Aronson and coworkers (1982) found that smoking was associated with an increased risk of acute respiratory tract illness. In addition, these investigators found that smoking increased the likelihood of having a lower respiratory tract illness and increased the duration of the symptom of cough. These findings corroborated the results of other investigations (Haynes, Krstulovic, Bell 1966; Peters and Ferris 1967; Parnell, Anderson, Kinnis 1966) that showed the same trend for increased respiratory infections among smokers compared with nonsmokers. In contrast, Pollard and associates (1975) found no difference in the incidence of respiratory illness observed among smokers compared with nonsmokers. Short follow-up of 9 weeks and selection of Naval recruits who had a high prevalence of acute respiratory disease as patients may explain the discrepancy in results.

Kark, Lebiush, and Rannon (1982) studied an outbreak of influenza among 336 men serving in a military unit in Israel. They found that 68.5 percent of 168 current and occasional smokers had clinically apparent influenza as compared with 47.2 percent of never and former smokers. Smokers and nonsmokers with influenza had comparable serologic response rates. Among smokers, the attributable risk percentage for severe influenza, defined as illness resulting in bedrest or loss of workdays, was 40.6 percent (95-percent confidence interval (CI), 21.6–54.8 percent). Similar results have also been reported by several other researchers (Finklea, Sandifer, Smith 1969; MacKenzie, Mackenzie, Holt 1976; Kark and Lebiush 1981).

Smoking Cessation and Respiratory Infection

The relationship between altered immune and inflammatory functions and the occurrence of respiratory infections among ex-smokers has not been extensively investigated. This Section reviews available relevant studies.

Studies of animals have shown a return to normal immune and inflammatory function after cessation of cigarette smoke exposure (Holt and Keast 1977). Investigations of humans have yielded similar findings. Specifically, among former smokers, serum concentrations of IgG, IgA, and IgM (Hersey, Prendergast, Edwards 1983) and bronchoalveolar lavage cell numbers and percentages return to those of never smokers (Holt 1987). Additionally, Miller and coworkers (1982) found that within 6 weeks of smoking cessation, the number and function of T lymphocytes reverted to normal. Finally, Raman, Swinburne, and Fedulla (1983) found that 3 years after smoking cessation, former smokers had pneumococcal oropharyngeal adherence values comparable with those of never smokers. The significance of these changes in specific components of host defenses to the risk of subsequent respiratory infections among former smokers has not been characterized.

Mortality from influenza and pneumonia with respect to cigarette smoking has been assessed in several cohort studies (Table 5). Mortality from influenza and pneumonia was increased in ever smokers relative to never smokers in the American Cancer Society Cancer Prevention Study I (ACS CPS-I) followup from 1959 through 1963 (Hammond 1965). In the British Physicians Study, current and former smokers had small excesses of mortality from pneumonia, but annual mortality rates from pneumonia increased with the amount smoked (47/100,000 for 1–14 g tobacco/day, 62/100,000 for 15–24 g tobacco/day, 91/100,000 for ≥25 g/day) (Doll and Peto 1976). A similar exposure–response relationship was found in the U.S. Veterans Study (Rogot and Murray 1980).

Findings from ACS CPS-II on age-adjusted mortality from influenza and pneumonia have been examined for the effects of active smoking and smoking cessation (Table 5). Male former smokers of fewer than 21 cigarettes per day have mortality ratios after 10 years of abstinence that are approaching unity. Male former smokers of more than 21 cigarettes per day have mortality ratios approaching unity after 15 years of abstinence, but much higher for shorter periods of abstinence. Female former smokers of any amount have mortality ratios that approach those of never smokers within 3 to 5 years of abstinence.

The association between cigarette smoking status and mortality from influenza and pneumonia may partially reflect the effects of smoking on respiratory defense mechanisms including immune responses. The vulnerability of persons with cigarette-related cardiopulmonary diseases to respiratory infections may also contribute to the association. For example, Glezen, Decker, and Perrotta (1987) studied underlying diagnoses in patients hospitalized with acute respiratory disease during influenza epidemics in Houston, TX. Chronic pulmonary conditions were the most common underlying condition, and cardiac conditions were the next most frequent.

PART II: PULMONARY FUNCTION AMONG FORMER SMOKERS

Cross-Sectional Population Studies of FEV_1

Epidemiologic studies have generally evaluated airflow obstruction based on FEV_1, a spirometric parameter sensitive to airways and parenchymal effects. Cross-sectional population studies, that is, studies in which lung function and cigarette smoking are measured at a single point in time, have demonstrated that cigarette smoking is a strong determinant of FEV_1 level (US DHHS 1984). In those studies in which results from former smokers have been reported, the level of FEV_1 has generally been between that of never smokers and current smokers (Table 6).

Several studies have shown that the level of FEV_1 declines with increasing cumulative smoking among former smokers as well as current smokers (Burrows et al. 1977; Beck, Doyle, Schachter 1981; Dockery et al. 1988). Burrows and colleagues (1977)

TABLE 5.—Age-standardized mortality ratios for influenza and pneumonia for current and former smokers compared with never smokers

Reference	Population	Followup	Cause of death	Standardized mortality ratios by smoking status
Hammond (1965)	1,045,087 US men and women (ACS CPS-I)	4 yr	Influenza and pneumonia	Gender, age group (yr) / Never smokers / History of smoking Men 45–64: 1.0 / 1.9 Men 65–79: 1.0 / 1.7 Women 45–64: 1.0 / 1.3
Doll and Peto (1976)	34,440 male British doctors	20 yr	Pneumonia	Never smokers: 1.0 / Former smokers: 1.1 Smoking amount (cig/day) — Current smokers by amount (g/day): <10: 0.9 10–20 (1–14): 0.9 21–39 (15–24): 1.1 ≥40 (≥25): 1.7
Rogot and Murray (1980)	293,958 US veterans	16 yr	Influenza and pneumonia	Former smokers[a]: 0.8 1.0 1.0 1.3 Current smokers: 1.2 1.7 2.2 2.4
Carstensen, Pershagen, Eklund (1987)	25,000 Swedish men	16 yr	Pneumonia	Never smokers: 1.0 / Former smokers: 0.6 Current smokers by amount (g/day): 1–7: 1.3 8–15: 1.0 >15: 1.7

TABLE 5.—Continued

Reference	Population	Followup	Cause of death		Total former smokers	Standardized mortality ratios by smoking status						Current smokers
						\<1	1–2	3–5	6–10	11–15	≥16	
American Cancer Society (unpublished tabulations)	1,080,555 US men and women (ACS CPS-II)	4 yr	Influenza and pneumonia									
				Men, total	1.3	—[b]	—	—	—	—	—	1.8
				Men <21 cig/day	1.3	3.4	2.1	1.8	1.8	1.1	1.1	2.0
				Men ≥21 cig/day	1.3	2.4	—	2.2	2.1	2.1	0.9	1.2
				Women total	1.2	—[b]	—	—	—	—	—	2.7
				Women <20 cig/day	1.0	—	—	1.3	0.6	0.3	1.2	3.4
				Women ≥20 cig/day	1.1	1.3	2.4	0.6	2.4	1.3	0.2	2.0

NOTE: ACS CPS-I and -II=American Cancer Society Cancer Prevention Studies I and II.
[a] Former cigarette smokers who stopped smoking for reasons other than a physician's orders.
[b] Not calculated.

TABLE 6.—Association between cigarette smoking status and FEV$_1$ levels in selected cross-sectional studies of adult populations

Reference	Year of study	Location	Population	Findings
Goldsmith et al. (1962)	1961	San Francisco, CA	3,311 longshoremen	Mean FEV$_1$ % of predicted value Never smokers 100 Former smokers 97 Current smokers 93
Edelman et al. (1966)		Baltimore, MD	410 male volunteers, aged 20–103	By partial regression analysis, significant reduction of FEV$_1$ among current and former cigarette smokers
Higgins and Kjelsberg (1967)	1959–60	Tecumseh, MI	5,140 men and women, aged 16–79	Age-adjusted mean FEV$_1$ (L) Men Women Never smokers 3.3 2.3 Former smokers 3.3 2.3 Current smokers 3.1 2.3
Higgins et al. (1968)	1963	Marion County, WV	926 white men, aged 20–69	Mean FEV$_1$ (L) Never smokers 3.6 Former smokers 3.3 Current smokers 3.5
Wilhelmsen, Orha, Tibblin (1969)	1963	Göteborg, Sweden	331 men, age 50	Mean FEV$_1$ (L) Never smokers 3.8 Former smokers 3.7 Current smokers 3.5

TABLE 6.—Continued

Reference	Year of study	Location	Population	Findings
Woolf and Suero (1971)		Toronto, Canada	298 female volunteers, aged 25–54, employed at commercial firms	Adjusted mean levels 　　　　　　　　FEV$_1$　FEV$_1$/FVC ratio Never smokers　2.7　86.7 Former smokers　2.6　85.0 Current smokers　2.5　84.6
Schlesinger et al. (1972)	1968	Israel	4,331 male civil servants, aged 45 and older	Mean value of the FEV$_1$/FVC ratio Never smokers　76.0 Former smokers　74.3 Current smokers　73.6
Fletcher et al. (1976)	1961	London, England	1,136 men, aged 30–59, employed at bank or in maintenance of transportation equipment	Adjusted FEV$_1$ (L) Never smokers　3.3 Former smokers　3.2 Current smokers　3.0
Higgins, Keller, Metzner (1977)	1962–65	Tecumseh, MI	4,669 men and women, aged 20–74	Mean normalized FEV$_1$ score 　　　　　　　　Men　Women Never smokers　10.2　10.1 Former smokers　9.9　10.0 Current smokers　9.6　9.8

TABLE 6.—Continued

Reference	Year of study	Location	Population	Findings
Anderson (1979)		Lufa, Papua New Guinea	733 men and women aged 25 and older	Age and height-adjusted mean FEV$_1$ (L)
				Men Women
				Never smokers 2.6 2.4
				Former smokers 2.6 2.3
				Current smokers 2.6 2.4
Higenbottam et al. (1980)		London, England	18,403 male civil servants, aged 40–64	Age and height-adjusted mean FEV$_1$ (L)
				Former smokers 3.2
				<7 yr abstinent 3.2
				7–12 yr abstinent 3.2
				≥13 yr abstinent 3.1
				Current smokers 3.1
Huhti and Ikkala (1980)	1961	Rural commune, Finland	473 men and 569 women, followed for 10 yr	FEV$_1$ at initial examination
				Men Women
				Never smokers 3.5 2.5
				Former smokers 3.5 2.5
				Current smokers[a] 3.3 2.8
Bossé et al. (1980)	1963	Boston, MA	703 healthy male veterans followed for 10 yr	Initial FEV$_1$ adjusted for age
				Never smokers 3.6
				Former smokers 3.6
				Current smokers 3.3

TABLE 6.—Continued

Reference	Year of study	Location	Population	Findings
Bossé et al. (1981)	1963	Boston, MA	850 healthy male veterans followed for 5 yr	Initial FEV$_1$ adjusted for age Never smokers 4.0 Former smokers 3.7 Current smokers 3.8
Beck, Doyle, Schachter (1981)	1972–74	Lebanon and Ansonia, CT; Winnsboro, SC	4,690 men and women, aged 7 and older	Residual FEV$_1$ (L) adjusted for age, height, weight Men Women Never smokers −0.02 −0.02 Former smokers −0.12 −0.20 Current smokers −0.22 −0.27
Tashkin et al. (1984)	1973–75	Los Angeles, CA	1,092 men and 1,309 women aged 25–64 followed for 5 yr	Initial adjusted level of FEV$_1$ Men Women Nonsmokers 3.9 2.7 Former smokers 3.8 2.7 Current smokers[a] 3.6 2.5
Taylor, Joyce et al. (1985)	1981–82	London, UK	227 men followed for 7.5 yr	FEV$_1$ as percentage of predicted All Reactors Nonreactors Nonsmokers 119.1 92.0 121.4 Former smokers 107.8 96.4 111.4 Current smokers 100.5 84.6 108.5

TABLE 6.—Continued

Reference	Year of study	Location	Population	Findings
Camilli et al. (1987)		Tucson, AZ	654 men and 893 women aged 20 and older, who had FEV_1 at baseline and followup exams	Initial FEV_1 as percentage of predicted Men Women Nonsmokers 99.8 97.8 Former smokers 93.7 95.6 Current smokers[a] 91.8 91.6
Dockery et al. (1988)	1974–77	6 US communities	8,191 men and women aged 25–74	Deficit of FEV_1 (L) compared with expected Men Women Nonsmokers −0.03 −0.02 Former smokers −0.26 −0.05 Current smokers −0.51 −0.23

NOTE: FEV_1=1-sec forced expiratory volume; FVC=forced vital capacity.

[a] At initial examination, which includes continuing smokers and those who subsequently quit.

reported that the level of FEV_1 had a highly significant quantitative relationship with pack-years in a general population sample of 2,369 subjects in Tucson, AZ, and that smokers and former smokers had comparable levels accounting for pack-years.

Higenbottam and coworkers (1980) assessed lung function in the 18,000 males in the Whitehall Civil Servants Study. Mean FEV_1 values among former smokers, adjusted for age and height, were lower than those for never smokers, but greater than those for current smokers. FEV_1 among former smokers decreased with increasing total consumption of cigarettes, but length of abstinence had little effect on FEV_1 among former smokers, although the minimum period considered was less than 6 years. The authors suggested that the depression of lung function associated with cigarette smoking has two components—an irreversible component related to total consumption and a component rapidly reversible on cessation.

Beck, Doyle, and Schachter (1981) analyzed FEV_1 data from 4,690 subjects, aged 7 years and older, in 3 separate U.S. communities. These investigators also found that the deficit in FEV_1 compared with that expected for never smokers increased with cumulative smoking as measured by pack-years and duration of smoking. After adjusting for cumulative smoking, FEV_1 was 147 mL lower among male smokers and 78 mL lower among female smokers compared with former smokers.

Dockery and coworkers (1988) studied 8,191 randomly selected adults in 6 U.S. communities. These researchers found that the deficit of observed FEV_1 compared with expected age-, height-, and sex-specific values increased linearly with cumulative pack-years among former smokers and current smokers (Figure 7) (Dockery et al. 1988). For the same pack-years, FEV_1 was 123 mL higher among male former smokers and 107 mL higher among female former smokers compared with current smokers.

In a followup study of 227 men, Taylor, Joyce, and coworkers (1985) reported that percent-predicted FEV_1 for former smokers (107.8 percent predicted) was between that of smokers (100.5) and never smokers (119.1). Within each smoking category, men with increased bronchial reactivity to inhaled histamine had lower levels of percent-predicted FEV_1 than did nonreactors. These differences were statistically significant among smokers (84.6 vs. 108.5 percent predicted for reactors and nonreactors, respectively) and former smokers (96.4 vs. 121.5 percent predicted for reactors and nonreactors, respectively).

The results of these studies suggest that permanent loss of FEV_1 occurs with smoking and that the extent of the loss is associated with the cumulative amount smoked. However, before the development of overt COPD, cessation is associated with an average improvement of 75 to 150 mL, implying that smoking also causes reversible decrements of function.

Pulmonary Function Studies After Smoking Cessation

Studies in which the lung function of smokers was measured before and after smoking cessation are reviewed in this Section; tests of pulmonary function included spirometry, nitrogen washout, and other techniques potentially sensitive to the effects of cessation. Inflammatory lesions of the small airways have been demonstrated to occur in young adult smokers before the appearance of clinically significant airflow obstruction

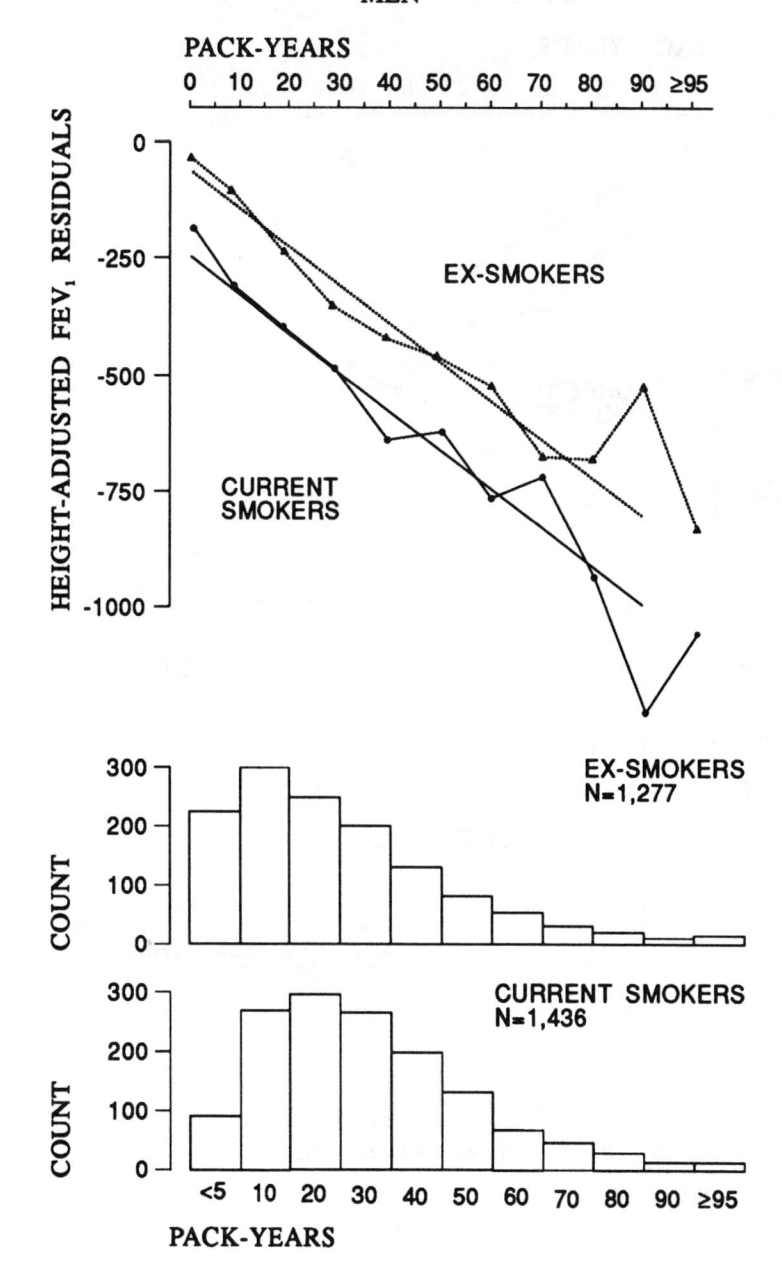

FIGURE 7.—Sex-specific mean height-adjusted FEV$_1$ residuals versus pack-years for current and ex-smokers, and distributions of number of subjects by pack-years

NOTE: FEV$_1$=1-sec forced expiratory volume.

SOURCE: Dockery et al. (1988).

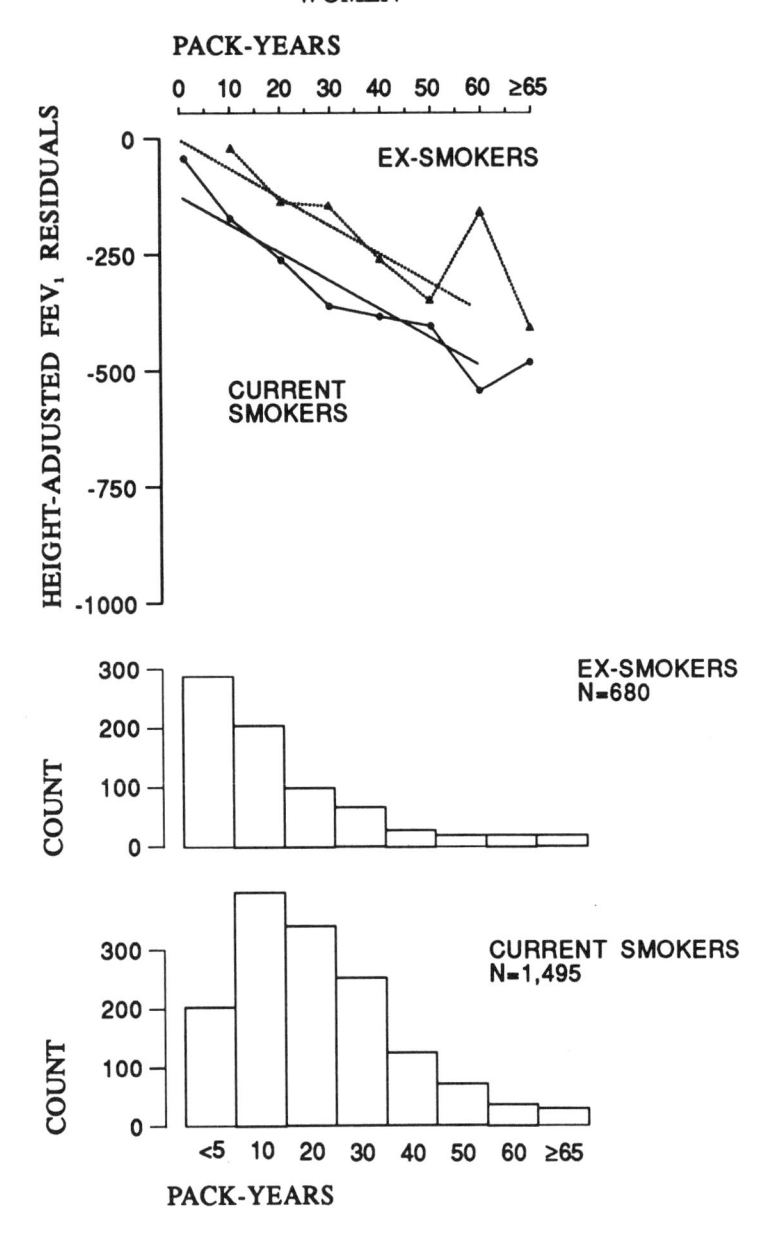

FIGURE 7. (Continued)—Sex-specific mean height-adjusted FEV_1 residuals versus pack-years for current and ex-smokers, and distributions of number of subjects by pack-years

NOTE: FEV_1=1-sec forced expiratory volume.

SOURCE: Dockery et al. (1988).

(Niewoehner, Kleinerman, Rice 1974). Tests sensitive to abnormalities of the small airways (e.g., helium-oxygen flow volume curves, the single breath nitrogen test or other tests of closing volume, and frequency dependence of compliance) would be expected to be particularly sensitive for detecting changes in function after cessation. In most of the studies reviewed in this Section, participants were enrolled through smoking cessation clinics and subsequently monitored for pulmonary function and smoking status. The data from these studies can assess reversible effects of smoking through documentation of functional change coincident with cessation; irreversible effects can be estimated by comparison of lung function level with predicted values for normal function.

Changes in Spirometric Parameters After Cessation

Studies of spirometric measurements of pulmonary function before and after smoking cessation are summarized in Table 7. Many of these studies suggested an improvement in pulmonary function following cessation, although the magnitude of the improvement was small in some of the studies.

Dirksen, Janzon, and Lindell (1974) studied a randomly selected sample of men born in 1914 in Malmö, Sweden. Fifty-eight heavy smokers were solicited to participate in a smoking cessation program, with 31 abstaining for 2 months. Vital capacity (VC) and FEV_1/FVC improved 8 to 10 days after cessation.

Bode and coworkers (1975) studied 10 healthy subjects who participated in a smoking cessation program and remained abstinent for 6 to 14 weeks. Small and nonsignificant improvements were found for VC (0.3 percent change) and FEV_1 (0.9 percent change). Maximum expiratory flow rates with helium at 50 and 25 percent of VC significantly increased.

Martin and colleagues (1975) observed 12 successful subjects from a smoking cessation clinic for 1 to 3 months. Changes of $\dot{V}_{max50}$ and $\dot{V}_{max25}$ after smoking cessation were variable and not statistically significant. Residual volume and total pulmonary resistance were also unchanged.

McCarthy, Craig, and Cherniack (1976) studied a group of smokers who volunteered to participate in a smoking cessation program. At 25 to 48 weeks after cessation, only 15 participants were still not smoking. Among these subjects, FVC increased from 3.92 L to 4.04 L (3.1 percent change), but FEV_1 (−0.3 percent change) and mid-maximum expiratory flow (MMEF) (−9.6 percent change) decreased. Fifty-nine subjects were evaluated between 6 and 24 weeks following cessation. Significant improvements were noted for FVC (2.3 percent of initial value) and the peak expiratory flow rate (6.7 percent of initial value). The FEV_1, $\dot{V}_{max50}$, and $\dot{V}_{max25}$ did not change significantly.

Bake and colleagues (1977) observed 17 subjects who were abstinent from cigarettes for at least 5 months. During this interval, VC and FEV_1 improved by 4.4 and 4.8 percent predicted, respectively, while $\dot{V}_{max50}$ and $\dot{V}_{max25}$ were reduced by 2.5 percent predicted and 7.3 percent predicted, respectively. At 2-year followup, only nine subjects were still smoking. No significant differences from baseline function were found in this group.

TABLE 7.—Spirometric studies of participants in smoking cessation programs

Reference	Population	Followup	Measure	TLC	FVC or VC	FEV$_1$	FEV$_1$/FVC	MMEF	$\dot{V}_{max50}$	$\dot{V}_{max75}$
Dirksen, Janzon, Lindell (1974)	31 men born in 1914, Malmö, Sweden	8–10 days 52–60 days	Change from initial		110 mL 20 mL		0.7% −1.3%			
Bode et al. (1975)	3 men and 7 women, aged 29–61, smoking clinic	6–14 wk	% change[a]	−0.8%	−0.2%	−0.7%		−2.7%	−2.0%	−10.6%
McCarthy, Craig, Cherniack (1976)	15 subjects, smoking clinic	25–48 wk	% change[b]		3.1%	0.3%		−9.6%		
Bake et al. (1977)	9 men and 8 women, aged 24–69, smoking clinic	5 mo 2 yr	Change in % predicted		4.4 2.2	4.8 −1.6			−2.5 0.7	−7.3 −11.1
Buist et al. (1976)	6 men and 7 women, aged 24–53, smoking clinic	1 mo 3 mo 6 mo 12 mo	Change from initial values	+10 mL −100 mL −240 mL −50 mL	−40 mL −310 mL −120 mL −70 mL	−40 mL −70 mL +30 mL +60 mL		−60 mL/sec −110 mL/sec +40 mL/sec −160 mL/sec		
Buist, Nagy, Sexton (1979)	3 men and 12 women, aged 24–52, smoking clinic	3–4 mo 6–8 mo 30 mo	Change in % predicted		2.4 6.5 6.5	1.5 4.6 3.3				

TABLE 7.—Continued

Reference	Population	Followup	Measure	TLC	FVC or VC	FEV_1	FEV_1/FVC	MMEF	$\dot{V}_{max50}$	$\dot{V}_{max75}$
Zamel, Leroux, Ramcharan (1979)	12 men and 14 women, mean age 36±9 yr	62±6 days	% change	1.2%	3.0%	4.0%				
Pride et al. (1980)	8 male smokers who thought easy to stop	4 yr		No improvement in spirometric tests or MMEF						

NOTE: TLC=total lung capacity; FVC=forced vital capacity; VC=vital capacity; FEV_1=1-sec forced expiratory volume; MMEF=mid-maximum expiratory flow.
[a]Average percentage change recalculated from individual values.
[b]Percentage change in reported mean values.

Buist and coworkers (1976) observed a group of six men and seven women who stopped smoking for at least 1 year after a smoking cessation program. Small changes were noted in spirometric parameters. The authors reported that MMEF distinguished between smokers and quitters in that over a 1-year period MMEF declined significantly among smokers but not among quitters.

Buist, Nagy, and Sexton (1979) supplemented this sample with participants from another smoking cessation program and extended followup to 30 months for both groups. Significant improvements were observed in VC, FEV$_1$, and MMEF among the quitters during the first 6 to 8 months (Figure 8). No further improvement was observed up to 30 months.

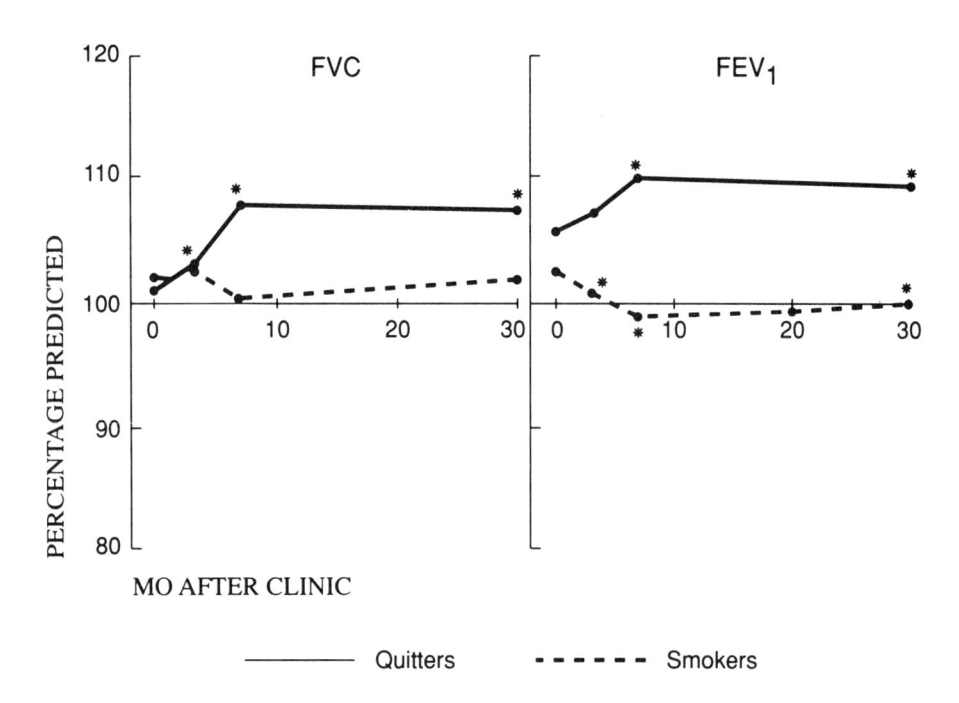

FIGURE 8.—Mean values for FVC and FEV$_1$, expressed as a percentage of predicted values, in 15 quitters and 42 smokers during 30 months after 2 smoking cessation clinics

NOTE: Asterisks (*) denote a significant difference from the initial value at p<0.05. FVC=forced vital capacity; FEV$_1$=1-sec forced expiratory volume.

SOURCE: Buist, Nagy, Sexton (1979).

Zamel, Leroux, and Ramcharan (1979) studied 26 healthy smokers for 2 months after cessation. They reported significant increases in VC and FEV$_1$ of 3.0 and 4.0 percent change, respectively. In contrast, Pride and coworkers (1980) in a 4-year study of eight male smokers "who thought they would find it easy to give up smoking," reported no improvement in spirometric tests of MMEF.

Taken together, these studies suggest that smoking cessation quickly results in small improvements in lung function, as assessed by spirometry. Although the changes were not uniformly statistically significant in the investigations reviewed in this Section, the number of subjects was small in most of the studies. Compared with baseline before cessation, FVC or VC and FEV_1 may improve by about 4 or 5 percent at 4 to 8 months after cessation. In absolute value, this improvement is comparable with the approximately 100-mL improvement reported by Beck, Doyle, and Schachter (1981) and Dockery and coworkers (1988) based on cross-sectional comparison of former smokers to current smokers.

Tests of Small Airways Function

Several investigators have studied the effects of smoking cessation using measures of small airways function as determined by the single breath nitrogen test (Table 8) and other tests. In the single breath nitrogen test, the subject breathes one breath of 100 percent oxygen from residual volume to total lung capacity (TLC). A concentration gradient of nitrogen is thus established with the highest concentrations at the apex. Subsequently, the subject exhales, and the nitrogen concentration of the exhaled air is monitored. The indices of small airways function provided by this test include the closing volume (CV) expressed as a percentage of the vital capacity (CV/VC percent), the closing capacity (CC) expressed as a percentage of TLC (CC/TLC percent), and the slope of the nitrogen concentration during the alveolar plateau (slope of phase III). Both CV and CC are increased by abnormalities of the small airways, whereas the slope of the nitrogen concentration reflects the evenness of the ventilation distribution.

Buist and colleagues (1976) studied a group of 25 cigarette smokers who attended a smoking cessation clinic. Cessation resulted in significant improvements in CV, CC, and the slope of alveolar plateau at 6 and 12 months after cessation. Participants in a second smoking cessation clinic were added, and the followup continued to 30 months (Buist, Nagy, Sexton 1979). At the 6- to 8-month followup, CV had improved by 33 percent predicted among those who quit, CC by 20 percent predicted, and the slope of the alveolar plateau by 52 percent. No further improvements were evident at the 30-month followup (Figure 9).

Similar improvements have been reported by several other investigators. Bode and coworkers (1975) found that CV improved by 20 percent 6 to 14 weeks after cessation compared with initial values among 10 subjects. These investigators reported that the slope of phase III was unchanged by cessation. McCarthy, Craig, and Cherniack (1976) observed 131 smokers aged 17 to 66 years who volunteered to attend a smoking cessation clinic. For 15 persons abstinent from 25 to 48 weeks, cessation resulted in a significant 13-percent reduction in CC and a 27-percent reduction in the slope of phase III.

Bake and coworkers (1977) showed a 33-percent reduction in the percent-predicted slope of phase III among 17 subjects at 5 months after cessation. On the other hand, only small changes in CV and CC were observed. Zamel, Leroux, and Ramcharan (1979) investigated 26 smokers for an average of 62 days after cessation. Similarly,

TABLE 8.—Studies of closing volume (CV/VC%), closing capacity (CC/TLC%), and slope of alveolar plateau (SBN$_2$/L) among participants in smoking cessation programs

Reference	Location	Population	Followup	Measure	CV/VC %	CC/TLC %	SBN$_2$/L
Dirksen, Janzon, Lindell (1974)	Malmö, Sweden	31 men born in 1914	8–10 days 52–60 days	Change from initial	+1.0% -0.6%	-1.0% -1.6%	
Bode et al. (1975)	Smoking clinic	3 men, 7 women	6–14 wk	% change[a]	-35.7%		5.9%
Martin et al. (1975)	Smoking clinic	12 subjects	1–3 mo	Plots, quantitative data unpublished			
McCarthy, Craig, Cherniack (1976)		15 subjects	25–48 wk	% change	0.0%	-13.2%	-26.6%
Buist et al. (1976)	Smoking clinic	6 men, 7 women	1 mo 3 mo 6 mo 12 mo	Change from initial	-1.6% -1.9% -4.1% -3.6%	-0.8% +1.6% -5.7% -2.6%	-0.3% 0.0% -0.4% -0.3%
Bake et al. (1977)	Smoking clinic	9 men, 8 women	5 mo 2 yr	Change in % predicted	2.8 -2.5	-1.8 0.3	-33.2 -43.8
Buist, Nagy, Sexton (1979)	Smoking clinic	3 men, 12 women	3–4 mo 6–8 mo 30 mo	Change in % predicted	-23.1 -33.0 -25.4	-1.6 -19.5 -15.4	-25.6 -51.9 -48.4

TABLE 8.—Continued

Reference	Location	Population	Followup	Measure	CV/VC %	CC/TLC %	SBN$_2$/L
Zamel, Leroux, Ramcharan (1979)		12 men, 14 women	62±6 days	% change	-4.1%	-1.9%	-10.3%
Pride et al. (1980)		8 male smokers who thought easy to stop	4 yr		No improvement		Significant decline

NOTE: CV=closing volume; VC=vital capacity; TLC=total lung capacity.
[a] Average percentage change recalculated from individual values.

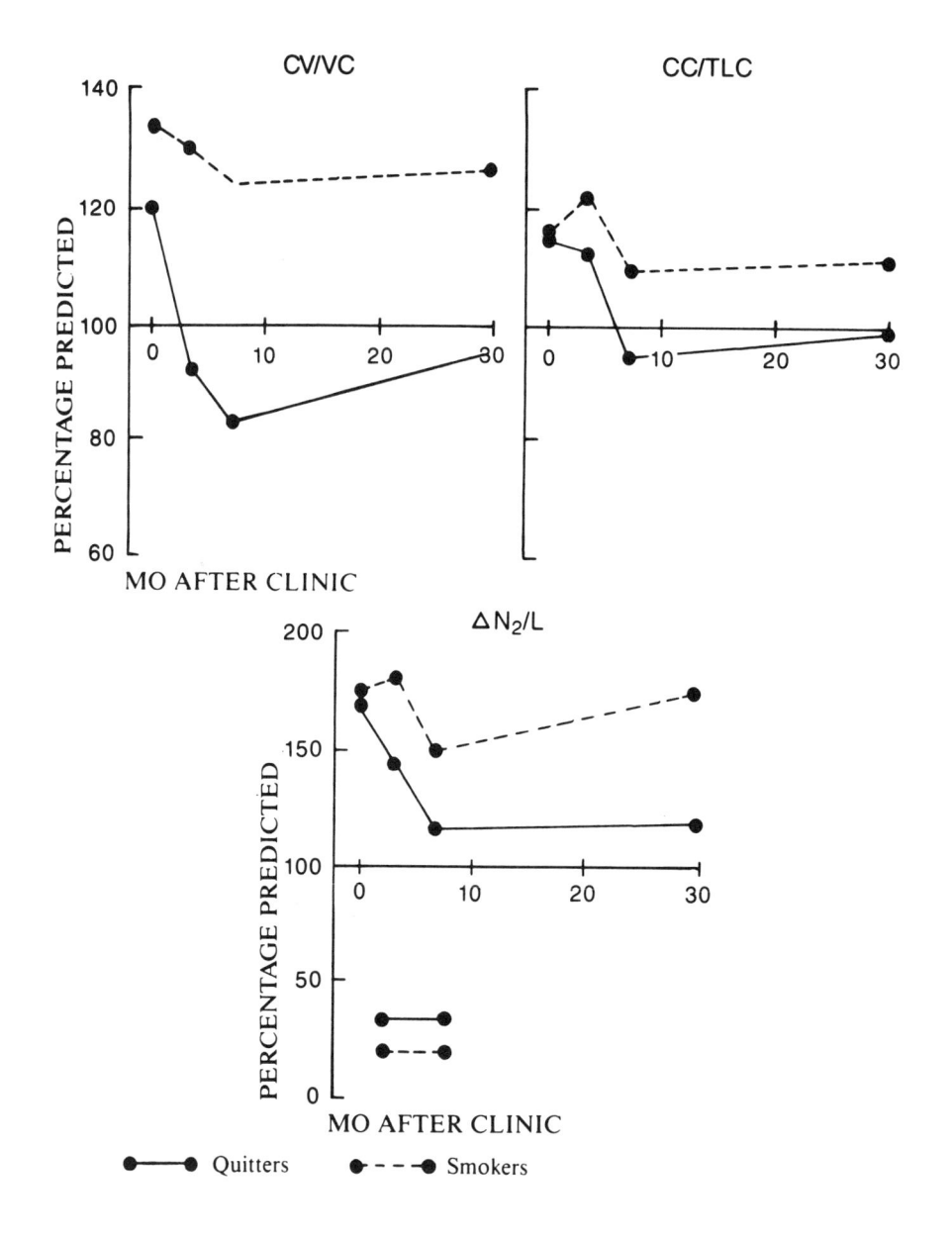

FIGURE 9.—Mean values for the ratio of CV/VC, of CC/TLC, and slope for phase III of the single breath N₂ test (ΔN₂/L), expressed as a percentage of predicted values in 15 quitters and 42 smokers during 30 months after 2 smoking cessation clinics

NOTE: Asterisks (*) denote a significant difference from the initial value at $p<0.05$. CV=closing volume; VC=vital capacity; CC=closing capacity; TLC=total lung capacity.

SOURCE: Buist, Nagy, Sexton (1979).

small improvements in CV and CC were observed, although slope of phase III improved by 10 percent.

Martin and coworkers (1975) stated that "CV did not improve with cessation" among 12 participants in a smoking cessation program tracked for 1 to 3 months. In a 4-year followup of eight men who successfully gave up smoking, Pride and colleagues (1980) reported no improvement in CV, but a significant decline in the slope of phase III within the first few months of cessation. Further improvement did not occur over subsequent years.

In summary, abnormalities in the small airways, as measured by CV, CC, and slope of phase III, are substantially reversible among smokers who have not developed significant airflow obstruction. Recovery occurs rapidly and appears to be complete for these measures between 6 months and 1 year after cessation, although the implications of these changes for morbidity and mortality are uncertain.

Abnormal frequency dependence of lung compliance (an increased reduction of lung compliance as respiratory frequency increases) also indicates abnormal function of the small airways. Ingram and O'Cain (1971) examined six smokers with abnormal frequency dependence of compliance who quit smoking. At 1 to 8 weeks after cessation, values in all six had returned to normal. Martin and coworkers (1975) studied 12 participants in a smoking cessation program. At 1 to 3 months after cessation, dynamic compliance was less frequency dependent among 8 of the 12 subjects. Zamel, Leroux, and Ramcharan (1979) also reported less frequency dependence of dynamic compliance among 26 healthy smokers at 2 months after cessation.

Diffusing Capacity Among Former Smokers

Numerous studies, using a variety of methods, have shown that pulmonary diffusing capacity is between 6 and 20 percent lower among smokers than among age-matched nonsmokers (Teculescu and Stanescu 1970; Van Ganse, Ferris, Cotes 1972; Krumholz and Hedrick 1973; Frans et al. 1975; Hyland et al. 1978; Enjeti et al. 1978; Bosisio et al. 1980; Miller et al. 1983; Knudson et al. 1984). Only a few studies, however, have assessed the effect of smoking cessation on diffusing capacity.

Marcq and Minette (1976) measured single breath carbon monoxide (CO) diffusing capacity ($DL_{co}SB$) in male subjects with normal values of FEV_1 and FEV_1 divided by FVC. Diffusing capacity was below normal in 13 of 54 (24 percent) of the current smokers compared with 1 of 17 (6 percent) of the former smokers of at least 6 months abstinence.

Miller and colleagues (1983) examined $DL_{co}SB$ in a survey of 511 randomly selected subjects from a population in Michigan. Among never smokers, the mean $DL_{co}SB$ was 32.5 mL CO per mm Hg per minute for males and 23.0 mL CO per mm Hg per minute for females. Compared with never smokers and adjusted for age and height, male current smokers had 17 percent lower (5.4 mL CO/mm Hg per minute), and female current smokers had 16 percent lower (3.6 mL CO/mm Hg per minute) $DL_{co}SB$. Male former smokers abstinent for at least 2 years were lower by 7 percent (2.3 mL CO/mm Hg per minute) compared with never smokers, whereas no difference was found between female current and former smokers.

Zamel, Leroux, and Ramcharan (1979) measured $DL_{co}SB$ among 26 healthy smokers before and 2 months after cessation. Although $DL_{co}SB$ improved slightly following cessation (0.8 mL CO/mm Hg per minute), the difference was not statistically significant.

Knudson, Kaltenborn, and Burrows (1989) measured $DL_{co}SB$ in the seventh population survey conducted in the longitudinal study of a population-based sample in Tucson, AZ. Among current and former smokers, $DL_{co}SB$ dropped as cumulative consumption of cigarettes increased (Figure 10). Current smokers had significantly lower $DL_{co}SB$ than either former smokers or never smokers; in persons with normal spirometry, former and never smokers had comparable $DL_{co}SB$; former smokers in the group with abnormal spirometry had significantly lower $DL_{co}SB$. The $DL_{co}SB$ quickly returned to normal as the duration of abstinence increased. Within 2 years of quitting, $DL_{co}SB$ had reached 100 percent of that predicted for women; after 3 years of abstinence, mean $DL_{co}SB$ was 100 percent of that predicted for men.

These data suggest that the effects of cigarette smoking on pulmonary diffusing capacity, as on other measures of lung function, include both irreversible and reversible components. The extent of irreversible change is predicted by cumulative consumption; the reversible component improves quickly after cessation.

Other Measures

Among 19 heavy smokers studied by Dirksen, Janzon, and Lindell (1974), ventilation distribution measured by open-circuit nitrogen clearance improved 1 week after smoking cessation. Regional lung function measured with ^{133}Xe showed improvement 1 to 3 months after cessation in the study by Martin and colleagues (1975). Zamel and Webster (1984) performed detailed studies of five men and five women before and 60 days after cessation. Although $\dot{V}_{max60percent\ TLC}$ with helium and air and the maximum flow-static recoil curve did not change, static recoil pressure at 60 percent TLC did decrease significantly 2 months after cessation in 18 of 22 smokers. Michaels and coworkers (1979) also observed a decrease in static recoil pressure at any lung volume after smoking cessation. These authors concluded that a decrease in small airway muscle tone might have accounted for these findings.

Longitudinal Population-Based Studies

The natural history of COPD has been described in longitudinal studies of up to two decades. Although a population has not been studied from childhood to the development of COPD during adulthood, the available data from existing separate investigations encompass the entire course of the disease and support the conceptual model presented earlier (Figure 2).

Measures of pulmonary function begin to decline after 25 to 30 years of age. For FEV_1, the annual rate of decline, as estimated from cross-sectional studies, is about 20 to 30 mL annually (US DHHS 1984). Faster loss of function over a sufficient period of time can lead to the development of clinically significant airflow obstruction (Figure 2). The available longitudinal data indicate that cigarette smoking is the primary risk

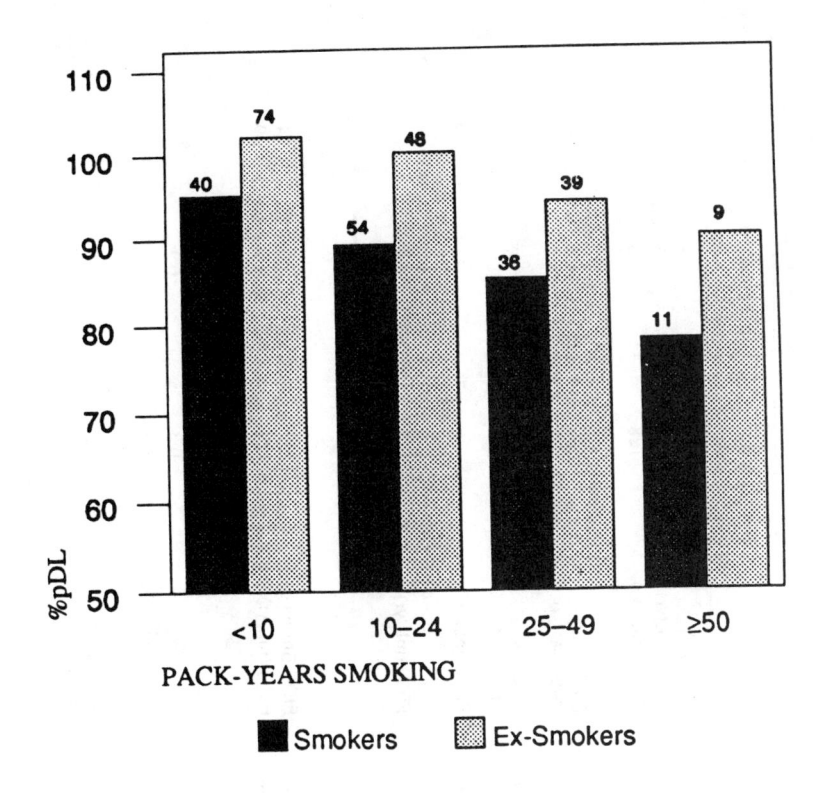

FIGURE 10.—Percent-predicted diffusing capacity (%pDL) by pack-years of smoking, current smokers and former smokers, in a study of adults in Tucson, AZ

NOTE: Numbers above bars represent sample sizes.

SOURCE: Knudson, Kaltenborn, Burrows (1989).

factor for excessive loss of FEV_1 (US DHHS 1984), and smokers have much faster rates of loss of FEV_1 than never smokers (Table 9). Table 9 describes rates of change in lung function in selected major longitudinal studies. In each, former smokers or quitters have less decline than current smokers during the followup period.

In many investigations, dose–response relationships have been found between the amount smoked during the followup interval and the rate of the FEV_1 decline (US DHHS 1984). For example, Fletcher and colleagues (1976) conducted a study of 792 employed men and performed pulmonary function measurements semiannually for 8 years. They reported that the annual loss of FEV_1 was 36 mL per year for never smokers. The rate of decline among cigarette smokers increased with amount smoked per day (44 mL/year for ≤4 cigarettes/day; 46 mL/year for 5 to 15 cigarettes/day; 54 mL/year for 15 to 25 cigarettes/day; and 54 mL/year for >25 cigarettes/day). The rate

TABLE 9.—Population-based longitudinal studies of annual decline in pulmonary function

Reference	Population	Followup	Gender	Measure	Never smokers	Former smokers	Quitters	Smokers
Wilhelmsen, Orha, Tibblin (1969)	Swedish men born in 1913	4 yr	Male	VC (mL/yr) FEV$_1$ (mL/yr) PEF (L/min/yr)	63 43 128	58 33 140	58 40 100	94 70 155
Ashley et al. (1975)	Framingham Study	10 yr 2 exams	Male Female	FVC (mL/yr) FEV$_1$/FVC (%/yr) FVC (mL/yr) FEV$_1$/FVC (%/yr)	39 0.3 33 4.2		46 -0.1 30 0.2	58 0.5 39 3.0
Fletcher et al. (1976)	British workers	8 yr Semiannual	Male	FEV$_1$ (mL/yr)	36	31	38	50
Kauffmann et al. (1979)	French workers	12 yr	Male	FEV$_1$ (mL/yr)[a]	42	44		49
Huhti and Ikkala (1980)	Middle-aged rural Finns	10 yr	Male Female	FEV$_1$ (mL/yr) FEV$_1$ (mL/yr)	33 27	45 27	44 39	51 35
Woolf and Zamel (1980)	Canadian volunteers aged 25–54	5 yr 2 exams	Female	FEV$_1$ (%/yr) FEV$_1$/FVC (%/yr)	0.3 1.3	0.2 1.4		0.7 1.7
Bossé et al. (1980)	Healthy US veterans	10 yr 3 exams	Male	FEV$_1$ (mL/yr) FVC (mL/yr)	52 69	57 72		62 73

TABLE 9.—Continued

Reference	Population	Followup	Gender	Measure	Never smokers	Former smokers	Quitters	Smokers
Bossé et al. (1981)	Healthy US veterans	5 yr 2 exams	Male	FEV_1 (mL/yr)[b] FVC (mL/yr)[b]	61 68		49 64	78 91
Van der Lende et al. (1981)	Random sample in the Netherlands, aged 15–39	9–13 yr 4 exams	Male and Female	FEV_1 (mL/yr)[c] VC (mL/yr)[c]	16.6 13.7	13.4 13.2		24.5 15.7
Tashkin et al. (1984)	Population sample in southern California	5 yr 2 exams	Male	FEV_1 (mL/yr)[d] FVC (mL/yr)[d]	56 60	52 60	62 68	70 64
			Female	FEV_1 (mL/yr) FVC (mL/yr)	42 44	38 42	38 44	54 54
Taylor et al. (1985)	Volunteer population in the United Kingdom	7.5 yr 2 exams	Male	FEV_1/H^3 (mL/yr/m^3)	6.6	8.0[e]		10.9

Rate of decline by smoking status

TABLE 9.—Continued

Reference	Population	Followup	Gender	Measure	Never smokers	Former smokers	Quitters	Smokers
Camilli et al. (1987)	Population sample in Tucson, AZ	Mean 9.4 yr 5.2 exams	Male	FEV_1 (mL/yr)[f]	12.9	10.8	13.2	25.8
			Female	FEV_1 (mL/yr)[g]	7.6	6.5	2.9	14.6
Burrows et al. (1987)	Population sample in Tucson, AZ	10.0 yr 5.4 exams	Male	FEV_1 (mL/yr)[h]		11.8		26.6
Townsend et al. (in press)	MRFIT	2–4 yr	Male	FEV_1 (mL/yr)	51	44	50	59

NOTE: Negative numbers indicate an increase. Former smokers stopped smoking prior to start of study; quitters stopped smoking after start of study. Mean values for all smokers have been calculated weighted by number of subjects, where published data was stratified by amount of smoking. VC=vital capacity; FEV_1=1-sec forced expiratory volume; PEF=peak expiratory flow; FVC=forced vital capacity; H^3=height cubed; MRFIT=Multiple Risk Factor Intervention Trial.

[a] Adjusted for initial level.
[b] Adjusted for age.
[c] Adjusted for initial level, height, sex, and area of residence. Weighted mean for smokers.
[d] Adjusted for age, height, and area of residence.
[e] Includes former smokers and quitters.
[f] Adjusted to age 50, height 172 cm.
[g] Adjusted to age 50, height 161 cm.
[h] Recalculated from FEV_1/FVC specific values.

of loss among former smokers (i.e., smokers who stopped before the first examination) was 31 mL per year, not significantly different from that of never smokers. In addition, smokers who stopped in the first 2 years of the followup had an annual decline of 38 mL per year. The authors concluded that smokers who stopped before or early in the study had FEV_1 declines similar to never smokers. In spite of FEV_1 levels having been reduced by previous smoking, further damage to FEV_1 due to smoking ceases within a few years of cessation. However, recovery of function was not documented in the study of Fletcher and colleagues (1976). These results have been confirmed in multiple population-based longitudinal studies of FEV_1 and other pulmonary function parameters (Table 9).

Camilli and associates (1987) examined longitudinal decline of FEV_1 in a population sample of 1,705 adults in Tucson, AZ. Mean followup was 9.4 years with an average of 5.2 examinations. Former smokers were defined as having stopped before enrollment and continuing to abstain at their last two followup examinations. Quitters smoked on entry into the program but stopped before their last two followup examinations. Rates of loss for former smokers and quitters were comparable with those for never smokers and less than those for smokers (Table 9). The age-specific rates of loss (Figure 11) suggest that the benefits of cessation may be greatest among the youngest smokers, that is those with the shortest smoking history. FEV_1 increased in the youngest group, a finding that the authors interpreted as indicating that the earliest effects of smoking are relatively reversible and could represent, in part, a bronchoconstrictive effect.

Among the males in the 50- to 69-year-old age group (Figure 12), 10 of the 24 subjects who quit did so before their second followup examination. For these 10 subjects, the revised annual loss of FEV_1 from the time of cessation returned to that of never smokers, and was much less than that among smokers. In several years, reduced lung function due to previous smoking was not recovered, except possibly among former smokers who had only been smoking a short time.

Taylor, Joyce, and coworkers (1985) examined the annual decline of height-corrected FEV_1 (FEV_1 divided by height^3) over 7.5 years in 227 men who were free of a clinical diagnosis of asthma and had not received bronchodilator treatment. Former smokers had an annual decline of FEV_1 divided by height^3 (8.0 ± 0.8 mL/year/m^3) that was not statistically different from that of never smokers (6.6 ± 0.6 mL/year/m^3) but was significantly less than that of continuing smokers (10.9 ± 0.7 mL/year/m^3). The 71 former smokers included 50 smokers who had stopped during the followup period. Smokers with bronchial reactivity to inhaled histamine had significantly accelerated annual decline of FEV_1, but an effect of bronchial reactivity was not found among former smokers or never smokers. The reactive former smokers had a lower level percent-predicted FEV_1 at the end of the followup (96.4 vs. 111.4 percent predicted). Because their annual rate of loss was not accelerated, the low level of former smokers must be attributed to either steeper decline while they were smoking, low level of FEV_1 before they started smoking, or both.

Townsend and colleagues (in press) have recently reported on FEV_1 decline in participants in the Multiple Risk Factor Intervention Trial. The analysis was limited to 4,926 subjects who had not used β-blocking agents or smoked cigars, cigarillos, or pipes

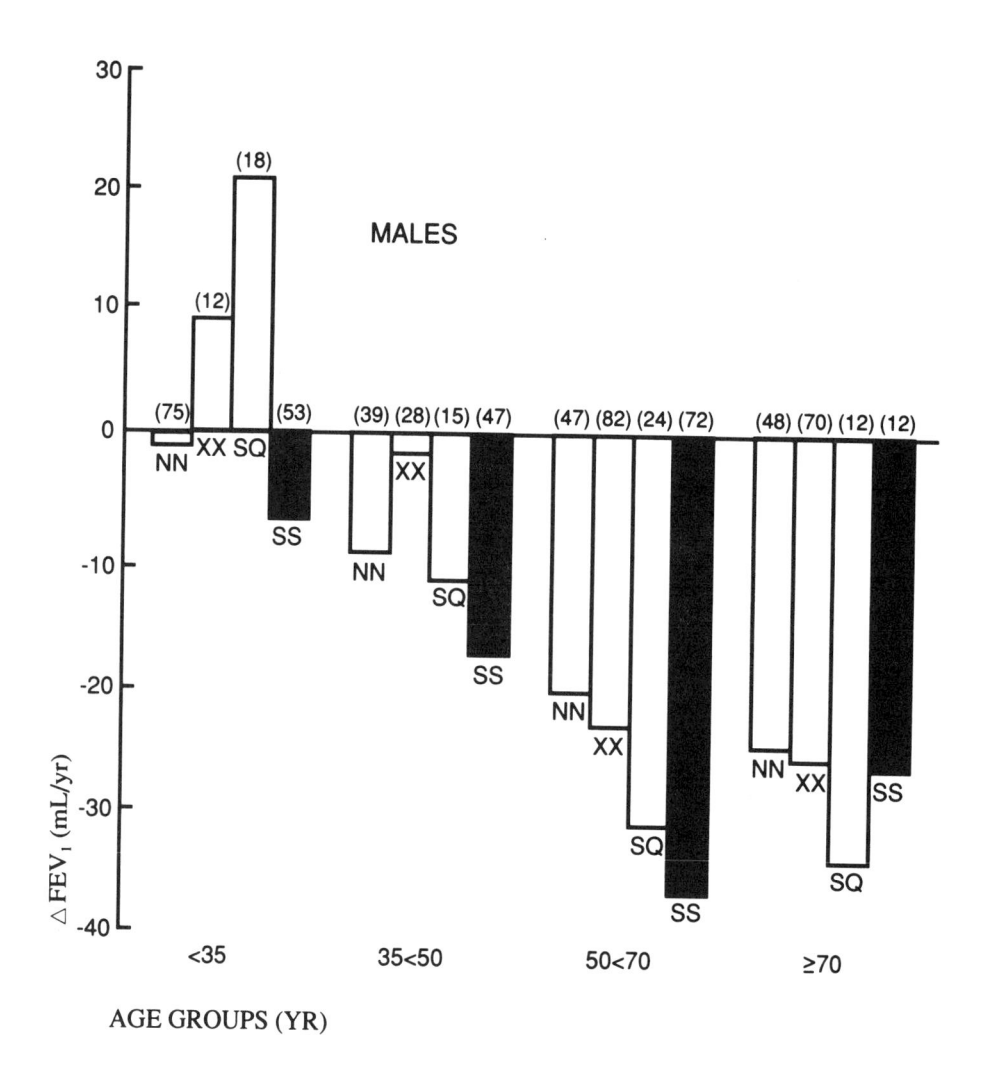

FIGURE 11.—Mean ΔFEV_1 values in never smokers (NN), consistent ex-smokers (XX), subjects who quit smoking during followup (SQ), and consistent smokers (SS) in several age groups

NOTE: Numbers of subjects in each category are shown in parentheses. FEV_1=1-sec forced expiratory volume.

SOURCE: Camilli et al. (1987)

during the trial and who were observed over 2 to 4 years during the latter half of the study. Subjects who quit smoking during the first 12 months of the study lost FEV_1 at a significantly lower rate than those reporting smoking throughout the trial. Cross-sectional analysis of data from the midpoint of the trial indicated the highest level of FEV_1 for never smokers and the lowest levels for continuing smokers at all ages; FEV_1 levels for former smokers at enrollment and those quitting during the first year were inter-

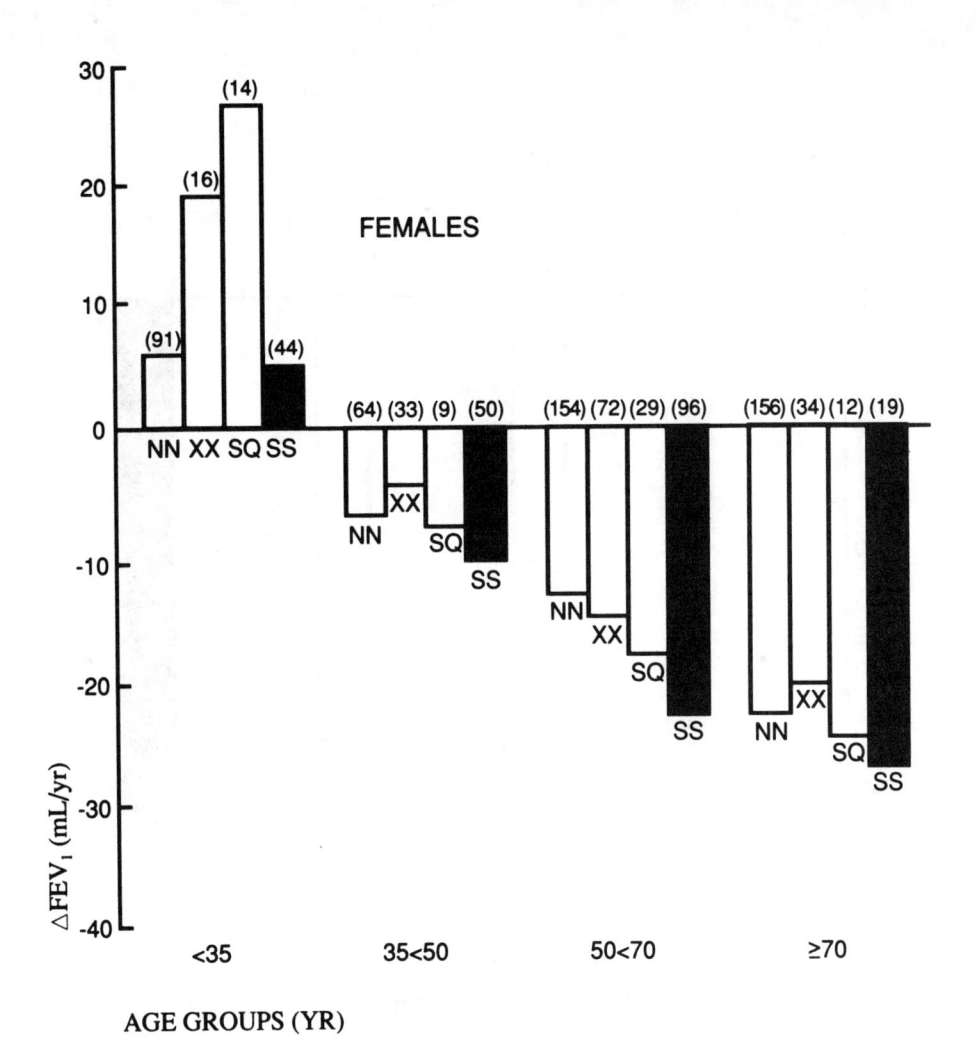

FIGURE 11. (Continued)—Mean ΔFEV_1 values in never smokers (NN), consistent ex-smokers (XX), subjects who quit smoking during followup (SQ), and consistent smokers (SS) in several age groups

NOTE: Numbers of subjects in each category are shown in parentheses. FEV_1=1-sec forced expiratory volume.

SOURCE: Camilli et al. (1987)

mediate. The findings in the group quitting smoking during the first 12 months may underestimate the benefits of cessation because of subsequent relapse within this group; 16 percent of the quitters had an elevated serum thiocyanate level (>100 μm/dL) indicative of smoking at the first examination compared with 6 percent of never smokers and 7 percent of former smokers.

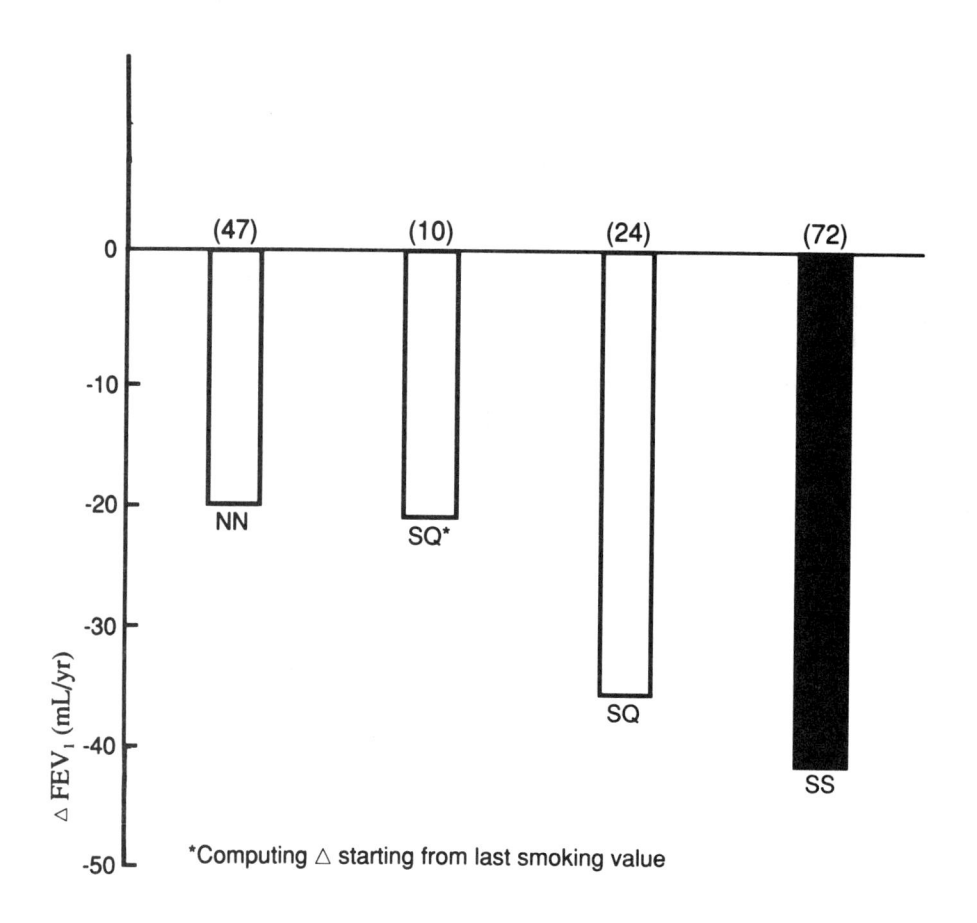

FIGURE 12.—Effects of quitting smoking during followup among men aged 50–69

NOTE: Subjects in the SQ* group are included in the SQ group.
SOURCE: Camilli et al. (1987).

In the Copenhagen City Heart Study, spirometry was performed on 2 occasions separated by 5 years for 12,698 adult residents of the city selected at random (Lange et al. 1989). In general, persons who stopped smoking during this interval experienced less decline of FEV_1 than those who continued to smoke (Table 10); the effect of cessation varied with subject age and amount smoked at the time of quitting.

In 1986, the National Heart, Lung, and Blood Institute (NHLBI) initiated a multicenter investigation, the Lung Health Study, to determine whether smoking cessation and bronchodilator therapy can influence the course of subjects without clinical illness who are at high risk for the development of COPD (Anthonisen 1989). Six thousand smokers, aged 35 to 59 years, with evidence of airways obstruction were recruited. They were randomly assigned to one of three groups: a group that received no intervention or usual care group; a group that received an intensive state-of-the-art

TABLE 10.— Decline of FEV_1 (mL/yr) in subjects in the Copenhagen City Heart Study

Smoking group	Women <55 yr	Women ≥55 yr	Men <55 yr	Men ≥55 yr
Never smokers	13 (722)	32 (754)	21 (302)	34 (151)
Former smokers	18 (321)	32 (307)	27 (306)	36 (430)
Continuing light smokers	17 (641)	39 (439)	22 (279)	52 (227)
Quitting light smokers	15 (80)	28 (77)	17 (51)	11 (31)
Continuing heavy smokers	30 (624)	48 (196)	42 (634)	56 (248)
Quitting heavy smokers	9 (17)	— (8)	36 (32)	43 (14)

NOTE: Numbers of subjects given in parentheses. Light smokers consumed <15 cig/day; heavy smokers consumed ≥15 cig/day. FEV_1=1-sec forced expiratory volume.
SOURCE: Abstracted from table 2 in Lange et al. (1989).

smoking cessation program and regular therapy with an inhaled bronchodilator (ipratropium bromide); and a third group that received the smoking cessation program and a placebo bronchodilator. Placebo/bronchodilator therapy was administered in double-blind fashion. All groups were studied at yearly intervals for 5 years, with rate of change of FEV_1 as the primary end point and respiratory morbidity as a secondary end-point.

In this investigation, a large number of smokers with early airways obstruction were characterized and will be studied closely for 5 years. An extensive data base will be created to test numerous hypotheses regarding smoking cessation. The question of airways reactivity as a risk factor for rapid lung function loss will be tested definitively in that methacholine sensitivity will have been measured both at the beginning and at the followup period.

The findings of the longitudinal studies on smoking cessation and decline of FEV_1 have important implications. Persons losing FEV_1 at a greater rate are at risk of developing COPD. After cessation, the return of the rate of decline of FEV_1 to that of never smokers implies that the process leading to COPD can be arrested by cessation.

PART III. AIRWAY RESPONSIVENESS, CIGARETTE SMOKING, AND SMOKING CESSATION

Population-based studies support a role for smoking as a cause of heightened airway responsiveness (Woolcock et al. 1987; Sparrow et al. 1987; Burney et al. 1987). Most cross-sectional studies that have evaluated this relationship have not adjusted for baseline airway caliber, which may be reduced among smokers (Woolcock et al. 1987; Burney et al. 1987; Welty et al. 1984; Van der Lende et al. 1981; Pham et al. 1984; Buczko et al. 1984), so that it is difficult to determine how much of the increase in airway responsiveness is accounted for by a direct smoking effect or by a reduction in prechallenge pulmonary function (Fanta and Ingram 1981). Atopy may modify the influence of smoking by further increasing nonspecific airway responsiveness. As noted by O'Connor, Sparrow, and Weiss (1989), this modification may be underestimated in most studies because those with an allergic predisposition and heightened nonspecific responsiveness may not begin smoking—or if they do begin, they may soon quit. The importance of smoking-induced heightened airway responsiveness in the pathogenesis of asthma is unknown, and airway hyperresponsiveness is a suspected risk factor for COPD.

Mechanisms of Heightened Airway Responsiveness Among Smokers and Former Smokers

In both clinical and population-based studies, smoking has been associated with increased airway epithelial permeability (Jones et al. 1980; Minty, Jordan, Jones 1981; Mason et al. 1983), elevated levels of IgE (Burrows et al. 1981; Warren et al. 1982; Zetterström et al. 1981; Hällgren et al. 1982; Bonini et al. 1982; Stein et al. 1983), and greater numbers of peripheral eosinophils (Burrows et al. 1980; Taylor, Gross et al. 1985; Tollerud et al. 1989; Kauffmann et al. 1986). These physiologic and immunologic alterations may partly explain the observed relationship between cigarette consumption and heightened airway responsiveness and/or asthma (Brown, McFadden, Ingram 1977; Malo, Filiatrault, Martin 1982; Cockcroft et al. 1979; Buczko et al. 1984; Casale et al. 1987; Van der Lende et al. 1981; Gerrard, Cockcroft et al. 1980; Kabiraj et al. 1982; Pham et al. 1984; Enarson et al. 1985; Taylor, Joyce et al. 1985; Woolcock et al. 1987; Sparrow et al. 1987; Rijcken et al. 1987; Burney et al. 1987). Allergy to environmental antigens is known to modify this relationship (Burrows, Lebowitz, Barbee 1976; Welty et al. 1984; Buczko et al. 1984; Schachter, Doyle, Beck 1984; Kiviloog, Irnell, Eklund 1974; Dodge and Burrows 1980). The complexity of these interrelationships is only partially explained by published findings, and additional clarifying studies are needed. This Section reviews studies that have addressed the above associations with respect to ex-smokers which may explain why airway responsiveness returns to normal with abstinence.

Smoking increases pulmonary epithelial permeability, which rapidly returns to normal among young smokers after cessation. Minty, Jordan, and Jones (1981) used a radiolabeled aerosol technique to study 10 young asymptomatic male smokers who had stopped smoking for 1, 3, 7, 14, and 21 days. They found that recovery of the epithelial integrity began within 24 hours and reached maximum at 7 days. Mason and colleagues (1983) later confirmed these findings in 10 young smokers. These studies included small numbers of subjects and had short followup periods after cessation, making interpretation and generalization of the findings difficult.

Cross-Sectional Studies

Cross-sectional population-based data have shown that former smokers have less airway responsiveness than current smokers. Burney and colleagues (1987) studied 511 randomly selected subjects aged 18 to 64 years using inhaled histamine challenge.

Of the population, 14 percent were histamine-responsive as defined by PD20 (the dose of histamine resulting in a 20-percent decline in FEV_1). Responsiveness was related to atopy in younger subjects (aged <40 years) and smoking in older participants (aged >40 years). Former smokers (N=116) had bronchial reactivity similar to never smokers but lower than current smokers across all age strata (12 vs. 10 vs. 24 percent, respectively). The increase in threshold dose of histamine with age for former smokers was 0.053 per year compared with 0.086 per year among current smokers and 0.027 per year among never smokers. However, for those aged 35 to 44 years, former smokers were more responsive than the other smoking groups (14 vs. 13 and 7 percent for current and never smokers, respectively). The criteria for classification of former smokers were not provided.

Cerveri and colleagues (1989) found similar results in their study of 295 normal never smokers, 70 normal current smokers, and 50 former smokers randomly selected from the general population of a small town in Lombardy, Italy. The daily amount smoked was a stronger predictor of airway responsiveness than the duration of cigarette use. Further, among ex-smokers, duration of abstinence did not significantly influence airway responsiveness; however, former smokers with longer abstinence tended to have less bronchial reactivity.

Longitudinal Studies

Longitudinal population-based studies have not been conducted specifically to evaluate temporal changes in airway responsiveness among former smokers. Several cohort studies designed to measure declines in spirometric function have included single measurements of airway reactivity. These studies generally confirmed lower responsiveness among former smokers than current smokers and suggested an association between bronchial reactivity and a more rapid decline in ventilatory function. Vollmer, Johnson, and Buist (1985) examined bronchodilator responsiveness among subjects from 2 cohorts, 351 members of the Portland Cohort, which included a random sample of 507 Multnomah County employees, and 444 adults from the Screening Center Cohort, consisting of 1,024 subjects screened for emphysema. Individuals were classified as responsive if they showed a 7.72-percent increase in FEV_1 after two puffs of an isoproterenol metered-dose inhaler. Although no data were presented, former smokers were reported to have a distribution of responsiveness similar to that of current smokers and skewed toward higher values. In case–control analysis conducted within the cohort, responsiveness in both current and former smokers was associated with lower baseline pulmonary function and more rapid ventilatory decline over 9 to 11 years. Former smokers in both cohorts had rates of decline that approximated or exceeded those for current smokers, especially among those subjects who were responsive.

In a 6-year study of 267 white male grain elevator workers, Tabona and coworkers (1984) found that the percentage of former smokers who were methacholine responsive, defined as a PC20 ≤8 mg/mL, was similar to that of never smokers (19.6 vs. 16.7 vs. 25.8 percent for former, never, and current smokers, respectively). In contrast to the Vollmer, Johnson, and Buist study (1985), former smokers showed the lowest ventilatory decline of all smoking groups across all age categories (Tabona et al. 1984).

However, former smokers who were methacholine responsive had greater FEV_1 loss over the 6 years of the study than those who were not methacholine responsive. Atopy, presence of symptoms, and initial lung function were not predictive of decline in lung function.

Finally, Taylor, Joyce, and coworkers (1985) conducted an investigation over a 7.5-year period of bronchial reactivity and FEV_1 annual rate of decline among 227 London men, aged 25 to 61 years. These investigators confirmed the results for current smokers of Vollmer, Johnson, and Buist (1985) and Tabona and coworkers (1984). Similarly, former smokers had intermediate levels of methacholine responsiveness compared with the other groups, and those former smokers who were responsive had lower rates of baseline ventilatory function. In contrast, however, former smokers had comparable rates of ventilatory decline, regardless of methacholine responsiveness.

In all of these longitudinal studies, bronchodilator or methacholine responsiveness was measured near the end of the study period. Furthermore, precise definitions of former smokers with regard to amount smoked, duration of abstinence, and reasons for quitting were not provided. As discussed previously, the prevalence of airway responsiveness may also lead to a decision to stop smoking. These limitations in study design must be considered in interpreting the associations among smoking cessation, nonspecific airway responsiveness, and annual decline in FEV_1.

Clinical Studies

Four small clinical studies have addressed airway responsiveness before and after smoking cessation. Buczko and coworkers (1984) studied 18 age- and sex-matched pairs of healthy nonatopic asymptomatic smokers and nonsmokers. Methacholine responsiveness was defined as the threshold dose causing a decrease in partial flows, measured at a volume of 40 percent of the VC above residual volumes (V_{40p}), below the 95-percent CI of CV. In the first part of the study, these researchers found that smokers had greater overall methacholine responsiveness than never smokers, but the difference was significant only for smokers with greater than 10 pack-years of cigarette consumption (Buczko et al. 1984). In the second part of the study, 17 smokers were studied with methacholine testing before and 3 months after smoking cessation. Threshold dose did not increase significantly for the group as a whole; however, airway responsiveness did decrease among a subset of five smokers with the greatest initial responsiveness.

Similar results were found by Simonsson and Rolf (1982) who measured methacholine responsiveness in 10 heavy smokers without symptoms or abnormal pulmonary function tests. They studied each subject 1 week before cessation and 1, 1.6, and 12 months after smoking cessation. Carboxyhemoglobin was measured to verify smoking abstinence. At baseline, only two subjects were responsive as determined by a 15-percent reduction in FEV_1 after inhalation of 0.1 percent methacholine. Within 1 month of abstinence, airways responsiveness decreased among four subjects. By 12 months, however, no further significant improvement in airway responsiveness was found for the group.

In contrast, Bolin, Dahms, and Slavin (1980) and Fennerty and coworkers (1987) found increases in airway responsiveness after cessation. Bolin, Dahms, and Slavin (1980) evaluated the effect of discontinuing smoking on methacholine sensitivity in seven asthmatic subjects. PC20 was measured before and 1 day after stopping smoking and was found to be 5.62 mg/mL and 1.56 mg/mL, respectively. This increase in airway responsiveness was seen among four of the seven subjects. Finally, Fennerty and colleagues (1987) recorded PD20 to histamine in 14 asthmatics before and 24 hours after smoking cessation. PD20 did not increase significantly. In seven subjects who abstained for 7 days, however, PD20 dose increased significantly (0.67 ± 0.43 mg/mL vs. 2.28 ± 2.03 mg/mL).

These studies are limited by short followup, small numbers of subjects, and a lack of adjustment for baseline airway caliber or pulmonary function. Additionally, the analyses did not control for seasonal variation in testing, and the latter three studies did not include a control group.

In summary, former smokers appear to have bronchial reactivity comparable with that of never smokers. The comparability of bronchial reactivity among former smokers and never smokers implies that smoking-induced changes in airway responsiveness may resolve with abstinence. Available data, however, are limited and not definitive. More research is needed to determine the interaction of smoking cessation with nonspecific airway responsiveness in altering rates of decline in ventilatory function.

PART IV. EFFECTS OF SMOKING CESSATION ON COPD MORTALITY

The Centers for Disease Control reported that 71,099 persons in the United States died in 1986 with COPD (ICD-9-CM 491-2, 496) as the underlying cause, and 164,049 persons died with COPD as the underlying cause or as a contributing cause (CDC 1989). It was estimated that 81.5 percent of COPD mortality was attributable to smoking (Table 11).

Data from both prospective and retrospective studies have consistently indicated an increased mortality from COPD in cigarette smokers compared with never smokers. In addition, the degree of tobacco exposure, as measured by the number of cigarettes smoked daily or duration of smoking, strongly affects the risk of death from COPD. This literature was reviewed in the 1984 Report of the Surgeon General (US DHHS 1984), in which cigarette smoking was identified as the major cause of COPD mortality for men and women in the United States. The proceedings of a recent workshop sponsored by NHLBI address the rise in mortality from COPD (Speizer et al. 1989).

Several prospective studies have shown that cessation of smoking leads to a decreased risk of mortality compared with that of continuing smokers (Table 12). In the British Physicians Study, Doll and Peto (1976) reported on a 20-year followup of 34,440 male British doctors who completed a questionnaire about their smoking behavior in 1951. Compared with never smokers, age-adjusted death rates for chronic bronchitis or emphysema were elevated for current smokers and for former smokers (mortality ratio=16.7 and 14.7, respectively).

TABLE 11.—Mortality attributable to COPD, United States, 1986

Smoking status	Crude prevalence (%)	Relative risk	Population attributable risk (%)	Estimated attributable deaths[a]
Current smokers				
Male	32.0	9.6	42.7	45,678
Female	24.0	10.5	54.3	31,049
Former smokers				
Male	34.9	8.7	41.7	44,604
Female	15.3	7.0	21.9	12,501
TOTAL			81.5	133,832

NOTE: COPD=chronic obstructive pulmonary disease.
[a] Includes deaths for which COPD was listed as either the underlying or a contributing cause of death.
SOURCE: CDC (1989).

A study of mortality among female British physicians has also been reported (Doll et al. 1980). A cohort of 6,194 female doctors who had responded to the 1951 questionnaire was studied for 22 years. The age-adjusted mortality ratio for chronic bronchitis and emphysema among continuing smokers increased with reported cigarettes smoked per day (Table 12). Former smokers had a mortality ratio of 5.0 compared with never smokers, which represented a reduction in mortality ratios of 52 percent (1 to 14 cigarettes/day) when compared with light smokers and of 84 percent when compared with heavy smokers (≥25 cigarettes/day).

Peto and coworkers (1983) reported COPD mortality based on a 20- to 25-year followup of 2,718 British men who had been enrolled in 5 different respiratory studies in the 1950s. There were no deaths attributed to COPD among never smokers. The ratio of observed to expected COPD deaths was 1.20 and 0.65 for current and former smokers, respectively, with expected deaths based on the entire cohort including smokers and nonsmokers. Thus, the mortality ratio for former smokers was 46 percent lower than that of continuing smokers (Peto et al. 1983).

Ebi-Kryston (1989) recently reported on chronic bronchitis mortality in a 15-year followup of 17,717 male British civil servants. Compared with never smokers, former smokers had a mortality ratio of 5.57 and continuing smokers had a ratio of 8.21. Thus, former smokers had a mortality ratio reduced by 32 percent compared with continuing smokers. Although the data were not presented for COPD, the author reported that the results were similar (Ebi-Kryston 1989).

In the United States, Rogot and Murray (1980) reported data on emphysema and bronchitis mortality among 293,958 U.S. veterans studied for 16 years. Former smokers were restricted to those who stopped smoking cigarettes for reasons other than a physician's orders. Current smokers had a mortality ratio of 12.07 compared with

TABLE 12.— Prospective studies of COPD mortality in relation to cigarette smoking status

| Reference | Population | Followup | Cause of death | Standardized mortality ratio by smoking status |||
				Never smokers	Former smokers	Current smokers
Doll and Peto (1976)	34,440 British male physicians	20 yr	Chronic bronchitis and emphysema	1.0	14.7	16.7
Doll et al. (1980)	6,194 British female physicians	22 yr	Chronic bronchitis and emphysema	1.0	5.0	1–14 cig/day 10.5 15–24 cig/day 28.5 ≥25 cig/day 32.0
Rogot and Murray (1980)	293,958 US veterans aged 31–84	16 yr	Bronchitis and emphysema	1.0	5.2[a]	12.1
Peto et al. (1983)	2,718 British men (5 cohorts)	20–25 yr	COPD	0[b]	0.7[b]	1.2[b]
Carstensen, Pershagen, Eklund (1987)	25,129 Swedish men		Chronic bronchitis and emphysema	1.0	1.8	1–7 cig/day 1.9 8–15 cig/day 2.9 >15 cig/day 5.3
Ebi-Kryston (1989)	17,717 British male civil servants aged 40–64	15 yr	Chronic bronchitis	1.0	5.6	8.2
ACS CPS-II (unpublished tabulations)			COPD Men Women	1.0 1.0	8.5 7.0	10.1 10.5

TABLE 12.—Continued

Reference	Population	Followup	Cause of death		Never smokers	Former smokers[a]	Current smokers
Tockman and Comstock (1989)	17,036 Washington County, MD, men aged 35-85 at start of followup periods	13 yr	COPD	1963-68 1969-75	1.00 0.0	2.5 1.5	2.5 3.6
	19,074 Washington County, MD, women aged 35-85 at start of followup periods	13 yr	COPD	1963-68 1969-75	1.00 1.31	1.6 1.0	3.1 7.5
Marcus et al. (1989)	11,136 Japanese-American men in Hawaii, aged 45-65 at enrollment	20 yr	COPD	1965-69 1970-74 1975-79 1980-84	1.00 1.4 2.0 1.7	7.0 4.3 1.9 1.1	3.9 1.8 2.7 5.7

Standardized mortality ratio by smoking status

NOTE: COPD=chronic obstructive pulmonary disease; ACS CPS-II=American Cancer Society Cancer Prevention Study II.
[a]Former smokers who stopped smoking cigarettes for reasons other than physician's orders.
[b]Observed deaths/expected deaths.

never smokers. Former smokers had a mortality ratio of 5.20 compared with never smokers.

The proceedings of the workshop sponsored by NHLBI on rising COPD mortality included several reports from population-based cohort studies (Speizer et al. 1989). Tockman and Comstock (1989) described mortality in more than 35,000 white residents of Washington County, MD, who were enrolled in 1963 and followed through 1975. Based on the 1963 smoking information, former smokers generally had lower mortality rates for COPD than did current smokers. Marcus and colleagues (1989) reported similar analyses for subjects in the Honolulu Heart Program cohort. Coding of death certificates for COPD differed substantially between the Honolulu Heart Program and the State Health Department. Mortality rates based on the Honolulu Heart Program coding showed a temporal pattern of declining mortality from COPD among former smokers with increasing mortality among the current smokers during the followup period 1965–1984.

Recent data from ACS CPS-II provide new evidence on mortality from COPD (ACS, unpublished tabulations). The age-adjusted death rates for COPD for men and women were approximately tenfold higher among current smokers compared with never smokers. The mortality ratios for male and female former smokers compared with never smokers were 8.5 and 7.0, lower than for current smokers (ACS, unpublished tabulations).

Several studies have reported on variation in COPD mortality by duration of abstinence (Table 13). In these studies, COPD mortality for former smokers initially increases after cessation above the rates for continuing smokers. The maximum mortality ratio for former smokers was found within the first 5 years of abstinence for ACS CPS-II and between 5 and 9 years after cessation for the British Physicians Study (Doll and Peto 1976). As discussed in Chapter 2, this initial increase in mortality probably reflects cessation by persons with smoking-related illnesses or symptoms. However, even in the U.S. Veterans Study (Rogot and Murray 1980), in which only former smokers who stopped for reasons other than a physician's orders were considered, death rates for emphysema and bronchitis among former smokers were higher than for those of current smokers after 5 to 9 years of abstinence.

Following this initial rise in COPD mortality after cessation, the mortality ratios drop with increasing duration of abstinence (Table 13). However, even after 20 years or more of abstinence, the risk of COPD mortality among former smokers remains elevated in comparison with never smokers.

PART V. FORMER SMOKERS WITH ESTABLISHED CHRONIC OBSTRUCTIVE PULMONARY DISEASE

Effect of Smoking Cessation on FEV_1 Decline Among COPD Patients

The beneficial effects of smoking cessation on reducing the annual loss of pulmonary function are clearly shown in population studies and followup of smoking cessation participants. These populations have been relatively young and largely free of

TABLE 13.—Standardized mortality ratios for COPD among current and former smokers broken down by years of abstinence

Study	Current smokers[a]	<1	1–2	3–5	6–10	11–15	≥16
ACS CPS-II (unpublished tabulations)							
Men <21 cig/day	9.7	15.8	21.3	16.7	12.1	9.1	2.7
≥21 cig/day	13.5	22.6	28.5	25.9	20.2	12.6	4.5
Women <20 cig/day	6.1	11.5	10.0	12.6	3.5	3.4	2.6
≥20 cig/day	17.1	25.8	32.8	21.3	9.8	8.3	3.9

Study	Current smokers	<5	5–9	10–14	15–20	≥15	
US Veterans Study (Rogot and Murray 1980)	12.1	11.7	14.4	10.2	5.7	7.6	

Study	Current smokers	<5	5–9	10–14	≥15		
British Physicians Study (men) (Doll and Peto 1976)	35.6	34.2	47.7	7.3	8.1		

NOTE: COPD=chronic obstructive pulmonary disease; ACS CPS-II=American Cancer Society Cancer Prevention Study II.

[a] The reference category, never smokers, has a standardized mortality ratio of 1.0 by definition.

respiratory disease. The question arises whether the course of the disease can be influenced by smoking cessation once clinically overt COPD becomes apparent.

Hughes and coworkers (1982) examined the annual change in lung function among 56 male patients with radiologic evidence of emphysema. Patients who had stopped smoking prior to entry into the study and who did not smoke subsequently had a lower initial level of FEV_1 compared with patients who were smoking (45 vs. 55 percent predicted), but the annual rate of loss of FEV_1 for the former smokers was less (16.4±8.8 mL/year vs. 53.5±5.4 mL/year). Similar results were reported for annual decline of VC (14.9±18.6 mL/year vs. 53.1±11.3 mL/year). Diffusing capacity was lower at the initial assessment among smokers, 57 percent predicted, compared with former smokers, 75 percent, but diffusing capacity did not change significantly during followup.

Postma and coworkers (1986) examined the change in lung function in a 2- to 21-year followup of 81 patients with chronic airflow obstruction. Fifty-nine of the patients smoked throughout the study, and 22 stopped at the start or some time during followup. Initial level of FEV_1 was lower among former smokers, but the annual loss of FEV_1 was smaller (49±7 mL/year) than for smokers (85±5 mL/year).

In the National Institutes of Health Intermittent Positive Pressure Breathing Trial, 985 patients with COPD but without chronic hypoxemia were enrolled and studied for almost 3 years (Anthonisen et al. 1986). Spirometry was performed at entry and repeated every 3 months. The mean annual decline of FEV_1 was 44 mL per year; the investigators reported that neither past nor present smoking behavior affected the decline of FEV_1 although the data were not provided.

In summary, two of the three studies suggested that cessation of smoking is followed by a reduction of the annual loss of pulmonary function, even among patients with advanced COPD or emphysema. However, a beneficial effect of smoking cessation was not found in the large Intermittent Positive Pressure Breathing Trial. Additional investigation of the effect of continuing to smoke on lung function decline in patients with COPD is warranted.

Effect of Smoking Cessation on Mortality Among COPD Patients

The evidence for an effect of smoking cessation on survival of patients with COPD is limited. Traver, Cline, and Burrows (1979) found no association between the smoking status and the survival of 2 patient groups, 200 COPD patients in Chicago, IL, who were studied for 15 years and 100 patients in Tucson, AZ, evaluated for up to 7 years.

In a followup of up to 13 years, Kanner and coworkers (1983) examined the survival of 100 patients with chronic airflow limitation, aged 32 to 55 at enrollment. Twelve-year survival probabilities were 86, 79, and 64 percent for never, former, and current smokers, respectively.

Postma and colleagues (1985) studied survival of 129 patients with severe chronic airflow obstruction (FEV_1 ≤1,000 mL) for up to 18 years. All nonrespiratory deaths were censored. Patients were classified by the degree of reversibility of airflow obstruction. For both smokers and former smokers, relative survival was highest among those with the greatest reversibility of airflow obstruction. Smokers who quit smoking before the start of followup had a higher survival rate than did continuing smokers (Figure 13). Within each stratum of reversibility, former smokers had lower mortality than current smokers.

In contrast, mortality in the 3-year followup period of the Intermittent Positive Pressure Breathing Trial was not significantly related to smoking status. The followup period was relatively brief, however. Patient age and the level of FEV_1 at enrollment were the strongest predictors of mortality.

In those prospective studies, smoking was evaluated on entry into the study. Subsequent changes in smoking status (i.e., smokers ceasing to smoke or former smokers reverting back to smoking) would reduce the estimated effects of smoking cessation compared with continued smoking. Overall, the extent of the evidence is limited, and a conclusion cannot yet be reached on the effect of smoking on mortality following diagnosis of COPD.

CONCLUSIONS

1. Smoking cessation reduces rates of respiratory symptoms such as cough, sputum production, and wheezing, and respiratory infections such as bronchitis and pneumonia, compared with continued smoking.

2. For persons without overt chronic obstructive pulmonary disease (COPD), smoking cessation improves pulmonary function about 5 percent within a few months after cessation.

3. Cigarette smoking accelerates the age-related decline in lung function that occurs among never smokers. With sustained abstinence from smoking, the rate of decline in pulmonary function among former smokers returns to that of never smokers.

4. With sustained abstinence, the COPD mortality rates among former smokers decline in comparison with continuing smokers.

References

ABBOUD, R.T., JOHNSON, A.J., RICHTER, A.M., ELWOOD, R.K. Comparison of in vitro neutrophil elastase release in nonsmokers and smokers. *American Review of Respiratory Disease* 128(3):507–510, 1983.

AMERICAN CANCER SOCIETY. Unpublished tabulations.

AMERICAN COLLEGE OF CHEST PHYSICIANS–AMERICAN THORACIC SOCIETY. Pulmonary terms and symbols. A report of the ACCP–ATS Joint Committee on Pulmonary Nomenclature. *Chest* 67(5):583–593, May 1975.

AMERICAN THORACIC SOCIETY. Standards for the diagnosis and care of patients with chronic obstructive pulmonary disease (COPD) and asthma. *American Review of Respiratory Disease* 136(1):225–244, July 1987.

ANDERSEN, P., CHRISTENSEN, K.M. Serum antibodies to pigeon antigens in smokers and nonsmokers. *Acta Medica Scandinavica* 213(3):191–193, 1983.

ANDERSEN, P., PEDERSEN, D.F., BACH, B., BONDE, G.J. Serum antibodies and immunoglobulins in smokers and nonsmokers. *Clinical and Experimental Immunology* 47(2):467–473, February 1982.

ANDERSEN, P., SCHONHEYDER, H. Antibodies to hen and duck antigens in poultry workers. *Clinical Allergy* 14(5):421–428, 1984.

ANDERSON, H.R. Chronic lung disease in the Papua, New Guinea highlands. *Thorax* 34:647–653, 1979.

ANDO, M., SUGIMOTO, M., NISHI, R., SUGA, M., HORIO, S., KOHROGI, H., SHIMAZU, K., ARAKI, S. Surface morphology and function of human pulmonary alveolar macrophages from smokers and non-smokers. *Thorax* 39(11):850–856, 1984.

ANTHONISEN, N.R. Lung Health Study. (Editorial.) *American Review of Respiratory Disease* 140(4):871–872, October 1989.

ANTHONISEN, N.R., WRIGHT, E.C., HODGKIN, J.E., IPPB TRIAL GROUP. Prognosis in chronic obstructive pulmonary disease. *American Review of Respiratory Disease* 133:14–20, 1986.

ASHLEY, F., KANNEL, W.B., SORLIE, P.D., MASSON, R. Pulmonary function: Relation to aging, cigarette habit, and mortality. The Framingham Study. *Annals of Internal Medicine* 82:739–745, 1975.

BABBOTT, F.L. JR., GUMP, D.W., SYLWESTER, D.L., MACPHERSON, B.V., HOLLY, R.C. Respiratory symptoms and lung function in a sample of Vermont dairymen and industrial workers. *American Journal of Public Health* 70(3):241–245, 1980.

BAHOUS, J., CARTIER, A., PINEAU, L., BERNARD, C., GHEZZO, H., MARTIN, R.R., MALO, J.L. Pulmonary function tests and airway responsiveness to methacholine in chronic bronchiectasis of the adult. *Bulletin Européen de Physiopathologie Respiratoire* 20(4):375–380, July/August 1984.

BAKE, B., OXHÖJ, H., SIXT, R., WILHELMSEN, L. Ventilatory lung function following two years of tobacco abstinence. *Scandinavian Journal of Respiratory Diseases* 58(6):311–318, December 1977.

BALLAL, S.G. Cigarette smoking and respiratory symptoms among Sudanese doctors. *East African Medical Journal* 61(2):95–103, February 1984.

BARTELIK, S., ZIOLO, H., BARTELIK, M. Physiological and biochemical blood parameters in non-smokers and tobacco smokers. *Polski Tygodnik Lekarski* 39(1):7–8, January 1984.

BECK, G.J., DOYLE, C.A., SCHACHTER, E.N. Smoking and lung function. *American Review of Respiratory Disease* 123(2):149–155, February 1981.

BECK, G.J., DOYLE, C.A., SCHACHTER, E.N. A longitudinal study of respiratory health in a rural community. *American Review of Respiratory Disease* 125(4):375–381, April 1982.

BECKLAKE, M.R., PERMUTT, S. Evaluation of tests of lung function for "screening" for early detection of chronic obstructive lung disease. In: Macklem, P.T., Permutt, S. (eds.) *The Lung in Transition Between Health and Disease.* New York: Marcel Decker, 1979, pp. 345-387.

BELL, D.Y., HASEMAN, J.A., SPOCK, A., MCLENNAN, G., HOOK, G.E.R. Plasma proteins of the bronchoalveolar surface of the lungs of smokers and nonsmokers. *American Review of Respiratory Disease* 124:72-79, 1981.

BEST, E.W.R. *A Canadian Study of Smoking and Health.* Department of National Health and Welfare, Epidemiology Division, Health Services Branch, Biostatistics Division, Research and Statistics Directorate, Ottawa, 1966, p. 137.

BODE, F.R., DOSMAN, J., MARTIN, R.R., MACKLEM, P.T. Reversibility of pulmonary function abnormalities in smokers. A prospective study of early diagnostic tests of small airways disease. *American Journal of Medicine* 59(1):43-52, July 1975.

BOLIN, J.F., DAHMS, T.E., SLAVIN, R.G. Effect of discontinuing smoking on Mecholyl sensitivity in asthmatic smokers. (Abstract.) *Journal of Allergy and Clinical Immunology* 64:207-208, 1980.

BONINI, S. Smoking, IgE and occupational allergy. (Letter.) *British Medical Journal* 284:512-513, February 13, 1982.

BOSISIO, E., GRISETTI, G.C., PANZUTI, F., SERGI, M. Pulmonary diffusing capacity and its components (DM and VC) in young, healthy smokers. *Respiration* 40(6):307-310, 1980.

BOSSÉ, R., SPARROW, D., GARVEY, A.J., COSTA, P.T. JR., WEISS, S.T., ROWE, J.W. Cigarette smoking, aging, and decline in pulmonary function: A longitudinal study. *Archives of Environmental Health* 35(4):247-252, July/August 1980.

BOSSÉ, R., SPARROW, D., ROSE, C.L., WEISS, S.T. Longitudinal effect of age and smoking cessation on pulmonary function. *American Review of Respiratory Disease* 123(4):378-381, 1981.

BOYD, G., MADKOUR, M., MIDDLETON, S., LYNCH, P. Effect of smoking on circulating antibody levels to avian protein in pigeon breeder's disease. *Thorax* 32:643-652, 1977.

BRIDGES, R.B., WYATT, R.J., REHM, S.R. Effect of smoking on peripheral blood leukocytes and serum antiproteases. *European Journal of Respiratory Diseases* 66(Supplement 139):24-33, 1985.

BRODER, I., MINTZ, S., HUTCHEON, M., COREY, P., SILVERMAN, F., DAVIES, G., LEZNOFF, A., PERESS, L., THOMAS, P. Comparison of respiratory variables in grain elevator workers and civic outside workers of Thunder Bay, Canada. *American Review of Respiratory Disease* 119(2):193-203, February 1979.

BROWN, N.E., MCFADDEN, E.R. JR., INGRAM, R.H. JR. Airway responses to inhaled histamine in asymptomatic smokers and nonsmokers. *Journal of Applied Physiology* 42(4):508-513, April 1977.

BUCZKO, G.B., DAY, A., VANDERDOELEN, J.L., BOUCHER, R., ZAMEL, N. Effects of cigarette smoking and short-term smoking cessation on airway responsiveness to inhaled methacholine. *American Review of Respiratory Disease* 129(1):12-14, January 1984.

BUIST, A.S., GHEZZO, H., ANTHONISEN, N.R., CHERNIACK, R.M., DUCIC, S., MACKLEM, P.T., MANFREDA, J., MARTIN, R.R., MCCARTHY, D., ROSS, B.B. Relationship between the single-breath N_2 test and age, sex, and smoking habit in three North American cities. *American Review of Respiratory Disease* 120(2):305-318, August 1979.

BUIST, A.S., NAGY, J.M., SEXTON, G.J. The effect of smoking cessation on pulmonary function: A 30-month follow-up of two smoking cessation clinics. *American Review of Respiratory Disease* 120(4): 953-957, October 1979.

BUIST, A.S., SEXTON, G.J., NAGY, J.M., ROSS, B.B. The effect of smoking cessation and modification on lung function. *American Review of Respiratory Disease* 114(1):115-122, July 1976.

BUIST, A.S., VOLLMER, W.M. Prospective investigations in asthma. What have we learned from longitudinal studies about lung growth and senescence in asthma? *Chest* 91(Supplement):119S–126S, June 1987.

BURNEY, P.G.J., BRITTON, J.R., CHINN, S., TATTERSFIELD, A.E., PAPACOSTA, A.O., KELSON, M.C., ANDERSON, F., CORFIELD, D.R. Descriptive epidemiology of bronchial reactivity in an adult population: Results from a community study. *Thorax* 42(1):38–44, January 1987.

BURROWS, B. An overview of obstructive lung diseases. *Medical Clinics of North America* 65(3):455–471, May 1981.

BURROWS, B., HALONEN, M., BARBEE, R.A., LEBOWITZ, M.D. The relationship of serum immunoglobulin E to cigarette smoking. *American Review of Respiratory Disease* 124(5):523–525, November 1981.

BURROWS, B., HASAN, F.M., BARBEE, R.A., HALONEN, M., LEBOWITZ, M.D. Epidemiologic observations on eosinophilia and its relation to respiratory disorders. *American Review of Respiratory Disease* 122(5):709–719, November 1980.

BURROWS, B., KNUDSON, R.J., CAMILLI, A.E., LYLE, S.K., LEBOWITZ, M.D. The "horse-racing effect" and predicting decline in forced expiratory volume in one second from screening spirometry. *American Review of Respiratory Disease* 135(4):788–793, April 1987.

BURROWS, B., KNUDSON, R.J., CLINE, M.G., LEBOWITZ, M.D. Quantitative relationships between cigarette smoking and ventilatory function. *American Review of Respiratory Disease* 115(2):195–205, February 1977.

BURROWS, B., LEBOWITZ, A.D., BARBEE, R.A. Respiratory disorders and allergy skin-test reactions. *Annals of Internal Medicine* 84(2):134–139, February 1976.

BURTON, R.C., FERGUSON, P., GRAY, M., HALL, J., HAYES, M., SMART, Y.C. Effects of age, gender, and cigarette smoking on human immunoregulatory T-cell subsets: Establishment of normal ranges and comparison with patients with colorectal cancer and multiple sclerosis. *Diagnostic Immunology* 1(3):216–223, 1983.

CAMILLI, A.E., BURROWS, B., KNUDSON, R.J., LYLE, S.K., LEBOWITZ, M.D. Longitudinal changes in forced expiratory volume in one second in adults. Effects of smoking and smoking cessation. *American Review of Respiratory Disease* 135(4):794–799, April 1987.

CAMNER, P., PHILIPSON, K., ARVIDSSON, T. Withdrawal of cigarette smoking: A study on tracheobronchial clearance. *Archives of Environmental Health* 26:90–92, February 1973.

CARSTENSEN, J.M., PERSHAGEN, G., EKLUND, G. Mortality in relation to cigarette and pipe smoking: 16 years' observation of 25,000 Swedish men. *Journal of Epidemiology and Community Health* 41:166–172, 1987.

CASALE, T.B., RHODES, B.J., DONNELLY, A.L., WEILER, J.M. Airway responses to methacholine in asymptomatic nonatopic cigarette smokers. *Journal of Applied Physiology* 62(5):1888–1892, 1987.

CENTERS FOR DISEASE CONTROL. Chronic disease reports: Chronic obstructive pulmonary disease mortality—United States, 1986. *Morbidity and Mortality Weekly Report* 38(32):549–552, August 18, 1989.

CERVERI, I., BRUSCHI, C., ZOIA, M.C., MACCARINI, L., GRASSI, M., LEBOWITZ, M.D., RAMPULLA, C., GRASSI, C. Smoking habit and bronchial reactivity in normal subjects. A population-based study. *American Review of Respiratory Disease* 140:191–196, 1989.

CHAN-YEUNG, M., VEDAL, S., KUS, J., MACLEAN, L., ENARSON, D., TSE, K.S. Symptoms, pulmonary function, and bronchial hyperreactivity in western red cedar workers compared with those in office workers. *American Review of Respiratory Disease* 130:1038–1041, 1984.

COCKCROFT, D.W., RUFFIN, R.E., FRITH, P.A., CARTIER, A., JUNIPER, E.F., DOLOVICH, J., HARGREAVE, F.E. Determinants of allergen-induced asthma: Dose of allergen, circulating IgE antibody concentration, and bronchial responsiveness to inhaled histamine. *American Review of Respiratory Disease* 120:1053–1058, 1979.

COMSTOCK, G.W., BROWNLOW, W.J., STONE, R.W., SARTWELL, P.E. Cigarette smoking and changes in respiratory findings. *Archives of Environmental Health* 21(1):50–57, July 1970.

CORMIER, Y., BÉLANGER, J. The fluctuant nature of precipitating antibodies in dairy farmers. *Thorax* 44:469–473, 1989.

CORRE, F., LELLOUCH, J., SCHWARTZ, D. Smoking and leucocyte-counts. Results of an epidemiological survey. *Lancet* 2:632–634, September 18, 1971.

COSIO, M., GHEZZO, H., HOGG, J.C., CORBIN, R., LOVELAND, M., DOSMAN, J., MACKLEM, P.T. The relations between structural changes in small airways and pulmonary-function tests. *New England Journal of Medicine* 298(23):1277–1281, June 8, 1977.

DALES, L.G., FRIEDMAN, G.D., SIEGELAUB, A.G., SELTZER, C.C. Cigarette smoking and serum chemistry tests. *Journal of Chronic Diseases* 27(6):293–307, August 1974.

DANIELE, R.P., DAUBER, J.H., ALTOSE, M.D., ROWLANDS, D.T. JR., GORENBERG, D.J. Lymphocyte studies in asymptomatic cigarette smokers. A comparison between lung and peripheral blood. *American Review of Respiratory Disease* 116:997–1005, 1977.

DAVIS, R.M., NOVOTNY, T.E. The epidemiology of cigarette smoking and its impact on chronic obstructive pulmonary disease. *American Review of Respiratory Disease* 140(Supplement):S82–S84, 1989.

DEAN, G., LEE, P.N., TODD, G.F., WICKEN, A.J., SPARKS, D.N. Factors related to respiratory and cardiovascular symptoms in the United Kingdom. *Journal of Epidemiology and Community Health* 32(2):86–96, June 1978.

DEMONCHY, J.G.R., KAUFFMAN, H.F., VENGE, P., KOËTER, G.H., JANSEN, H.M., SLUITER, H.J., DE VRIES, K. Bronchoalveolar eosinophilia during allergen-induced late asthmatic reactions. *American Review of Respiratory Disease* 131(3):373–376, March 1985.

DESHAZO, R.D., BANKS, D.E., DIEM, J.E., NORDBERG, J.A., BASER, Y., BEVIER, D., SALVAGGIO, J.E. Bronchoalveolar lavage cell–lymphocyte interactions in normal non-smokers and smokers. Analysis with a novel system. *American Review of Respiratory Disease* 127:545–548, 1983.

DIRKSEN, H., JANZON, L., LINDELL, S.E. Influence of smoking and cessation of smoking on lung function. A population study of closing volume and nitrogen wash-out. *Scandinavian Journal of Respiratory Diseases* 85(Supplement):266–274, 1974.

DOCKERY, D.W., SPEIZER, F.E., FERRIS, B.G. JR., WARE, J.H., LOUIS, T.A., SPIRO, A. III. Cumulative and reversible effects of lifetime smoking on simple tests of lung function in adults. *American Review of Respiratory Disease* 137:286–292, 1988.

DODGE, R.R., BURROWS, B. The prevalence and incidence of asthma and asthma-like symptoms in a general population sample. *American Review of Respiratory Disease* 122:567–575, 1980.

DOLL, R., GRAY, R., HAFNER, B., PETO, R. Mortality in relation to smoking: 22 years' observations on female British doctors. *British Medical Journal* 280(6219):967–971, April 5, 1980.

DOLL, R., PETO, R. Mortality in relation to smoking: 20 years' observations on male British doctors. *British Medical Journal* 2(6051):1525–1536, December 25, 1976.

DOPICO, G.A., REDDAN, W., TSIATIS, A., PETERS, M.E., RANKIN, J. Epidemiologic study of clinical and physiologic parameters in grain handlers of northern United States. *American Review of Respiratory Disease* 130:759–765, 1984.

EBI-KRYSTON, K.L. Predicting 15 year chronic bronchitis mortality in the Whitehall study. *Journal of Epidemiology and Community Health* 43(2):168–172, June 1989.

EDELMAN, N.H., MITTMAN, C., NORRIS, A.H., COHEN, B.H., SHOCK, N.W. The effects of cigarette smoking upon spirometric performance of community dwelling men. *American Review of Respiratory Disease* 94(3):421–429, September 1966.

ENARSON, D.A., CHAN-YEUNG, M., TABONA, M., KUS, J., VEDAL, S., LAM, S. Predictors of bronchial hyperexcitability in grainhandlers. *Chest* 87(4):452–455, April 1985.

ENJETI, S., HAZELWOOD, B., PERMUTT, S., MENKES, H., TERRY, P. Pulmonary function in young smokers: Male–female differences. *American Review of Respiratory Disease* 118:667–676, 1978.

FANTA, C.H., INGRAM, R.H. JR. Airway responsiveness and chronic airway obstruction. *Medical Clinics of North America* 65(3):473–487, May 1981.

FEINLEIB, M., ROSENBERG, H.M., COLLINS, J.G., DELOZIER, J.E., POKRAS, R., CHEVARLEY, F.M. Trends in COPD morbidity and mortality in the United States. *American Review of Respiratory Disease* 140(Supplement):S9–S18, 1989.

FENNERTY, A.G., BANKS, J., EBDEN, P., BEVAN, C. The effect of cigarette withdrawal on asthmatics who smoke. *European Journal of Respiratory Diseases* 71(5):395–399, November 1987.

FERRIS, B.G. JR., ANDERSON, D.O. The prevalence of chronic respiratory disease in a New Hampshire town. *American Review of Respiratory Diseases* 86:165–177, 1962.

FERRIS, B.G. JR., HIGGINS, I.T.T., HIGGINS, M.W., PETERS, J.M., VAN GANSE, W.F., GOLDMAN, M.D. Chronic nonspecific respiratory disease, Berlin, New Hampshire, 1961–1967: A cross-sectional study. *American Review of Respiratory Disease* 104(2):232–244, 1971.

FERSON, M., EDWARDS, A., LIND, A., MILTON, G.W., HERSEY, P. Low natural killer-cell activity and immunoglobulin levels associated with smoking in human subjects. *International Journal of Cancer* 23:603–609, 1979.

FINKLEA, J.F., HASSELBLAD, V., RIGGAN, W.B., NELSON, W.C., HAMMER, D.I., NEWILL, V.A. Cigarette smoking and hemagglutination inhibition response to influenza after natural disease and immunization. *American Review of Respiratory Disease* 104(3):368–376, September 1971.

FINKLEA, J.F., SANDIFER, S.H., SMITH, D.D. Cigarette smoking and epidemic influenza. *American Journal of Epidemiology* 90(5):390–399, November 1969.

FISHER, G.L., MCNEILL, K.L., FINCH, G.L., WILSON, F.D., GOLDE, D.W. Functional evaluation of lung macrophages from cigarette smokers and nonsmokers. *Journal of the Reticuloendothelial Society* 32(4):311–321, October 1982.

FLETCHER, C., PETO, R. The natural history of chronic airflow obstruction. *British Medical Journal* 1(9):1645–1648, June 1, 1977.

FLETCHER, C.M., ELMES, P.C., FAIRBAIRN, A.S., WOOD, C.H. The significance of respiratory symptoms and the diagnosis of chronic bronchitis in a working population. *British Medical Journal* 5147:258–266, August 29, 1959.

FLETCHER, C.M., PETO, R., TINKER, C., SPEIZER, F.G. *The Natural History of Chronic Bronchitis and Emphysema. An Eight-Year Study of Early Chronic Obstructive Lung Disease in Working Men in London.* New York: Oxford University Press, 1976.

FLETCHER, C.M., TINKER, C.M. Chronic bronchitis: A further study of simple diagnostic methods in a working population. *British Medical Journal* 5238:1491–1498, May 27, 1961.

FRANS, A., STANESCU, D.C., VERITER, C., CLERBAUX, T., BRASSEUR, L. Smoking and pulmonary diffusing capacity. *Scandinavian Journal of Respiratory Diseases* 56(3):165–183, September 1975.

FRIEDMAN, G.D., SIEGELAUB, A.B. Changes after quitting cigarette smoking. *Circulation* 61(4):716–723, 1980.

FRIEDMAN, G.D., SIEGELAUB, A.B., SELTZER, C.C., FELDMAN, R., COLLEN, M.F. Smoking habits and the leukocyte count. *Archives of Environmental Health* 26:137–143, March 1973.

GADEK, J.E., FELLS, G.A., CRYSTAL, R.G. Cigarette smoking induces functional antiprotease deficiency in the lower respiratory tract of humans. *Science* 206(4424):1315–1316, December 1979.

GADEK, J.E., FELLS, G.A., ZIMMERMAN, R.L., RENNARD, S.I., CRYSTAL, R.G. Antielastases of the human alveolar structures: Implications for the protease-antiprotease theory of emphysema. *Journal of Clinical Investigation* 68(4):889–898, October 1981.

GALDSTON, M., LEVYTSKA, V., SCHWARTZ, M.S., MAGNÚSSON, B. Ceruloplasmin. Increased serum concentration and impaired antioxidant activity in cigarette smokers, and ability to prevent suppression of elastase inhibitory capacity of alpha$_1$-proteinase inhibitor. *American Review of Respiratory Disease* 129:258–263, 1984.

GERRARD, J.W., COCKCROFT, D.W., MINK, J.T., COTTON, D.J., POONAWALA, R., DOSMAN, J.A. Increased nonspecific bronchial reactivity in cigarette smokers with normal lung function. *American Review of Respiratory Disease* 122(4):577–581, October 1980.

GERRARD, J.W., HEINER, D.C., KO, C.G., MINK, J., MEYERS, A., DOSMAN, J.A. Immunoglobulin levels in smokers and non-smokers. *Annals of Allergy* 44(5):261–262, May 1980.

GINNS, L.C., GOLDENHEIM, P.D., MILLER, L.G., BURTON, R.C., GILLICK, L., COLVIN, R.B., GOLDSTEIN, G., KUNG, P.C., HURWITZ, C., KAZEMI, H. T-lymphocyte subsets in smoking and lung cancer. Analysis by monoclonal antibodies and flow cytometry. *American Review of Respiratory Disease* 126:265–269, 1982.

GLEZEN, W.P., DECKER, M., PERROTTA, D.M. Survey of underlying conditions of persons hospitalized with acute respiratory disease during influenza epidemics in Houston, 1978–1981. *American Review of Respiratory Disease* 136:550–555, 1987.

GOLDSMITH, J.R., HECHTER, H.H., PERKINS, N.M., BORHANI, N.O. Pulmonary function and respiratory findings among longshoremen. *American Review of Respiratory Disease* 86(6):867–874, December 1962.

GOODMAN, R.M., YERGIN, B.M., LANDA, J.F., GOLINVAUX, M.H., SACKNER, M.A. Relationship of smoking history and pulmonary function tests to trachael mucous velocity in nonsmokers, young smokers, ex-smokers, and patients with chronic bronchitis. *American Review of Respiratory Disease* 117(2):205–214, February 1978.

GOTOH, T., UEDA, S., NAKAYAMA, T., TAKISHITA, Y., YASOUKA, S., TSUBURA, E. Protein components of bronchoalveolar lavage fluids from non-smokers and smokers. *European Journal of Respiratory Diseases* 64(5):369–377, July 1983.

GREENING, A.P., LOWRIE, D.B. Extracellular release of hydrogen peroxide by human alveolar macrophages: The relationship to cigarette smoking and lower respiratory tract infections. *Clinical Science* 65:661–664, 1983.

GROSS, P., PFITZER, E.A., TOLKER, E., BABYAK, M.A., KASCHAK, M. Experimental emphysema. Its production with papain in normal and silicotic rats. *Archives of Environmental Health* 11(1):50–58, July 1965.

GRUCHOW, H.W., HOFFMANN, R.G., MARX, J.J. JR., EMANUEL, D.A., RIMM, A.A. Precipitating antibodies to farmer's lung antigens in a Wisconsin farming population. *American Review of Respiratory Disease* 124:411–415, 1981.

GULSVIK, A., FAGERHOL, M.K. Smoking and immunoglobulin levels. (Letter.) *Lancet* 1:449, February 24, 1979.

HÄLLGREN, R., NOÛ, E., ARRENDAL, H., HIESCHE, K. Smoking and circulating IgE in bronchial carcinoma. *Acta Medica Scandinavica* 211:269–273, 1982.

HAMMOND, E.C. Evidence on the effects of giving up cigarette smoking. *American Journal of Public Health* 55(5):682–691, May 1965.

HAMMOND, E.C., HORN, D. Smoking and death rates—Report on forty-four months of followup of 187,783 men. *Journal of the American Medical Association* 166(11):1294–1308, March 15, 1958.

HARRIS, J.O., OLSEN, G.N., CASTLE, J.R., MALONEY, A.S. Comparison of proteolytic enzyme activity in pulmonary alveolar macrophages and blood leukocytes in smokers and nonsmokers. *American Review of Respiratory Disease* 111(6):579–586, May 1975.

HARRIS, J.O., SWENSON, E.L.W., JOHNSON, J.E. Human alveolar macrophages: Comparison of phagocytic ability, glucose utilization, and ultrastructure in smokers and nonsmokers. *Journal of Clinical Investigations* 49(11):2086–2096, November 1970.

HAWTHORNE, V.M., FRY, J.S. Smoking and health: The association between smoking behaviour, total mortality, and cardiorespiratory disease in west central Scotland. *Journal of Epidemiology and Community Health* 32:260–266, 1978.

HAYNES, W.F. JR., KRSTULOVIC, V.J., BELL, A.L. JR. Smoking habit and incidence of respiratory tract infections in a group of adolescent males. *American Review of Respiratory Disease* 93(5):780–785, May 1966.

HEISKELL, C.L., MILLER, J.N., ALDRICH, H.J., CARPENTER, C.M. Smoking and serologic abnormalities. *Journal of the American Medical Association* 181:88–91, 1962.

HERSEY, P., PRENDERGAST, D., EDWARDS, A. Effects of cigarette smoking on the immune system. Follow-up studies in norma subjects after cessation of smoking. *Medical Journal of Australia* 2(9):425–429, October 29, 1983.

HIGENBOTTAM, T., SHIPLEY, M.J., CLARK, T.J.H., ROSE, G. Lung function and symptoms of cigarette smokers related to tar yield and number of cigarettes smoked. *Lancet* 1(8165):409–412, February 23, 1980.

HIGENBOTTAM, T.W., FEYERABAND, C., CLARK, T.J.H. Cigarette smoking in asthma. *British Journal of Diseases of the Chest* 74:279–284, 1980.

HIGGINS, I.T.T., HIGGINS, M.W., LOCKSHIN, M.D., CANALE, N. Chronic respiratory diseases in mining communities in Marion County, West Virginia. *British Journal of Industrial Medicine* 25:165, 1968.

HIGGINS, M.W., KELLER, J.B., METZNER, H.L. Smoking, socioeconomic status and chronic respiratory disease. *American Review of Respiratory Disease* 116(3):403–410, September 1977.

HIGGINS, M.W., KJELSBERG, M. Characteristics of smokers and nonsmokers in Tecumseh, Michigan. II. The distribution of selected physical measurements and physiologic variables and the prevalence of certain diseases in smokers and nonsmokers. *American Journal of Epidemiology* 86(1):60–77, 1967.

HILLERDAHL, G., RYLANDER, R. Asthma and cessation of smoking. *Clinical Allergy* 14:45–47, 1984.

HOIDAL, J.R., FOX, R.B., LEMARBRE, P.A., TAKIFF, H.E., REPINE, J.E. Oxidative metabolism of alveolar macrophages from young asymptomatic cigarette smokers. Increased superoxide anion release and its potential consequences. *Chest* 77(2, Supplement):270–271, February 1980.

HOIDAL, J.R., FOX, R.B., TAKIFF, H.E., REPINE, J.E. Alveolar macrophages (AM) from young, asymptomatic cigarette smokers (CS) and nonsmokers (NS) use equal amounts of oxygen (O_2-) and glucose ($1-^{14}C$), but smoker AM make more superoxide anion. (Abstract.) *American Review of Respiratory Disease* 119(4, Supplement):222A, April 1979.

HOIDAL, J.R., NIEWOEHNER, D.E. Lung phagocyte recruitment and metabolic alterations induced by cigarette smoke in humans and in hamsters. *American Review of Respiratory Disease* 126:548–552, 1982.

HOLT, P.G. Immune and inflammatory function in cigarette smokers. *Thorax* 42:241–249, 1987.

HOLT, P.G., KEAST, D. Environmentally induced changes in immunological function: Acute and chronic effects of inhalation of tobacco smoke and other atmospheric contaminants in man and experimental animals. *Bacteriological Reviews* 41(1):205–216, March 1977.

HORN, B.R., ROBIN, E.D., THEODORE, J., VAN KESSEL, A. Total eosinophil counts in the management of bronchial asthma. *New England Journal of Medicine* 292(22):1152–1155, May 29, 1975.

HUGHES, D.A., HASLAM, P.L., TOWNSEND, P.J., TURNER-WARWICK, M. Numerical and functional alterations in circulatory lymphocytes in cigarette smokers. *Clinical and Experimental Immunology* 61(2):459–466, August 1985.

HUGHES, J.A., HUTCHISON, D.C.S., BELLAMY, D., DOWD, D.E., RYAN, K.C., HUGH-JONES, P. The influence of cigarette smoking and its withdrawal on the annual change of lung function in pulmonary emphysema. *Quarterly Journal of Medicine* 51(202):115–124, Spring 1982.

HUHTI, E., IKKALA, J. A 10-year follow-up study of respiratory symptoms and ventilatory function in a middle-aged rural population. *European Journal of Respiratory Diseases* 61(1): 33–45, February 1980.

HUNNINGHAKE, G.W., CRYSTAL, R.G. Cigarette smoking and lung destruction. Accumulation of neutrophils in the lungs of cigarette smokers. *American Review of Respiratory Disease* 128(5):833–838, November 1983.

HUNNINGHAKE, G.W., GADEK, J.E., KAWANAMI, O., FERRANS, V.J., CRYSTAL, R.G. Inflammatory and immune processes in the human lung in health and disease: Evaluation by bronchoalveolar lavage. *American Journal of Pathology* 97:149–206, 1979.

HYLAND, R.H., KRASTINS, R.R., ASPIN, N., MANSELL, A., ZAMEL, N. Effect of body position on carbon monoxide diffusing capacity in asymptomatic smokers and nonsmokers. *American Review of Respiratory Disease* 117(6):1045–1053, June 1978.

INGRAM, R.H. JR., O'CAIN, C.F. Frequency dependence of compliance in apparently healthy smokers versus nonsmokers. *Bulletin de Physiopathologie Respiratoire* 7(1):195–210, January–February 1971.

INGRAM, R.H. JR., SCHILDER, D.P. Association of a decrease in dynamic compliance with a change in gas distribution. *Journal of Applied Physiology* 23(6):911–916, December 1967.

JANOFF, A., WHITE, R., CARP, H., HAREL, S., DEARING, R., LEE, D. Lung injury induced by leukocytic proteases. *American Journal of Pathology* 97(1):111–129, October 1979.

JONES, J.G., MINTY, B.D., LAWLER, P., HULANDS, G.L., CRAWLEY, J.C.W., VEALL, N. Increased alveolar epithelial permeability in cigarette smokers. *Lancet* 1(8159):66–68, January 12, 1980.

JOSEPH, M., TONNEL, A.B., CAPRON, A., VOISIN, C. Enzyme release and superoxide anion production by human alveolar macrophages stimulated with immunoglobulin E. *Clinical and Experimental Immunology* 40:416–422, 1980.

KABIRAJ, M.U., SIMONSSON, B.G., GROTH, S., BJÖRKLUND, A., BÜLOW, K., LINDELL, S.E. Bronchial reactivity, smoking, and alpha-1-antitrypsin. A population-based study of middle-aged men. *American Review of Respiratory Disease* 126:864–869, 1982.

KANNER, R.E., RENZETTI, A.D., STANISH, W.M., BARKMAN, H.W., KLAUBER, M.R. Predictors of survival in subjects with chronic airflow limitation. *American Journal of Medicine* 74:249–255, February 1983.

KARK, J.D., LEBIUSH, M. Smoking and epidemic influenza-like illness in female military recruits: A brief survey. *American Journal of Public Health* 71(5):530–532, May 1981.

KARK, J.D., LEBIUSH, M., RANNON, L. Cigarette smoking as a risk factor for epidemic A(H_1N_1) influenza in young men. *New England Journal of Medicine* 307(17):1042–1046, October 21, 1982.

KASZUBOWSKI, P., WYSOCKI, J., MACHALSKI, M. T-lymphocytes and their T-gamma and T-mu subpopulations in cigarette smokers. *Polskie Archiwum Medycyny Wewnetrznej* 65(2):101–105, February 1981.

KAUFFMANN, F., NEUKIRCH, F., KOROBAEFF, M., MARNE, M.-J., CLAUDE, J.-R., LELLOUCH, J. Eosinophils, smoking, and lung function. An epidemiologic survey among 912 working men. *American Review of Respiratory Disease* 134(6):1172–1175, December 1986.

KAUFFMANN, F., QUERLEUX, E., DROUET, D., LELLOUCH, J., BRILLE, D. Evolútion du vems en 12 ans et tabagisme chez 556 travailleurs de la region parisienne. [Twelve year FEV_1 changes and the smoking habits among 556 workers in the Paris area.] *Bulletin Européen de Physiopathologie Respiratoire* 15:723–737, 1979.

KILBURN, K.H., WARSHAW, R., THORNTON, J.C. Asbestos diseases and pulmonary symptoms and signs in shipyard workers and their families in Los Angeles. *Archives of Internal Medicine* 146:2213–2220, November 1986.

KIVILOOG, J., IRNELL, L., EKLUND, G. The prevalence of bronchial asthma and chronic bronchitis in smokers and non-smokers in a representative local Swedish population. *Scandinavian Journal of Respiratory Diseases* 55:262–276, 1974.

KLEIN, R.C., SALVAGGIO, J.E. Nonspecificity of the bronchoconstricting effect of histamine and acetyl-beta-methylcholine in patients with obstructive airway disease. *Journal of Allergy* 37(3):158–168, March 1966.

KNOWLES, G.K., TAYLOR, P., TURNER-WARWICK, M. A comparison of antibody responses to admune inactivated influenza vaccine in serum and respiratory secretions of healthy non-smokers, healthy cigarette-smokers and patients with chronic bronchitis. *British Journal of Diseases of the Chest* 75:283–290, 1981.

KNUDSON, R.J., BLOOM, J.W., KNUDSON, D.E., KALTENBORN, W.T. Subclinical effects of smoking. Physiologic comparison of healthy middle-aged smokers and nonsmokers and interrelationships of lung function measurements. *Chest* 86:20–29, July 1984.

KNUDSON, R.J., BURROWS, B., LEBOWITZ, M.D. The maximal expiratory flow-volume curve: Its use in the detection of ventilatory abnormalities in a population study. *American Review of Respiratory Disease* 114(3):871–879, November 1976.

KNUDSON, R.J., KALTENBORN, W.T., BURROWS, B. The effects of cigarette smoking and smoking cessation on the carbon monoxide diffusing capacity of the lung in asymptomatic subjects. *American Review of Respiratory Disease* 140(3):645–651, 1989.

KORN, R.J., DOCKERY, D.W., SPEIZER, F.E., WARE, J.H., FERRIS, B.G. JR. Occupational exposures and chronic respiratory symptoms. A population-based study. *American Review of Respiratory Disease* 136:298–304, 1987.

KOSMIDER, S., FELUS, E., WYSOCKI, J. Evaluation of some humoral resistance determinants in cigarette smokers. *Polski Tygodnik Lekarski* 28(2):47–50, January 8, 1973.

KRUMHOLZ, R.A., HEDRICK, E.C. Pulmonary function differences in normal smoking and nonsmoking, middle-aged, white-collar workers. *American Review of Respiratory Disease* 107(2):225–230, February 1973.

KUSAKA, H., HOMMA, Y., OGASAWARA, H., MUNAKATA, M., TANIMURA, K., UKITA, H., DENZUMI, N., KAWAKAMI, Y. Five-year follow-up of *Micropolyspora faeni* antibody in smoking and nonsmoking farmers. *American Review of Respiratory Disease* 140(3):695–699, 1989.

LABEDZKI, L., MAGNUSSEN, H., HARTMANN, V., LOOS, U., MACKES, G., SCHWABE, H., BRAUMSCHWEIG, D., TIPPELMANN, G., FROST-HENSEL, E. Bronchoalveolar lavage in persons with lung disease: Cytology and macrophage function. *Praxis und Klinik der Pneumologie* 37(1):832–835, October 1983.

LANGE, P., GROTH, S., NYBOE, J., MORTENSEN, J., APPLEYARD, M., JENSEN, G., SCHNOHR, P. Effects of smoking and changes in smoking habits on the decline of FEV_1. *European Respiratory Journal* 2:811–816, 1989.

LAURELL, C.-B., ERIKSSON, S. The electrophoretic $_1$-globulin pattern of serum in $_1$-antitrypsin deficiency. *Scandinavian Journal of Clinical and Laboratory Investigation* 15(2):132–140, 1963.

LEBOWITZ, M.D., BURROWS, B. Quantitative relationships between cigarette smoking and chronic productive cough. *International Journal of Epidemiology* 6(2):107–113, 1977.

LEEDER, S.R., COLLEY, J.R.T., CORKHILL, R., HOLLAND, W.W. Change in respiratory symptom prevalence in adults who alter their smoking habits. *American Journal of Epidemiology* 105(6):522–529, 1977.

LEITCH, A.G., LUMB, E.M., KAY, A.B. Mediators of hypersensitivity in the sputum of young, symptomatic cigarette smokers. *Clinical Allergy* 11:257–262, 1981.

LOURENÇO, R.V., KLIMEK, M.F., BOROWSKI, C.J. Deposition and clearance of 2% particles in the tracheobronchial tree of normal subjects—Smokers and nonsmokers. *Journal of Clinical Investigation* 50:1411–1420, 1971.

MACKENZIE, J.S., MACKENZIE, I.H., HOLT, P.G. The effect of cigarette smoking on susceptibility to epidemic influenza and on serological responses to live attenuated and killed subunit influenza vaccines. *Journal of Hygiene* 77(3):409–417, December 1976.

MALO, J.L., FILIATRAULT, S., MARTIN, R.R. Bronchial responsiveness to inhaled methacholine in young asymptomatic smokers. *Journal of Applied Physiology* 52(6):1464–1470, June 1982.

MANFREDA, J., NELSON, N., CHERNIACK, R.M. Prevalence of respiratory abnormalities in a rural and an urban community. *American Review of Respiratory Disease* 117:215–226, 1978.

MARCQ, M., MINETTE, A. Lung function changes in smokers with normal conventional spirometry. *American Review of Respiratory Disease* 114:723–738, 1976.

MARCUS, E.B., BUIST, A.S., MACLEAN, C.J., YANO, K. Twenty-year trends in mortality from chronic obstructive pulmonary disease: The Honolulu heart program. *American Review of Respiratory Disease* 140(Supplement):S64–S68, 1989.

MARTIN, R.R., LINDSAY, D., DESPAS, P., BRUCE, D., LEROUX, M., ANTHONISEN, N.R., MACKLEM, P.T. The early detection of airway obstruction. *American Review of Respiratory Disease* 111:119–125, 1975.

MARTIN, R.R., WARR, G.A. Cigarette smoking and human pulmonary macrophages. *Hospital Practice* 12(9):97–104, September 1977.

MARTINEZ, F.D., ANTOGNONI, G., MACRI, F., BONCI, E., MIDULLA, F., DE CASTRO, G., RONCHETTI, R. Parental smoking enhances bronchial responsiveness in nine-year-old children. *American Review of Respiratory Disease* 138:518–523, 1988.

MASON, G.R., USZLER, J.M., EFFROS, R.M., REID, E. Rapidly reversible alterations of pulmonary epithelial permeability induced by smoking. *Chest* 83(1):6–11, January 1983.

MCCARTHY, D.S., CRAIG, D.B., CHERNIACK, R.M. Effect of modification of the smoking habit on lung function. *American Review of Respiratory Disease* 114(1):103–113, July 1976.

MCSHARRY, C., BANHAM, S.W., BOYD, G. Effect of cigarette smoking on the antibody response to inhaled antigens and the prevalence of extrinsic allergic alveolitis among pigeon breeders. *Clinical Allergy* 15(5):487–494, September 1985.

MCSHARRY, C., BANHAM, S.W., LYNCH, P.P., BOYD, G. Antibody measurement in extrinsic allergic alveolitis. *European Journal of Respiratory Diseases* 65(4):259–265, May 1984.

MCSHARRY, C., WILKINSON, P.C. Cigarette smoking and the antibody response to inhaled antigens. *Immunology Today* 7:98–102, 1986.

MICHAELS, R., SIGURDSON, M., THURLBECK, S., CHERNIACK, R. Elastic recoil of the lung in cigarette smokers: The effect of nebulized bronchodilator and cessation of smoking. *American Review of Respiratory Disease* 119(5):707–716, May 1979.

MILLER, A., THORNTON, J.C., ANDERSON, H.A., SELIKOFF, I.J. Clinical respiratory abnormalities in Michigan. Prevalence by sex and smoking history in a representative sample of the adult population. *Chest* 94(6):1187–1194, December 1988.

MILLER, A., THORNTON, J.C., WARSHAW, R., ANDERSON, H., TEIRSTEIN, A.S., SELIKOFF, I.J. Single breath diffusing capacity in a representative sample of the population of Michigan, a large industrial state. *American Review of Respiratory Disease* 127(3):270–277, March 1983.

MILLER, L.G., GOLDSTEIN, G., MURPHY, M., GINNS, L.C. Reversible alterations in immunoregulatory T cells in smoking. Analysis by monoclonal antibodies and flow cytometry. *Chest* 82(5):526–529, 1982.

MINTY, B.D., JORDAN, C., JONES, J.G. Rapid improvement in abnormal pulmonary epithelial permeability after stopping cigarettes. *British Medical Journal* 282:1183–1186, April 11, 1981.

MORGAN, D.C., SMYTH, J.T., LISTER, R.W., PETHYBRIDGE, R.J. Chest symptoms and farmer's lung: A community survey. *British Journal of Industrial Medicine* 30(3):259–265, July 1973.

MORGAN, D.C., SMYTH, J.T., LISTER, R.W., PETHYBRIDGE, R.J., GILSON, J.C., CALLAGHAN, P., THOMAS, G.O. Chest symptoms in farming communities with special reference to farmer's lung. *British Journal of Industrial Medicine* 32(3):228–234, August 1975.

MUELLER, R.E., KEBLE, D.L., PLUMMER, J., WALKER, S.H. The prevalence of chronic bronchitis, chronic airway obstruction, and respiratory symptoms in a Colorado city. *American Review of Respiratory Disease* 103:209–228, 1971.

NAGAI, A., WEST, W.W., THURLBECK, W.M. The National Institutes of Health intermittent positive-pressure breathing trial: Pathology studies. II. Correlation between morphologic findings, clinical findings, and evidence of expiratory air-flow obstruction. *American Review of Respiratory Disease* 132(5):946–953, November 1985.

NIELSEN, H. A quantitative and qualitative study of blood monocytes in smokers. *European Journal of Respiratory Diseases* 66(5):327–332, May 1985.

NIEWOEHNER, D.E., KLEINERMAN, J., RICE, D.B. Pathologic changes in the peripheral airways of young cigarette smokers. *New England Journal of Medicine* 291(15):755–758, October 10, 1974.

NOBLE, R.C., PENNY, B.B. Comparison of leukocyte count and function in smoking and nonsmoking young men. *Infection and Immunity* 12(3):550–555, September 1975.

O'CONNOR, G.T., SPARROW, D., WEISS, S.T. The role of allergy and nonspecific airway hyperresponsiveness in the pathogenesis of chronic obstructive pulmonary disease. *American Review of Respiratory Disease* 140:225–252, 1989.

ONARI, K., SADAMOTO, K., TAKAISHI, M., INAMIZU, T., IKUTA, T., YORIOKA, N., ISHIOKA, S., YAMAKIDO, M., NISHIMOTO, Y. Immunological studies on cigarette smokers. Part II. Cell mediated immunity in cigarette smokers and the influence of the water-soluble fraction of cigarette smoke (WSF) on the immunity of mice. *Hiroshima Journal of Medical Science* 29(2):29–34, June 1, 1980.

PAOLETTI, P., CAMILLI, A.E., HOLBERG, C.J., LEBOWITZ, M.D. Respiratory effects in relation to estimated tar exposure from current and cumulative cigarette consumption. *Chest* 88(6):849–855, December 1985.

PARKER, C.D., BILBO, R.E., REED, C.E. Methacholine aerosol as test for bronchial asthma. *Archives of Internal Medicine* 115(4):452–458, April 1965.

PARNELL, J.L., ANDERSON, D.O., KINNIS, C. Cigarette smoking and respiratory infections in a class of student nurses. *New England Journal of Medicine* 274(18):980–984, May 5, 1966.

PAYNE, M., KJELSBERG, M. Respiratory symptoms, lung function, and smoking habits in an adult population. *American Journal of Public Health* 54(2):261–277, February 1964.

PEAT, J.K., WOOLCOCK, A.J., CULLEN, K. Rate of decline of lung function in subjects with asthma. *European Journal of Respiratory Diseases* 70(3):171–179, March 1987.

PETERS, J.M., FERRIS, B.G. JR. Smoking and morbidity in a college-age group. *American Review of Respiratory Disease* 95(5):783–789, May 1967.

PETO, R., SPEIZER, F.E., COCHRANE, A.L., MOORE, F., FLETCHER, C.M., TINKER, C.M., HIGGINS, I.T.T., GRAY, R.G., RICHARDS, S.M., GILLILAND, J., NORMAN-SMITH, B. The relevance in adults of air-flow obstruction, but not of mucus hypersecretion, to mortality from chronic lung disease. Results from 20 years of prospective observation. *American Review of Respiratory Disease* 128(3):491–500, 1983.

PHAM, Q.T., MUR, J.M., CHAU, N., GABIANO, M., HENQUEL, J.C., TECULESCU, D. Prognostic value of acetylcholine challenge test: A prospective study. *British Journal of Industrial Medicine* 41:267–271, 1984.

POLLARD, R.B., MELTON, L.J. III, HOEFFLER, D.F., SPRINGER, G.L., SCHEINER, E.F. Smoking and respiratory illness in military recruits. *Archives of Environmental Health* 30:533–537, 1975.

POSTMA, D.S., DE VRIES, K., KOËTER, G.H., SLUITER, H.J. Independent influence of reversibility of air-flow obstruction and nonspecific hyperreactivity on the long-term course of lung function in chronic air-flow obstruction. *American Review of Respiratory Disease* 134(2):276–280, August 1986.

POSTMA, D.S., GIMENO, F., VAN DER WEELE, L.T., SLUITER, H.J. Assessment of ventilatory variables in survival prediction of patients with chronic airflow obstruction: The importance of reversibility. *European Journal of Respiratory Diseases* 67(5):360–368, November 1985.

POUKKULA, A., HUHTI, E., MÄKARÄINEN, M. Chronic respiratory disease among workers in a pulp mill. A ten-year follow-up study. *Chest* 81(3):285–289, March 1982.

PRE, J.M., BLADIER, D., BATTESTI, J.-P. Cytological and immunochemical reactions of human alveoli to tobacco aggression: Importance and characteristics. *IRCS Journal of Medical Science: Biochemistry* 8(9):637–638, 1980.

PRIDE, N.B., TATTERSALL, S.F., BENSON, M.K., HUNTER, D., MANSELL, A., FLETCHER, C.M., PETO, R. Peripheral lung function and spirometry in male smokers and exsmokers. *Chest* 77(2, Supplement):289–290, February 1980.

RAMAN, A.S., SWINBURNE, A.J., FEDULLA, A.J. Pneumococcal adherence to the buccal epithelial cells of cigarette smokers. *Chest* 83:23–27, 1983.

RAMSDALE, E.H., MORRIS, M.M., ROBERTS, R.S., HARGREAVE, F.E. Bronchial responsiveness to methacholine in chronic bronchitis: Relationship to airflow obstruction and cold air responsiveness. *Thorax* 39(12):912–918, December 1984.

RAMSDELL, J.W., NACHTWEY, F.J., MOSER, K.M. Bronchial hyperreactivity in chronic obstructive bronchitis. *American Review of Respiratory Disease* 126(5):829–832, November 1982.

RAZMA, A.G., LYNCH, J.P. III, WILSON, B.S., WARD, P.A., KUNKEL, S.L. Human alveolar macrophage activation and DR antigen expression in cigarette smokers. *Chest* 85(6, Supplement):41S–43S, June 1984.

REYNOLDS, H.Y., NEWBALL, H.H. Aalysis of proteins and respiratory cells obtained from human lungs by bronchial lavage. *Journal of Laboratory and Clinical Medicine* 84(4):559–573, October 1974.

RICHARDS, S.W., PETERSON, P.K., VERBRUGH, H.A., NELSON, R.D., HAMMER-SCHMIDT, D.E., HOIDAL, J.R. Chemotactic and phagocytic responses of human alveolar macrophages to activated complement components. *Infection and Immunity* 43(2):775–778, February 1984.

RIJCKEN, B., SCHOUTEN, J.P., WEISS, S.T., SPEIZER, F.E., VAN DER LENDE, R. The relationship of nonspecific bronchial responsiveness to respiratory symptoms in a random population sample. *American Review of Respiratory Disease* 136:62–68, 1987.

ROBERTSON, J., CALDWELL, J.R., CASTLE, J.R., WALDMAN, R.H. Evidence for the presence of components of the alternative (properdin) pathway of complement activation in respiratory secretions. *Journal of Immunology* 117(3):900–903, September 1976.

ROBERTSON, M.D., BOYD, D.E., FERNIE, J.M., DAVIS, J.M.G. Some immunological studies on coalworkers with and without pneumonoconiosis. *American Journal of Industrial Medicine* 4(3):467–476, 1983.

ROGOT, E., MURRAY, J.L. Smoking and causes of death among U.S. veterans: 16 years of observation. *Public Health Reports* 95(3):213–222, May–June 1980.

SAETTA, M., GHEZZO, H., KIM, W.D., KING, M., ANGUS, G.E., WANG, N.-S., COSIO, M.G. Loss of alveolar attachments in smokers: A morphometric correlate of lung function impairment. *American Review of Respiratory Disease* 132:894–900, 1985.

SCHACHTER, E.N., DOYLE, C.A., BECK, G.J. A prospective study of asthma in a rural community. *Chest* 85(5):623–630, May 1984.

SCHENKER, M.B., SAMET, J.M., SPEIZER, F.E. Effect of cigarette tar content and smoking habits on respiratory symptoms in women. *American Review of Respiratory Disease* 125:684–690, 1982.

SCHLESINGER, Z., GOLDBOURT, U., MEDALIE, J.H., RISS, E., NEUFELD, H.N., ORON, D. Pulmonary function and respiratory disease among adult male Israelis. Variations by age and birth place. *Israel Journal of Medical Sciences* 8(7):957–964, July 1972.

SHARP, J.T., PAUL, O., MCKEAN, H., BEST, W.R. A longitudinal study of bronchitic symptoms and spirometry in a middle-aged, male, industrial population. *American Review of Respiratory Disease* 108(5):1066–1077, November 1973.

SIMANI, A.S., INOUE, S., HOGG, J.C. Penetration of the respiratory epithelium of guinea pigs following exposure to cigarette smoke. *Laboratory Investigation* 31(1):75–81, July 1974.

SIMONSSON, B.G., ROLF, C. Bronchial reactivity to methacholine in ten non-obstructive heavy smokers before and up to one year after cessation of smoking. *European Journal of Respiratory Diseases* 63:526–534, 1982.

SMART, Y.C., COX, J., ROBERTS, T.K., BRINSMEAD, M.W., BURTON, R.C. Differential effect of cigarette smoking on recirculating T lymphocyte subsets in pregnant women. *Journal of Immunology* 137(1):1–3, July 1, 1986.

SNIDER, G.L. Chronic bronchitis and emphysema. In: Murray, J.F., Nadel, J.A. (eds.) *Textbook of Respiratory Medicine*. Philadelphia: W.B. Saunders Co., 1988, pp. 1069–1106.

SNIDER, G.L. Chronic obstructive pulmonary disease: A definition and implications of structural determinants of airflow obstruction for epidemiology. *American Review of Respiratory Disease*, 140(3, Supplement):S3–S8, September 1989.

SPARROW, D., O'CONNOR, G., COLTON, T., BARRY, C.L., WEISS, S.T. The relationship of nonspecific bronchial responsiveness to the occurrence of respiratory symptoms and decreased levels of pulmonary function. *American Review of Respiratory Disease* 135:1255–1260, 1987.

SPEIZER, F.E., FAY, M.E., DOCKERY, D.W., FERRIS, B.G. JR. Chronic obstructive pulmonary disease mortality in six U.S. cities. *American Review of Respiratory Disease* 140:S49–S55,1989.

SPEIZER, F.E., TAGER, I.B. Epidemiology of chronic mucus hypersecretion and obstructive airways disease. *Epidemiologic Reviews* 1:124–142, 1979.

STEIN, R., EVANS, S., MILNER, R., RAND, C., DOLOVICH, J. Isotopic and enzymatic IgE assays in non-allergic subjects. *Allergy* 38(6):389–398, August 1983.

SUCIU-FOCA, N., MOLONARO, A., BUDA, J., REEMTSMA, K. Cellular immune responsiveness in cigarette smokers. (Letter.) *Lancet* 1:1062, May 25, 1974.

TABONA, M., CHAN-YEUNG, M., ENARSON, D., MACLEAN, L., DORKEN, E., SCHULZER, M. Host factors affecting longitudinal decline in lung spirometry among grain elevator workers. *Chest* 85(6):782–786, June 1984.

TAGER, I.B., SEGAL, M.R., SPEIZER, F.E., WEISS, S.T. The natural history of forced expiratory volumes—Effect of cigarette smoking and respiratory symptoms. *American Review of Respiratory Disease* 138:837–838, 1988.

TAGER, I.B., WEISS, S.T., MUÑOZ, A., ROSNER, B., SPEIZER, F.E. Longitudinal study of the effects of maternal smoking on pulmonary function in children. *New England Journal of Medicine* 309:699–703, September 22, 1983.

TASHKIN, D.P., CLARK, V.A., COULSON, A.H., SIMMONS, M., BOURQUE, L.B., REEMS, C., DETELS, R., SAYRE, J.W., ROKAW, S.N. The UCLA population studies of chronic obstructive respiratory disease. VIII. Effects of smoking cessation on lung function: A prospective study of a free-living population. *American Review of Respiratory Disease* 130(5):707–715, November 1984.

TAYLOR, R.G., GROSS, E., JOYCE, H., HOLLAND, F., PRIDE, N.B. Smoking, allergy, and the differential white blood cell count. *Thorax* 40:17–22, 1985.

TAYLOR, R.G., JOYCE, H., GROSS, E., HOLLAND, F., PRIDE, N.B. Bronchial reactivity to inhaled histamine and annual rate of decline in FEV_1 in male smokers and ex-smokers. *Thorax* 40:9–16, 1985.

TECULESCU, D.B., STANESCU, D.C. Lung diffusing capacity. Normal values in male smokers and non-smokers using the breath-holding technique. *Scandinavian Journal of Respiratory Diseases* 51(3):137–149, 1970.

THOMSON, M.L., PAVIA, D. Long-term tobacco smoking and mucociliary clearance from the human lung in health and respiratory impairment. *Archives of Environmental Health* 26: 86–89, February 1973.

THURLBECK, W.M. Chronic airflow obstruction in lung disease. In: Bennington, J.L. (ed.) *Major Problems in Pathology*, Volume 5. Philadelphia: W.B. Saunders Company, 1976, pp. 235–287.

TOCKMAN, M.S., COMSTOCK, G.W. Respiratory risk factors and mortality: Longitudinal studies in Washington County, Maryland. *American Review of Respiratory Disease* 140(Spplement):S56S63, 1989.

TOLLERUD, D.J., CLARK, J.W., BROWN, L.M., NEULAND, C.Y., MANN, D.L., PANKIWTROST, L.K., BLATTNER, W.A., HOOVER, R.N. The effects of cigarette smoking on T cell subsets. A population-based survey of healthy Caucasions. *American Review of Respiratory Disease* 139:1446–1451, 1989.

TOWNSEND, M.C., DUCHENE, A.G., MORGAN, J., BROWNER, W.S. Cigarette smoking intervention in the Multiple Risk Factor Intervention Trial: Results and relationships to other outcomes. Pulmonary function in relation to cigarette smoking and smoking cessation. *Preventive Medicine*, in press.

TRAVER, G.A., CLINE, M.G., BURROWS, B. Predictors of mortality in chronic obstructive pulmonary disease: A 15-year follow-up study. *American Review of Respiratory Disease* 119(6):895–902, June 1979.

U.S. DEPARTMENT OF HEALTH AND HUMAN SERVICES. *The Health Consequences of Smoking: Chronic Obstructive Lung Disease. A Report of the Surgeon General.* U.S. Department of Health and Human Services, Public Health Service, Office on Smoking and Health. DHHS Publication No. (PHS) 84-50205, 1984.

U.S. DEPARTMENT OF HEALTH AND HUMAN SERVICES. *The Health Consequences of Smoking: Cancer and Chronic Lung Disease in the Workplace. A Report of the Surgeon General.* U.S. Department of Health and Human Services, Public Health Service, Office on Smoking and Health. DHHS Publication No. (PHS) 85-50207, 1985.

U.S. DEPARTMENT OF HEALTH AND HUMAN SERVICES. *The Health Consequences of Involuntary Smoking. A Report of the Surgeon General.* U.S. Department of Health and Human Services, Public Health Service, Centers for Disease Control. DHHS Publication No. (CDC) 87-8398, 1986.

U.S. DEPARTMENT OF HEALTH AND HUMAN SERVICES. *Reducing the Health Consequences of Smoking: 25 Years of Progress. A Report of the Surgeon General.* U.S. Department of Health and Human Services, Public Health Service, Centers for Disease Control, Center for Chronic Disease Prevention and Health Promotion, Office on Smoking and Health. DHHS Publication No. (CDC) 89-8411, 1989.

U.S. DEPARTMENT OF HEALTH, EDUCATION, AND WELFARE. *The Health Consequences of Smoking. A Report of the Surgeon General: 1971.* U.S. Department of Health, Education, and Welfare, Public Health Service, Health Services and Mental Health Administration. DHEW Publication No. (HSM) 71-7513, 1971.

U.S. DEPARTMENT OF HEALTH, EDUCATION, AND WELFARE. *Smoking and Health: A Report of the Surgeon General.* U.S. Department of Health, Education, and Welfare, Public Health Service, Office of the Assistant Secretary for Health, Office on Smoking and Health. DHEW Publication No. (PHS) 79-50066, 1979.

U.S. PUBLIC HEALTH SERVICE. *Smoking and Health. Report of the Advisory Committee to the Surgeon General of the Public Health Service.* U.S. Department of Health, Education, and Welfare, Public Health Service, Center for Disease Control. PHS Publication No. 1103, 1964.

VAN DER LENDE, R., KOK, T.J., REIG, R.P., QUANJER, P.H., SCHOUTEN, J.P., ORIE, N.G.M. Diminutions de cv et de vems avec le temps: Index des effets du tabagisme et de la pollution de l'air. [Decreases in VC and FEV_1 with time: Indicators for effects of smoking and air pollution.] *Bulletin Européen de Physiopathologie Respiratoire* 17:775–792, 1981.

VAN GANSE, W.F., FERRIS, B.G. JR., COTES, J.E. Cigarette smoking and pulmonary diffusing capacity (transfer factor). *American Review of Respiratory Disease* 105(1):30–41, January 1972.

VELLUTI, G., CAPELLI, O., LUSUARDI, M., BRAGHIROLI, A., PELLEGRINO, M., MILANTI, G., BENEDETTI, L. Bronchoalveolar lavage in the normal lung. First of three parts: Protein, enzymatic and ionic features. *Respiration* 44(6):403–410, November–December 1983.

VILLIGER, B., BROEKELMANN, T., KELLEY, D., HEYMACH, G.J. III, MCDONALD, J.A. Bronchoalveolar fibronectin in smokers and non-smokers. *American Review of Respiratory Disease* 124(5):652–654, November 1981.

VOLLMER, W.M., JOHNSON, L.R., BUIST, A.S. Relationship of response to a bronchodilator and decline in forced expiratory volume in one second in population studies. *American Review of Respiratory Disease* 132:1186–1193, 1985.

VOS-BRAT, L.C., RUMKE, P.H. Immunoglobuline concentraties. PHA reacties van lymfocyten in vittro en enkele antistof titers van gezonde rokers. *Jaarboek Van Kankeronderzoek en Kankerbestrijding in Nederland* 19:49–53, 1969.

WARR, G.A., MARTIN, R.R. Chemotactic responsiveness of human alveolar macrophages: Effects of cigarette smoking. *Infection and Immunity* 9(4):769–771, April 1974.

WARR, G.A., MARTIN, R.R. Immune receptors of human alveolar macrophages: Comparison between cigarette smokers and nonsmokers. *Journal of the Reticuloendothelial Society* 22(3):181–187, September 1977.

WARREN, C.P.W., HOLFORD-STREVENS, V., WONG, C., MANFREDA, J. The relationship between smoking and total immunoglobulin E levels. *Journal of Allergy and Clinical Immunology* 69(4):370–375, 1982.

WEISS, S.T., TAGER, I.B., MUNOZ, A., SPEIZER, F.E. The relationship of respiratory infections in early childhood to the occurrence of increased levels of bronchial responsiveness and atopy. *American Review of Respiratory Disease* 131(4):573–578, April 1985.

WEISS, W., BOUCOT, K.R., COOPER, D.A., CARNAHAN, W.J. Smoking and the health of older men. II. Smoking and ventilatory function. *Archives of Environmental Health* 7:538–553, November 1963.

WELTY, C., WEISS, S.T., TAGER, I.B., MUÑOZ, A., BECKER, C., SPEIZER, F.E., INGRAM, R.H. JR. The relationship of airways responsiveness to cold air, cigarette smoking, and atopy to respiratory symptoms and pulmonary function in adults. *American Review of Respiratory Disease* 130:198–203, 1984.

WHITEHEAD, R.H., HOOPER, B.E., GRIMSHAW, D.A., HUGHES, L.E. Cellular immune responsiveness in cigarette smokers. *Lancet* 1(7868):1232–1233, June 15, 1974.

WILHELMSEN, L., ORHA, I., TIBBLIN, G. Decrease in ventilatory capacity between ages of 50 and 54 in representative sample of Swedish men. *British Medical Journal* 3:553–556, September 1969.

WILHELMSEN, L., TIBBLIN, G. Tobacco smoking in fifty-year-old men. I. Respiratory symptoms and ventilatory function tests. *Scandinavian Journal of Respiratory Diseases* 47:121–130, 1966.

WINGERD, J., SPONZILLI, E.E. Concentrations of serum protein fractions in white women: Effects of age, weight, smoking, tonsillectomy, and other factors. *Clinical Chemistry* 23(7): 1310–1317, 1977.

WOOLCOCK, A.J., PEAT, J.K., SALOME, C.M., YAN, K., ANDERSON, S.D., SCHOEFFEL, R.E., MCCOWAGE, G., KILLALEA, T. Prevalence of bronchial hyperresponsiveness and asthma in a rural adult population. *Thorax* 42:361–368, 1987.

WOOLF, C.R., SUERO, J.T. The respiratory effects of regular cigarette smoking in women. *American Review of Respiratory Disease* 103(1):26–37, January 1971.

WOOLF, C.R., ZAMEL, N. The respiratory effects of regular cigarette smoking in women. A five-year prospective study. *Chest* 78(5):707–713, November 1980.

WRIGHT, J.L. Small airway disease: Structure and function. In: Hensley, M.J., Saunders, N.A. (eds.) *Clinical Epidemiology of Chronic Obstructive Pulmonary Disease*. New York: Marcel Dekker, Inc., 1989, p. 55.

WYATT, R.J., BRIDGES, R.B., HALATEK, D.G. Complement levels in cigarette smokers: Elevations of serum concentrations of C5, C9 and C1-inhibitor. *Journal of Clinical and Laboratory Immunology* 6:131–135, 1981.

ZAMEL, N., LEROUX, M., RAMCHARAN, V. Decrease in lung recoil pressure after cessation of smoking. *American Review of Respiratory Disease* 119(2):205–211, February 1979.

ZAMEL, N., WEBSTER, P.M. Amelioration de la dynamique du debit expiratoire apres arret du tabac. [Improved expiratory airflow dynamics with smoking cessation.] *Bulletin Europeen de Physiopathologie Respiratoire* 20:19–23, 1984.

ZETTERSTRÖM, O., OSTERMAN, K., MACHADO, L., JOHANSSON, S.G.O. Another smoking hazard: Raised serum IgE concentration and increased risk of occupational allergy. *British Medical Journal* 283:1215–1217, November 7, 1981.

CHAPTER 8
SMOKING CESSATION AND REPRODUCTION

CONTENTS

Part I. Female 371
  Pregnancy and Pregnancy Outcome 371
    Introduction 371
    Pathophysiologic Framework 371
    Nonexperimental Studies 374
      Fertility and Infertility 374
      Ectopic Pregnancy and Spontaneous Abortion 375
      Fetal, Neonatal, and Perinatal Mortality 376
      Birthweight and Gestational Duration 379
        Introduction 379
        Continued Smoking 381
        Cessation Before Conception 382
        Cessation After Conception 383
          Birthweight 383
          Preterm Delivery 386
      Complications of Pregnancy 387
    Randomized Trials of Smoking Cessation During Pregnancy 387
    Prevalence of Smoking and Smoking Cessation During Pregnancy and Time
      Trends in Prevalence and Cessation 390
      Introduction 390
      Prevalence of Smoking and Smoking Cessation 390
      Time Trends in Smoking and Smoking Cessation 393
    Estimates of Attributable Risk Percent 393
  Age at Natural Menopause 396
    Introduction 396
    Pathophysiologic Framework 396
    Studies of Former Smokers 398

Part II. Male 400
  Introduction 400
  Pathophysiologic Framework 400
  Sexual Activity and Performance 401
  Sperm Density and Quality 404

Conclusions 410

References 411

PART I. FEMALE

Pregnancy and Pregnancy Outcome

Introduction

Since the late 1940s, cigarette smoking during pregnancy has been linked with poor pregnancy outcome (Bernhard 1949; Athayde 1948). Adverse effects of smoking on pregnancy began to receive considerable attention after publication of the results of a study of 7,499 pregnant women in San Bernardino County, CA, in which the rate of prematurity, defined as birthweight less than 2,500 g, was found to be about twice as high among smokers as among nonsmokers during pregnancy (Simpson 1957).

Early reports of the Surgeon General (US DHEW 1971, 1973, 1978) concluded that maternal smoking during pregnancy retards fetal growth and is a probable cause of late fetal and infant mortality (US DHEW 1973). The 1977 Report of the Surgeon General (US DHEW 1978) concluded that smoking during pregnancy has dose–response relationships with abruptio placentae, placenta previa, bleeding during pregnancy, premature and prolonged rupture of the membranes, and preterm delivery. The 1979 and 1980 Reports of the Surgeon General (US DHEW 1979; US DHHS 1980) comprehensively reviewed information on the association of maternal smoking with pregnancy outcome and further concluded that the risk of spontaneous abortion increases with the amount of smoking and that the risk of sudden infant death syndrome (SIDS) is increased by maternal smoking during pregnancy. The 1980 Report (US DHHS 1980) also indicated the possibility of a link between cigarette smoking and impaired fertility.

Two earlier reports of the Surgeon General (US DHEW 1979; US DHHS 1980) concluded that mean gestational duration is not affected by maternal smoking and that data are not sufficient to support a conclusion that maternal smoking increases, decreases, or has no association with risk of congenital malformations.

This Section reviews observational studies of smoking cessation and the following reproductive outcomes: fertility and infertility; ectopic pregnancy and spontaneous abortion; fetal, neonatal, and perinatal mortality; birthweight and gestational duration; and complications of pregnancy. Three randomized trials of smoking cessation and pregnancy outcome are described and discussed in detail. Information on the prevalence of smoking during pregnancy and time trends in prevalence is presented, along with estimates of the attributable risk of several pregnancy outcomes. SIDS and congenital malformations are not considered because of the limited information on smoking cessation.

Pathophysiologic Framework

The effects of smoking that might mediate adverse effects on the developing fetus and on fertility, fetal loss, and pregnancy complications have been reviewed in other publications (Longo 1982; Mattison 1982; US DHHS 1980). These reviews are summarized with attention to the temporal course of the relation between exposure to cigarette smoking and pregnancy outcome as well as the distinction between reversible and irreversible effects of smoking. Reversible effects would be expected to result in similar risks for never smokers and former smokers, whereas irreversible effects would be expected to lead to different risks in both current and former smokers compared with never smokers.

Several pathways have been postulated by which tobacco smoke might adversely affect fertility (Mattison 1982) (Table 1). These include disturbance of hypothalamic–pituitary function, interference with motility in the female reproductive tract (Chow et al. 1988), and impairment of implantation, all of which are thought to be reversible consequences of exposure to absorbed chemicals in tobacco smoke (principally nicotine). It has also been suggested that smoking results in oocyte depletion through direct toxicity (Mattison 1980), which would have irreversible consequences for fertility. Chow and colleagues (1988) postulated that altered immune function (Hersey, Prendergast, Edwards 1983) may predispose smokers to pelvic inflammatory disease, which in turn can result in permanent scarring and occlusion of the fallopian tubes. Alterations in the neuroendocrine control of ovulation have been suggested to account for increased amenorrhea reported among smokers (Pettersson, Fries, Nillius 1973); this mechanism, as an effect of smoking on fertility, would be reversible.

TABLE 1.—Possible mechanisms for the effect of smoking on pregnancy and pregnancy outcome

Outcome	Possible mechanism
Reduced fertility	Hormonal effects
	Impaired tubal motility
	Impaired implantation
	Oocyte depletion
	Altered immunity leading to pelvic inflammatory disease
Spontaneous abortion	Nicotine toxicity
Reduced birthweight	Impaired weight gain
	Nicotine toxicity
	CO toxicity
	Increased cyanide leading to impaired vitamin B_{12} metabolism
	Hypoxia due to increased levels of CO or to vasoconstriction of umbilical artery

NOTE: CO=carbon monoxide.

Mechanisms for an effect of cigarette smoking on spontaneous abortion have not been clearly defined, partly because so little is known about the pathophysiologic basis for spontaneous abortion. The causes of spontaneous abortion are broadly divided into genetic and nongenetic causes (Kline 1984). Because smoking seems to have its primary impact on chromosomally normal spontaneous abortions (Kline 1984; Alberman et al. 1976), nongenetic pathways are implicated for smoking (Table 1).

Most attention has been focused on the mechanisms mediating a reduction of fetal growth among smokers (Table 1). An indirect, nutritionally based mechanism in which smokers are postulated to eat less and gain less weight during pregnancy, thus delivering smaller infants, has been prominent in discussions of fetal growth retardation in smokers (Papoz et al. 1982; Rush 1974; Meyer 1978; Davies and Abernethy 1976). This subject has been reviewed in depth in previous reports of the Surgeon General (US DHEW 1979; US DHHS 1980) and more recently by other researchers (Werler, Pober, Holmes 1985). Differences in weight gain do not entirely explain fetal growth retardation in smokers because differences in weight gain during pregnancy between smokers and nonsmokers are very small and have not been observed consistently and because a relationship between growth retardation and smoking persists after adjusting for maternal weight gain.

In this context, however, the studies of weight gain in women who quit smoking during pregnancy are of interest. Pulkkinen (1985) found that women who quit smoking during the first trimester gained more weight than nonsmokers or continuing smokers (1.0 vs. 1.3 kg average difference, respectively). Kuzma and Kissinger (1981) also found that women who quit smoking during pregnancy gained more weight compared with women who did not smoke during pregnancy (average difference of 4.7 kg) and women who smoked throughout pregnancy (average difference of 5.6 kg). Also, women who quit smoking before the onset of pregnancy were reported to gain more weight during pregnancy than nonsmokers or smokers (1.3 kg and 0.9 kg average difference, respectively) (Anderson et al. 1984). Rush (1974) reported a reduction in weight gain of 0.12 pounds per week among continuing smokers compared with those who quit. This pattern may reflect the well-established tendency to gain weight following smoking cessation (Manley and Boland 1983; Rabkin 1984), as discussed further in Chapter 11.

There are several hypotheses that attempt to explain the mechanism by which fetal growth is affected by cigarette smoking (Table 1), but cigarette smoking is believed to impact on fetal growth through intrauterine hypoxia (Longo 1977). Carbon monoxide, a component of cigarette smoke, has the ability to cross the placenta and bind with the hemoglobin in both the mother and the fetus producing carboxyhemoglobin. Carboxyhemoglobin reduces the ability of the blood to carry adequate levels of oxygen to the fetus. Smoking is also believed to cause vasoconstriction of the umbilical arteries, and therefore, impact on placental blood flow (Lehtovirta and Forss 1978; Naeye and Tafari 1983; Longo 1982). Cigarette smoking during pregnancy decreases the availability of oxygen to the fetus by both mechanisms.

These mechanisms imply a reversible effect of cigarette smoking for fetal growth because normal function would resume shortly after nicotine or CO is cleared from the system. Support for the suggestion that these effects are reversible is derived from several sources. Davies and coworkers (1979) found that 48 hours of smoking cessation late in pregnancy increased oxygen availability to the fetus. Višnjevac and Mikov (1986) found similarly low levels of carboxyhemoglobin (COHb) in mothers and newborns when the mother was a former smoker or never smoker; mothers who smoked during pregnancy and their newborns had high levels of COHb.

Mechanisms for the effects of smoking on neonatal, perinatal, and infant mortality are poorly understood, although the reduction in birthweight is often considered to be the mediating process. However, smoking appears to cause a shift in the distribution of birthweight without having much effect on mean gestational age (US DHEW 1979; US DHHS 1980), and shifts in birthweight distribution across different populations do not always produce corresponding shifts in mortality (Wilcox 1983; Wilcox and Russell 1983a,b).

That gestational age is little affected by smoking, whereas birthweight is reduced at every gestational age, explains why small infants of smokers have a better prognosis than small infants of nonsmokers (Yerushalmy 1971; MacMahon, Alpert, Salber 1966). Increases in perinatal mortality among smokers may result not from the reduction in birthweight, but rather from the modest increases in preterm delivery, very low birthweight, and specific pathologic conditions such as placenta previa and abruptio placentae. However, this has not been addressed explicitly in any study. Because the smaller smoking-related increases in less frequent, more severe outcomes parallel the pronounced smoking-related reduction in birthweight, birthweight serves as a useful empirical marker of smoking's harmful consequences, even if it is not the direct mediator of those effects.

Nonexperimental Studies

Fertility and Infertility

Consistent evidence indicates that smokers have lower fertility than nonsmokers (Daling et al. 1987; Howe et al. 1985; Baird and Wilcox 1985; Hartz et al. 1987), as noted in the 1989 Report of the Surgeon General (US DHHS 1989). The studies that have assessed indicators of fertility in former smokers are summarized in Table 2.

Pettersson, Fries, and Nillius (1973) studied secondary amenorrhea, one mechanism for reduced fertility, and found an increased prevalence among smokers. However, prevalence among former smokers was even higher than among continuing smokers. Hammond (1961) found that irregular menstrual cycles were more common among smokers than never smokers and that former smokers were at slightly lower risk than never smokers.

Howe and colleagues (1985) analyzed data on more than 4,000 women in a British cohort study, which assessed the safety of oral contraceptives. Compared with never smokers, women who smoked 20 cigarettes or more at entry into the study were twice as likely to be undelivered 5 years after ceasing contraceptive use with the intention of becoming pregnant, whereas former smokers had the same likelihood of being undelivered as never smokers. Baird and Wilcox (1985) reported that the time period until pregnancy was the same for 31 women who quit smoking in the year prior to attempting to conceive as it was for never smokers.

Daling and coworkers (1987) conducted a large case–control study in Washington State and found that, compared with never smokers, the relative risk of primary tubal infertility was 2.7 among current smokers and 1.1 among former smokers. Information

TABLE 2.—Summary of studies of fertility among smokers and former smokers

Reference	Location	Measure of fertility	Relative risk of measure of fertility[a] Smokers	Former smokers
Pettersson, Fries, Nillius (1973)	Sweden	Secondary amenorrhea	1.3	1.6
Howe et al. (1985)	England	Not pregnant 5 yr after ceasing contraceptive use	2.0[b]	1.0
Baird and Wilcox (1985)	Minnesota	Time to pregnancy >1 yr	3.4	1.0
Daling et al. (1987)	Seattle	Primary tubal infertility	2.7	1.0
Daling et al. (1985)	Seattle	Secondary tubal infertility	1.6	1.3

[a]Compared with never smokers.
[b]Smokers of >20 cig/day.

on secondary tubal infertility from the same study (Daling et al. 1985) revealed a smaller difference between current and former smokers. Although the study focused on prior induced abortion, data are presented that allow computation of crude odds ratios for current and former cigarette smokers. Current smokers had a 1.6-fold increase in the risk of secondary tubal infertility, and former smokers had a 1.3-fold increase in risk. It is difficult to assess the causal effect of smoking on tubal infertility independent of the effects of sexually transmitted diseases (STDs) known to co-vary with smoking in many populations.

In summary, the data suggest that impairment of fertility measured as delay in time to conception is related to smoking near the time of attempting to conceive and that smoking cessation prior to conception returns fertility to that of never smokers. Conclusions about smoking and the risk of tubal infertility cannot be drawn because of concern about uncontrolled confounding.

Ectopic Pregnancy and Spontaneous Abortion

Tubal (ectopic) pregnancy occurs at about the same time in the reproductive process as fetal loss. However, the mechanisms are thought to be similar to those operating in tubal infertility and largely concern tubal motility and patency. Several reports indicate an increased risk of ectopic pregnancy in smokers (Campbell and Gray 1987; Matsunaga and Shiota 1980), but only Chow and associates (1988) examined the association with prior smoking in detail. In a case–control study in western Washington State, 155 cases of tubal pregnancy were compared with 456 controls who had given birth. Current smokers had an estimated 2.2-fold increased risk of ectopic pregnancy compared with never smokers. All former smokers had a 1.6-fold increase, but this increase was limited to those who had quit within the preceding 8 years. Longer durations of abstinence yielded an odds ratio of 1.0.

Concerns about the possibility of differences in sexual activity between smokers and nonsmokers and the occurrence of STDs limit the ability to draw firm conclusions about the association of smoking with ectopic pregnancy. There is little information about former smokers, and consequently, no conclusion can be drawn.

Some data suggest an association between smoking and increased risk of spontaneous abortion (US DHHS 1989). Data on smoking cessation are very sparse. Kline (1984) noted that the adverse effect of smoking observed in a case–control study of smoking and spontaneous abortion (Kline et al. 1977) was limited to current, not former, smokers. Alberman and colleagues (1976) found that the proportion of spontaneous abortions with abnormal karyotypes decreased with increased smoking but was identical for never smokers and women who stopped smoking prior to pregnancy (Alberman et al. 1976). The interpretation of this finding is uncertain.

Fetal, Neonatal, and Perinatal Mortality

Information linking cigarette smoking with an increased risk of the various measures of mortality used to assess pregnancy outcome has been reviewed in previous reports of the Surgeon General and other publications (US DHEW 1979; US DHHS 1980; US DHHS 1986). Table 3 provides data on perinatal and neonatal mortality from the earlier reports of the Surgeon General (US DHEW 1979; US DHHS 1980) and adds information from a more recent publication on the topic (Rush and Cassano 1983). The studies are consistent in indicating higher mortality in children born to women who smoke. The high risk of mortality is independent of various factors, such as education and social class, that are also associated with mortality.

Kleinman and colleagues (1988) assessed the effect of smoking on fetal and infant mortality in 362,621 births in Missouri during 1979–1983. Using multivariate statistical techniques, these investigators estimated the effects of smoking on fetal and infant mortality among black and white primiparous and multiparous women. After adjustment for marital status, education, and age, fetal plus infant mortality rates were 25 to 56 percent higher in smokers for all categories of maternal race and parity. The elevations in the estimated risks of fetal plus infant mortality were statistically significant in all categories. In further analyses of data from the Missouri births and deaths, Malloy and coworkers (1988) showed that the relative risk of fetal plus infant mortality among whites was significantly elevated for the infants of women who smoked in all categories of low birthweight, even after adjustment for marital status, education, age, and parity (Table 4). This data set is unique in its size, consisting of more than 350,000 births. The data indicate that even in the normal birthweight infants of smokers—those that weighed 2,500 g or more—mortality was significantly elevated for infants of mothers who smoked.

Information on fetal, neonatal, and perinatal mortality in former smokers is sparse (Table 5). Butler, Goldstein, and Ross (1972) analyzed data from the British Perinatal Mortality Survey and estimated that perinatal mortality was the same for women who

TABLE 3.—Summary of studies of perinatal and neonatal mortality in smokers and nonsmokers during pregnancy

Reference	Number of births	Category	Perinatal mortality[a] Smokers	Perinatal mortality[a] Nonsmokers	Neonatal mortality[a] Smokers	Neonatal mortality[a] Nonsmokers
Yerushalmy (1964)	6,800	Whites Blacks			13.9 22.0	12.4 23.4
Comstock and Lundin (1967)	12,287				23.6[b]	15.6[b]
		Amount smoked				
Meyer and Tonascia (1977)	51,490	<1 ppd ≥1 ppd	28.0 33.4	23.0		
		Social class[c]				
Rantakallio (1978)	12,068	I+II III+IV Farmers Unknown	28.1[d] 25.1 25.5[d] 29.4[d]	22.4[d] 19.6 39.0[d] 36.8[d]		
		Amount smoked				
Rush and Cassano (1983)		<5 cig/day 5–14 cig/day >15 cig/day	15.9 26.1 28.3	18.7		
Butler, Goldstein, Ross 1972)	21,788		41.1	32.0	17.6	13.7
		Amount smoked				
Andrews and McGarry (1972)	18,631	1–4 cig/day 5–9 cig/day 10–19 cig/day ≥20 cig/day	25 20 32 36	24		
		Race and Amount smoked				
Niswander and Gordon (1972)	37,912	White 1–10 cig/day ≥11 cig/day Black 1–10 cig/day ≥11 cig/day	 31.5 38.2 41.5 57.4	31.4 38.5		

TABLE 3.—Continued

Reference	Number of births	Category	Perinatal mortality[a] Smokers	Nonsmokers	Neonatal mortality[a] Smokers	Nonsmokers
		Race				
Rush and Kass (1972)	3,266	White Black	31.4 54.1	29.2 28.6		
		Maternal age				
Fabia (1973)	6,879	<25 yr 25–34 yr ≥35 yr	16.1 13.2 41.7	12.1 12.6 23.0		

NOTE: ppd= packs/day.
[a]Per 1,000; definition of mortality as in paper cited.
[b]Adjusted for sex of infant and father's education.
[c]Defined in paper cited.
[d]Rate based on five deaths or fewer.

TABLE 4.—Estimated relative risk of fetal plus infant mortality for maternal smoking in several birthweight groups, adjusting for maternal marital status, education, age, and parity

Birthweight group (g)	Estimated relative risk	95% CI
500–999	1.71	1.46–2.00
1,000–1,499	1.78	1.58–2.01
1,500–1,999	2.00	1.84–2.18
2,000–2,499	2.44	2.33–2.55
≥2,500	1.24	1.10–1.39

NOTE: Figures are for whites only. CI=confidence interval.
SOURCE: Malloy et al. (1988).

smoked prior to conception and who stopped before the fourth month of pregnancy as it was for never smokers. However, perinatal mortality was higher for continuing smokers than for never smokers for all categories of amount smoked. Andrews and McGarry (1972) examined mortality in the Cardiff birth survey of more than 18,631 births. Perinatal mortality was 29 per 1,000 in those who quit smoking before pregnancy or in the early months of pregnancy; 29 per 1,000 in continuing smokers; and 24 per 1,000 in "nonsmokers." Rush and Cassano (1983) analyzed data from the 1970 British birth cohort, consisting of all births in Great Britain during a single week in 1970.

Perinatal mortality among those who smoked before pregnancy but quit during pregnancy (15.0/1,000) was lower than for either nonsmokers during pregnancy (18.7/1,000) or smokers of 5 cigarettes or more per day throughout pregnancy (26.9/1,000).

TABLE 5. —Summary of studies of perinatal mortality in smokers throughout pregnancy, smokers who quit in the early months of pregnancy, and nonsmokers during pregnancy

Reference	Number of births	Perinatal mortality[a] Nonsmokers	Former smokers		Smoked throughout pregnancy	
Butler, Goldstein, Ross (1972)	21,788	32.2	1–4 cig/day	31.7[b]	1–4 cig/day	38.5
			5–9 cig/day	31.1	5–9 cig/day	42.2
			10–19 cig/day	28.1	10–19 cig/day	41.6
			20–30 cig/day	35.2	20–30 cig/day	41.2
Andrews and McGarry (1972)	18,631	24		29[c]		29
Rush and Cassano (1983)	16,688	18.7		15.0[d]		26.9

[a] Late fetal and neonatal deaths/total births × 1,000.
[b] Women who quit smoking before the fourth month of pregnancy.
[c] Women who quit smoking before pregnancy or during early pregnancy.
[d] Women who quit smoking during early pregnancy.

Fetal, neonatal, and perinatal mortality are rare events. This limits the study of their association with smoking cessation. Lack of data makes it impossible to draw a firm conclusion about the association of smoking cessation with the risk of fetal, neonatal, or perinatal mortality. However, the limited available data are consistent with the conclusion that perinatal and neonatal mortality are lower among infants of women who quit smoking than among those women who smoke throughout pregnancy. The possibility must be considered that differences between women who quit smoking and those who continue to smoke account for the lower rate of perinatal and neonatal mortality in the studies in which this has been observed.

Birthweight and Gestational Duration

Introduction

Fetal, neonatal, and perinatal mortality are the most direct measures of pregnancy outcome. Mortality is relatively uncommon, and very large samples are needed for study. This has led to the widespread study of birthweight and the percentage of births that are low birthweight (<2,500 g) as surrogates for the study of mortality. This strategy has been justified by the extremely strong association between birthweight and the percent of low birthweight and each of the measures of mortality (Figure 1). Equally important is weight at birth as a determinant of infant health (McCormick 1985).

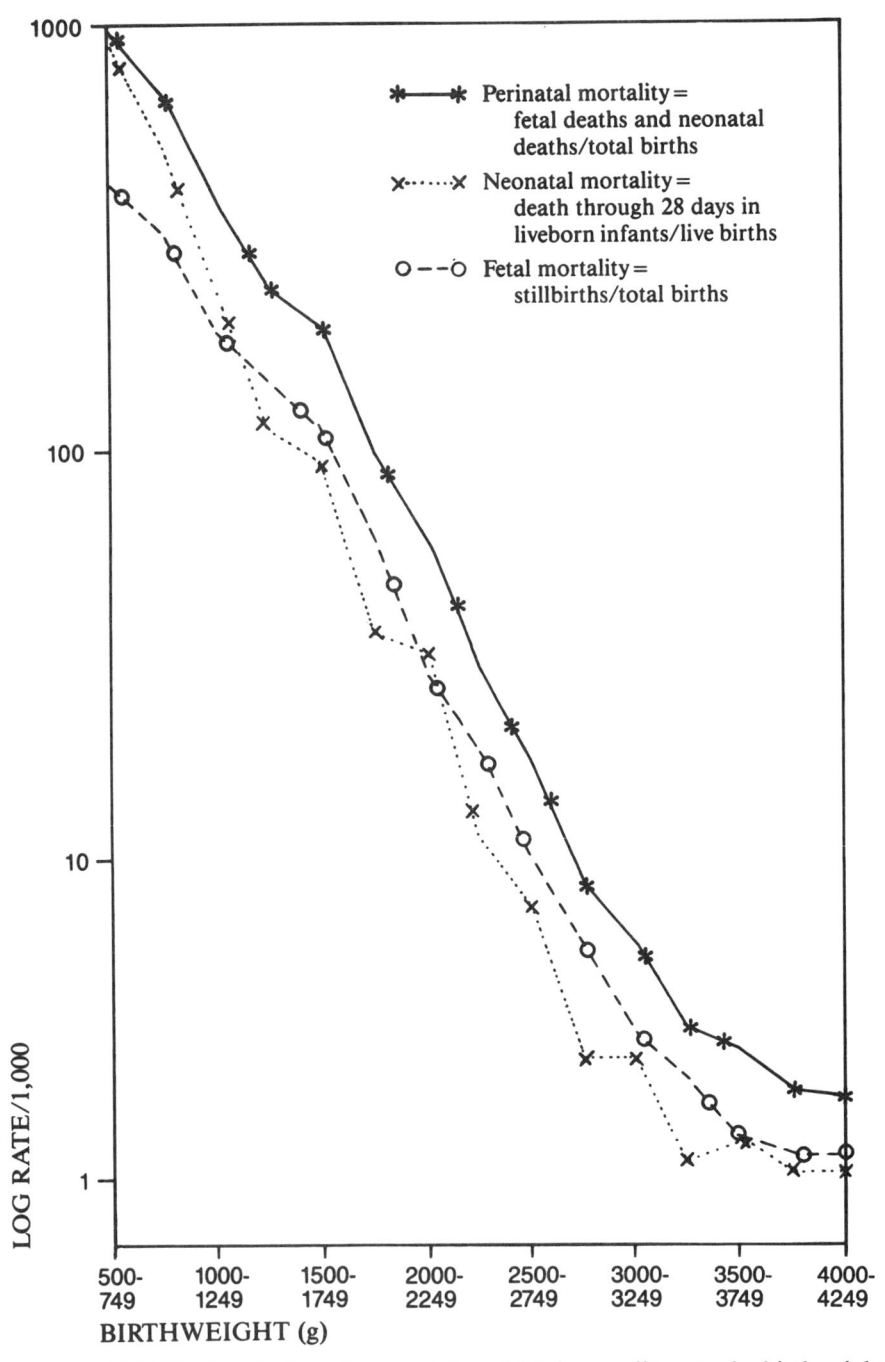

FIGURE 1.—Perinatal, neonatal, and fetal mortality rates by birthweight in singleton white males, 1980

SOURCE: Williams and Chen (1982).

Birthweight is, however, a result of gestational age at birth and the rate of fetal growth. Recognition of the complex relationships among gestational duration, rate of fetal growth, birthweight, and mortality has led to attempts to classify infants according to gestational duration or joint distribution of birthweight and gestational duration. Generally, births are categorized as preterm (<37 weeks gestation) and/or as small for gestational age (SGA) (<10th percentile of weight for a given gestational age). Joint classification is thought to provide a more discriminating basis for the study of etiologic agents.

Preterm delivery is strongly associated with increases in the risk of fetal, neonatal, and perinatal mortality and with significant childhood morbidity. Both preterm delivery and SGA increase the risk of cerebral palsy, although the risk is much greater for preterm delivery (Ellenberg and Nelson 1979). SGA is associated with increased risk of neonatal and perinatal mortality at every gestational age (Koops, Morgan, Battaglia 1982; Lubchenco, Searls, Brazie 1972); with SIDS (Buck et al. 1989); and with neurocognitive deficits, short stature, and small head circumference in childhood (Fitzhardinge and Steven 1972; Hill et al. 1984; Westwood et al. 1983; Ounsted and Taylor 1971; Harvey et al. 1982; Ounsted, Moar, Scott 1984, 1988; Fancourt et al. 1976).

Continued Smoking

As reviewed in previous Surgeon General's reports (US DHEW 1979; US DHHS 1980) and in other literature (Landesman-Dwyer and Emanuel 1979; Longo 1982; Werler, Pober, Holmes 1985; Kramer 1987), smoking during pregnancy decreases mean birthweight and increases the proportion of low birthweight births. Estimates vary among studies, but birthweight is reduced by an average of approximately 200 g, and the proportion of low birthweight is approximately doubled by cigarette smoking (Meyer, Jonas, Tonascia 1976; US DHHS 1980; US DHEW 1979; McIntosh 1984; Committee to Study the Prevention of Low Birthweight 1985; Kramer 1987). Mean birthweight decreases and the percent low birthweight increases with increasing number of cigarettes smoked daily. The relationship between cigarette smoking and decreased birthweight is considered to be causal (US DHEW 1979; US DHHS 1980, 1989).

Smoking affects birthweight and the percentage of babies who are born of low birthweight by retarding fetal growth. A measure of fetal growth retardation is the probability of delivering an infant who is in the less than 10th percentile for gestational age. The relative risk of SGA is about 3.5- to 4.0-fold higher among the infants of smokers than for the infants of nonsmokers (Ounsted, Moar, Scott 1985). Preterm birth is also associated with maternal smoking, although not as strongly. Estimates of the relative risk of delivering before 37 weeks of gestation are typically about 1.5 for smoking during pregnancy (Committee to Study the Prevention of Low Birthweight 1985; Kramer 1987; Shiono, Klebanoff, Rhoads 1986). Mean gestational duration among smokers is not significantly shorter than it is among nonsmokers (US DHEW 1979; US DHHS 1980). This finding is consistent with the observation that the risk of delivering early is greater among smokers than nonsmokers, but the percentage of preterm deliveries is so small that the mean would not be affected unless the shift were very large (US DHEW 1979; US DHHS 1980).

Cessation Before Conception

Most studies of cigarette smoking and birthweight have failed to separate never smokers from women who quit smoking prior to conception. MacMahon, Alpert, and Salber (1966) first examined the association of pre-pregnancy smoking with birthweight and found no significant difference in the mean birthweight of infants whose mothers smoked before but not during pregnancy compared with never smokers. Subsequent research has confirmed the absence of an association between smoking prior to conception and reduced birthweight (Table 6). In all of these studies, smokers who quit before conception had mean birthweight values that were equivalent or higher than those of never smokers. Other studies in which information on mean birthweight could not be derived (Kline, Stein, Hutzler 1987; Anderson et al. 1984; Wainright 1983), with the exception of Zabriskie (1963), have also consistently shown no association between birthweight and smoking that ceased prior to conception. Zabriskie (1963) failed, however, to adjust for smoking during pregnancy, and these results are not directly pertinent in a comparison of birthweight in never smokers and smokers who quit before conception.

TABLE 6.—Summary of studies of mean birthweight, by smoking status

	Mean birthweight (g)		
Reference	Never smoked	Smoked before but not during pregnancy	Smoked during pregnancy
Cope, Lancaster, Stevens (1973)	3,376	3,395	3,200
Van den Berg (1977)	3,463	3,457	3,255
Rush and Cassano (1983)	3,357	3,384	NR
Višnjevac and Mikov (1986)	3,327	3,331	3,097

NOTE: NR=not reported.

In interpreting these data, misclassification of exposure needs to be considered. MacArthur and Knox (1988) reported that women who quit smoking during pregnancy, and possibly those who quit before pregnancy, were more often living with a partner who smoked. Passive smoke exposure may adversely affect the fetus (Martin and

Bracken 1986). Furthermore, for whatever reason, some women may misrepresent their smoking status, denying that they have continued smoking, thus leading to an underestimation of the benefit of smoking cessation prior to conception.

More important, women who quit smoking prior to conception differ in other respects from women who continue to smoke. Women who quit may have smoked fewer cigarettes per day prior to quitting. Studies of smoking cessation prior to conception have not accounted fully for other differences between women who quit and those who continue to smoke.

Cessation After Conception

Birthweight

Table 7 summarizes nonexperimental studies in which information on mean birthweight in nonsmokers, smokers throughout pregnancy, and smokers who quit after conception could be derived. The data from each of these studies are consistent in two important ways. First, women who smoked throughout pregnancy delivered infants who weighed less than the infants of nonsmokers. Second, women who quit smoking delivered infants who weighed more than the infants of smokers throughout pregnancy. In most of these studies, mean birthweight values among infants whose mothers stopped smoking were the same or higher than those of infants of nonsmokers.

Table 8 summarizes nonexperimental studies estimating the relative risk of low birthweight for continuing smokers and quitters some time during pregnancy compared with nonsmokers during pregnancy. These studies are consistent with those examining mean birthweight. Compared with nonsmokers, the risk of low birthweight is elevated among smokers throughout pregnancy, and the risk is about 1.0 for women who quit. In addition, Kleinman and Madans (1985) reported no association between the risk of low birthweight for women who quit smoking during pregnancy compared with those who had not smoked in the 12 months prior to conception among participants in the 1980 National Natality Survey (NNS).

An important aspect of smoking cessation and pregnancy outcome is the timing of cessation during pregnancy and its relation to birthweight. How early in pregnancy cessation must occur to avoid the adverse effects of smoking on birthweight is a key issue with important implications for counseling pregnant smokers.

In most of the studies examining this question, only information on cessation in the early months of pregnancy is presented. However, Rush and Cassano (1983) found that mean birthweight among women who quit as late as the seventh to eighth month of pregnancy was higher than for women who smoked throughout pregnancy, but lower than for nonsmokers and for women who quit earlier in gestation. MacArthur and Knox (1988) concluded that quitting any time before the 30th week of gestation increases birthweight when compared with continuing to smoke. Cooper (1989) assessed patterns of cigarette smoking by trimester of pregnancy. Women who reported smoking during the "first trimester of pregnancy only" had a 30-percent increased risk of having a low birthweight baby, while women who reported smoking during the "first and second trimester of pregnancy only" had a 70-percent higher risk of a low

TABLE 7.—Summary of nonexperimental studies of smoking cessation after conception, mean increase (+) or decrease (−) in birthweight (g) according to timing of cessation

Reference	1	2	3	4	5	6	7	8	9	Unknown	Smoked throughout
Lowe (1959)				+14							−182
Underwood et al. (1967)		−108			−152						−230
Butler, Goldstein, Ross (1972)				+46							−160
Andrews and McGarry (1972)			−80								−170
Papoz et al. (1982)						+10					−70
Rush and Cassano (1983)	+98				+43		+36	−90			−155
Pulkkinen (1985)			−61								−225
Counsilman and MacKay (1985)			−40								−235
Kline, Stein, Hutzler (1987)										+12	−202
MacArthur and Knox (1988)	+22			−58							−242

NOTE: Mean increases or decreases are relative to nonsmokers during pregnancy.

birthweight baby. Women who reported smoking throughout their pregnancy had a 90-percent increased risk of having a low birthweight baby in contrast to nonsmokers.

Most fetal growth occurs late in pregnancy, and the primary smoke constituents considered as candidates in mediating the effect of smoking on fetal growth (i.e., CO and nicotine leading to intrauterine hypoxia) have short-term reversible effects. The data in Tables 6 and 7 support the conclusion that the adverse effect of smoking on birthweight occurs in the latter part of gestation, primarily during the third trimester, and that cessation at any time during gestation is likely to mitigate the adverse effect of smoking on fetal growth.

Because it is difficult to persuade all pregnant smokers to quit smoking entirely, the benefit of reducing the number of cigarettes smoked per day becomes a public health issue. The observation that cigarette smoking retards fetal growth in a dose–response

TABLE 8.—Summary of nonexperimental studies of relative risk of low birthweight for smoking cessation after conception

		Relative risk[a]	
Reference		Ceased smoking after conception	Smoked throughout pregnancy
Frazier et al. (1961)		1.0	1.7
Van den Berg (1977)[b]		1.6	3.0
Petitti and Coleman (in press)			
Whites	<1 mo	0.5	2.7
	1–2 mo	1.0	
	2–3 mo	0.6	
Blacks	<1 mo	1.4	3.8
	1–2 mo	1.0	
	2–3 mo	1.1	
Andrews and McGarry (1972)		1.3	2.0

[a]Compared with nonsmokers during pregnancy.
[b]Whites only.

fashion supports the benefit of reducing the number of cigarettes smoked per day. Hebel, Fox, and Sexton (1988) used data from their randomized trial of smoking cessation to examine this question. These researchers found that the benefit of decreased smoking for birthweight during pregnancy was almost entirely restricted to those who achieved total cessation, perhaps because women who reduce the number of cigarettes smoked compensate by inhaling more deeply, by puffing more frequently, or by smoking the cigarette to a shorter butt length. Findings from another randomized trial support the conclusion that abstinence, not reduction, should be the goal in pregnancy (MacArthur, Newton, Knox 1987). In this latter study, the intervention led to a considerable reduction in the reported mean number of cigarettes smoked per day but almost no difference in the percentage of women who quit entirely; there was no difference in birthweight between the treatment and control groups (MacArthur, Newton, Knox 1987). Because of the social stigma associated with smoking during pregnancy, it is possible that some women in this intervention trial falsely reported a reduction in smoking; if so, this underreporting would lead to an underestimation of possible benefits of reducing cigarette consumption.

Whether quitting only during the first half of pregnancy will prevent a reduction in birthweight is another important consideration. Most fetal growth takes place in the last trimester; early quitting virtually eliminates the effect of smoking on birthweight. Thus, smoking late in pregnancy may have an adverse effect on birthweight even if there is abstinence in the first trimester. Lowe (1959) found that the mean birthweight of infants of smokers who quit early in pregnancy but resumed smoking was between that of smokers throughout pregnancy and that of never smokers. Infants of women who gave up cigarettes by the fifth month of pregnancy and who did not resume smoking had a mean birthweight identical to that of never smokers. MacArthur and Knox (1988) also found that infants born to women who quit smoking early in their pregnancy but started again before delivery had a mean birthweight value between that of smokers throughout pregnancy and those of both early quitters and never smokers. These data indicate that abstinence throughout the third trimester of pregnancy is necessary to realize the full benefit of smoking cessation for birthweight.

Preterm Delivery

The effect of smoking on birthweight is principally due to a reduction in size for a given gestational age rather than to a large decrease in gestational duration (US DHEW 1979; US DHHS 1980). Thus, it would be expected that pregnancy outcome in women who quit would reflect a predominant effect on size for gestational age.

Andrews and McGarry (1972) considered preterm delivery as a distinct endpoint in continuing smokers and quitters; the latter group included a mixture of women who quit prior to conception and women who quit during their pregnancy. The rate of preterm delivery among nonsmokers was 6.7 per 100 compared with 7.5 per 100 for ex-smokers and 9.2 per 100 for women who continued to smoke throughout pregnancy (Andrews and McGarry 1972).

Berkowitz, Holford, and Berkowitz (1982) examined the association between smoking during each trimester of pregnancy and the risk of preterm delivery in a case–control study of 175 mothers of singleton, preterm infants and 313 mothers of singleton, term infants. The risk of preterm delivery was increased among women who smoked in the third trimester of pregnancy, especially if they smoked heavily (>10 cigarettes per day).

Using data from a longitudinal study of pregnant women, Van den Berg and Oechsli (1984) reported rates of preterm delivery (≤ 37 weeks) among never smokers, smokers who stopped at the beginning of pregnancy, and continuing smokers for 10,947 white women whose singleton pregnancies progressed beyond 22 weeks. The rate of preterm delivery was 5.4 percent in never smokers, 6.8 percent in quitters, and 7.6 percent in continuing smokers. The difference in the rate of preterm delivery between never smokers and quitters was not statistically significant ($p>0.05$); however, the difference between never smokers and continuing smokers was significant.

In a population-based case–control study of white and black women delivering singleton infants without congenital anomalies in a large urban county, Petitti and Coleman (in press) reported that the estimated relative risk of very low birthweight (<1,500 g) or of other preterm births among black and white women who quit smoking prior to the fourth month of gestation was not increased in comparison with those of nonsmokers. The estimated relative risk of very low birthweight (<1,500 g) in continuing smokers was 2.5 for whites and 3.1 for blacks and that of other preterm births was 2.0 for whites and 3.7 for blacks.

MacArthur and Knox (1988) examined gestational duration according to smoking during pregnancy. Mean gestational length was 1.7 days shorter among continuing smokers than nonsmokers. Compared with nonsmokers, gestational periods were 0.4 days shorter for women who quit smoking by the 6th week of pregnancy, 1.5 days longer for women who quit between the 6th and 16th weeks of pregnancy, and 0.3 days longer for women who quit after the 16th week of pregnancy.

Because of the limited data on the risk of preterm delivery among women who quit smoking after conception, a firm conclusion about benefit, or lack of benefit, attributable to smoking cessation for this pregnancy outcome cannot be drawn.

Complications of Pregnancy

Women who smoke during pregnancy are at increased risk of bleeding during pregnancy and of placenta previa and abruptio placentae (US DHEW 1979; US DHHS 1980; Naeye 1978; Naeye 1980). These women are probably at decreased risk of preeclampsia (US DHEW 1979; US DHHS 1980; Marcoux, Brisson, Fabia 1989). Few data on these pregnancy complications among former smokers are available.

In Naeye's (1980) analysis of data from the Collaborative Perinatal Project, smoking for more than 6 years (but not short-term smoking) was found to be associated with a relative risk of 1.6 to 1.9 for abruptio placentae and a relative risk of 2.4 to 2.8 for placenta previa. Women who had stopped smoking by their first prenatal visit were not at increased risk of abruptio placentae, but were still at twofold increased risk of placenta previa if they were long-term smokers. However, the latter result was based on only 18 exposed cases.

Marcoux, Brisson, and Fabia (1989) found that, compared with women who had never smoked, those who smoked at the time of conception were protected from preeclampsia (estimated relative risk (RR)=0.51), whereas women who smoked but quit prior to conception had the same risk of preeclampsia as never smokers (RR=0.97). Women who smoked at conception but quit prior to 20 weeks' gestation were not as protected from development of preeclampsia as were continuing smokers. Because of the otherwise serious adverse effects of smoking on the fetus, this minor "benefit" of smoking during pregnancy probably has no public health consequence.

Randomized Trials of Smoking Cessation During Pregnancy

Three randomized trials have been conducted on pregnancy outcome in relation to advice to stop smoking (Donovan 1977; Sexton and Hebel 1984; MacArthur, Newton, Knox 1987). Table 9 summarizes the studies and birthweight results. Two other randomized trials have also been conducted on the effect of various programs on smoking cessation rates among pregnant women (Ershoff, Mullen, Quinn 1989; Windsor et al. 1985), and other trials are in progress. Information on pregnancy outcome is not available, and these studies are not reviewed.

Donovan (1977) studied smokers in three maternity units in England. Women aged 35 years or younger at the start of pregnancy, who smoked more than 5 cigarettes per day, who had less than 30 weeks of gestation at the first prenatal visit, and who had no prior perinatal deaths, were randomly assigned to a control group that received usual prenatal care or to a test group that was given intense individual antismoking advice by a physician at each prenatal care unit. There were 263 women in the test group and 289 in the control group. Mean daily cigarette consumption decreased from 17.1 cigarettes per day early in pregnancy to 9.2 cigarettes per day late in pregnancy in the intervention

TABLE 9.—Summary of birthweight outcome in randomized trials of smoking cessation in pregnancy

Reference	Number of subjects I	Number of subjects C	Smoking at end of pregnancy I	Smoking at end of pregnancy C	Birthweight (g) I	Birthweight (g) C	Difference (g)[a]
Donovan (1977)	263	289	9.2 cig/day	16.4 cig/day	3,172	3,184	−12
Sexton and Hebel (1984)	463	472	57.0%	80.0%	3,278	3,186	+92
MacArthur, Newton, Knox (1987)	493	489	91%	94%	3,164	3,130	+34

NOTE: I=intervention group; C=control group.
[a] Mean in intervention minus mean in control.

group, but increased slightly from 14.7 to 16.4 in the control group. Mean birthweight was 3,172 g in the test group and 3,184 g in the control group. In the test group 10 percent of the infants had low birthweight (<2,500 g) compared with 9 percent in the control group. There were four perinatal deaths in the test group and one in the control group. None of the differences in birth outcome between the test and control groups were statistically significant.

Although this trial might be regarded as evidence against a benefit of smoking cessation during pregnancy, a number of limitations of the study must be considered. First, no data are presented concerning the percentage of pregnant smokers who quit smoking entirely. Reducing cigarette consumption almost certainly has a smaller benefit for pregnancy outcome than complete cessation. Second, the time at which smoking behavior changed during pregnancy is unclear; data on cigarette consumption for three periods during pregnancy were obtained postnatally, and may have been affected by recall bias. Data from observational studies discussed in the previous section strongly suggest that smoking during the last trimester of pregnancy is a critical mediator of reduction in fetal growth among smokers.

Information from another British randomized trial (MacArthur, Newton, Knox 1987) also questions the benefit of smoking cessation during pregnancy. In this study, women who smoked at the time they were scheduled for a prenatal visit at a large hospital were assigned randomly to a control group that received routine care or to an intervention group that received supplementary health education about smoking during pregnancy. The planned intervention consisted of advice to stop smoking and information about the effects of smoking on the fetus, presented visually by a booklet or verbally by the obstetrician. There were 489 women in the control group and 493 in the intervention group. Mean birthweight for infants in the control group was 3,130 g compared with 3,164 g for the intervention group. The percentages of low birthweight and perinatal mortality in the two groups were not reported. The difference in mean birthweight was not statistically significant as determined by the conventional 0.05 probability value and a two-sided test.

In this trial, only 9 percent of the women in the intervention group quit smoking entirely, compared with 6 percent of the women in the control group. The failure of the intervention to cause smoking cessation makes this trial essentially uninformative concerning the benefit, or lack of benefit, of smoking cessation during pregnancy. In the intervention group, 28 percent of the women reduced the number of cigarettes smoked per day, compared with 19 percent of the women in the control group. The greater reduction in cigarette consumption in the intervention group, in the absence of a difference in mean birthweight between the intervention and control groups, suggests that reducing smoking does not entirely prevent the adverse effects of smoking on birthweight.

The third randomized trial (Sexton and Hebel 1984) recruited women in a large metropolitan area from various sources. Smokers of at least 10 cigarettes per day at the beginning of pregnancy, who had not passed the 18th week of gestation, were randomly assigned to a control group that received routine advice or to a treatment group that received intensive, ongoing advice throughout pregnancy from specially trained professional staff. There were 472 women in the control group and 463 women in the treatment group. The mean birthweight of infants born to women in the control group was 3,186 g compared with 3,278 g for infants of women in the treatment group. The percentage of low birthweight infants was 8.9 in the control group and 6.8 in the treatment group. There were 11 stillbirths in the control group and 9 in the treatment group. The difference in mean birthweight was statistically significant ($p<0.05$, two-tailed test); the differences in the percentages of low birthweight and in fetal mortality were not statistically significant.

In this trial, 43 percent of the women in the treatment group had ceased smoking entirely by the eighth month of pregnancy, compared with 20 percent of the women in the control group. The intervention was, therefore, highly successful in causing substantial changes in smoking that exceeded changes in the comparison group. The investigators ruled out concomitant changes in consumption of alcohol and coffee as explanations for the increase in birthweight. Weight gain was 1.0 kg greater among the treatment group than the control group, but at least part of the difference in weight gain was a result of the higher birthweight of the infant (Sexton and Hebel 1984).

Review of these three randomized trials leads to two conclusions. First, to prevent entirely the adverse consequences of smoking on birthweight, it is necessary for women to cease smoking completely. Second, intensive interventions spanning the entire period of gestation may be necessary to effect large changes among the percentage of women who abstain from smoking entirely.

Prevalence of Smoking and Smoking Cessation During Pregnancy and Time Trends in Prevalence and Cessation

Introduction

Ideally, conclusions about the prevalence of smoking during pregnancy and trends in prevalence would be based on representative samples of pregnant women performed at regular intervals using the same methodology. Assessment of smoking cessation during pregnancy and time trends in smoking cessation should be based on representative samples of women who start pregnancy as smokers and who are monitored for smoking behavior throughout gestation. Available data fall short of these ideals.

Furthermore, available information on smoking and smoking cessation in pregnancy is based almost exclusively on self-reported behavior. Few data on the quality of self-reported smoking specifically in relation to pregnancy have been collected, and it is possible that the societal pressures against smoking during pregnancy would make underreporting more problematic than for other populations (Chapter 2). Similarly, pregnant smokers who admit to smoking might underreport their daily cigarette consumption, perhaps to a greater extent than nonpregnant smokers. The effect of underreporting of smoking and overreporting of cessation would make the data from former smokers more similar to that of continuing smokers with respect to their reproductive health outcomes. Also, smokers who reduce the amount of nicotine in their cigarettes by changing brands or those who reduce the number of cigarettes they smoke per day without quitting may compensate to maintain the same nicotine dose (US DHHS 1988).

Prevalence of Smoking and Smoking Cessation

Pertinent data on smoking during pregnancy from the 1985 National Health Interview Survey (NHIS) (NCHS 1988) are presented in Table 10. The 1985 survey focused on health promotion and disease prevention. The survey involved nearly 35,000 households and more than 90,000 persons, and the response rate was 95.7 percent. Information concerning smoking during pregnancy was obtained from all female household members aged 18 to 44 years who had had a live birth in the 5 years prior to the survey. The proportion of women who had smoked at any time during the year preceding pregnancy was 32 percent overall. Of women with less than 12 years of education, 46 percent smoked in the year preceding pregnancy, compared with 13 percent of women with 16 or more years of education. Thirty percent of married women had smoked, compared with 40 percent of formerly married women.

Patterns of smoking cessation or reduction were reported in detail for some demographic subgroups. Overall, 21 percent of women who smoked prior to pregnancy quit upon learning of their pregnancy, and an additional 36 percent reduced the number of cigarettes they smoked. Cessation (but not reduction) was strongly related to education and family income. Among women with less than 12 years of education, 12 years of education, and more than 12 years of education, 15, 20, and 32 percent quit,

TABLE 10.—Smoking and smoking cessation during pregnancy, summary of results of two surveys of national probability samples

Study (yr)	Percentage of pregnant women					
	Smoked before pregnancy	Reduced amount smoked	Quit upon learning of pregnancy				
			All	Educational attainment (yr)		
				<12	12	≥13
National Health Interview Survey[a] (1980–1985)	32	36	21	15	20	32
National Natality Survey[b] (1980)	31	27	18	10	15	22

[a]NCHS (1988).
[b]Prager et al. (1984).

respectively. The proportions for reduction in smoking were 34, 38, and 36 percent, respectively. Younger mothers were slightly more likely to quit than older mothers, and white mothers quit slightly more often than black mothers (21 vs. 18 percent). More married mothers (23 percent) than never married (19 percent) or formerly married (14 percent) mothers quit, although the proportions reducing their smoking levels were similar (36, 37, and 35 percent, respectively).

Fingerhut, Kleinman, and Kendrick (1990) also reported data on smoking in whites before and during pregnancy based on the Linked Telephone Survey, which reinterviewed 1,550 women aged 20 to 44 years who were respondents to the 1985 NHIS. This analysis confirmed the previous findings that smoking prior to pregnancy and quitting during pregnancy were strongly related to age and educational attainment. Information on amount smoked prior to pregnancy was obtained in this survey. Fifty-nine percent of women who smoked less than 1 pack per day prior to pregnancy quit smoking, compared with 25 percent of those who smoked 1 pack or more per day. Of the white women who smoked prior to pregnancy, 39 percent quit during pregnancy (27 percent when they found out they were pregnant and 12 percent later in pregnancy). This estimate of quitting during pregnancy is higher than the previous estimate of quitting from whites in this survey because it includes as quitters both women who quit upon learning that they were pregnant and those who quit later in pregnancy.

Smoking during pregnancy was also assessed in the 1980 NNS (Prager et al. 1984) (Table 10). Questionnaires were distributed to a national probability sample of married women who had had live births in 1980; the response rate was 56 percent. The restriction to married women severely compromises the generalizability of results, especially for subgroups such as blacks and youth because smoking during pregnancy is consistently more common among unmarried mothers (Schramm 1980; Rush and Cassano 1983) and nearly one-half of black infants are born to unmarried mothers (NCHS 1982). The low response rate might have also affected the validity of the study.

Prager and associates (1984) asked women how many cigarettes they smoked per day before and after they found out they were pregnant. Among all married respondents, 31 percent smoked before pregnancy. Whites were more likely to smoke than blacks (32 vs. 25 percent). These investigators reported a strong association of smoking with age, with younger mothers more likely to smoke than older mothers. There were even more pronounced gradients with education. Among women with less than a high school education, 50 percent smoked before pregnancy, and this percentage diminished monotonically to 15 percent among women with 16 or more years of education.

Among the women in the study (Prager et al. 1984) who smoked prior to pregnancy, 18 percent quit after realizing they were pregnant. White women were somewhat more likely to quit than black women (18 vs. 13 percent). Mothers older than 35 years of age were markedly less likely to quit; only 7 percent did. Again, education had a strong association with quitting; 10 percent of mothers with less than 12 years of education quit, and the percentage increased monotonically to 24 percent among mothers with 16 or more years of education. The patterns of cessation by amount of smoking are also of interest. Women who were smoking 1 to 10 cigarettes per day at the time of pregnancy recognition were far more likely to quit than women smoking 11 or more cigarettes per day (31 vs. 12 percent). Among the heavier smokers, 27 percent reduced their consumption to 10 or fewer cigarettes per day even though they did not quit.

Williamson and associates (1989) used data from the Behavioral Risk Factor Surveillance System in 1985 and 1986 to compare smoking patterns among pregnant and nonpregnant women. Data were collected through 19,124 telephone interviews of a population-based sample of women in 26 States, with ascertainment of current pregnancy status, smoking history, and current smoking practices. Women pregnant at the time of interview were less likely to be current smokers than nonpregnant women (21 vs. 30 percent), but had a similar likelihood of ever having smoked (43 vs. 45 percent). The proportion of former smokers was thus greater among pregnant women (22 vs. 15 percent), largely accounting for the difference in current smoking patterns. This study (Williamson et al. 1989) suggests that if 30 percent of women pregnant at the time of the survey smoked prior to pregnancy, then 30 percent of smokers would have had to quit after becoming pregnant to account for the reported smoking rate of 21 percent. Among pregnant women who smoked, the mean number of cigarettes consumed per day was 12, compared with 20 cigarettes per day among nonpregnant women who smoked. These data suggest that smokers who do not quit upon becoming pregnant tend to reduce their cigarette consumption (Williamson et al. 1989).

Patterns of smoking were generally similar across demographic subgroups, with one important exception. Among unmarried women, smoking was slightly more common in pregnant than nonpregnant women (36 vs. 34 percent), implying no change in smoking among unmarried pregnant women. The absence of pregnancy-related reduction in smoking for unmarried women was due exclusively to a markedly higher smoking prevalence for white unmarried pregnant women. The results suggest that data on married mothers cannot be generalized to unmarried mothers.

A number of investigators reported smoking patterns in selected populations, such as women delivering in a particular hospital or geographic region or those receiving prenatal care at a specific clinic. Table 11 summarizes several of these studies. Although none are true probability samples, these studies provide an indication of the diversity of smoking and smoking cessation among different populations. The proportion quitting during pregnancy ranges from 6 to 49 percent.

Time Trends in Smoking and Smoking Cessation

Kleinman and Kopstein (1987) compared the pattern of smoking cessation during pregnancy from the similarly designed 1967 and 1980 NNS. Although there were some changes in the proportion of mothers who were married at the time of each of the two surveys and the characteristics of nonrespondents might have varied, the surveys provide a unique opportunity to assess temporal trends in smoking and smoking cessation during pregnancy. The percentage of mothers who smoked prior to pregnancy decreased markedly during that period, from 45 to 30 percent for white mothers and 40 to 25 percent for black mothers. The percentage of white mothers who quit after pregnancy rose from 11 to 17 percent between the two surveys, whereas the percentage of black mothers who quit decreased from 17 to 11 percent over that interval. During the interval between the surveys, the diminution of smoking during pregnancy was more pronounced for highly educated women, increasing the differential exposure to tobacco by educational status (Kleinman and Kopstein 1987).

Estimates of Attributable Risk Percent

Although several measures of attributable risk are commonly used to describe the burden of disease associated with an exposure, the most recent report of the Surgeon General (US DHHS 1989) has focused on attributable risk percent, frequently termed etiologic fraction, as the most relevant measure of the likely public health impact of smoking cessation. Calculation of the attributable risk percent uses the formula as follows:

$$ARpercent = \frac{(RR-1)p}{[(RR-1)p]+1}$$

where p is the proportion of persons with the exposure and RR is an estimate of the relative risk of the outcome in those who are exposed compared with those unexposed.

At least three different studies (Meyer, Jonas, Tonascia 1976; McIntosh 1984; Kramer 1987) estimated the relative risk of several pregnancy outcomes after reviewing the research literature. Table 12 summarizes these studies and provides estimates of attributable risk for prevalences of smoking of 20, 30, 40, and 50 percent based on the relative risk estimates from the three studies. As noted earlier, demographic subgroups of women differ markedly in smoking prevalence. Of those women with less than a high school education, 50 percent smoked during pregnancy; of those women with some college education, 20 percent smoked during pregnancy (NCHS 1988). Approximately 30 percent of married women and 40 percent of unmarried women smoked prior to

TABLE 11.—Patterns of smoking cessation during pregnancy among selected populations

Reference	Location	Source	Years	% Smoking initially	% Smokers quitting[a]	% Smokers reducing[a]
Lowe (1959)	Birmingham, UK	Maternity hospitals	1958	43	20	NR
Schwartz et al. (1972)	Paris	Hospitals	1963–69	17	31	10
Butler, Goldstein, Ross (1972)	United Kingdom	National survey	1958	38	18	NR
Hook (1976)	New York State	Not stated	NR	50	NR	24
Papoz et al. (1982)	Paris	Maternity hospital	1976–79	37	49	NR
Ershoff et al. (1983)	Southern California	HMO	1980	22	38	NR
Pulkkinen (1985)	Finland	Prenatal care clinic	1980	NR	28	NR
Windsor et al. (1985)	Birmingham, AL	Maternity hospital	1981–82	29	22	NR
MacArthur, Newton, Knox (1987)	West Midlands, UK	Maternity hospital	1981–82	29	6	19
MacArthur and Knox (1988)	West Midlands, UK	Maternity hospital	NR	32	17	NR

NOTE: NR=not reported; HMO=health maintenance organization.
[a] Quitting or reducing by the end of the fourth month (16 wk).

TABLE 12.—Summary of studies that estimated relative risk of various pregnancy outcomes for smoking based on a "synthesis" of the literature, and attributable risk percent based on several estimates of the prevalence of smoking during pregnancy

		Perinatal mortality		Low birthweight		Preterm delivery	
Reference	p[a]	RR	AR%	RR	AR%	RR	AR%
Meyer, Jonas, Tonascia (1976)	0.20	1.21[b]	4	1.99[b]	17	1.32[b]	6
	0.30		6		23		9
	0.40		8		28		11
	0.50		10		33		14
McIntosh (1984)	0.20	1.25	5	1.81	14	1.45	8
	0.30		7		19		12
	0.40		9		24		15
	0.50		11		29		18
Kramer (1987)	0.20	NR	—	2.42	22	1.41	8
	0.30		—		30		11
	0.40		—		36		14
	0.50		—		42		17

NOTE: RR=relative risk; AR=attributable risk; NR=not reported.
[a]Prevalence of smoking.
[b]Averaging across studies.

pregnancy (NCHS 1988). The most recent estimates suggest that about 25 percent of U.S. women smoke throughout pregnancy (NCHS 1988).

The relative risk estimates for perinatal mortality and preterm delivery are remarkably consistent, especially considering that these authors conducted independent syntheses of the literature. Estimates of the relative risk of low birthweight ranged from 1.81 (McIntosh 1984) to 2.42 (Kramer 1987), probably because of differences in the number of studies used to derive the estimate. For this reason, attributable risk percent for a given prevalence of smoking is more variable for low birthweight than for perinatal mortality and preterm delivery.

Based on data that indicate that about 25 percent of U.S. women smoke throughout pregnancy, it can be estimated that 5 to 6 percent of perinatal deaths, 17 to 26 percent of low birthweight births, and 7 to 10 percent of preterm deliveries could be prevented by elimination of smoking during pregnancy. In groups with a 50-percent prevalence of smoking, such as women with less than a high school education, approximately 10 to 11 percent of perinatal deaths, 29 to 42 percent of low birthweight births, and 14 to 18 percent of preterm deliveries might be prevented by elimination of smoking during pregnancy. These contributions to adverse pregnancy outcome are sizable, and smoking is probably the most important modifiable cause of poor pregnancy outcome among women in the United States (Kramer 1987).

Age at Natural Menopause

Introduction

The significance of menopause extends beyond marking the end of female reproductive potential. The age at which menopause occurs also may have implications for the risks of osteoporotic fractures, ischemic heart disease, and cancers of the reproductive system. Thus, the effect of smoking on the age of menopause could have potentially broad health implications.

In fact, an early natural menopause has been observed consistently among women who smoke cigarettes. As summarized in Table 13, the major studies addressing this topic have indicated that currently smoking women cease menstruating from 1 to 2 years earlier than otherwise similar nonsmokers. Expressed as relative risk, women aged 44 to 54 years who smoke become menopausal at about twice the rate of never smokers (Willett et al. 1983; Bailey, Robinson, Vessey 1977; Hartz et al. 1987; Andersen, Transbol, Christiansen 1982; Baron 1990).

Several features of the data suggest that this is a causal relationship. By using both cohort and cross-sectional methodology with a variety of subject populations, the results have been replicated repeatedly in studies in several areas of the United States and Europe. Dose–response effects have generally been found, with heavy smokers experiencing an even earlier menopause on average than light smokers. However, these trends have not always been assessed with formal tests of statistical significance in the reports describing the data. Several studies demonstrating this association have controlled for potential covariates. That premenopausal smokers may be more likely than nonsmokers to have a hysterectomy does not appear to explain the relationship (Krailo and Pike 1983).

Pathophysiologic Framework

There are at least three ways in which cigarette smoking could lead to an early natural menopause. Experiments with laboratory rodents indicate that the polycyclic aromatic hydrocarbons found in cigarette smoke may be directly toxic to ovarian follicles (Mattison 1980). Mattison and colleagues found that intraperitoneal injection of benzo(a)pyrene, 3-methylcholanthrene, or 7,12-dimethylbenz(a)anthracene led to ovarian follicular atresia (Mattison and Thorgeirsson 1978, 1979; Gulyas and Mattison 1979). Earlier uncontrolled studies of prolonged exposure of mice to cigarette smoke led to similar findings (Essenberg, Fagan, Malerstein 1951), which were also seen in a later controlled study of rats (Subbarao 1988). However, other investigators failed to find ovarian atrophy in rodents chronically exposed to cigarette smoke (Haag, Larson, Weatherby 1960; Dontenwill et al. 1973a), and in most studies, parenteral nicotine or tobacco extract has had minimal effect on the ovaries of experimental animals (Essenberg, Fagan, Malerstein 1951; Thienes 1960; Larson, Haag, Silvette 1961; Larson and Silvette 1968).

The other two postulated mechanisms for premature menopause do not involve direct ovarian toxicity. Cigarette smoking may interfere with luteinizing hormone release at

TABLE 13.—Summary of studies reporting relationship of cigarette smoking and age at natural menopause

Reference	Source and number of subjects	Covariates considered	Difference in median menopausal ages[a] (yr)
Jick, Porter, Morrison (1977)	2,143 hospital patients in Boston area	Parity, marital status, coffee/tea/alcohol, hospital service, diagnosis	1.7
	1,391 hospital patients in 7 countries	Same as above	1.3[b]
Daniell (1978)	500 patients	Weight	2.0[c]
Bailey, Robinson, Vessey (1977)	733 health screenees	None	1.3[b]
McNamara et al. (1978)	1,553 general population subjects	None	0.8[c]
Lindquist and Bengtsson (1979)	873 general population subjects	Weight	1.2[b]
Kaufman et al. (1980)	656 hospital patients	Parity, ponderal index, age first smoked, geographic region	1.7[c]
Adena and Gallagher (1982)	10,995 health screenees	Weight, alcohol intake, drug taking	1.0
Willett et al. (1983)	66,663 nurses	Height, weight, diabetes, hypertension, age of menarche, nulliparity	1.4
McKinlay, Bifano, McKinlay (1985)	5,350 general population subjects	None	1.7
Everson et al. (1986)	261 population subjects	Passive smoking	1.1
Hiatt and Fireman (1986)	5,346 HMO health screenees	None	0.95[c]
Stanford et al. (1987)	3,545 breast cancer screenees	None	0.3
Brambilla and McKinlay (1989)	2,565	Education, income	1.5

NOTE: HMO=health maintenance organization.
[a] Median menopausal age among nonsmokers minus median menopausal age among smokers.
[b] Computed by Adena and Gallagher (1982).
[c] Difference in mean menopausal ages.

least in rodents exposed to parenteral nicotine or cigarette smoke (Andersson et al. 1980; Andersson et al. 1984; Andersson et al. 1988; Eneroth et al. 1977a,b; Kanematsu and Sawyer 1973; Blake, Norman, Sawyer 1974; Blake 1974; Blake et al. 1972a,b; McLean, Rubel, Nikitovitch-Winer 1977). This effect appears to be due to a nicotinic effect on neurotransmitter release. A return to a more normal function after the end of exposure to smoke or nicotine has not been documented, but it seems likely that such a nicotinic effect on the brain would not be permanent. Therefore, it is possible that in humans, smoking could cause a reversible interference in the pituitary-ovarian axis, which could lead to a cessation of menses. Several investigators found that smoking has been associated with menstrual irregularity earlier in reproductive life (Wood 1978; Pettersson, Fries, Nillius 1973; Brown, Vessey, Stratton 1988; Hammond 1961).

Smoking has also been associated with disturbances of estradiol metabolism. Michnovicz and colleagues (1986) found that premenopausal smokers tend to metabolize estradiol through pathways producing more catechol-estrogen metabolites than nonsmokers. This change would be expected to result in a relative antiestrogenic influence because of the lack of estrogenic potency of the catechol-estrogens compared with the estrogenic metabolites, such as estriol, which are produced in larger amounts in nonsmokers. There is also evidence that nicotine may inhibit aromatase, an enzyme important in the synthesis of estrogens (Barbieri, McShane, Ryan 1986; Barbieri, Gochberg, Ryan 1986). Again, the recovery of normal enzymatic function after cessation of smoking has not been studied. However, it is postulated that these or similar disturbances could result in enough antagonism of estrogen effect to cause an early cessation of menstrual cycling in women already in the perimenopausal years (Baron, LaVecchia, Levi 1990).

Studies of Former Smokers

Former smokers experience menopause only slightly earlier than never smokers (Table 14). In a study of hospitalized women, Jick, Porter, and Morrison (1977) found that former smokers had a median age at menopause between that of never smokers and that of women currently smoking half a pack of cigarettes per day. Kaufman and coworkers (1980) reported on hospitalized women aged 60 to 69 years. Data from 10 women who stopped smoking before age 35 indicated that the mean age at menopause was 0.2 years earlier than in never smokers, after adjustment for parity and body habitus (Kaufman et al. 1980). In a cross-sectional study of women attending a screening clinic, Adena and Gallagher (1982) found ex-smokers to have a median age of natural menopause 0.3 years earlier than never smokers. Finally, Hiatt and Fireman (1986) found among a group of enrollees in a prepaid health plan attending a screening clinic that ex-smokers reached menopause about 0.5 years earlier than never smokers. Thus, natural menopause appears to occur, at most, 6 months earlier in ex-smokers than in never smokers.

Limited findings on relative risk of early menopause in former smokers are available (Willett et al. 1983; Baron, LaVecchia, Levi 1990). From data presented by Lindquist and Bengtsson (1979) regarding 50-year-old women, it can be calculated that compared with never smokers, former smokers had a relative risk of early menopause of 1.8

TABLE 14.—Summary of studies of age at natural menopause among former smokers

Reference	Number of ex-smokers	Covariates considered	Findings
Jick, Porter, Morrison (1977)	439	None	Ex-smokers had menopause between those of current light smokers and never smokers
Lindquist and Bengtsson (1979)	30	None	Odds ratio of being menopausal for ex-smokers vs. never smokers was 1.8
Kaufman et al. (1980)	10	Parity, region, Quetelet's Index	Mean age at menopause was 0.2 yr earlier among ex-smokers than among never smokers
Adena and Gallagher (1982)	NR	None	Median age of menopause was 0.3 yr earlier among ex-smokers than among never smokers
Willett et al. (1983)	16,034	Age, weight, nulliparity	Odds ratio of being menopausal for current smokers vs. never smokers was 1.10
Hiatt and Fireman (1986)	576	None	Mean age at menopause was 0.5 yr earlier among ex-smokers than among never smokers

NOTE: NR=not reported.

(95-percent confidence interval, (CI), 1.1–4.7). In a prospective study of American nurses, Willett and coworkers (1983) found ex-smokers to have a relative risk of early menopause of 1.1 (95-percent CI, 0.98–1.23) compared with never smokers after adjustment for age, weight, and nulliparity. In this study, those who stopped smoking in the 2 years previously retained a modest increase in risk of early menopause (RR=1.4); after a longer period of abstinence, there was no effect associated with previous smoking (Willett et al. 1983).

All the investigations of smoking and menopause have relied on self-report of menstrual status and smoking history. It is unlikely that misclassification with regard to these features would seriously distort the findings regarding current smoking, but the results for former smoking may be more susceptible to artifact. In particular, some of the study participants who claimed to be former smokers might actually have continued to smoke, or they might have quit for health reasons related to an early natural menopause. Like current smokers, former smokers may be more likely to be passively exposed to passive smoking than never smokers, thus possibly affecting menopausal age. These factors would tend to lead to an exaggeration of the apparent impact of former smoking on menopausal age (Chapter 2). Therefore, the results summarized above may overstate the degree to which former smoking is associated with any disturbance in menopausal age.

It appears that age at menopause in former smokers is closer to that of never smokers than to current smokers, and the data are consistent with a decline in the risk of early menopause with the cessation of smoking. The effect of smoking on menopausal age may be partly or wholly reversible with cessation of smoking during the premenopausal years. However, some pertinent data are lacking. Most of the studies did not consider how long it takes after cessation of smoking for the risk of early natural menopause to decrease. No studies have verified that the women who stopped smoking had a lifetime smoking exposure similar to that of women who continued smoking.

PART II. MALE

Introduction

Cigarette smoking has been considered to be associated with impairment of male sexual functioning, and tobacco abstinence has been recommended for men attempting to maximize sexual performance (Larson, Haag, Silvette 1961; Sterling and Kobayashi 1975; Ochsner 1971a,b). An association between smoking and impaired sexual performance among men has been publicized in the lay press (Reuben 1988). Although some data provide evidence for this association, they are inconclusive.

Pathophysiologic Framework

Three general types of mechanisms have been proposed to explain the harmful effect of cigarette smoking on sexual performance, impotence, and sperm quality. First, smoking may expose the testes to compounds that are directly toxic to the sperm-producing germinal epithelium, to early sperm forms, or to the hormone-producing Leydig cells. The effects on sperm may be a manifestation of a genotoxic effect of cigarette smoke constituents (Obe and Herha 1978; DeMarini 1983).

Second, smoking causes atherosclerotic peripheral vascular disease (Chapter 6); this may translate into a diminished vascular supply to the genitals, as reflected by the penile brachial index (PBI) and other vascular measurements. A diminished vascular supply to the genitals would compromise sexual performance and spermatogenesis and hormone production. Although atherosclerosis is often considered a fixed lesion, several studies have suggested that atherosclerotic plaques may regress with appropriate lifestyle changes (Barndt et al. 1977; Nikkilä 1980; Kramsch et al. 1981; Chapter 6). However, no studies have been conducted on the effect of smoking cessation on regression of atherosclerotic lesions.

Nonatherosclerotic vascular changes may also mediate the effect of smoking on genital function. The vasoconstrictive effects of nicotine in cigarette smoke may impair the complicated vascular processes involved in erection (Benowitz 1988). This may be due in part to disturbances of prostaglandin production in the vascular endothelium or to an enhancement of platelet aggregation noted by several investigators (Nadler, Velasco, Horton 1983; Alster et al. 1986; Taylor et al. 1987; Lassila et al. 1988; Jeremy et al. 1986; FitzGerald, Oates, Nowak 1988; Chapter 6).

Finally, hormonal effects of cigarette smoking could alter sexual responsiveness and spermatogenesis. Alterations in the secretion of luteinizing hormone releasing hormone (Moss, Riskind, Dudley 1979) or catecholamines (Patra, Sanyal, Biswas 1979; Klaiber and Broverman 1988) are two such possibilities, but disturbances in sex hormones, particularly low testosterone or high estradiol, have been suggested more often. In general, men who smoke cigarettes have similar or higher testosterone levels than nonsmokers; thus, it is difficult to associate low testosterone with sexual dysfunction among men who smoke (Briggs 1973; Shaarawy and Mahmoud 1982; Andersen, Semczuk, Tabor 1984; Handelsman et al. 1984; Deslypere and Vermeulen 1984; Vermeulen and Deslypere 1985; Vogt, Heller, Borelli 1986; Barrett-Connor and Khaw 1987; Dai et al. 1988; Lichtenstein et al. 1987; Meikle et al. 1987; Klaiber and Broverman 1988). The adrenal androgens (i.e., androstenedione, dehydroepiandrosterone, and dehydroepiandrosterone sulfate) are elevated in male smokers (Barrett-Connor, Khaw, Yen 1986; Barrett-Connor and Khaw 1987; Dai et al. 1988). Aromatization of these hormones may explain the elevated levels of estradiol among males who currently smoke (Entrican, Mackie, Douglas 1978; Lindholm et al. 1982; Klaiber, Broverman, Dalen 1984; Barrett-Connor and Khaw 1987; Lichtenstein et al. 1987; Dai et al. 1988; Klaiber and Broverman 1988). Elevations in circulating estrogens may interfere with spermatogenesis and sexual behavior (Klaiber and Broverman 1988); such an explanation remains speculative.

Several studies have suggested that the estradiol and testosterone levels of former smokers are comparable with those of never smokers (Deslypere and Vermeulen 1984; Vogt, Heller, Borelli 1986; Barrett-Connor and Khaw 1987; Lichtenstein et al. 1987). This observation implies that smoking cessation is likely to reverse any effect mediated by disturbances of these hormones. Alternatively, former smokers may have had a lower total dose. Androstenedione and dehydroepiandrosterone sulfate levels may be modestly higher in former smokers compared with those of never smokers (Barrett-Connor, Khaw, Yen 1986; Barrett-Connor and Khaw 1987; Lichtenstein et al. 1987). However, the relevance of these findings to sexual capabilities is unlikely to be significant. These hormones appear to have little intrinsic potency, and are important because of their capacity for conversion to more active hormones such as testosterone and estradiol (Baxter and Tyrrell 1987).

Sexual Activity and Performance

Surveys of the relationship between smoking and frequency of sexual episodes (intercourse or masturbation) have generally found smokers to be as sexually active as nonsmokers. In two studies of elderly men, sexual activity in smokers was comparable with that of nonsmokers (Tsitouras, Martin, Harman 1982; Diokno, Brown, Herzog 1990); in a cross-sectional study of younger men, no differences were indicated (Vogt, Heller, Borelli 1986). Adolescent smokers are more sexually active than nonsmokers (Russell 1971; Malcolm and Shephard 1978). In contrast, Cendron and Vallery-Masson (1971), in studying 70 men older than age 45, found that those who reported smoking between ages 25 to 40 also reported being less sexually active at those ages than those who denied smoking. Overall, it appears that the relation between current cigarette smoking and the level of male sexual activity is not very strong. Among younger males, personality differences between smokers and nonsmokers may dominate any adverse physiologic effects (Russell 1971).

If, as the aforementioned studies suggest, current smokers (or ever smokers) are similar in sexual habits to never smokers, then no differences would be expected for former smokers. Vogt, Heller, and Borelli (1986) evaluated 239 healthy male volunteers aged 19 to 40 without genital abnormalities or diseases and taking no medications. The study results indicated that the 36 former smokers among them were comparable with both never smokers and current smokers in sexual activity (Vogt, Heller, Borelli 1986).

Impotence, the inability to maintain an erection sufficient for intercourse, has been more extensively investigated in relation to smoking. Among treated hypertensives aged 40 to 64, cigarette smokers were more likely to report impotence, although the differences were modest and not statistically significant (Bühler et al. 1988). A statistically significant association was reported among men undergoing radiation therapy for prostatic cancer (Goldstein et al. 1984). However, in both studies, potentially important covariates, such as alcohol intake and age, were not considered. Two other studies of men undergoing impotence evaluation indicated a high prevalence of smoking and suggested an association between smoking with impotence (Virag, Bouilly, Frydman 1985; Condra et al. 1986). Unfortunately, neither study included a sexually functional control group, and both studies based their conclusions on questionable comparisons of the smoking rate in their clinic patients with that of the general population. Vogt, Heller, and Borelli (1986) studied a group of young volunteers without selecting for impotence. These investigators found that smokers reported more difficulties with decreased libido and erection than nonsmokers (Vogt, Heller, Borelli 1986). This analysis did not consider former smokers separately.

An acute effect of smoking on sexual performance is suggested by a study of smokers monitored while viewing erotic films (Gilbert, Hagen, D'Agostino 1986). The successive smoking of 2 cigarettes high in nicotine content significantly impaired the rate of penile diameter change compared with that observed after smoking 1 cigarette or eating candy. However, the clinical relevance of these observations is unknown because frank impotence was not studied.

An important clinical measurement in the evaluation of impotence is the PBI, which indicates the systolic blood pressure in the penis divided by systolic blood pressure in the arm. A low value is considered to be evidence of compromise of the penile blood supply, a factor which may interfere with erection. Several studies of men undergoing evaluation of impotence reported an association between smoking and low PBI (Jacobs et al. 1983; Condra et al. 1986; Bornman and Du Plessis 1986; DePalma et al. 1987).

Among impotent diabetics, evidence of nocturnal erections was found less in smokers compared with nonsmokers, thus suggesting an increased risk of vascular compromise in smokers (Takahashi and Hirata 1988). However, other studies of impotent men have not reported differences between smokers and nonsmokers in vascular measurements (Wabrek et al. 1983; Virag, Bouilly, Frydman 1985; Kaiser et al. 1988). Most of these investigations did not consider covariates such as alcohol use, although one study suggested that smoking in isolation had little effect and that an association of smoking with an abnormal PBI may be due to the association of smoking with other arterial risk factors (Virag, Bouilly, Frydman 1985).

In many of the studies relating smoking and impotence, the investigators did not distinquish nonsmokers as ex-smokers or never smokers. However, two investigations considered former smokers separately (Table 15). Wabrek and associates (1983) studied 120 men who were referred to a hospital-based erectile dysfunction program. The percentage of former smokers was approximately the same among men with impaired, borderline, and normal PBI. Condra and colleagues (1986) reported on 178 patients also referred for impotence. Former smokers were not separated for analysis, but this study suggests that the PBI for ex-smokers is more normal than in current smokers (Condra et al. 1986). However, neither study considered important covariates, such as age and alcohol use (Wabrek et al. 1983; Condra et al. 1986).

Two recent investigations considered the effect of smoking cessation on impotence. Forsberg and colleagues (1979) noted that two smoking men who were impotent improved their functioning after smoking cessation at the same time that measures of penile blood flow improved. However, it is not clear how these two men were selected for this study, and control subjects were lacking. Elist, Jarman, and Edson (1984) reported on the treatment of 60 impotent men. Twenty nonsmokers were treated with the vasodilator isoxsuprine, and 40 smokers were either advised to stop smoking or advised to stop smoking and also given isoxsuprine. There was no mention of randomization, and there was no untreated control group. Similar proportions improved whether given isoxsuprine, convinced to stop smoking, or both (Elist, Jarman, Edson 1984).

Animal data have not elucidated the relation between smoking and either sexual activity or impotence. Soulairac and Soulairac (1972) studied the sexual activity of male rats given either a 0.6 mg/kg or a 1.2 mg/kg dose of nicotine subcutaneously. The sexual activity of the rats after the nicotine administration was compared with that before treatment. Sexual activity was markedly increased with the 0.6 mg/kg dose, and at 1.2 mg/kg there was trembling and twitching and no sexual behavior for 2 to 3 hours. In contrast, exposure to smoke from 1 cigarette has been shown to interfere with the physiology of erection in male dogs (Juenemann et al. 1987).

In summary, the level of sexual activity does not appear to be affected by cigarette smoking. Cigarette smoking may be associated with impaired male sexual performance. Among impotent men, smokers are more likely to have an underlying vascular problem. These associations have been more commonly noted in groups already at high risk of impotence, such as hypertensives and diabetics. However, these associations have not been consistently observed, and the positive findings may be due to the association of smoking with other factors such as alcohol use. Moreover, because the

TABLE 15.—Sexual performance among male former smokers

Reference	Study population	Findings	Comments
Vogt, Heller, Obe (1984)	Volunteers	No differences in sexual activity between former, current, and never smokers	No consideration of covariates
Wabrek et al. (1983)	Impotent patients	Proportion of former smokers similar in men with abnormal, impaired, and normal PBI	No consideration of covariates
Condra et al. (1986)	Impotent patients	Indications that former smokers had more normal PBI than current smokers	No consideration of covariates
Forsberg et al. (1979)	Impotent patients	Two smokers improved sexual performance after smoking cessation	No controls
Elist, Jarman, Edson (1984)	Impotent patients	Smoking cessation improved sexual performance as well as vasodilator	No untreated and controls

NOTE: PBI=penile brachial index.

studies of PBI are generated entirely in referral populations, it is unclear if these findings can be generalized. Because of limited and uncontrolled data, no conclusions can be drawn regarding sexual performance or PBI among former smokers.

Sperm Density and Quality

Measurements of sperm density, morphology, and motility are commonly used assessments of sperm quality (Rogers and Russell 1987). Over 20 studies have dealt with the relation of cigarette smoking to sperm density, motility, and morphology (Viczian 1968a; Schirren and Gey 1969; Campbell and Harrison 1979; Vogel, Broverman, Klaiber 1979; Stekhun 1980; Nebe and Schirren 1980; Evans et al. 1981; Godfrey 1981; Rodriguez-Rigau, Smith, Steinberger 1982; Shaarawy and Mahmoud 1982; Buiatti et al. 1984; Andersen, Semczuk, Tabor 1984; Nordenson, Abramsson, Duchek 1984; Handelsman et al. 1984; Hoidas et al. 1985; Kulikauskas, Blaustein, Ablin 1985; Ablin 1986; Rantala and Koskimies 1987; Vogt, Heller, Borelli 1986; Klaiber et al. 1987; Dikshit, Buch, Mansuri 1987; Saaranen et al. 1987; Klaiber and Broverman 1988; Saaranen et al. 1989; Rui, Oldereid, Purvis 1989; Marshburn, Sloan, Hammond 1989; Oldereid et al. 1989). Table 16 summarizes the findings of those studies that reported mean values for smokers and nonsmokers. In most studies, men smoking cigarettes had lower sperm density, although many of these studies indicated differences that were not statistically significant. The smokers' average sperm density was at least 80 percent that of the nonsmokers. In several studies sperm morphology or motility was impaired in smokers compared with nonsmokers, but this was a less consistent finding. Few studies have considered the spermatic chromosomal characteristics of smokers compared with nonsmokers. Nordenson, Abramsson, and Duchek (1984) found smokers to have more chromosome breaks than nonsmokers, but Oldereid and coworkers (1989) reported no differences in DNA condensation as assessed by flow cytometry.

Although differences in mean values of any of these measurements suggest an effect of smoking, the most relevant parameter may be the percentage of smokers and nonsmokers who exhibit deficiencies in sperm density, morphology, or motility. Several researchers have investigated the relative risk of azoospermia (no sperm in the ejaculate) or oligospermia (reduced number of sperm) in smokers versus nonsmokers or never smokers (Table 17). Although the range of relative risks is wide, there is a clear pattern of increased risk among smokers. However, the clinical significance of oligospermia is uncertain. Most studies have used one ejaculate per man, although the within-man coefficient of variation can be as much as 60 percent (Schenker et al. 1988).

The available information suggests that current smoking is related to low sperm density. However, these data are limited. Many studies investigated men visiting infertility clinics, limiting generalization. Moreover, if male smokers with poor sperm quality are most likely to attend these clinics, selection biases may distort the results. Also, many of these studies were relatively informal. Few of the studies accounted for potentially confounding factors such as alcohol use and age. Less than half of the studies documented that a period of sexual abstinence was required for subjects before giving the sperm sample, and few of the studies analyzed multiple semen specimens as some authorities recommend (Zaneveld and Jeyendran 1988). Most studies have a small number of subjects, and their statistical power is limited for this reason. In some of the studies, it is not clear whether former smokers were included in the smoker or nonsmoker group.

A few studies investigated ex-smokers (Table 18). One was a case–control study of male infertility in Italy (Buiatti et al. 1984). The cases were azoospermic or oligospermic men being treated for infertility at the University of Florence. Controls were University outpatients who had normal sperm counts. There were no significant differences between smoking categories in the percentage of men with low sperm counts. Vogt, Heller, and Borelli (1986) evaluated 239 male volunteers. Among former smokers (those who had smoked for at least 1 year and those who had stopped smoking for at least 1 year), percent normal spermatozoa, percent young forms, percent old forms, and percent degenerate forms were comparable with those of never smokers. Stekhun (1980) reported that 42 percent of former smokers had oligospermia compared with 18 percent of never smokers. Schirren and Gey (1969) reported that three men with low sperm density and motility showed substantial increases in these parameters 3 to 6 months after smoking cessation. However, there were no controls defined in this analysis. Because of the limitations of the four studies, no conclusions are possible regarding the effects of smoking cessation on sperm quality in humans.

Animal studies have not been particularly informative. In some studies, rodents that were heavily exposed to nicotine or cigarette smoke demonstrated testicular atrophy, but this has not been a general finding (Larson, Haag, Silvette 1961; Larson and Silvette 1968; Dontenwill et al. 1973b; Essenberg, Fagan, Malerstein 1951; Thienes 1960;

TABLE 16.—Sperm quality among smokers and nonsmokers

Reference	Study population (number of nonsmokers/number of smokers)	Sperm density	% Normal sperm	% Motile sperm	Comments
Viczian (1968a)	Obstetrics clinic (smokers only) (50/120)	0.82	0.90	0.77	No decrease in sperm density with increasing amounts smoked; controls were fertile men
Vogel, Broverman, Klaiber (1979)	Unstated (39/17)	0.60[a]	NS	0.87[a]	
Nebe and Schirren (1980)	Andrology clinic (455/451)	1.01	—	—	
Evans et al. (1981)	Subfertility clinic (43/43)	—	0.92[a]	—	Smokers and nonsmokers matched on sperm density
Godfrey (1981)	Infertility clinic (74/75)	—	0.94	—	Oligospermic[b] men omitted (<1 × 10^6/mL)
Spira et al. (1981)	Vasectomy candidates (173/122)	0.75[a]	0.94	0.93[a]	
	Infertility clinic (228/292)	0.86	0.91[a]	0.97	
Rodriguez-Rigau, Smith, Steinberger (1982)	Infertility clinic (101/58)	0.95	1.00	1.00	
Shaarawy and Mahmoud (1982)	Volunteers (20/25)	0.93	0.69[a]	0.67[a]	All subjects were fertile
Andersen, Semczuk, Tabor (1984)	Infertility clinic (86/137)	0.99	1.07	1.08	10 azoospermic[c] smokers omitted from analysis
Handelsman et al. (1984)	Semen donors (71/23)	0.67	0.98	0.93[a]	
Kulikauskas, Blaustein, Ablin (1985)	Fertility clinic (135/103)	0.43[a]	1.00	0.78[a]	
Rantala and Koskimies (1987)	Infertility clinic (50/60)	0.90	0.98	0.95	Oligospermic[b] men omitted (<1 × 10^6/mL)
Vogt, Heller, Borelli (1986)	Volunteers (52/150)	0.81[a]	1.01	0.99	

TABLE 16.—Continued

Reference	Study population (number of nonsmokers/number of smokers)	Sperm density	% Normal sperm	% Motile sperm	Comments
Saaranen et al. (1987)	Infertility clinic (110/54)	0.81	1.00	0.97	Azoospermic[c] men omitted
Klaiber et al. (1987)	Paid volunteers (90/60)	0.77[a]	0.98	0.89[a]	
	Males from infertile couples (43/51)	0.52[a]	0.94	0.80[a]	
Dikshit, Buch, Mansuri (1987)	Infertility clinic (288/219)	0.96	0.99	1.01	
Klaiber and Broverman (1988)	Volunteers (21/22)	0.93	1.02	0.97	
Saaranen et al. (1989)	Semen donors and fertile men (32/28)	0.83	0.95	1.01	
Marshburn, Sloan, Hammond (1989)	Infertility clinic (294/152)	0.92	0.99	0.94	
Rui, Oldereid, Purvis (1989)	Infertility clinic (203/147)	1.17	1.05	0.96	Azoospermic[c] men omitted
Effendy and Krause (1987)	Infertility clinic (61/31)	1.13	1.06	1.12	

[a]Statistically significant difference (p<0.05) between smokers and nonsmokers.
[b]Oligospermia is a low sperm count.
[c]Azoospermia is the absence of sperm.

Thompson et al. 1973; Patra, Sanyal, Biswas 1979; Biswas and Patra 1981). Some studies have noted a disturbance of spermatogenesis, a decrease in the interstitium, or a destruction of the seminiferous epithelium (Larson, Haag, Silvette 1961; Larson and Silvette 1968; Essenberg, Fagan, Malerstein 1951; Viczian 1968b; Wyrobeck and Bruce 1975; Biswas and Patra 1981; Alwachi et al. 1986; El-Sayad et al. 1987). The results may depend on the duration and dose of exposure, as well as on the ages at which exposure takes place. Moreover, the relevance to humans of the large doses given to the animals is uncertain. None of these investigations considered spermatogenesis after exposure ended; thus, few conclusions may be drawn regarding the effect of cessation of exposure even within the limitations of the animal studies.

TABLE 17.—Estimated relative risk of azoospermia or oligospermia among smokers versus nonsmokers or never smokers

Reference	Study population (number of nonsmokers/ number of smokers)	Contrast	Estimated relative risk in smokers	Comments
Schirren and Gey (1969)	Andrology clinic (580/1377)	Azoospermia; smokers vs. nonsmokers	1.2	
		Oligospermia; smokers vs. nonsmokers	1.2	Oligospermia not defined
Campbell and Harrison (1979)	Fertility clinic (119/134)	Oligospermia ($<40 \times 10^6$/mL); smokers vs. nonsmokers	1.6[a]	Azoospermic men omitted
Stekhun (1980)	Not stated (33/105)	Oligospermia; current smokers vs. never smokers	3.2[a]	Oligospermia not defined
Rodriguez-Rigau, Smith, Steinberger (1982)	Fertility clinic (101/58)	Oligospermia; ($<20 \times 10^6$/mL); current smokers vs. nonsmokers	0.9	
Buiatti et al. (1984)	Fertility clinic (80/135)	Oligospermia ($<20 \times 10^6$/mL); smokers vs. nonsmokers	1.0	
Andersen, Semczuk, Tabor (1984)	Fertility clinic (86/147)	Azoospermia; current smokers vs. nonsmokers	∞[a]	
Ablin (1986)	Not stated (135/238)	Oligospermia ($<40 \times 10^6$/mL); smokers vs. nonsmokers	2.9[a]	
Vogt, Heller, Borelli (1986)	Volunteers (52/150)	Oligospermia ($<1 \times 10^6$/mL); current smokers vs. never smokers	∞	
		Azoospermia; current smokers vs. never smokers	∞	
Klaiber et al. (1987)	Volunteers with varicocele (11/9)	Oligospermia ($<20 \times 10^6$/mL); current smokers vs. never smokers	∞	
	Volunteers without varicocele (79/61)	Oligospermia ($<20 \times 10^6$mL); current smokers vs. never smokers	1.3	
	Fertility clinic with varicocele (8/21)	Oligospermia ($<20 \times 10^6$/mL); current smokers vs. never smokers	7.7	

TABLE 17.—Continued

Reference	Study population (number of nonsmokers/ number of smokers)	Contrast	Estimated relative risk in smokers	Comments
Klaiber et al. (1987) (continued)	Fertility clinic without varicocele (35/30)	Oligospermia (<20 × 10^6/mL); current smokers vs. never smokers	1.5	
Dikshit, Buch, Mansuri (1987)	Fertility clinic (219/288)	Oligospermia (<20 × 10^6/mL); current smokers vs. never smokers	1.2	
		Azoospermia; current smokers vs. never smokers	1.1	

NOTE: Azoospermia is the absence of sperm; oligospermia is a low sperm count.
[a]Estimated relative risk statistically significantly ($p<0.05$) different from 1.0.

TABLE 18.—Sperm quality among former smokers

Reference	Study population	Findings	Comments
Schirren and Gey (1969)	Andrology patients	Smoking cessation improved sperm density and motility in 3 smokers	No control
Stekhun (1980)	Not stated	Former smokers had RR of 2.3 for oligospermia	Oligospermia not defined
Buiatti et al. (1984)	Male partners of infertile couples	No difference between current, former, and never smokers in prevalence of azoo-/oligospermia	
Vogt, Heller, Borelli (1986)	Healthy volunteers	No difference between current, former, and never smokers in sperm morphology	No consideration of covariates

NOTE: RR=relative risk.

CONCLUSIONS

1. Women who stop smoking before becoming pregnant have infants of the same birthweight as those born to never smokers.
2. Pregnant smokers who stop smoking at any time up to the 30th week of gestation have infants with higher birthweight than do women who smoke throughout pregnancy. Quitting in the first 3 to 4 months of pregnancy and abstaining throughout the remainder of pregnancy protect the fetus from the adverse effects of smoking on birthweight.
3. Evidence from two intervention trials suggests that reducing daily cigarette consumption without quitting has little or no benefit for birthweight.
4. Recent estimates of the prevalence of smoking during pregnancy, combined with an estimate of the relative risk of low birthweight outcome in smokers, suggest that 17 to 26 percent of low birthweight births could be prevented by eliminating smoking during pregnancy; in groups with a high prevalence of smoking (e.g., women with less than a high school education), 29 to 42 percent of low birthweight births might be prevented by elimination of cigarette smoking during pregnancy.
5. Approximately 30 percent of women who are cigarette smokers quit after recognition of pregnancy, with greater proportions quitting among married women and especially among women with higher levels of educational attainment.
6. Smoking causes women to have natural menopause 1 to 2 years early. Former smokers have an age at natural menopause similar to that of never smokers.

References

ABLIN, R.J. Cigarette smoking and quality of sperm. (Letter.) *New York State Journal of Medicine* 86(2):108, February 1986.

ADENA, M.A., GALLAGHER, H.G. Cigarette smoking and the age at menopause. *Annals of Human Biology* 9(2):121-130, 1982.

ALBERMAN, E., CREASY, M., ELLIOTT, M., SPICER, C. Maternal factors associated with fetal chromosomal anomalies in spontaneous abortions. *British Journal of Obstetrics and Gynaecology* 83(3):621-627, August 1976.

ALSTER, P., BRANDT, R., KOUL, B.L., NOWAK, J., SONNENFELD, T. Effect of nicotine on prostacyclin formation in human endocardium *in vitro*. *General Pharmacology* 17(4):441-444, 1986.

ALWACHI, S.N., AL-KOBAISI, M.F., MAHMOUD, F.A., ZAHID, Z.R. Possible effect of nicotine on the spermatogenesis and testicular activity of the mature male albino mice. *Journal of Biological Science Research* 17(3):185-194, 1986.

ANDERSEN, A.N., SEMCZUK, M., TABOR, A. Prolactin and pituitary-gonadal function in cigarette smoking infertile patients. *Andrologia* 16(5):391-396, 1984.

ANDERSEN, F.S., TRANSBOL, I., CHRISTIANSEN, C. Is cigarette smoking a promoter of the menopause? *Acta Medica Scandinavica* 212:137-139, 1982.

ANDERSON, G.D., BLIDNER, I.N., MCCLEMONT, S., SINCLAIR, J.C. Determinants of size at birth in a Canadian population. *American Journal of Obstetrics and Gynecology* 150(3):236-244, October 1, 1984.

ANDERSSON, K., ENEROTH, P., FUXE, K., HÄRFSTRAND, A. Effects of acute intermittent exposure to cigarette smoke on hypothalamic and preoptic catecholamine nerve terminal systems and on neuroendocrine function in the diestrous rat. *Archives of Pharmacology* 337:131-139, 1988.

ANDERSSON, K., FUXE, K., ENEROTH, P., AGNATI, L. Differential effects of mecamylamine on the nicotine induced changes in amine levels and turnover in hypothalamic dopamine and noradrenaline nerve terminal systems and in the secretion of adenohypophyseal hormones in the castrated female rat. Evidence for involvement of cholinergic nicotine-like receptors. *Acta Physiologica Scandinavica* 120:489-498, 1984.

ANDERSSON, K., FUXE, K., ENEROTH, P., GUSTAFSSON, J.-A., AGNATI, L.F. Mecamylamine induced blockade of nicotine induced inhibition of gonadotrophin and TSH secretion and of nicotine induced increases of catecholamine turnover in the rat hypothalamus. *Acta Physiologica Scandinavica* 479(Supplement):27-29, 1980.

ANDREWS, J., MCGARRY, J.M. A community study of smoking in pregnancy. *Journal of Obstetrics and Gynaecology of the British Commonwealth* 79(12):1057-1073, December 1972.

ATHAYDE, E. Incidencia de abortos e mortinalidade nas operarias da industria de fumo. (Inquirito realizada na regiao fumageira da Bahia). *Brasil-Med* 62:237-239, 1948.

BAILEY, A., ROBINSON, D., VESSEY, M. Smoking and age of natural menopause. (Letter.) *Lancet* 2(8040):722, October 1, 1977.

BAIRD, D.D., WILCOX, A.J. Cigarette smoking associated with delayed conception. *Journal of the American Medical Association* 253(20):2979-2983, May 24-31, 1985.

BARBIERI, R.L., GOCHBERG, J., RYAN, K.J. Nicotine, cotinine, and anabasine inhibit aromatase in human trophoblast in vitro. *Journal of Clinical Investigation* 77:1727-1733, June 1986.

BARBIERI, R.L., MCSHANE, P.M., RYAN, K.J. Constituents of cigarette smoke inhibit human granulosa cell aromatase. *Fertility and Sterility* 46(2):232-236, August 1986.

BARNDT, R. JR., BLANKENHORN, D.H., CRAWFORD, D.W., BROOKS, S.H. Regression and progression of early femoral atherosclerosis in treated hyperlipoproteinemic patients. *Annals of Internal Medicine* 86:139–146, 1977.
BARON, J.A. Cigarette smoking and age at natural menopause. In: Wald, N., Baron, J.A. (eds.) *Smoking and Hormone-Related Disorders.* Oxford: Oxford University Press, 1990, pp. 57–63.
BARON, J.A., LA VECCHIA, C., LEVI, F. The anti-estrogenic effect of cigarette smoking in women. *American Journal of Obstetrics and Gynecology* 162(2):502–514, February 1990.
BARRETT-CONNOR, E., KHAW, K.-T. Cigarette smoking and increased endogenous estrogen levels in men. *American Journal of Epidemiology* 126(2):187–192, 1987.
BARRETT-CONNOR, E., KHAW, K.-T., YEN, S.S.C. A prospective study of dehydroepiandrosterone sulfate, mortality, and cardiovascular disease. *New England Journal of Medicine* 315(24):1519–1524, 1986.
BAXTER, J.D., TYRRELL, J.B. The adrenal cortex. In: Felig, P., Baxter, J.D., Broadus, A.E., Frohman, L.A. (eds.) *Endocrinology and Metabolism.* Second Edition. New York: McGraw-Hill, 1987, pp. 511–573.
BENOWITZ, N.L. Pharmacologic aspects of cigarette smoking and nicotine addiction. *New England Journal of Medicine* 319(20):1318–1330, November 17, 1988.
BERKOWITZ, G.S., HOLFORD, T.R., BERKOWITZ, R.L. Effects of cigarette smoking, alcohol, coffee and tea consumption on preterm delivery. *Early Human Development* 7(3):239–250, 1982.
BERNHARD, P. Sichere schaden des Zigarettenrauchens bei der Frau. [Certain injurious effects of cigarette smoking on women.] *Medizinische Monatsschrift* 3:58–60, 1949.
BISWAS, N.M., PATRA, P.B. Role of testosterone propionate on spermatogenesis following chronic nicotine administration in immature rats. *Indian Journal of Experimental Biology* 19:604–606, July 1981.
BLAKE, C.A. Parallelism and divergence in luteinizing hormone and follicle-stimulating hormone release in nicotine-treated rats. *Proceedings of the Society for Experimental Biology and Medicine* 145:716–720, 1974.
BLAKE, C.A., NORMAN, R.L., SAWYER, C.H. Localization of the inhibitory actions of estrogen and nicotine on release of luteinizing hormone in rats. *Neuroendocrinology* 16:22–35, 1974.
BLAKE, C.A., SCARAMUZZI, R.J., NORMAN, R.L., KANEMATSU, S., SAWYER, C.H. Effect of nicotine on the proestrous ovulatory surge of LH in the rat. *Endocrinology* 91(5):1253–1258, November 1972a.
BLAKE, C.A., SCARAMUZZI, R.J., NORMAN, R.L., KANEMATSU, S., SAWYER, C.H. Nicotine delays the ovulatory surge of luteinizing hormone in the rat. *Proceedings of the Society for Experimental Biology and Medicine* 141(3):1014–1016, December 1972b.
BORNMAN, M.S., DU PLESSIS, D.J. Smoking and vascular impotence. *South African Medical Journal* 70(6):329–330, September 13, 1986.
BRAMBILLA, D.J., MCKINLAY, S.M. A prospective study of factors affecting age at menopause. *Journal of Clinical Epidemiology* 42(11):1031–1039, 1989.
BRIGGS, M.H. Cigarette smoking and infertility in men. *Medical Journal of Australia* 1(12):616–617, March 24, 1973.
BROWN, S., VESSEY, M., STRATTON, I. The influence of method of contraception and cigarette smoking on menstrual patterns. *British Journal of Obstetrics and Gynaecology* 95:905–910, September 1988.
BUCK, G.M., COOKFAIR, D.L., MICHALEK, A.M., NASCA, P.C., STANDFAST, S.J., SEVER, L.E., KRAMER, A.A. Intrauterine growth retardation and risk of sudden infant death syndrome (SIDS). *American Journal of Epidemiology* 129(5):874–884, May 1989.

BÜHLER, F.R., VESANEN, K., WATTERS, J.T., BOLLI, P. Impact of smoking on heart attacks, strokes, blood pressure control, drug dose, and quality of life aspects in the International Prospective Primary Prevention Study in Hypertension. *American Heart Journal* 115 (1):282–288, January 1988.
BUIATTI, E., BARCHIELLI, A., GEDDES, M., NASTASI, L., KRIEBEL, D., FRANCHINI, M., SCARSELLI, G. Risk factors in male infertility: A case–control study. *Archives of Environmental Health* 39(4):266–270, July–August 1984.
BUTLER, N.R., GOLDSTEIN, H., ROSS, E.M. Cigarette smoking in pregnancy: Its influence on birth weight and perinatal mortality. *British Medical Journal* 2:127–130, April 15, 1972.
CAMPBELL, J.M., HARRISON, K.L. Smoking and infertility. (Letter.) *Medical Journal of Australia* 1:342–343, April 21, 1979.
CAMPBELL, O.M., GRAY, R.H. Smoking and ectopic pregnancy: A multinational case–control study. In: Rosenberg, M.J. (ed.) *Smoking and Reproductive Health*. Littleton, Massachusetts: PSG Publishing, 1987, pp. 70–75.
CENDRON, N., VALLERY-MASSON, J. Tabac et comportement sexuel chez l'homme. *Vie Médicale* 25:3027–3030, July 1971.
CHOW, W.-H., DALING, J.R., WEISS, N.S., VOIGT, L.F. Maternal cigarette smoking and tubal pregnancy. *Obstetrics and Gynecology* 71(2):167–170, February 1988.
COMMITTEE TO STUDY THE PREVENTION OF LOW BIRTHWEIGHT. *Preventing Low Birthweight*. Washington, D.C.: National Academy Press, 1985.
COMSTOCK, G.W., LUNDIN, F.E. JR. Parental smoking and perinatal mortality. *American Journal of Obstetrics and Gynecology* 98(5):708–718, July 1, 1967.
CONDRA, M., MORALES, A., OWEN, J.A., SURRIDGE, D.H., FENEMORE, J. Prevalence and significance of tobacco smoking in impotence. *Urology* 27(6):495–498, June 1986.
COOPER, L. An Epidemiologic Assessment of Low Birth Weight and Smoking Behavior in a Black Urban Population. Doctoral Dissertation. University of Maryland, 1989.
COPE, I., LANCASTER, P., STEVENS, L. Smoking in pregnancy. *Medical Journal of Australia* 1:673–677, April 7, 1973.
COUNSILMAN, J.J., MACKAY, E.V. Cigarette smoking by pregnant women with particular reference to their past and subsequent breast feeding behaviour. *Australian and New Zealand Journal of Obstetrics and Gynaecology* 25(2):101–106, May 1985.
DAI, W.S., GUTAI, J.P., KULLER, L.H., CAULEY, J.A. Cigarette smoking and serum sex hormones in men. *American Journal of Epidemiology* 128(4):796–805, 1988.
DALING, J., WEISS, N., SPADONI, L., MOORE, D.E., VOIGT, L. Cigarette smoking and primary tubal infertility. In: Rosenberg, M.J. (ed.) *Smoking and Reproductive Health*. Littleton, Massachusetts: PSG Publishing, 1987, pp. 40–46.
DALING, J.R., WEISS, N.S., VOIGT, L., SPADONI, L.R., SODERSTROM, R., MOORE, D.E., STADEL, B.V. Tubal infertility in relation to prior induced abortion. *Fertility and Sterility* 43(3):389–394, March 1985.
DANIELL, H.W. Smoking, obesity, and the menopause. (Letter.) *Lancet* 2(8085):373, August 12, 1978.
DAVIES, D.P., ABERNETHY, M. Cigarette smoking in pregnancy: Associations with maternal weight gain and fetal growth. *Lancet* 1(7956):385–387, February 21, 1976.
DAVIES, J.M., LATTO, I.P., JONES, J.G., VEALE, A., WARDROP, C.A.J. Effects of stopping smoking for 48 hours on oxygen availability from the blood: A study on pregnant women. *British Medical Journal* 2:355–356, August 11, 1979.
DEMARINI, D.M. Genotoxicity of tobacco smoke and tobacco smoke condensate. *Mutation Research* 114:59–89, 1983.
DEPALMA, R.G., EMSELLEM, H.A., EDWARDS, C.M., DRUY, E.M., SHULTZ, S.W., MILLER, H.C., BERGSRUD, D. A screening sequence for vasculogenic impotence. *Journal of Vascular Surgery* 5(2):228–236, February 1987.

DESLYPERE, J.P., VERMEULEN, A. Leydig cell function in normal men: Effect of age, life-style, residence, diet, and activity. *Journal of Clinical Endocrinology and Metabolism* 59(5):955–962, 1984.
DIKSHIT, R.K., BUCH, J.G., MANSURI, S.M. Effect of tobacco consumption on semen quality of a population of hypofertile males. *Fertility and Sterility* 48(2):334–336, August 1987.
DIOKNO, A.C., BROWN, M.B., HERZOG, A.R. Sexual function in the elderly. *Archives of Internal Medicine* 150(1):197–200, January 1990.
DONOVAN, J.W. Randomised controlled trial of anti-smoking advice in pregnancy. *British Journal of Preventive and Social Medicine* 31:6–12, 1977.
DONTENWILL, W., CHEVALIER, H.-J., HARKE, H.-P., LAFRENZ, U., RECKZEH, G., SCHNEIDER, B. Investigations on the effects of chronic cigarette-smoke inhalation in Syrian golden hamsters. *Journal of the National Cancer Institute* 51(6):1781–1807, December 1973a.
DONTENWILL, W., CHEVALIER, H.-J., HARKE, H.-P., LAFRENZ, U., RECKZEH, G., SCHNEIDER, B. Experimental investigations of the effect of cigarette smoke exposure on testicular function of Syrian golden hamsters. *Toxicology* 1:309–320, 1973b.
EFFENDY, I., KRAUSE, W. Environmental risk factors in the history of male patients of an infertility clinic. *Andrologia* 19 (Special number):262–265, June 1987.
EL-SAYAD, H.I., GHANIM, A.E., GAMAL EL DIN, A., SWEDAN, N., EL-SHERIF, F.A. Testicular damage in rats after subcutaneous administration of cigarette smoking residues. *Journal of the Egyptian Society of Parasitology* 17(1):179–188, 1987.
ELIST, J., JARMAN, W.D., EDSON, M. Evaluating medical treatment of impotence. *Urology* 23(4):374–375, April 1984.
ELLENBERG, J.H., NELSON, K.B. Birth weight and gestational age in children with cerebral palsy or seizure disorders. *American Journal of Diseases of Children* 133(10):1044–1048, October 1979.
ENEROTH, P., FUXE, K., GUSTAFSSON, J.-Å., HÖKFELT, T., LÖFSTRÖM, A., SKETT, P., AGNATI, L. The effect of nicotine on central catecholamine neurons and gonadotropin secretion. II. Inhibitory influence of nicotine on LH, FSH and prolactin secretion in the ovariectomized female rat and its relation to regional changes in dopamine and noradrenaline levels and turnover. *Medical Biology* 55:158–166, 1977a.
ENEROTH, P., FUXE, K., GUSTAFSSON, J.-Å., HÖKFELT, T., LÖFSTRÖM, A., SKETT, P., AGNATI, L. The effect of nicotine on central catecholamine neurons and gonadotropin secretion. III. Studies on prepubertal female rats treated with pregnant mare serum gonadotropin. *Medical Biology* 55:167–176, 1977b.
ENTRICAN, J., MACKIE, M., DOUGLAS, A.S. Oestrogens, myocardial infarction, and smoking. (Letter.) *Lancet* 2(8098):1048, November 11, 1978.
ERSHOFF, D.H., AARONSON, N.K., DANAHER, B.G., WASSERMAN, F.W. Behavioral, health, and cost outcomes of an HMO-based prenatal health education program. *Public Health Reports* 98(6):536–547, November–December 1983.
ERSHOFF, D.H., MULLEN, P.D., QUINN, V.P. A randomized trial of a serialized self-help smoking cessation program for pregnant women in an HMO. *American Journal of Public Health* 79(2):182–187, February 1989.
ESSENBERG, J.M., FAGAN, L., MALERSTEIN, A.J. Chronic poisoning of the ovaries and testes of albino rats and mice by nicotine and cigarette smoke. *Western Journal of Surgical Obstetrics and Gynecology* 59:27–32, 1951.
EVANS, H.J., FLETCHER, J., TORRANCE, M., HARGREAVE, T.B. Sperm abnormalities and cigarette smoking. *Lancet* 1(8221):627–629, March 21, 1981.

EVERSON, R.B., SANDLER, D.P., WILCOX, A.J., SCHREINEMACHERS, D., SHORE, D.L., WEINBERG, C. Effect of passive exposure to smoking on age at natural menopause. *British Medical Journal* 293:792, September 27, 1986.

FABIA, J. Cigarettes pendant la grossesse, poids de naissance et mortalité perinatale. *Canadian Medical Association Journal* 109(11):1104–1107, December 1, 1973.

FANCOURT, R., CAMPBELL, S., HARVEY, D., NORMAN, A.P. Follow-up study of small-for-dates babies. *British Medical Journal* 1:1435–1437, June 12, 1976.

FINGERHUT, L.A., KLEINMAN, J.C., KENDRICK, J.S. Smoking before, during, and after pregnancy. *American Journal of Public Health* 80(5):541–544, May 1990.

FITZGERALD, G.A., OATES, J.A., NOWAK, J. Cigarette smoking and hemostatic function. *American Heart Journal* 115(1, Part II):267–271, 1988.

FITZHARDINGE, P.M., STEVEN, E.M. The small-for-date infant. I. Later growth patterns. *Pediatrics* 49(5):671–681, May 1972.

FORSBERG, L., GUSTAVII, B., HÖJERBACK, T., OLSSON, A.M. Impotence, smoking, and β-blocking drugs. *Fertility and Sterility* 31(5):589–591, May 1979.

FRAZIER, T.M., DAVIS, G.H., GOLDSTEIN, H., GOLDBERG, I.D. Cigarette smoking and prematurity: A prospective study. *American Journal of Obstetrics and Gynecology* 81(5):988–996, May 1961.

GILBERT, D.G., HAGEN, R.L., D'AGOSTINO, J.A. The effects of cigarette smoking on human sexual potency. *Addictive Behaviors* 11:431–434, 1986.

GODFREY, B. Sperm morphology in smokers. (Letter.) *Lancet* 1(8226):948, April 25, 1981.

GOLDSTEIN, I., FELDMAN, M.I., DECKERS, P.J., BABAYAN, R.K., KRANE, R.J. Radiation-associated impotence. *Journal of the American Medical Association* 251(7):903–910, February 17, 1984.

GULYAS, B.J., MATTISON, D.R. Degeneration of mouse oocytes in response to polycyclic aromatic hydrocarbons. *Anatomical Record* 193:863–882, 1979.

HAAG, H.B., LARSON, P.S., WEATHERBY, J.H. The effect on rats of chronic exposure to cigarette smoke. *Annals of the New York Academy of Science* 90:227–238, 1960.

HAMMOND, E.C. Smoking in relation to physical complaints. *Archives of Environmental Health* 3:28–46, August 1961.

HANDELSMAN, D.J., CONWAY, A.J., BOYLAN, L.M., TURTLE, J.R. Testicular function in potential sperm donors: Normal ranges and the effects of smoking and varicocele. *International Journal of Andrology* 7:369–382, 1984.

HARTZ, A.J., KELBER, S., BORKOWF, H., WILD, R., GILLIS, B.L., RIMM, A.A. The association of smoking with clinical indicators of altered sex steroids—A study of 50,145 women. *Public Health Reports* 102(3):254–259, May–June 1987.

HARVEY, D., PRINCE, J., BUNTON, J., PARKINSON, C., CAMPBELL, S. Abilities of children who were small-for-gestational-age babies. *Pediatrics* 69(3):296–300, March 1982.

HEBEL, J.R., FOX, N.L., SEXTON, M. Dose–response of birth weight to various measures of maternal smoking during pregnancy. *Journal of Clinical Epidemiology* 41(5):483–489, 1988.

HERSEY, P., PRENDERGAST, D., EDWARDS, A. Effects of cigarette smoking on the immune system. Follow-up studies in normal subjects after cessation of smoking. *Medical Journal of Australia* 2:425–429, October 29, 1983.

HIATT, R.A., FIREMAN, B.H. Smoking, menopause, and breast cancer. *Journal of the National Cancer Institute* 76(5):833–838, May 1986.

HILL, R.M., VERNIAUD, W.M., DETER, R.L., TENNYSON, L.M., RETTIG, G.M., ZION, T.E., VORDERMAN, A.L., HELMS, P.G., MCCULLEY, L.B., HILL, L.L. The effects of intrauterine malnutrition on the term infant: A 14-year progressive study. *Acta Paediatrica Scandinavica* 73:482–487, 1984.

HOIDAS, S., WILLIAMS, A.E., TOCHER, J.L., HARGREAVE, T.B. Scoring sperm morphology from fertile and infertile cigarette smokers using the scanning electron microscope and image analysis. *Fertility and Sterility* 43(4):595–598, April 1985.

HOOK, E.B. Changes in tobacco smoking and ingestion of alcohol and caffeinated beverages during early pregnancy: Are these consequences, in part, of feto-protective mechanisms diminishing maternal exposure to embryotoxins? In: Kelly, S., Hook, E.B., Janerich, D.P., Porter, I.H. (eds.) *Birth Defects: Risks and Consequences.* New York: Academic Press, 1976, pp. 173–183.

HOWE, G., WESTHOFF, C., VESSEY, M., YEATES, D. Effects of age, cigarette smoking, and other factors on fertility: Findings in a large prospective study. *British Medical Journal* 290:1697–1700, June 8, 1985.

JACOBS, J.A., FISHKIN, R., COHEN, S., GOLDMAN, A., MULHOLLAND, S.G. A multidisciplinary approach to the evaluation and management of male sexual dysfunction. *Journal of Urology* 129:35–37, January 1983.

JEREMY, J.Y., MIKHAILIDIS, D.P., THOMPSON, C.S., DANDONA, P. The effect of cigarette smoke and diabetes mellitus on muscarinic stimulation of prostacyclin synthesis by the rat penis. *Diabetes Research* 3:467–469, 1986.

JICK, H., PORTER, J., MORRISON, A.S. Relation between smoking and age of natural menopause. *Lancet* 1(8026):1354–1355, June 25, 1977.

JUENEMANN, K.-P., LUE, T.F., LUO, J.-A., BENOWITZ, N.L., ABOZEID, M., TANAGHO, E.A. The effect of cigarette smoking on penile erection. *Journal of Urology* 138:438–441, August 1987.

KAISER, F.E., VIOSCA, S.P., MORLEY, J.E., MOORADIAN, A.D., DAVIS, S.S., KORENMAN, S.G. Impotence and aging: Clinical and hormonal factors. *Journal of the American Geriatric Society* 36:511–519, 1988.

KANEMATSU, S., SAWYER, C.H. Inhibition of the progesterone-advanced LH surge at proestrus by nicotine. *Proceedings of the Society for Experimental Biology and Medicine* 143:1183–1186, 1973.

KAUFMAN, D.W., SLONE, D., ROSENBERG, L., MIETTINEN, O.S., SHAPIRO, S. Cigarette smoking and age at natural menopause. *American Journal of Public Health* 70(4):420–422, April 1980.

KLAIBER, E.L., BROVERMAN, D.M. Dynamics of estradiol and testosterone and seminal fluid indexes in smokers and nonsmokers. *Fertility and Sterility* 50(4):630–634, October 1988.

KLAIBER, E.L., BROVERMAN, D.M., DALEN, J.E. Serum estradiol levels in male cigarette smokers. *American Journal of Medicine* 77:858–862, November 1984.

KLAIBER, E.L., BROVERMAN, D.M., POKOLY, T.B., ALBERT, A.J., HOWARD, P.J. JR., SHERER, J.F. JR. Interrelationships of cigarette smoking, testicular varicoceles, and seminal fluid indexes. *Fertility and Sterility* 47(3):481–486, March 1987.

KLEINMAN, J.C., KOPSTEIN, A. Smoking during pregnancy, 1967–80. *American Journal of Public Health* 77(7):823–825, July 1987.

KLEINMAN, J.C., MADANS, J.H. The effects of maternal smoking, physical stature, and educational attainment on the incidence of low birth weight. *American Journal of Epidemiology* 121(6):843–855, June 1985.

KLEINMAN, J.C., PIERRE, M.B. JR., MADANS, J.H., LAND, G.H., SCHRAMM, W.F. The effects of maternal smoking on fetal and infant mortality. *American Journal of Epidemiology* 127(2):274–281, 1988.

KLINE, J. Environmental exposures and spontaneous abortion. In: Gold, E. (ed.) *The Changing Risk of Disease in Women: An Epidemiologic Approach.* Lexington, Massachusetts: D.C. Heath and Company, 1984, pp. 127–138.

KLINE, J., STEIN, Z., HUTZLER, M. Cigarettes, alcohol and marijuana: Varying associations with birthweight. *International Journal of Epidemiology* 16:44–51, 1987.
KLINE, J., STEIN, Z.A., SUSSER, M., WARBURTON, D. Smoking: A risk factor for spontaneous abortion. *New England Journal of Medicine* 297(15):793–796, October 13, 1977.
KOOPS, B.L., MORGAN, L.J., BATTAGLIA, F.C. Neonatal mortality risk in relation to birth weight and gestational age: Update. *Journal of Pediatrics* 101(6):969–977, December 1982.
KRAILO, M.D., PIKE, M.C. Estimation of the distribution of age at natural menopause from prevalence data. *American Journal of Epidemiology* 117(3):356–361, 1983.
KRAMER, M.S. Determinants of low birth weight: Methodological assessment and meta-analysis. *Bulletin of the World Health Organization* 65(5):663–737, 1987.
KRAMSCH, D.M., ASPEN, A.J., ABRAMOWITZ, B.M., KREIMENDAHL, T., HOOD, W.B. JR. Reduction of coronary atherosclerosis by moderate conditioning exercise in monkeys on an atherogenic diet. *New England Journal of Medicine* 305(25):1483–1489, December 17, 1981.
KULIKAUSKAS, V., BLAUSTEIN, D., ABLIN, R.J. Cigarette smoking and its possible effects on sperm. *Fertility and Sterility* 44(4):526–528, October 1985.
KUZMA, J.W., KISSINGER, D.G. Patterns of alcohol and cigarette use in pregnancy. *Neurobehavioral Toxicology and Teratology* 3:211–221, 1981.
LANDESMAN-DWYER, S., EMANUEL, I. Smoking during pregnancy. *Teratology* 19(1):119–125, 1979.
LARSON, P.S., HAAG, H.B., SILVETTE, H. *Tobacco: Experimental and Clinical Studies*. Baltimore: Williams and Wilkins Company, 1961.
LARSON, P.S., SILVETTE, H. *Tobacco: Experimental and Clinical Studies, Supplement I*. Baltimore: Williams and Wilkins Company, 1968.
LASSILA, R., SEYBERTH, H.W., HAAPANEN, A., SCHWEER, H., KOSKENVUO, M., LAUSTIOLA, K.E. Vasoactive and atherogenic effects of cigarette smoking: A study of monozygotic twins discordant for smoking. *British Medical Journal* 297:955–957, October 15, 1988.
LEHTOVIRTA, P., FORSS, M. The acute effect of smoking on intervillous blood flow of the placenta. *British Journal of Obstetrics and Gynaecology* 85:729–731, October 1978.
LICHTENSTEIN, M.J., YARNELL, J.W.G., ELWOOD, P.C., BESWICK, A.D., SWEETNAM, P.M., MARKS, V., TEALE, D., RIAD-FAHMY, D. Sex hormones, insulin, lipids, and prevalent ischemic heart disease. *American Journal of Epidemiology* 126(4):647–657, 1987.
LINDHOLM, J., WINKEL, P., BRODTHAGEN, U., GYNTELBERG, F. Coronary risk factors and plasma sex hormones. *American Journal of Medicine* 73(5):648–651, November 1982.
LINDQUIST, O., BENGTSSON, C. Menopausal age in relation to smoking. *Acta Medica Scandinavica* 205:73–77, 1979.
LONGO, L.D. The biological effects of carbon monoxide on the pregnant woman, fetus, and newborn infant. *American Journal of Obstetrics and Gynecology* 129(1):69–103, September 1, 1977.
LONGO, L.D. Some health consequences of maternal smoking: Issues without answers. In: Nyhan, W.L. and Jones, K.L. (eds.) *Prenatal Diagnosis and Mechanisms of Teratogenesis* Birth Defects: Original article series, volume 18(3A). New York: Alan R. Liss, Inc., 1982, pp. 13–31.
LOWE, C.R. Effect of mothers' smoking habits on birth weight of their children. *British Medical Journal* 2(1):673–676, October 10, 1959.
LUBCHENCO, L.O., SEARLS, D.T., BRAZIE, J.V. Neonatal mortality rate: Relationship to birth weight and gestational age. *Journal of Pediatrics* 81(4):814–822, October 1972.

MACARTHUR, C., KNOX, E.G. Smoking and pregnancy: Effects of stopping at different stages. *British Journal of Obstetrics and Gynaecology* 95(6):551–555, June 1988.

MACARTHUR, C., NEWTON, J.R., KNOX, E.G. Effect of anti-smoking health education on infant size at birth: A randomized controlled trial. *British Journal of Obstetrics and Gynaecology* 94:295–300, April 1987.

MACMAHON, B., ALPERT, M., SALBER, E.J. Infant weight and parental smoking habits. *American Journal of Epidemiology* 82(3):247–261, November 1966.

MALCOLM, S., SHEPHARD, R.J. Personality and sexual behavior of the adolescent smoker. *American Journal of Drug and Alcohol Abuse* 5(1):87–96, 1978.

MALLOY, M.H., KLEINMAN, J.C., LAND, G.H., SCHRAMM, W.F. The association of maternal smoking with age and cause of infant death. *American Journal of Epidemiology* 128(1):46–55, July 1988.

MANLEY, R.S., BOLAND, F.J. Side-effects and weight gain following a smoking cessation program. *Addictive Behaviors* 8:375–380, 1983.

MARCOUX, S., BRISSON, J., FABIA, J. The effect of cigarette smoking on the risk of preeclampsia and gestational hypertension. *American Journal of Epidemiology* 130(5):950–957, 1989.

MARSHBURN, P.B., SLOAN, C.S., HAMMOND, M.G. Semen quality and association with coffee drinking, cigarette smoking, and ethanol consumption. *Fertility and Sterility* 52(1):162–165, July 1989.

MARTIN, T.R., BRACKEN, M.B. Association of low birth weight with passive smoke exposure in pregnancy. *American Journal of Epidemiology* 124(4):633–642, 1986.

MATSUNAGA, E., SHIOTA, K. Ectopic pregnancy and myoma uteri: Teratogenic effects and maternal characteristics. *Teratology* 21:61–69, 1980.

MATTISON, D.R. Morphology of oocyte and follicle destruction by polycyclic aromatic hydrocarbons in mice. *Toxicology and Applied Pharmacology* 53:249–259, 1980.

MATTISON, D.R. The effects of smoking on fertility from gametogenesis to implantation. *Environmental Research* 28(2):410–433, August 1982.

MATTISON, D.R., THORGEIRSSON, S.S. Smoking and industrial pollution, and their effects on menopause and ovarian cancer. *Lancet* 1(8057):187–188, July 28, 1978.

MATTISON, D.R., THORGEIRSSON, S.S. Ovarian aryl hydrocarbon hydroxylase activity and primordial oocyte toxicity of polycyclic aromatic hydrocarbons in mice. *Cancer Research* 39:3471–3475, September 1979.

MCCORMICK, M. The contribution of low birth weight to infant mortality and childhood morbidity. *New England Journal of Medicine* 312(2):82–90, January 10, 1985.

MCGARRY, J.M., ANDREWS, J. Smoking in pregnancy and vitamin B_{12} metabolism. *British Medical Journal* 2(5805):74–77, April 8, 1972.

MCINTOSH, I.D. Smoking and pregnancy: Attributable risks and public health implications. *Canadian Journal of Public Health* 75:141–148, March–April 1984.

MCLEAN, B.K., RUBEL, A., NIKITOVITCH-WINER, M.B. The differential effects of exposure to tobacco smoke on the secretion of luteinizing hormone and prolactin in the proestrous rat. *Endocrinology* 100(6):1566–1570, June 1977.

MCNAMARA, P.M., HJORTLAND, M.C., GORDON, T., KANNEL, W.B. Natural history of menopause: The Framingham Study. *Journal of Continuing Education in Obstetrics and Gynecology* 20:27–35, 1978.

MEIKLE, A.W., BISHOP, D.T., STRINGHAM, J.D., FORD, M.H., WEST, D.W. Cigarette smoking alters plasma sex-steroid levels. *Clinical Research* 35(1):183A, 1987.

MEYER, M.B. How does maternal smoking affect birth weight and maternal weight gain? *American Journal of Obstetrics and Gynecology* 131(8):888–893, August 15, 1978.

MEYER, M.B., JONAS, B.S., TONASCIA, J.A. Perinatal events associated with maternal smoking during pregnancy. *American Journal of Epidemiology* 103(5):464–476, 1976.

MEYER, M.B., TONASCIA, J.A. Maternal smoking, pregnancy complications, and perinatal mortality. *American Journal of Obstetrics and Gynecology* 128:494–502,1977.

MICHNOVICZ, J.J., HERSHCOPF, R.J., NAGANUMA, H., BRADLOW, H.L., FISHMAN, J. Increased 2-hydroxylation of estradiol as a possible mechanism for the anti-estrogenic effect of cigarette smoking. *New England Journal of Medicine* 315(21):1305–1309, November 20, 1986.

MOSS, R.L., RISKIND, P., DUDLEY, C.A. Effects of LH–RH on sexual activities in animal and man. In: Colla et al. (eds.) *Central Nervous System Effects of Hypothalamic Hormones and Other Peptides.* New York: Raven Press, 1979.

NADLER, J.L., VELASCO, J.S., HORTON, R. Cigarette smoking inhibits prostacyclin formation. *Lancet* 1(8336):1248–1250, June 4, 1983.

NAEYE, R.L. Effects of maternal cigarette smoking on the fetus and placenta. *British Journal of Obstetrics and Gynaecology* 85(10):732–737, October 1978.

NAEYE, R.L. Abruptio placentae and placenta previa: Frequency, perinatal mortality, and cigarette smoking. *Obstetrics and Gynecology* 55(6):701–704, June 1980.

NAEYE, R.L., TAFARI, N. *Risk Factors in Pregnancy and Diseases of the Fetus and Newborn.* Baltimore, Maryland: Williams and Wilkins, 1983.

NATIONAL CENTER FOR HEALTH STATISTICS. Advance report of final natality statistics, 1980. *Monthly Vital Statistics Report* 31(Supplement 8):1–8, November 30, 1982.

NATIONAL CENTER FOR HEALTH STATISTICS. Health promotion and disease prevention: United States, 1985. *Vital and Health Statistics,* Series 10, No. 163, Public Health Service. DHHS Publication No. (PHS) 88-1591, February 1988.

NEBE, K.H., SCHIRREN, C. Statistische untersuchungen bei andrologischen patienten. III. Nikotin und ejakulatparameter. *Andrologia* 12(6):493–502, November–December 1980.

NIKKILÄ, E.A. Is human atherosclerosis reversible? In: Miller, N.E., Lewis, B. (eds.) *Lipoproteins, Atherosclerosis and Coronary Heart Disease.* Amsterdam: Elsevier/North-Holland Biomedical Press, 1980, pp. 155–164.

NISWANDER, K.R., GORDON, M. Demographic characteristics. Cigarette smoking. In: *The Women and Their Pregnancies.* The Collaborative Perinatal Study of the National Institute of Neurological Diseases and Stroke. U.S. Department of Health, Education, and Welfare, Public Health Service, National Institutes of Health. Philadelphia: W.B. Saunders Co., 1972, pp.72–80.

NORDENSON, I., ABRAMSSON, L., DUCHEK, M. Somatic chromosomal aberrations and male infertility. *Human Heredity* 34:240–245, 1984.

OBE, G., HERHA, J. Chromosomal aberrations in heavy smokers. *Human Genetics* 41:259–263, 1978.

OCHSNER, A. The health menace of tobacco. *Medical Aspects of Human Sexuality* 59:246–252, November 1971a.

OCHSNER, A. Influence of smoking on sexuality and pregnancy. *Medical Aspects of Human Sexuality* 5(11):82–92, November 1971b.

OLDEREID, N.B., RUI, H., CLAUSEN, O.P.F., PURVIS, K. Cigarette smoking and human sperm quality assessed by laser-Doppler spectroscopy and DNA flow cytometry. *Journal of Reproduction and Fertility* 86:731–736, 1989.

OUNSTED, M., MOAR, V.A., SCOTT, A. Risk factors associated with small-for-dates and large-for-dates infants. *British Journal of Obstetrics and Gynaecology* 92:226–232, March 1985.

OUNSTED, M., TAYLOR, M.E. The postnatal growth of children who were small-for-dates or large-for-dates at birth. *Developmental Medicine and Child Neurology* 13:421–434, 1971.

OUNSTED, M.K., MOAR, V.A., SCOTT, A. Children of deviant birth weight at the age of seven years: Health, handicap, size and developmental status. *Early Human Development* 9:323–340, 1984.

PAPOZ, L., ESCHWEGE, E., PEQUIGNOT, G., BARRAT, J., SCHWARTZ, D. Maternal smoking and birth weight in relation to dietary habits. *American Journal of Obstetrics and Gynecology* 142(7):870–876, April 1, 1982.
PATRA, P.B., SANYAL, S., BISWAS, N.M. Possible alpha-adrenergic involvement in nicotine induced alteration of spermatogenesis in rat. *Andrologia* 11(4):273–278, 1979.
PETITTI, D.B., COLEMAN, C. Cigarette smoking and the risk of low birth weight: A comparison in black and white women. *Epidemiology*, in press.
PETTERSSON, F., FRIES, H., NILLIUS, S.J. Epidemiology of secondary amenorrhea. I. Incidence and prevalence rates. *American Journal of Obstetrics and Gynecology* 117(1):80–86, September 1, 1973.
PRAGER, K., MALIN, H., SPIEGLER, D., VAN NATTA, P., PLACEK., P.J. Smoking and drinking behavior before and during pregnancy of married mothers of live-born infants and stillborn infants. *Public Health Reports* 99(2):117–127, March–April 1984.
PULKKINEN, P. Smoking and pregnancy: The influence of maternal and gestational factors on the outcome of pregnancy and the newborn. *Annales Chirurgiae et Gynaecologiae* 74(Supplement 197):55–59, 1985.
RABKIN, S. Relationship between weight change and the reduction or cessation of cigarette smoking. *International Journal of Obesity* 8:665–673, 1984.
RANTAKALLIO, P. Relationship of maternal smoking to morbidity and mortality of the child up to the age of five. *Acta Paediatrica Scandinavica* 67(5):621–631, September 1978.
RANTALA, M.-L., KOSKIMIES, A.I. Semen quality of infertile couples—Comparison between smokers and non-smokers. *Andrologia* 19(1):42–46, January–February 1987.
REUBEN, D. Warning: Smoking endangers your sex life. *Reader's Digest*, April 1988, pp. 98–100.
RODRIGUEZ-RIGAU, L.J., SMITH, K.D., STEINBERGER, E. Cigarette smoking and semen quality. *Fertility and Sterility* 38(1):115–116, July 1982.
ROGERS, B.J., RUSSELL, L.D. Semen analysis, sperm functional abnormalities, and enhancement of semen parameters. In: Gondos, B., Riddick, D.H. (eds.) *Pathology of Infertility*. New York: Thieme Medical Publishers, 1987, pp. 335–352.
RUI, H., OLDEREID, N.B., PURVIS, K. Røyking og spermiekvalitet hos menn under fertilitetsutredning. *Tidsskr Nor Laegeforen* 109(5):573–575, 1989.
RUSH, D. Examination of the relationship between birthweight, cigarette smoking during pregnancy and maternal weight gain. *Journal of Obstetrics and Gynaecology of the British Commonwealth* 81:746–752, October 1974.
RUSH, D., CASSANO, P. Relationship of cigarette smoking and social class to birth weight and perinatal mortality among all births in Britain, 5–11 April 1970. *Journal of Epidemiology and Community Health* 37(4):249–255, December 1983.
RUSH, D., KASS, E.H. Maternal smoking: A reassessment of the association with perinatal mortality. *American Journal of Epidemiology* 96(3):183–196, September 1972.
RUSSELL, M.A.H. Cigarette smoking: Natural history of a dependence disorder. *British Journal of Medical Psychology* 44(1):1–16, May 1971.
SAARANEN, M., KANTOLA, M., SAARIKOSKI, S., VANHA-PERTTULA, T. Human seminal plasma cadmium: Comparison with fertility and smoking habits. *Andrologia* 21(2): 140–145, 1989.
SAARANEN, M., SUONIO, S., KAUHANEN, O., SAARIKOSKI, S. Cigarette smoking and semen quality in men of reproductive age. *Andrologia* 19(6):670–676, 1987.
SCHENKER, M.B., SAMUELS, S.J., PERKINS, C., LEWIS, E.L., KATZ, D.F., OVERSTREET, J.W. Prospective surveillance of sperm quality in the workplace. *Journal of Occupational Medicine* 30(4):336–344, April 1988.
SCHIRREN, C., GEY, G. Der einfluss des rauchens auf die fortpflanzungsfähigkeit bei mann und frau. *Zeitschrift für Haut- und Geschlechtskrankheiten* 44(5):175–182, 1969.

SCHRAMM, W. Smoking and pregnancy outcome. *Missouri Medicine* 77(10):619–626, October 1980.
SCHWARTZ, D., GOUJARD, J., KAMINSKI, M., RUMEAU-ROUQUETTE, C. Smoking and pregnancy. Results of a prospective study of 6,989 women. *Revue Européenne d'Études Cliniques et Biologiques* 17:867–879, 1972.
SEXTON, M., HEBEL, J.R. A clinical trial of change in maternal smoking and its effect on birth weight. *Journal of the American Medical Association* 251(7):911–915, February 17, 1984.
SHAARAWY, M., MAHMOUD, K.Z. Endocrine profile and semen characteristics in male smokers. *Fertility and Sterility* 38(2):255–257, August 1982.
SHIONO, P.H., KLEBANOFF, M.A., RHOADS, G.G. Smoking and drinking during pregnancy. *Journal of the American Medical Association* 255(1):82–86, January 3, 1986.
SIMPSON, W.J. A preliminary report on cigarette smoking and the incidence of prematurity. *American Journal of Obstetrics and Gynecology* 73(4):808–815, April 1957.
SOULAIRAC, M.-L., SOULAIRAC, A. Action de la nicotine sur le comportement sexuel du rat mâle. *Comptes Rendus Société de Biologie* 166:798–802, June 20, 1972.
SPIRA, A., DUCOT, B., JOUANNET, P., SOUMAH, A., FENEUX, D., ALBERT, M. Consommation de tabac, d'alcool, et fertilité masculine. *INSERM* 103:363–378, 1981.
STANFORD, J.L., HARTGE, P., BRINTON, L.A., HOOVER, R.N., BROOKMEYER, R. Factors influencing the age at natural menopause. *Journal of Chronic Diseases* 40(11):995–1002, 1987.
STEKHUN, F.I. [Effect of tobacco smoking on spermatogenesis indices.] *Vrach Delo* 7:93–94, July 1980.
STERLING, T.D., KOBAYASHI, D. A critical review of reports on the effect of smoking on sex and fertility. *Journal of Sex Research* 11(2):201–217, August 1975.
SUBBARAO, V.V. Effects of smoking on female reproductive functions and the onset of menopause. In: Aoki, M., Hisamichi, S., Tominaga, S. (eds.) *Smoking and Health 1987*. Amsterdam: Elsevier Science Publishers, 1988, pp. 537–539.
TAKAHASHI, Y., HIRATA, Y. Nocturnal penile tumescence monitoring with stamps in impotent diabetics. *Diabetes Research and Clinical Practice* 4:197–201, 1988.
TAYLOR, R.R., STURM, M., VANDONGEN, R., STROPHAIR, J., BEILIN, L.J. Whole blood platelet aggregation is not affected by cigarette smoking but is sex-related. *Clinical and Experimental Pharmacology and Physiology* 14:665–671, 1987.
THIENES, C.H. Chronic nicotine poisoning. *Annals of the New York Academy of Sciences* 90:239–248, 1960.
THOMPSON, J.H., IRWIN, F.D., KANEMATSU, S., SERAYDARIAN, K., SUH, M. Effects of chronic nicotine administration and age in male Fischer-344 rats. *Toxicology and Applied Pharmacology* 26:606–620, 1973.
TSITOURAS, P.D., MARTIN, C.E., HARMAN, S.M. Relationship of serum testosterone to sexual activity in healthy elderly men. *Journal of Gerontology* 37(3):288–293, 1982.
UNDERWOOD, P.B., KESLER, K.F., O'LANE, J.M., CALLAGAN, D.A. Parental smoking empirically related to pregnancy outcome. *Journal of Obstetrics and Gynecology* 29(1):1–8, January 1967.
U.S. DEPARTMENT OF HEALTH AND HUMAN SERVICES. *The Health Consequences of Smoking for Women. A Report of the Surgeon General.* U.S. Department of Health and Human Services, Public Health Service, Office of the Assistant Secretary for Health, Office on Smoking and Health, 1980.
U.S. DEPARTMENT OF HEALTH AND HUMAN SERVICES. *Report of the Secretary's Task Force on Black and Minority Health. Vol 6: Infant Mortality and Low Birthweight.* U.S. Department of Health and Human Services. January 1986.

U.S. DEPARTMENT OF HEALTH AND HUMAN SERVICES. *The Health Consequences of Smoking: Nicotine Addiction. A Report of the Surgeon General, 1988.* U.S. Department of Health and Human Services, Public Health Service, Centers for Disease Control, Center for Health Promotion and Education, Office on Smoking and Health. DHHS Publication No. (CDC) 88-8406, 1988.

U.S. DEPARTMENT OF HEALTH AND HUMAN SERVICES. *Reducing the Health Consequences of Smoking: 25 Years of Progress. A Report of the Surgeon General.* U.S. Department of Health and Human Services, Public Health Service, Centers for Disease Control, Center for Chronic Disease Prevention and Health Promotion, Office on Smoking and Health. DHHS Publication No. (CDC) 89-8411, 1989.

U.S. DEPARTMENT OF HEALTH, EDUCATION, AND WELFARE. *The Health Consequences of Smoking. A Report of the Surgeon General: 1971.* U.S. Department of Health, Education, and Welfare, Public Health Service, Health Services and Mental Health Administration. DHEW Publication No. (HSM) 71-7513, 1971.

U.S. DEPARTMENT OF HEALTH, EDUCATION, AND WELFARE. *The Health Consequences of Smoking.* U.S. Department of Health, Education, and Welfare, Public Health Service, Health Services and Mental Health Administration. DHEW Publication No. (HSM) 73-8704, 1973.

U.S. DEPARTMENT OF HEALTH, EDUCATION, AND WELFARE. *The Health Consequences of Smoking, 1977–1978.* U.S. Department of Health, Education, and Welfare, Public Health Service, Office of the Assistant Secretary for Health, Office on Smoking and Health. DHEW Publication No. (PHS) 79-50065, 1978.

U.S. DEPARTMENT OF HEALTH, EDUCATION, AND WELFARE. *Smoking and Health. A Report of the Surgeon General.* U.S. Department of Health, Education, and Welfare, Public Health Service, Office of the Assistant Secretary for Health, Office on Smoking and Health. DHEW Publication No. (PHS) 79-50066, 1979.

VAN DEN BERG, B.J. Epidemiologic observations of prematurity: Effects of tobacco, coffee and alcohol. In: Reed, D.M., Stanley, F.J. (eds.) *Epidemiology of Prematurity.* Baltimore, Maryland: Urban and Schwarzenberg, 1977, pp. 157–176.

VAN DEN BERG, B.J., OECHSLI, F.W. Prematurity in perinatal epidemiology. In: Bracken, M.B. (ed.), Oxford University Press, New York, 1984, pp. 69–85.

VERMEULEN, A., DESLYPERE, J.P. Testicular endocrine function in the ageing male. *Maturitas* 7:273–279, 1985.

VICZIAN, M. Dohanyosokon vegzett ondo-vizsgalatok tapasztalatai. [Experiences with the sperm examination of smokers.] *Orvosi Hetilap* 109:1077–1079, May 19, 1968a.

VICZIAN, M. The effect of cigarette smoke inhalation on spermatogenesis in rats. *Experientia* 24:511–513, 1968b.

VIRAG, R., BOUILLY, P., FRYDMAN, D. Is impotence an arterial disorder? *Lancet* 1(8422): 181–184, January 26, 1985.

VIŠNJEVAC, V., MIKOV, M. Smoking and carboxyhaemoglobin concentrations in mothers and their newborn infants. *Human Toxicology* 5:175–177, 1986.

VOGEL, W., BROVERMAN, D.M., KLAIBER, E.L. Gonadal, behavioral and electroencephalographic correlates of smoking. In: Remond, A., Izard, C. (eds.) *Electrophysiological Effects of Nicotine.* Amsterdam: Elsevier/North-Holland Biomedical Press, 1979, pp. 201–214.

VOGT, H.-J., HELLER, W.-D., BORELLI, S. Sperm quality of healthy smokers, ex-smokers, and never-smokers. *Fertility and Sterility* 45(1):106–110, January 1986.

VOGT, H.-J., HELLER, W.-D., OBE, G. Spermatogenesis in smokers and non-smokers: An andrological and genetic study. In: Obe, G. (ed.) *Mutations in Man.* Berlin: Springer-Verlag, 1984, pp. 247–291.

WABREK, A.J., SHELLEY, M.M., HOROWITZ, L.M., BASTARACHE, M.M., GIUCA, J.E. Noninvasive penile arterial evaluation in 120 males with erectile dysfuntion. *Urology* 22(3): 230–234, September 1983.
WAINRIGHT, R.L. Change in observed birth weight associated with change in maternal cigarette smoking. *American Journal of Epidemiology* 117(6):668–675, June 1983.
WERLER, M.M., POBER, B.R., HOLMES, L.B. Smoking and pregnancy. *Teratology* 32(3): 473–481, December 1985.
WESTWOOD, M., KRAMER, M.S., MUNZ, D., LOVETT, J.M., WATTERS, G.V. Growth and development of full-term nonasphyxiated small-for-gestational-age newborns: Follow-up through adolescence. *Pediatrics* 71(3):376–382, March 1983.
WILCOX, A.J. Intrauterine growth retardation: Beyond birthweight criteria. (Editorial.) *Early Human Development* 8:189–193, October 1983.
WILCOX, A.J., RUSSELL, I.T. Birthweight and perinatal mortality. I. On the frequency distribution of birthweight. *International Journal of Epidemiology* 12(3):314–318, September 1983a.
WILCOX, A.J., RUSSELL, I.T. Birthweight and perinatal mortality. II. On weight-specific mortality. *International Journal of Epidemiology* 12(3):319–325, 1983b.
WILLETT, W., STAMPFER, M.J., BAIN, C., LIPNICK, R., SPEIZER, F.E., ROSNER, B., CRAMER, D., HENNEKENS, C.H. Cigarette smoking, relative weight, and menopause. *American Journal of Epidemiology* 117(6):651–658, 1983.
WILLIAMS, R.L., CHEN, P.M. *California Perinatal Statistics, 1978–1980.* Prepared by University of California, Santa Barbara Community and Organization Research Institute. Department of Health Services, State of California, Maternal and Child Health Services. June 1982, p. 11.
WILLIAMSON, D.F., SERDULA, M.K., KENDRICK, J.S., BINKIN, N.J. Comparing the prevalence of smoking in pregnant and nonpregnant women, 1985 to 1986. *Journal of the American Medical Association* 261(1):70–74, January 6, 1989.
WINDSOR, R.A., CUTTER, G., MORRIS, J., REESE, Y., MANZELLA, B., BARTLETT, E.E., SAMUELSON, C., SPANOS, D. The effectiveness of smoking cessation methods for smokers in public health maternity clinics: A randomized trial. *American Journal of Public Health* 75(12):1389–1392, December 1985.
WOOD, C. The association of psycho-social factors and gynaecological symptoms. *Australian Family Physician* 7:471–478, April 1978.
WYROBEK, A.J., BRUCE, W.R. Chemical induction of sperm abnormalities in mice. *Proceedings of the National Academy of Science* 72:4425–4429, 1975.
YERUSHALMY, J. Mother's cigarette smoking and survival of infant. *American Journal of Obstetrics and Gynecology* 88(4):505–518, February 15, 1964.
YERUSHALMY, J. The relationship of parents' cigarette smoking to outcome of pregnancy— Implications as to the problem of inferring causation from observed associations. *American Journal of Epidemiology* 93(6)443–456, 1971.
ZABRISKIE, J.R. Effect of cigarette smoking during pregnancy: Study of 2000 cases. *Obstetrics and Gynecology* 21(4):405–411, April 1963.
ZANEVELD, L.J.D., JEYENDRAN, R.S. Modern assessment of semen for diagnostic purposes. *Seminars in Reproductive Endocrinology* 6(4):323–336, 1988.

CHAPTER 9
SMOKING, SMOKING CESSATION, AND OTHER NONMALIGNANT DISEASES

CONTENTS

Part I. Peptic Ulcer Disease 429
  Introduction 429
  Impact of Smoking and Smoking Cessation on Ulcer Occurrence 429
    Smoking and Gastrointestinal Physiology 429
    Trends in Peptic Ulcer Disease 430
    Morbidity From Peptic Ulcers 431
    Mortality From Peptic Ulcers 432
  Effects of Smoking on Ulcer Healing and Recurrence 432
    Healing of Duodenal Ulcers 432
    Recurrence of Duodenal Ulcers 433
    Healing of Gastric Ulcers 440
    Recurrence of Gastric Ulcers 440
  Summary 441
Part II. Osteoporosis and Skin Wrinkling 443
  Osteoporosis 443
    Introduction 443
    Pathophysiologic Framework 443
    Bone Mineral Content in Smokers Compared With Nonsmokers 444
    Smoking as a Risk Factor for Osteoporotic Fractures 449
    Smoking Cessation and Osteoporosis and Fracture 453
    Summary 453
  Skin Wrinkling 453
    Introduction 453
    Pathophysiologic Framework 453
    Smoking and Skin Wrinkling 455
    Smoking Cessation and Skin Wrinkling 456
    Summary 457
Conclusions 457
References 459

PART I. PEPTIC ULCER DISEASE

Introduction

Numerous studies have demonstrated the association between smoking and the occurrence of peptic ulcer disease. This association was noted in the 1964, 1971, and 1972 Surgeon General's Reports (US PHS 1964; US DHEW 1971, 1972). The 1979 Report stated that the evidence of an association between cigarette smoking and peptic ulcer was strong enough to suggest a causal relationship (US DHEW 1979). That Report concluded that cigarette smoking was associated with the incidence of peptic ulcer disease and with increased risk of dying from peptic ulcer disease; the evidence that smoking retards healing of peptic ulcers was regarded as highly suggestive. The 1989 Report (US DHHS 1989) stated that smoking cessation may reduce peptic ulcer incidence and is an important component of peptic ulcer treatment, even with the effective drug therapy presently available. This Section focuses on smoking cessation and the occurrence and course of peptic ulcer disease.

Impact of Smoking and Smoking Cessation on Ulcer Occurrence

Smoking and Gastrointestinal Physiology

Kikendall, Evaul, and Johnson (1984) reviewed the effect of cigarette smoking on aspects of gastrointestinal physiology relevant to peptic ulcer disease. The literature available at the time of their review supported the following concepts. Chronic cigarette smokers have higher maximal acid output than nonsmokers. Smoking 1 cigarette or more has no consistent immediate effect on acid secretion. Smoking 1 cigarette immediately decreases alkaline pancreatic secretion and immediately results in a pronounced fall in duodenal bulb pH, especially in subjects with gastric acid hypersecretion. Smoking has a variable effect on gastric emptying, depending on experimental design. Smoking increases duodenogastric reflux. Smoking decreases gastric mucosal blood flow. Smoking during waking hours inhibits the antisecretory effects of a nocturnal dose of cimetidine, ranitidine, or poldine.

Subsequent to this review, the two latter concepts have been seriously challenged. Robert, Leung, and Guth (1986) found that neither nicotine nor smoking inhibited basal gastric mucosal blood flow in rats. Several investigators could not confirm that smoking antagonized the antisecretory effect of cimetidine or ranitidine (Deakin, Ramage, Williams 1988; Bianchi Porro et al. 1983; Bauerfeind et al. 1987).

However, several of the findings from this earlier review (Kikendall, Evaul, Johnson 1984) have been confirmed by more recent reports. Parente and associates (1985) confirmed higher pentagastrin-stimulated acid secretion among chronic heavy smokers than among nonsmokers. Smokers also had higher basal serum pepsinogen-I levels. These differences were statistically significant and large enough to be of clinical importance. Higher maximal gastric acid secretory rates among smokers compared with nonsmokers were also demonstrated by Whitfield and Hobsley (1985) in a study of 201 patients with duodenal ulcer.

Additionally, Mueller-Lissner (1986) noted that chronic smokers who abstained from smoking for 12 hours had more duodenogastric bile reflux than nonsmokers and confirmed that smoking cigarettes acutely augments the already elevated rate of bile reflux. Quimby and coworkers (1986) reported that active smoking transiently decreased gastric mucosal prostaglandin synthesis.

In summary, the known effects of smoking on gastroduodenal physiology provide multiple potential mechanisms for enhancement of an ulcer diathesis by active smoking. Several of the effects of smoking, most notably the inhibition of alkaline pancreatic secretion, the reduction of duodenal bulb pH, and the reduction of prostaglandin synthesis, are transient effects that could be reversed quickly by abstinence from smoking.

Trends in Peptic Ulcer Disease

During the past several decades, the rates of hospitalization for and mortality from peptic ulcer disease in the United States have declined dramatically (Kurata et al. 1983). Although changes in coding practices and/or diagnostic procedures could explain some of the decline, the trends in mortality from peptic ulcer have paralleled the decreasing prevalence of smoking. Kurata and coworkers (1986) studied trends in ulcer mortality and smoking in the United States between 1920 and 1980 and estimated that the portion of duodenal-ulcer-related mortality attributable to smoking was between 43 and 63 percent for men and 25 and 50 percent for women. In contrast, Sonnenberg (1986) concluded that smoking was not the main determinant of the birth cohort phenomenon of declining peptic ulcer mortality in the United Kingdom. This study descriptively compared the death rates for duodenal and gastric ulcer with the annual cigarette consumption in the United Kingdom according to birth cohorts and found a lack of correlation between ulcer mortality and cigarette consumption (Sonnenberg 1986). Thus, factors in addition to cigarette smoking may also underlie the recent trends in these indicators of peptic ulcer disease.

Two factors that have received considerable attention in recent years are *Helicobacter pylori* gastritis (Graham 1989) and the use of nonsteroidal anti-inflammatory drugs (Griffin, Ray, Schaffner 1988). Martin and associates (1989), in an endoscopic study, found that smoking was a risk factor for peptic ulcer disease among patients who had *Helicobacter pylori* gastritis. Willoughby and colleagues (1986) found that smoking was associated with peptic ulcer disease among subjects with rheumatoid arthritis, most of whom were taking nonsteroidal anti-inflammatory drugs. Ehsanullah and colleagues (1988) and Yeomans and associates (1988) also showed an association of smoking with the acute gastric erosions and submucosal hemorrhages induced by these drugs. These studies demonstrated that smoking is associated with ulcer disease related to both *Helicobacter pylori* and nonsteroidal anti-inflammatory drugs.

Morbidity From Peptic Ulcers

In an analysis of prospective cohort data on ulcer incidence in women from the National Health and Nutrition Examination Survey I Epidemiologic Followup Study, the relative risk for developing peptic ulcer was 1.3 among former smokers (95-percent confidence interval (CI), 0.7–2.9) and 1.9 among current smokers (95-percent CI, 1.2–2.6) compared with lifetime nonsmokers (Anda et al. 1990). In this study, former smokers were defined as persons who had smoked at least 100 cigarettes in their lifetime but who were not smoking at the time of the baseline interview. The mean length of followup in this cohort was 9 years. This analysis used the Cox proportional hazards model to adjust for the potential confounding effects of age, sex, socioeconomic status, regular aspirin use, alcohol intake, and coffee consumption.

Ainley and associates (1986) surveyed the smoking behavior of 1,217 patients undergoing endoscopy. This study did not include "normal" or community controls as all patients had indications for endoscopy. Of the smokers, 11.9 percent had gastric ulcers, a diagnosis shared by 7.7 percent of ex-smokers ($p<0.025$) and 4.6 percent of never smokers ($p<0.001$). Of the smokers, 12.8 percent had duodenal ulcer compared with 6.8 percent of ex-smokers ($p<0.01$) and 6.1 percent of never smokers ($p<0.001$).

In a study of nearly 6,000 Japanese men living in Hawaii (Stemmermann et al. 1989), 243 developed gastric ulcers and 99 developed duodenal ulcers in 20 years of followup. Gastric ulcer developed among 6.7 percent of current smokers compared with 3.8 percent of former smokers and 3.2 percent of lifetime nonsmokers ($p<0.0001$). Duodenal ulcer developed more often ($p<0.0001$) among current smokers than among former smokers or never smokers (2.7 vs. 1.4 vs. 0.9 percent, respectively).

These three studies show that smokers are more likely than never smokers and former smokers to develop peptic ulcer disease. Two of the studies show higher frequencies among smokers for both duodenal and gastric ulcer. All three studies demonstrate that the risk of peptic ulcer for former smokers is between that for current smokers and for never smokers. The tendency of symptomatic smokers to stop smoking would bias the results of such studies toward reducing the apparent benefit of cessation (Chapter 2). These studies strongly suggest that the smoker's risk of developing either gastric or duodenal ulcer is diminished after smoking cessation.

In an early analysis of cross-sectional survey data among men aged 20 to 79 in Tecumseh, MI (Higgins and Kjelsberg 1967), the age-adjusted prevalences of self-reported peptic ulcer among nonsmokers (presumably never smokers), ex-smokers, and current smokers were 5.2, 8.0, and 7.1 percent, respectively. The definitions of smoking status were not presented, and the differences were not statistically significant. In this study, the prevalences of peptic ulcer among women who were nonsmokers, ex-smokers, or current smokers were 1.4, 1.5, and 2.8 percent, respectively; these differences were reported as statistically significant between smokers and nonsmokers (Higgins and Kjelsberg 1967). Earlier studies such as this, which were conducted before the advent of endoscopy, had relatively poor diagnostic accuracy and may consequently have been biased toward underestimating the effects of smoking.

Additional reports linked smoking to some of the complications of peptic ulcer disease. For example, 86 percent of 128 patients presenting with perforated duodenal ulcer were cigarette smokers compared with 51 percent (p<0.01) of retrospectively matched controls (Smedley et al. 1988). Other reports noted that smokers comprised 87 percent (Heuman, Larsson, Norrby 1983) and 86 percent (Hodnett et al. 1989) of patients with perforated duodenal ulcers and 83 percent of males undergoing surgery for peptic ulcer (Ross et al. 1982). These latter studies were uncontrolled, and the high percentages of smokers have not been confirmed in some other surgical series. Nevertheless, these latter studies support the findings of Smedley and associates (1988) and suggest that smokers with peptic ulcer who continue to smoke may be at greater risk for ulcer complications than nonsmokers.

Mortality From Peptic Ulcers

The American Cancer Society Cancer Prevention Study I (ACS CPS-I) found that the relative risk of mortality for peptic ulcer among men was 3.1 for current smokers (95-percent CI, 2.2–4.2) and 1.5 for former smokers (95-percent CI, 1.0–2.3) compared with lifetime nonsmokers (US DHHS 1989).

In the U.S. Veterans Study, the duodenal ulcer mortality ratios for current and ex-smokers compared with never smokers were 3.2 and 1.8, respectively (Kahn 1966). Ex-smokers in this report were persons who stopped smoking for reasons other than physician's orders but were otherwise not clearly defined. The mortality ratios for gastric ulcer among current and ex-smokers were 4.1 and 3.4, respectively. Although these differences in mortality were not statistically significant, the trends were similar to those in ACS CPS-I and supported the results of that study.

Effects of Smoking on Ulcer Healing and Recurrence

Healing of Duodenal Ulcers

Numerous trials evaluating ulcer therapy have suggested that smoking adversely affects ulcer healing. Kikendall, Evaul, and Johnson (1984) reviewed the results of 18 studies that assessed the impact of smoking on healing of duodenal ulcers. In most of these studies, the percentage of healed ulcers was lower among current smokers than among nonsmokers (Table 1). These studies were not explicitly designed to study smoking, and the nonsmoking category presumably included never as well as former smokers. When the data from these studies were subjected to meta-analysis, the percentage of healed ulcers was lower among smokers than among nonsmokers in patients treated with H_2-blockers (p<0.0001) and in patients given placebo (p<0.0001) (Table 2). The median difference in percentage of subjects completely healed was 22 percentage points in favor of nonsmokers in groups treated with H_2-blockers, 21.5 percentage points in groups receiving other active therapy, and 22 percentage points in groups receiving placebo. The data for groups receiving active therapy other than H_2-blockers were not subjected to statistical analysis because the data were not homogeneous, but the data in Table 1 show that nonsmokers in most of these other treatment groups fared better than their smoking peers. Most trials published since this

1984 review show similar trends toward greater likelihood of healing of duodenal ulcers in nonsmokers.

Recently, several reports have suggested that sucralfate (Lam et al. 1987) and misoprostol (Lam et al. 1986) may have particular value in treating duodenal ulcers among patients who smoke. Lam (1989) has compiled a list of six studies showing comparable duodenal ulcer healing rates for smokers and nonsmokers treated with sucralfate. Although a few studies offer contrary data (Van Deventer, Schneidman, Walsh 1985; Martin 1989), much of the evidence suggests that sucralfate heals duodenal ulcers in smokers and nonsmokers at comparable rates.

The claim that the efficacy of prostaglandins for duodenal ulcer healing is unaffected by smoking is based on the results of a single study (Lam et al. 1986). The design of this study is unusual because patients who smoked were encouraged to abstain from smoking during the study; therefore, healing efficacy in smokers may have been due to the combined effects of misoprostol and smoking cessation. Other duodenal ulcer treatment trials (Bianchi Porro and Parente 1988; Brand et al. 1985; Nicholson 1985) showed improved healing among nonsmokers. Nicholson (1985) treated duodenal ulcer patients with 200 µg misoprostol 4 times daily and documented healing in 73 of 138 smokers (53 percent) and 66 of 93 nonsmokers (71 percent, $p<0.01$). Thus, the evidence is tenuous at best that oral prostaglandins can overcome the adverse effects of smoking on the healing of duodenal ulcers.

Other recently reported clinical trials are not systematically reviewed in this Chapter. Most of the recent trials that have analyzed the effects of smoking on duodenal ulcer healing show lower healing rates among smokers than among nonsmokers.

In contrast to the numerous comparisons of duodenal ulcer healing rates among smokers and nonsmokers, only one study has examined specifically the effect of smoking cessation on duodenal ulcer healing (Hull and Beale 1985). In this study, 70 male smokers with duodenal ulcers were advised to stop smoking and were treated with cimetidine for 3 months. Those who stopped were no more likely than those who continued smoking to have healed their ulcers on endoscopic exam at 3 months (75 vs. 81 percent, respectively, not significant). Cimetidine treatment was then stopped. Three months later, 72 percent of those who quit smoking and 39 percent of smokers were ulcer-free at repeat endoscopy ($p<0.05$) (Hull and Beale 1985). Although these results require confirmation, the findings suggest either that some of the adverse effects of smoking on duodenal ulcer disease may persist for a few weeks after cessation of smoking or that cimetidine therapy may mitigate these effects.

Recurrence of Duodenal Ulcers

A number of prospective clinical trials of maintenance therapy for duodenal ulcer have assessed the impact of smoking on ulcer recurrence. In one of the larger trials (Sontag et al. 1984), 370 subjects with previously documented duodenal ulcer, who had no active ulcer at enrollment endoscopy, were randomized to placebo or cimetidine. Endoscopy was repeated at 6 and 12 months or whenever dyspepsia occurred during the 12 months of followup. In the placebo group, smokers were more likely than nonsmokers to experience recurrence (72 vs. 21 percent, $p<0.001$). In addition,

TABLE 1.—Percentage of healed duodenal ulcers among smoking and nonsmoking patients

Reference	Drug	Duration of Rx (wk)	Smokers N[a]	Smokers %[b]	Nonsmokers N[a]	Nonsmokers %[b]	p-value	Difference in % healed
Exclusively H₂-blocker therapy								
Bianchi Porro et al. (1981)	H₂-blockers	4	76	66	36	86	<0.05	20
Korman et al. (1983)	H₂-blockers	4–6	71	63	64	95	<0.01	32
Korman, Hansky et al. (1982)	Ranitidine	4	13	62	12	100	<0.05	38
Hetzel et al. (1978)	Cimetidine	6	43	86	43	80	NS	-6
Korman et al. (1981)	Cimetidine	6	10	50	15	100	<0.05	50
Marks et al. (1980)	Cimetidine	6	19	78	10	60	NS	-18
Bardhan et al. (1979)	Cimetidine	4	94	65	40	65	NS	0
Gugler et al. (1982)	Cimetidine	8	34	64	16	94	<0.05	29
Gugler et al. (1982)	Oxmetidine	8	35	71	14	93	NS	22
Korman, Hetzel et al. (1982)	Oxmetidine	4	27	70	15	87	NS	17
Korman, Hetzel et al. (1982)	Cimetidine	4	28	68	13	92	<0.05	24

TABLE 1.—Continued

Reference	Drug	Duration of Rx (wk)	Smokers N[a]	Smokers %[b]	Nonsmokers N[a]	Nonsmokers %[b]	p-value	Difference in % healed
Active therapy other than H$_2$-blockers								
Bianchi Porro et al. (1980)	Cimetidine or pirenzepine	4	63	71	27	81	NS	10
Sonnenberg et al. (1981)	Cimetidine, pirenzepine, or placebo	4	66	54	68	73	<0.05	19
Barbara et al. (1979)	Pirenzepine	4	16	69	28	43	NS	-26
Vantrappen et al. (1982)	Arbaprostil	4	68	65	14	79	NS	14
Peterson et al. (1977)	Antacid	4	28	75	8	88	NS	13
Korman et al. (1981)	Antacid	6	13	39	12	67	<0.05	28
Marks et al. (1980)	Sucralfate	6	20	90	9	67	NS	-23
Nagy (1978)	Carbenoxolone	—	11	55	10	80	NS	25
Young and St. John (1982)	Carbenoxolone	6	14	50	6	83	NS	33
Lam et al. (1979)	Antacid ± sulpiride	—	17	59	34	91	<0.05	32
Lam et al. (1979)	Placebo or sulpiride	—	15	27	35	51	NS	24
Massarrat and Eisenmann (1981)	Antacid	8	56	48	24	75	<0.05	27

TABLE 1.—Continued

Reference	Drug	Duration of Rx (wk)	Smokers N[a]	Smokers %[b]	Nonsmokers N[a]	Nonsmokers %[b]	p-value	Difference in % healed
Placebo therapy								
Bianchi Porro et al. (1980)	Placebo	4	55	31	15	53	NS	22
Nagy (1978)	Placebo	—	11	25	11	30	NS	5
Young and St. John (1982)	Placebo	6	15	20	5	40	NS	20
Hetzel et al. (1978)	Placebo	4	42	37	42	42	NS	5
Peterson et al. (1977)	Placebo	4	25	32	13	69	<0.03	37
Vantrappen et al. (1982)	Placebo	4	65	28	26	65	<0.05	37
Barbara et al. (1979)	Placebo	4	25	28	10	50	NS	22
Korman, Hansky et al. (1982)	Placebo	4	14	0	11	36	<0.05	36
Bianchi Porro et al. (1981)	Placebo	4	62	24	20	50	<0.01	26
Bardhan et al. (1979)	Placebo	4	33	24	13	38	NS	14

NOTE: NS=not statistically significant.
[a]N=total followed in smoking category.
[b]%=percentage of total who experienced healed ulcers within specified time; p-values calculated by chi-square when not provided in paper.
SOURCE: Kikendall, Evaul, Johnson (1984).

TABLE 2.—Results of statistical analysis of pooled data from Table 1

	\multicolumn{4}{c	}{Percentage healed}	Test statistic	
	\multicolumn{2}{c	}{Smokers}	\multicolumn{2}{c	}{Nonsmokers}	Z	p-value
	N[a]	%[b]	N[a]	%[b]		
All patient groups						
H_2-blockers	449	70	278	90	7.1	<0.0001
Placebo	347	28	166	49	4.6	<0.0001
Subset of large patient groups						
H_2-blockers	284	70	183	89	5.3	<0.0001
Placebo	149	29	88	51	3.4	<0.0012

[a]N=total followed in smoking category.
[b]%=percentage of total who experienced healed ulcers within specified time.
SOURCE: Kikendall, Evaul, Johnson (1984).

smokers receiving cimetidine were as likely to experience recurrence as nonsmokers receiving placebo, leading the authors to conclude that for smokers, quitting smoking may be more important in the prevention of ulcer recurrence than receiving cimetidine treatment (Sontag et al. 1984). Table 3 displays the results of similar prospective, controlled trials of the recurrence of duodenal ulcer identified in a literature search performed in March 1990. Trials or treatment groups with fewer than 12 smokers or 12 nonsmokers and reports that did not provide the raw data relative to smoking were omitted. Smokers had more recurrences than nonsmokers in every trial or every treatment group, regardless of the treatment (even surgery) and prophylactic therapy used to achieve healing. The difference was statistically significant in about half of the studies.

The only study of larger size that failed to show even a nonsignificant advantage for nonsmokers was an Australian community-based study, not included in Table 3 because the requisite raw data were not published (Nasiry et al. 1987). This study differed from most of those listed in Table 3 in several ways, including larger numbers of exclusions, 41-percent withdrawals, primary reliance on symptoms rather than endoscopy to document recurrences, and lack of systematic effort to control the use of medications that may affect ulcer recurrence. Factors such as these may explain the disparate results.

One trial listed in Table 3 found that incremental increases of cigarette consumption were significantly associated with greater risk of duodenal ulcer recurrence (Korman et al. 1983). Massarrat, Müller, and Schmitz-Moormann (1988) and Piper, McIntosh and Hudson (1985) also found that the number of cigarettes smoked per day was a significant predictor for ulcer recurrence. Although these studies were designed to assess risk factors for recurrence of duodenal ulcer, the latter two studies are not listed in Table 3 because one did not present the necessary raw data (Massarrat, Müller, Schmitz-Moormann 1988) and the other (Piper, McIntosh, Hudson 1985) had a study design that differed from that of the studies listed in Table 3.

TABLE 3.—Recurrences of duodenal ulcer in smokers and nonsmokers in clinical trials

Reference	Prophylaxis	Followup (mo)	Smokers N[a]	Smokers %[b]	Nonsmokers N[a]	Nonsmokers %[b]	p-value
Sontag et al. (1984)	Cimetidine	12	186	34	114	18	<0.01
Bianchi Porro et al. (1982)	Cimetidine	12	66	59	40	42	NS[c]
Lauritsen et al. (1987)	Ranitidine	12	48	33	21	19	NS
Gibinski et al. (1984)	Ranitidine	12	62	45	123	11	<0.005
Cerulli et al. (1987)	Nizatidine	3	139	17	118	4	0.001
Brunner (1988)	Roxatidine acetate	6	48	48	41	20	<0.01
Lauritsen et al. (1987)	Enprostil	12	52	65	14	50	NS
Sonnenberg et al. (1981)	Various	12	33	52	33	33	NS
Battaglia et al. (1984)	Various	12	46	30	24	21	NS
Paakkonen et al. (1989)	Sucralfate	12	13	69	19	47	NS
Bynum and Koch (1989)	Sucralfate	4	58	45	64	39	NS
Classen et al. (1983)	Sucralfate	6	37	25	51	18	NS
Graffner and Lindell (1988)	Parietal cell vagotomy	60–168	190	24	116	7	<0.01
Rydning et al. (1982)	Diet	6	55	69	18	39	<0.05
Sontag et al. (1984)	Placebo	12	39	72	31	21	<0.001
Bolin et al. (1987)	Placebo	12	13	85	13	77	NS
Marks et al. (1989)	Placebo	12	21	95	12	67	<0.05
Paakkonen et al. (1989)	Placebo	12	16	88	24	67	NS
Bynum and Koch (1989)	Placebo	4	50	81	67	50	<0.01
Classen et al. (1983)	Placebo	6	39	62	45	41	NS
Cerulli et al. (1987)	Placebo	3	146	37	110	25	0.05

TABLE 3.—Continued

Reference	Prophylaxis	Followup (mo)	Smokers N[a]	Smokers %[b]	Nonsmokers N[a]	Nonsmokers %[b]	p-value
Hallerback et al. (1987)[d]	None	12	111	80	147	58	<0.001
Korman et al. (1983)	None	12	45	84	60	53	<0.01
Lam et al. (1987)	None	24	60	100	178	74[e]	<0.05
Lee, Samloff, Hardman (1985)	None	4	58	69	49	45	<0.05
Koelz and Halter (1989)	None	12	25	64	28	50	NS

NOTE: NS=not statistically significant.
[a]N=total followed in smoking category.
[b]%=percentage of total who experienced recurrence within the specified time; p-values calculated by chi-square when not provided in paper.
[c]p<0.01 when heavy smokers were compared with nonsmokers.
[d]23% of subjects in this study had gastric ulcer.
[e]Estimated from figure in paper.

Healing of Gastric Ulcers

Doll, Jones, and Pygott (1958) studied 80 smokers hospitalized with gastric ulcer. Of these, 40 randomly chosen patients were advised to stop smoking; the remaining 40 did not receive advice regarding smoking. As assessed by barium examination, the average reduction in ulcer crater size at 28 days was 78.1 percent among those advised to stop smoking and 56.6 percent among those not advised to stop ($p<0.05$). The reduction in crater size was 83.2 percent among smokers who stopped smoking completely versus 71.8 percent among those advised to stop but who did not do so. Most of the latter group substantially reduced their tobacco consumption during the trial. This study indicates that gastric ulcer patients who stopped or reduced smoking after receiving medical advice responded much better to treatment than smokers who were not advised to stop (Doll, Jones, Pygott 1958). This study, performed in the era before the availability of potent antisecretory agents, suggests that smoking cessation alters the natural history of gastric ulcer among smokers.

These findings have been confirmed by Tatsuta, Iishi, and Okuda (1987). Sixty-four Japanese outpatients with endoscopically proven gastric ulcer were treated with antacids and dicyclomine hydrochloric acid. Additionally, half of the 40 smokers were advised to stop smoking or to reduce smoking by at least one-half. Advice regarding smoking was not given to the remaining smokers. Endoscopy was repeated in 12 weeks by an endoscopist who was unaware of the patients' symptoms or smoking status. Ulcers had healed in 11 of 12 smokers (92 percent) who stopped or reduced smoking and in 7 of 28 smokers (25 percent) who continued to smoke at their pretreatment level ($p<0.001$). Ulcers also healed in 60 percent of nonsmokers (Tatsuta, Iishi, Okuda 1987).

A retrospective study (Herrmann and Piper 1973) that employed air contrast radiography to assess ulcer presence and size in 101 gastric ulcer patients found mean decreases in ulcer size at 3 weeks of 69, 73, and 84 percent, for smokers who continued to smoke, smokers who stopped smoking, and nonsmokers, respectively. Although seeming to support the findings of Doll, Jones, and Pygott (1958) and Tatsuta, Iishi, and Okuda (1987), these differences were not statistically significant (Hermann and Piper 1973). The ulcer size at entry into this study was three times as great among smokers as among nonsmokers, rendering inappropriate a comparison of the time required for complete healing among groups.

Only these three clinical studies have assessed the benefits of smoking cessation on the healing of gastric ulcer; all three demonstrate or suggest a benefit. In contrast, recent randomized therapeutic clinical trials have generally shown no advantage in gastric ulcer healing for nonsmokers compared with smokers (Wright et al. 1982; Kellow et al. 1983; Farley et al. 1985; Euler et al. 1989; McCullough et al. 1989).

Recurrence of Gastric Ulcers

Tatsuta, Iishi, and Okuda (1987) evaluated the effect of smoking cessation on the recurrence of gastric ulcers for 47 participants who had an endoscopically proven gastric ulcer within the previous 6 months but who were ulcer-free at entry into the trial.

All were treated as outpatients with antacids and dicyclomine hydrochloric acid. Half of the smokers were advised to stop smoking or to reduce cigarette consumption by at least one-half. The remainder were not given this advice. Endoscopy was repeated at 3 and 6 months or whenever symptoms recurred. Data for seven patients who failed to complete the trial were not presented or analyzed. Ulcers recurred among 9 of 12 patients who continued to smoke at their previous level and in 3 of 13 patients who quit or substantially reduced their smoking (75 vs. 23 percent, p<0.05). An ulcer recurred in 1 of 15 (7 percent) nonsmokers (Tatsuta, Iishi, Okuda 1987).

This is the only prospective, controlled study that has evaluated the effect of smoking cessation on gastric ulcer recurrence. However, the reports of several clinical trials of maintenance therapy for gastric ulcer have provided data on the impact of smoking on the trial results. All such prospective, controlled clinical trials are displayed in Table 4. Although several of these trials or treatment groups are small, every treatment group shows an advantage for nonsmokers. In two trials, the difference was statistically significant. The median percentage difference in recurrences for smokers compared with nonsmokers is 20 percentage points.

Summary

The known effects of smoking on gastroduodenal physiology include several mechanisms that might enhance an ulcer diathesis. Most of these mechanisms are rapidly reversible upon cessation of smoking. The association of smoking with increased maximal gastric acid secretory capacity has not been assessed for reversibility.

Epidemiologic studies consistently demonstrate that current smokers compared with nonsmokers are at increased risk for occurrence of and death from duodenal and gastric ulcer. The risks for former smokers are generally found to be between those of current smokers and nonsmokers.

Duodenal ulcers are less likely to heal within specific time intervals among smokers than among nonsmokers, regardless of whether patients are treated with placebo or most active therapies. Both gastric and duodenal ulcers are more likely to recur within specified periods of observation among smokers compared with nonsmokers.

A limited number of clinical trials have been performed to assess the effect of smoking cessation on the course of peptic ulcer disease. These show that smoking cessation, or in some trials, substantial reduction of daily cigarette consumption, is associated with fewer duodenal ulcers at 6 months but not at 3 months, with improved short-term healing of gastric ulcers, and with reduced recurrence of gastric ulcers.

TABLE 4.—Recurrences of gastric ulcer in smokers and nonsmokers in clinical trials

			Recurrences				
			Smokers		Nonsmokers		
Reference	Prophylaxis	Followup (mo)	N[a]	%[b]	N[a]	%[b]	p-value
Barr et al. (1983)	Cimetidine	24	10	40	14	29	NS
Gibinski et al. (1984)	Ranitidine	12	35	37	43	14	<0.025
Borsch (1988)	Roxatidine acetate	6	31	35	36	28	NS
Marks et al. (1987)	Sucralfate	6	21	33	8	13	NS
Marks et al. (1985)	Sucralfate	6	27	19	4	0	NS
Marks et al. (1987)	Placebo	6	18	67	9	33	NS
Barr et al. (1983)	Placebo	24	15	60	10	40	NS
Marks et al. (1985)	Placebo	6	23	78	7	43	NS
Lauritsen et al. (1989)	None	6	144	45	73	25	<0.05

NOTE: NS=not statistically significant.
[a] N=total followed in smoking category.
[b] %=percentage of total who experienced recurrence within the specified time; p-values calculated by chi-square when not provided in paper.

PART II. OSTEOPOROSIS AND SKIN WRINKLING

Osteoporosis

Introduction

Osteoporosis is a condition of reduced bone mass that increases the risk of fractures, especially of the hip, distal forearm, and vertebrae, after minimal trauma (Consensus Conference 1984). The most devastating outcome of osteoporosis is hip fracture, occurring in over 200,000 persons each year in the United States (Haupt and Graves 1982; Lewinnek et al. 1980). Mortality in the first years after hip fracture is increased 15 to 20 percent (Cummings and Black 1986; Gallagher et al. 1980; Jensen and Tøndevold 1979; Lewinnek et al. 1980; Miller 1978). Results from three studies indicate that approximately 15 to 25 percent of previously functionally independent persons who sustained a hip fracture remained in a long-term facility after 1 year, and 25 to 35 percent of those who returned home after a hip fracture required help in performing daily activities (Campbell 1976; Jensen and Bagger 1982; Thomas and Stevens 1974).

Osteoporotic forearm and vertebral fractures also have been found common among the elderly. Most cases do not require hospitalization or result in long-term disability (Garraway et al. 1979; Owen et al. 1982); however, the cost of caring for these fractures has been estimated to be $140 million per year (Melton and Riggs 1983).

Established risk factors for osteoporotic fractures include advanced age, white race, female sex, number of years since natural or surgical menopause, slender body build, prolonged immobilization, alcohol use, and use of certain medications (Cummings et al. 1985). Postmenopausal estrogen replacement therapy decreases the risk of osteoporotic fractures; this risk reduction is greater with longer duration of treatment (Weiss et al. 1980).

Pathophysiologic Framework

Smoking may alter risk of osteoporosis and fracture through several mechanisms. First, bone loss accelerates at menopause (Lindquist and Bengtsson 1979; Lindquist et al. 1981; Paganini-Hill et al. 1981; Richelson et al. 1984; Mazess 1982), and smokers undergo menopause 1 to 2 years earlier than never smokers (Chapter 8). Second, a thin body build increases risk of osteoporotic fracture (Daniell 1976; Hutchinson, Polansky, Feinstein 1979; Kiel et al. 1987; Paganini-Hill et al. 1981; Williams et al. 1982; Wyshak 1981), and smokers generally weigh less than nonsmokers (Chapter 10). Third, smoking has been reported to reduce the endogenous production of estrogen (MacMahon et al. 1982) and increase its metabolism (Jensen, Christiansen, Rødbro 1985; Michnovicz et al. 1986).

Smoking also may decrease the effectiveness of exogenous estrogens (Daniell 1987). Endogenous estrogen metabolism is widely believed to affect the risk of osteoporosis and fracture, and exogenous estrogen use is firmly linked with lower rates of postmenopausal bone loss and lower risk of hip, forearm, and vertebral fracture among women (Ettinger, Genant, Cann 1985; Hutchinson, Polansky, Feinstein 1979; Kreiger et al. 1982; Paganini-Hill et al. 1981; Weiss et al. 1980; Riis, Thomsen, Christiansen 1987; Kiel et al. 1987). However, a 1- to 2-year shift in age at menopause probably does not alter the risk of osteoporotic fracture substantially. Not all researchers have found differences in endogenous estrogen levels between smokers and nonsmokers (Crawford et al. 1981; Friedman, Ravnikar, Barbieri 1987). Although therapy with exogenous estrogen reduces the risk of osteoporotic fractures among women (Ettinger, Genant, Cann 1985; Hutchinson, Polansky, Feinstein 1979; Kreiger et al. 1982; Paganini-Hill et al. 1981; Weiss et al. 1980; Riis, Thomsen, Christiansen 1987; Kiel et al. 1987), it is not certain whether levels of endogenous estrogen are lower in women with osteoporosis than in women without osteoporosis (Cauley et al. 1986; Davidson et al. 1983). The likely effects on osteoporosis and fracture risk of smoking-related changes in circulating levels of male sex hormones, if such changes occur (Chapter 8, Part I), are impossible to predict.

Bone Mineral Content in Smokers Compared With Nonsmokers

Susceptibility to fractures is increased by a reduction in bone mass. Smoking has been studied extensively in relation to various measurements of bone mass.

Using radiographs of the hand, Daniell (1976) measured percent cortical area (PCA) of the second metacarpal midpoint in 103 women aged 40 to 49 years and in 208 women aged 60 to 69 years. Smoking was associated with lower PCA among older women, but there was no difference in PCA between smokers and nonsmokers among younger women. PCA loss was estimated in 80 of the women aged 60 to 69 by comparison with averages for the younger women. Smokers had significantly greater PCA loss per year after menopause compared with nonsmokers (1.02 vs. 0.69 percent/ year, respectively, $p<0.001$). Nonobese smokers had greater PCA loss per year compared with nonobese nonsmokers, but obese smokers and obese nonsmokers did not differ in PCA loss. In both smokers and nonsmokers, nonobese women lost more PCA per year after menopause than obese women. None of these comparisons controlled for age or years since menopause.

Since this first report describing "osteoporosis of the slender smokers," at least 21 other studies comparing bone mass in smokers and nonsmokers have been published (Table 5). Nine of the nineteen studies found lower bone mass in smokers compared with nonsmokers (Aloia et al. 1988; Holló, Gergely, Boross 1979; Jensen, Christiansen, Rødbro 1985; McNair et al. 1980; Mellström et al. 1982; Rundgren and Mellström 1984; Sparrow et al. 1982; Suominen et al. 1984; Slemenda et al. 1989), and the difference was statistically significant in all but one of these nine studies (Suominen et al. 1984). The population-based studies by Mellström and associates (1982) and Rundgren and Mellström (1984) are noteworthy because they controlled for potentially confounding variables. In both studies, bone mass was measured by dual photon densitometry of the heel. Mellström and colleagues (1982) reported that bone mass of the heel was significantly lower in smokers than in nonsmokers. Rundgren and Mellström (1984) reported 10 to 20 percent lower bone mass in male smokers and 15 to 30 percent lower bone mass in female smokers.

TABLE 5.—Summary of studies of smoking and bone mass

Reference	Population	Bone measurement	Findings	Comments
Daniell (1976)	103 women aged 40–49 208 women aged 60–69	PCA from x ray of the right 2nd metacarpal	Women aged 40–49 yr: no association of smoking ≥10 cig/day for ≥5 yr and PCA; women aged 60–69 yr: smokers had lower PCA than nonsmokers[a]	Using the 40–49-year-old women as baseline, the 60–69-year-old smokers lost more PCA/yr than nonsmokers, but this finding was statistically significant only among nonobese women; no control for confounding
Holló, Gergely Boross (1979)	95 men aged 61–75 49 men aged 76–90 66 women aged 61–75	BM by SPA of radius of the nondominant forearm	BM was significantly less in heavy smokers (≥20 cig/day) compared to never smokers in each age, sex strata[a]	Controlled age and sex only
McNair et al. (1980)	163 insulin-dependent diabetics aged 21–70	BM by SPA at 6 forearm sites	Mean BM compared to normal nondiabetics: Smoker <11 cig/day 9.3% less 11–15 cig/day 10.1% less >15 cig/day 12.7% less Nonsmoker 5.4% less Mean BM in smokers significantly less than mean BM in nonsmokers	All subjects were diabetic, and findings may not generalize to all smokers; no control for confounders
Lindquist et al. (1981)	130 women in a population-based study in Sweden	BM by DPA at 3rd lumbar vertebrae	Stratifying by age and menopausal status, no difference in BM between smokers and nonsmokers	Controlled for age, race, sex, menopausal status
Lindergård (1981)	136 healthy volunteers aged 20–69	BM by SPA of midshaft of forearm	No association of smoking and BM	No control for confounders

TABLE 5.—Continued

Reference	Population	Bone measurement	Findings	Comments
Mellström et al. (1982)	357 men in a population-based study in Sweden	BM by DPA at heel	BM lower in smokers vs. nonsmokers[a]	No control for confounders
Lindquist (1982)	1,462 women in a population-based study in Sweden	BM by DPA at 3rd lumbar vertebrae	Stratifying by age and menopausal status, no difference in BM between smokers and nonsmokers	Controlled for age, race, sex, menopausal status; data may include that reported in Lindquist (1981)
Sparrow et al. (1982)	341 men aged 40–80 followed for 3–5 yr	PCA x ray of right 2nd metacarpal performed at baseline and 3–5 yr later	At baseline, no difference between PCA in smokers and nonsmokers; over the 3–5-yr period, smokers lost more PCA than nonsmokers[a] ($B = -0.148$, $p = 0.03$)	Controlled only for age
Rundgren and Mellström (1984)	409 men and 559 women born in 1901–02 or 1906–07 from a population-based study in Sweden	BM by DPA at heel	BM in women was 15–30% lower in smokers vs. nonsmokers[a] and in men 10–20% lower in smokers vs. nonsmokers[a]; no difference between ex-smokers and smokers	Controlled for age, race, sex, weight, but not for menopausal status or estrogen use
Suominen et al. (1984)	142 men aged 31–75	BM by γ ray attenuation in the calcaneums	BM in smokers lower than that in nonsmokers, but not statistically significant	Multiple tests performed; controlled for age only
Johnell and Nilsson (1984)	395 49-yr-old white women randomly selected from participants in a population-based study in Sweden	BM by γ absorptiometry at the radius 1 cm and 6 cm proximal to the ulnar styloid	No association of smoking and BM in univariate or multivariate analysis	Controlled for age, race (white), sex, height, weight, age at menarche, menopausal status, number of children breast feeding, oral contraceptive use, physical activity, and calcium intake

TABLE 5.—Continued

Reference	Population	Bone measurement	Findings	Comments
Jensen, Christiansen, Rødbro (1985)	136 postmenopausal women volunteers from Sweden randomly assigned to different estrogen doses and followed for 1 yr	BM by SPA at distal radius performed at baseline and after 1 yr of estrogen treatment	At baseline, no difference in BM between smokers (smoked in prior 6 mo) and nonsmokers (no smoking in prior 6 mo); in 28 smokers treated with high doses estrogen, the mean % increase in BM was less than the mean % increase in 28 treated nonsmokers[a]	No control for confounders
Sowers, Wallace, Lemke (1985)	86 women volunteers from 2 rural communities in Iowa	BM by SPA at distal radius	No association of smoking and BM	Small study with poor power; subjects were young, limiting generalizability; no control for confounders
Cauley et al. (1986)	78 white postmenopausal women not on estrogen therapy	BM CT scan of the dominant radius at 30% of distance from wrist to elbow	No association of smoking and BM in univariate analysis	Small study with poor power; no control of confounders
Slemenda et al. (1987)	84 peri- and postmenopausal women evaluated every 4 mo for 3 yr; none on estrogen therapy	BM SPA at midshaft and distal radius	No association of smoking and BM overall in peri- and postmenopausal groups	Small study with poor power; no control of confounders
McDermott and Witte (1988)	35 smokers (≥1 ppd for ≥14 yr and currently smoking) 35 nonsmokers (never smoked); matched for age, sex, weight, height, calcium intake, menopausal status, and estrogen use	BM SPA of midradius	No association of smoking and BM	Authors state that power to detect a 5% difference between groups at $\alpha = 0.05$ was >80% in both men and women; confounding controlled by matching

TABLE 5.—Continued

Reference	Population	Bone measurement	Findings	Comments
Aloia et al. (1988)	26 menstruating white women volunteers	BM SPA of the radius and DPA of the spine	Smoking was associated with lower BM in the radius ($p<0.01$) and of the spine ($p<0.03$)	Controlled for physical activity and height only
Picard et al. (1988)	183 healthy French-Canadian women aged 40–50	BM by DPA of 2nd–4th lumbar vertebrae and by SPA of the distal radius	No association of smoking with either BM of the lumbar vertebrae or distal radius	No control for confounders
Bilbrey, Weix, Kaplan (1988)	1,069 women referred for osteoporosis screening to 18 centers in 11 States	BM by SPA of distal and midradius	No association of smoking with BM of radius	
Stevenson et al. (1989)	284 healthy women (112 premenopausal, 172 postmenopausal) volunteers aged 21–68	BM by DPA of femoral neck, Wards triangle, trochanteric region and 2nd–4th lumbar vertebrae	In premenopausal women, correlation of ppd smoked and BM of vertebrae=−0.24[a]; no association at other sites; in postmenopausal women, no association of ppd smoked and BM at any site	Controlled for menopausal status only
Slemenda et al. (1989)	84 peri- and postmenopausal women	BM by SPA of distal and midradius, DPA of lumbar spine	Significantly low BM in heavy smokers compared with nonsmokers, no difference in rates of change in BM between smokers and nonsmokers	Controlled for menopausal status (by design) and adjusted for age and body mass index

NOTE: PCA=percent cortical area; BM=bone mass; SPA=single photon absorptiometry; DPA=dual photon absorptiometry; ppd= packs/day.

[a] $p<0.05$.

Eleven other published studies reported no association between smoking and bone mineral content (Bilbrey, Weix, Kaplan 1988; Cauley et al. 1986; Johnell and Nilsson 1984; Lindergård 1981; Lindquist 1982; Lindquist et al. 1981; McDermott and Witte 1988; Picard et al. 1988; Slemenda et al. 1987; Sowers, Wallace, Lemke 1985; Stevenson et al. 1989). In addition, one study that found differences in bone mass between heavy smokers and nonsmokers reported no differences in longitudinally measured rates of bone loss (Slemenda et al. 1989). Some of these studies were small, and the findings of no association may be due to type II statistical errors, that is, the failure to find a true association (Cauley et al. 1986; Slemenda et al. 1987; Sowers, Wallace, Lemke 1985); other studies were large and had excellent statistical power (Bilbrey, Weix, Kaplan 1988; Johnell and Nilsson 1984; Lindquist 1982; McDermott and Witte 1988).

One study evaluated the effect of smoking on bone mass among women taking estrogen (Jensen, Christiansen, Rødbro 1985). Among 56 postmenopausal women who underwent replacement therapy with high doses of estrogen for 1 year, the mean percentage increase in bone mass of the distal radius was 1.01 in 28 smokers compared with 2.58 in nonsmokers. This difference was statistically significant.

Smoking as a Risk Factor for Osteoporotic Fractures

Daniell (1976) reported that 76 percent of women with osteoporotic vertebral fractures smoked 10 cigarettes or more per day for 5 years or more, compared with 43 percent of controls with no vertebral fracture. Smoking is strongly associated with age, alcohol use, and, among some populations, use of exogenous estrogens. These are potentially strong confounders of the relationship between smoking and vertebral fracture, but Daniell's comparison between cases and controls did not consider them.

Since Daniell's 1976 study, seven other case–control studies have examined the association between smoking and fracture of the hip or vertebrae (Table 6). Five of the seven case–control studies reported an increased risk of these osteoporotic fractures among smokers (Aloia et al. 1985; Cooper, Barker, Wickham 1988; Paganini-Hill et al. 1981; Seeman et al. 1983; Williams et al. 1982), and this association was statistically significant in three of the studies (Aloia et al. 1985; Cooper, Barker, Wickham 1988; Williams et al. 1982). In the study by Williams and coworkers (1982), smokers were compared with obese nonsmokers, making it difficult to assess the independent association of smoking with the risk of osteoporotic fractures. A second analysis of smoking and the risk of hip or forearm fracture among the same subjects who were studied by Williams and colleagues (1982) showed no overall association of smoking and fractures (Alderman et al. 1986). In only two case–control studies were statistical adjustments made for age and exogenous estrogen use, which are potentially strong confounding variables; in both of these studies, there was no statistically significant association of smoking and fracture risk (Paganini-Hill et al. 1981; Kreiger et al. 1982; Kreiger and Hilditch 1986).

In five cohort studies (Table 7), there was no increase in the risk of fracture among smokers (Farmer et al. 1989; Felson et al. 1988; Hemenway et al. 1988; Holbrook, Barrett-Connor, Wingard 1988; Jensen 1986). Three of these reports were based on

TABLE 6.—Summary of case–control studies of smoking and fractures

Vertebral fractures

Reference	Population	Comparison	Estimated relative risk	Comments
Daniell (1976)	Cases: 38 women aged 40–69 with acute symptomatic vertebral fractures after minimal trauma Controls: 572 women outpatient volunteers aged 50–69	≥10 cig/day for ≥5 yr vs. less	4.2[a],[b]	No control for confounders; no statistical analysis
Seeman et al. (1983)	Cases: 105 men aged 44–84 with vertebral fractures Controls: 105 men aged 44–83 with Paget's disease matched for age and length of followup	Nonobese, nondrinking, nonsmokers vs. nonobese, nondrinking smokers with no underlying disease: aged <60 aged 60–69 aged ≥70	0.8 1.6 3.1	One-third of the cases had a medical condition associated with bone loss; controls with Paget's disease may not be representative of men without vertebral fractures; design controls for age, obesity, and alcohol use
Aloia et al. (1985)	Cases: 58 white women (mean age 64.5) volunteers with vertebral fractures Controls: 58 white women volunteers matched for age	Smokers vs. nonsmokers	3.2[a],[b]	Controlled for age only; multiple other risk factors examined using univariate tests

TABLE 6.—Continued

Reference	Population	Comparison	Estimated relative risk	Comments
Paganini-Hill et al. (1981)	Cases: 91 postmenopausal women aged >80 with hip fractures Controls: 182 age, race-matched postmenopausal women	1–10 cig/day vs. none ≥11 cig/day vs. none	1.05 1.96	Adjusted for age, age at menopause, Quetelet's Index, physical activity, alcohol consumption, and exogenous estrogen use
Kreiger et al. (1982); Kreiger and Hilditch (1986)	Cases: 98 postmenopausal women aged 45–74 yr hospitalized with hip fracture Trauma Controls: 83 postmenopausal women hospitalized for trauma Nontrauma Controls: 884 postmenopausal women hospitalized for medical illness	Ever vs. never smokers Trauma controls Nontrauma controls	1.27 1.29	Adjusted for age, Quetelet's Index, months breast feeding, ovariectomy, and estrogen use
Williams et al. (1982); Alderman et al. (1986)	Cases: 344 (355) white women aged 50–74 with hip or forearm fracture Controls: 567 (562) white women from a household survey	Among estrogen nonusers Hip fractures Average weight ever smoker vs. obese never smoker Thin ever smoker vs. obese never smoker Forearm fracture Thin ever smoker vs. obese never smoker ≤1 ppd vs. never >1 ppd vs. never	6.5[b] 13.5[b] 5.4[b] 1.0 1.2	Smokers and nonsmokers were not directly compared; the comparison group for all analyses was obese nonsmokers who had used estrogen for ≥1 yr; controlled for sex and race only

TABLE 6.—Continued

Reference	Population	Comparison	Estimated relative risk	Comments
			Hip and/or forearm fractures	
Cooper, Barker, Wickham (1988)	Cases: 300 men and women aged ≥50 hospitalized for hip fracture in England Controls: 600 community volunteers matched for age and sex	Smokers vs. nonsmokers	1.7[b]	Controlled for age and sex only
Lau et al. (1988)	Cases: 400 men and women hospitalized for hip fracture in Hong Kong Controls: 400 hospitalized and 400 community volunteers matched for age and sex	Smokers vs. nonsmokers	1.3	Controlled for age and sex only

NOTE: ppd=packs/day.
[a]Calculated from data in paper cited.
[b]$p<0.05$.

large samples from the Framingham Heart Study, the Nurses Health Study, and the first National Health and Nutrition Examination Survey. In the largest study by Hemenway and colleagues (1988), 96,508 nurses reported 975 hip or forearm fractures during an average 4 years of observation. The relative risk of fracture was 1.0 in each smoking category (former smokers, smokers of 1–14 cigarettes/day, 15–25 cigarettes/day, and >25 cigarettes/day) compared with never smokers.

Smoking Cessation and Osteoporosis and Fracture

No studies have evaluated the effect of smoking cessation on osteoporosis and fracture, nor are there studies of the risk of osteoporosis or fracture in former smokers compared with continuing smokers.

Summary

There is insufficient evidence to conclude that smoking decreases bone mineral content and the risk of osteoporotic fractures. Some studies have found lower bone mineral content in smokers compared with nonsmokers, but others have not. Some, but not all, case–control studies have found a higher risk of osteoporotic fracture among smokers. Most negative studies were limited by small sample size, and most positive studies were not designed to control for potentially strong confounding variables. Analysis of data in five cohort studies has found no association of smoking with increased risk of fracture.

Skin Wrinkling

Introduction

Although wrinkling of the facial skin is nearly universal among elderly persons, it is rarely mentioned in textbooks of dermatology or medicine, and little research has been published concerning its etiology or risk factors. Skin wrinkling is associated with sun exposure (Kligman 1969; Allen, Johnson, Diamond 1973; Daniell 1971; Knox, Cockerell, Freeman 1962; Rook, Wilkinson, Ebling 1979). Wrinkling occurs with increasing age (Daniell 1971; Knox, Cockerell, Freeman 1962; Rook, Wilkinson, Ebling 1979), but even among the elderly, wrinkling usually is confined to sun-exposed areas (Kligman 1969; Allen, Johnson, Diamond 1973; Knox, Cockerell, Freeman 1962). There is limited evidence that dramatic weight loss is associated with skin wrinkling (Daniell 1971).

Pathophysiologic Framework

It is not clear how cigarette smoking may promote skin wrinkling. Some investigators have concluded that a localized finding such as wrinkling of the face and hands could not be caused by a systemic factor such as the absorbed components of cigarette smoke.

TABLE 7.—Summary of cohort studies of smoking and fractures

Reference	Population/outcome	Comparison	Relative risk	Comments
Jensen (1986)	Population-based study of 70-year-old women in Copenhagen, Denmark: 77 smoked daily for ≥20 yr; 103 never smoked. Outcome: all fractures	% smokers with fracture vs. % nonsmokers with fracture; All postmenopausal fractures Osteoporotic fractures[b]	0.9[a] 0.7[a]	All subjects were 70-yr-old women; no control for other confounders
Hemenway et al. (1988)	96,508 nurses aged 35–59 at baseline (1980) followed for 4 yr. Outcome: self-report of 975 fractures of hip or forearm	Age-adjusted fracture rate compared to: never smokers Ex-smokers Smokers 1–14 cig/day 15–24 cig/day ≥25 cig/day	1.0 1.0 1.0 1.0	A very large cohort study producing narrow CIs (upper limit 1.25), but most women were middle-aged or younger; controlled for age only
Felson et al. (1988)	5,209 men and women in the Framingham Heart Study followed retrospectively for about 30 yr. Outcome: 217 documented hip fractures	Based on cig/day	No increase	No data given, but reported no association in any analysis
Holbrook, Barrett-Connor, Wingard (1988)	975 men and women aged 50–79 at baseline, followed for 14 yr. Outcome: 33 documented hip fractures	Smokers vs. nonsmokers	1.1	Cox regression model, adjusted for age, sex, body mass index, dietary calcium, and alcohol consumption
Farmer et al. (1989)	3,595 white women in NHANES-I aged 40–77 at baseline (1971–75) followed for an average of 10 yr. Outcome: 84 documented hip fractures	Based on number of yr smoked at baseline exam	No increase	No data given, but reported no significant association; analysis adjusted for age, body mass index, menopausal status, calcium consumption, and activity

NOTE: CI=confidence interval; NHANES-I=National Health and Nutrition Examination Survey I.
[a] Calculated from data in reference.
[b] Femoral neck, proximal humerus, lower forearm, vertebral crush.

However, facial skin, and to a lesser extent, the skin of the hands contain an intradermal elastic tissue mesh that is denser and more complex than in other areas (Shelley and Wood 1974). Thus, the toxic effect of both sunlight and smoking may be most damaging in these more susceptible areas. Alternatively, damage from sunlight and smoking may simply be additive, and the threshold for clinically apparent changes from smoking may not be reached in sun-protected areas of the skin. Histopathologic examination of sun-exposed skin commonly shows abnormalities of collagen in the dermis that decrease the elastic properties of the skin, a condition known as elastosis (Marks 1976; Shelley and Wood 1974). However, the mechanism by which sunlight might cause these changes is uncertain, and there is no evidence that smoking is associated with elastosis. Cigarette smoking has been shown to decrease capillary and arteriolar blood flow in the skin acutely (Klemp, Staberg, Thomsen 1982; Reus et al. 1984; Richardson 1987), and hence, may cause tissue hypoxia. However, there is no evidence that this causes changes in skin transparency and turgor or produces wrinkles.

Smoking and Skin Wrinkling

Several studies have reported that smoking is associated with prominent skin wrinkling, particularly in the periorbital or "crow's foot" area of the face.

Ippen and Ippen (1965) defined "cigarette skin" as appearing pale, grayish, and wrinkled, especially on the cheeks, with thick skin between the wrinkles. In an examination of women aged 35 to 84, 66 of the 84 smokers had cigarette skin compared with 27 of the 140 nonsmokers (relative risk=4.1, p<0.01). This study did not adjust for differences in age or sun exposure between the smokers and nonsmokers (Ippen and Ippen 1965).

Daniell (1971) examined facial wrinkles and smoking status among 1,104 subjects, most of whom were patients or visitors to his medical practice in Redding, CA. Skin wrinkling was assessed in the crow's foot area and the adjacent areas of the forehead and cheeks and graded as one of six categories of severity. Potential confounders such as age, race (98 percent of the subjects were white), sex, sun exposure, and body weight were also measured. Smokers were more often prominently wrinkled (wrinkle score 4–6) than nonsmokers. Prominent skin wrinkling was also more common in relation to increasing age and sun exposure. The association between smoking and prominent wrinkling was found in each age, sex, and sun exposure subgroup and was statistically significant in most of the subgroups. The most heavily wrinkled class in each age–sex group was composed entirely of smokers. Wrinkling increased with duration of smoking and number of cigarettes smoked daily. Prominent skin wrinkling was more common among smokers aged 40 to 49 than among nonsmokers aged 60 to 69 years. This study provided strong evidence that smoking is associated with skin wrinkling (Daniell 1971). However, the measurements of wrinkling are not very precise, and although an attempt was made to blind the wrinkle assessment, the subjects were patients and friends of the investigator, who may have known their smoking status.

Allen, Johnson, and Diamond (1973), reported on a study that they claimed refuted the above findings, but the data presented actually supported an association between smoking and skin wrinkling in whites (Boston 1973; Daniell 1973; Weiss 1973). Using

Daniell's 6 categories of wrinkling severity, Allen, Johnson, and Diamond (1973) examined 650 persons and obtained information on age, race, sex, smoking status, and sun exposure. Biopsies of the crow's foot area also were performed on some subjects. As evidence that there is no association between smoking and skin wrinkling, the researchers reported that among 137 black subjects, only 2 had prominent wrinkling, regardless of sun exposure or smoking status. Although only fragmentary data are presented, wrinkle scores among white smokers who were exposed to the sun less than 2 hours daily were significantly higher than wrinkle scores for white nonsmokers with limited sun exposure.

In a survey of 122 new patients attending a general medical practice in England, all but 1 of whom was white, wrinkling and other skin changes were found to be much more common among smokers than nonsmokers (Model 1985). "Smoker's face" was defined as exhibiting one or more of the following: lines or wrinkles on the face, typically radiating from the corners of the lips or eyes; gaunt facial features; grayish skin; and a plethoric complexion. Smoker's face was found among 46 percent of smokers, and none of the nonsmokers were classified as having smoker's face. The association of smoking and smoker's face was statistically significant ($p<0.001$) and remained so after controlling for age, social class, sun exposure, and recent weight change. Although this study shows a striking difference between smokers and nonsmokers, it is not clear that prominent skin wrinkling is the major or most common criterion for the diagnosis of smoker's face. Thus, the association reported may not be specific for wrinkling.

Smoking Cessation and Skin Wrinkling

No studies have assessed the effect of smoking cessation on skin wrinkling. Daniell (1971) noted that prominent wrinkling was common in former smokers, but supporting data were not presented. Model (1985) reported that 8 percent of former smokers had smoker's face compared with 46 percent of smokers.

Summary

There is limited but consistent evidence that smoking is associated with prominent facial skin wrinkling among whites (Allen, Johnson, Diamond 1973; Daniell 1971; Ippen and Ippen 1965; Model 1985) but not among blacks (Allen, Johnson, Diamond 1973). It is not clear whether former smokers are less wrinkled than smokers (Daniell 1971; Model 1985).

CONCLUSIONS

1. Smokers have an increased risk of development of both duodenal and gastric ulcer, and this increased risk is reduced by smoking cessation.

2. Ulcer disease is more severe among smokers than among nonsmokers. Smokers are less likely to experience healing of duodenal ulcers and are more likely to have

recurrences of both duodenal and gastric ulcers within specified timeframes. Most ulcer medications fail to alter these tendencies.

3. Smokers with gastric or duodenal ulcers who stop smoking improve their clinical course relative to smokers who continue to smoke.

4. The evidence that smoking increases the risk of osteoporotic fractures or decreases bone mass is inconclusive, with many conflicting findings. Data on smoking cessation are extremely limited at present.

5. There is evidence that smoking is associated with prominent facial skin wrinkling in whites, particularly in the periorbital ("crow's foot") and perioral areas of the face. The effect of cessation on skin wrinkling is unstudied.

References

AINLEY, C.C., FORGACS, I.C., KEELING, P.W.N., THOMPSON, R.P.H. Outpatient endoscopic survey of smoking and peptic ulcer. *Gut* 27:648–651, 1986.

ALDERMAN, B.W., WEISS, N.S., DALING, J.R., URE, C.L., BALLARD, J.H. Reproductive history and postmenopausal risk of hip and forearm fracture. *American Journal of Epidemiology* 124(2):262–267, 1986.

ALLEN, H.B., JOHNSON, B.L., DIAMOND, S.M. Smoker's wrinkles? *Journal of the American Medical Association* 225(9):1067–1069, August 27, 1973.

ALOIA, J.F., COHN, S.H., VASWANI, A., YEH, J.K., YUEN, K., ELLIS, K. Risk factors for postmenopausal osteoporosis. *American Journal of Medicine* 78:95–100, January 1985.

ALOIA, J.F., VASWANI, A.N., YEH, J.K., COHN, S.H. Premenopausal bone mass is related to physical activity. *Archives of Internal Medicine* 148:121–123, January 1988.

ANDA, R.F., WILLIAMSON, D.F., ESCOBEDO L.G., REMINGTON, P.L. Smoking and the risk of peptic ulcer disease among women in the United States. *Archives of Internal Medicine* 150:1437–1441, July 1990..

BARBARA, L., BELSASSO, E., BIANCHI PORRO, G., BLASI, A., CAENAZZO, E., CHIERICHETTI, S.M., DI FEBO, G., DI MARIO, F., FARINI, R., GIORGI-CONCIATO, M., GROSSI, E., MANGIAMELI, A., MIGLIOLI, M., NACCARATO, R., PETRILLO, M. Pirenzepine in duodenal ulcer. A multicentre double-blind controlled clinical trial. First of two parts. *Scandinavian Journal of Gastroenterology* 11 (Supplement 57):11–15, 1979.

BARDHAN, K.D., SAUL, D.M., EDWARDS, J.L., SMITH, P.M., FETTES, M., FORREST, J., HEADING, R.C., LOGAN, R.F.A., DRONFIELD, M.W., LANGMAN, M.J., LARKWORTHY, W., HAGGIE, S.J., WYLLIE, J.H., CORBETT, C., DUTHIE, H.L., FUSSEY, I.B., HOLDSWORTH, C.D., BALMFORTH, G.V., MARUYAMA, T. Comparison of two doses of cimetidine and placebo in the treatment of duodenal ulcer: A multicentre trial. *Gut* 20(1):68–74, January 1979.

BARR, G.D., KANG, J.Y., CANALESE, J., PIPER, D.W. A two-year prospective controlled study of maintenance cimetidine and gastric ulcer. *Gastroenterology* 85(1):100–104, July 1983.

BATTAGLIA, G., FARINI, R., DI MARIO, F., PICCOLI, A., PLEBANI, M., VIANELLO, F., BURLINA, A., NACCARATO, R. Recurrence of duodenal ulcer under continuous antisecretory treatment: An approach to the detection of predictive markers. *American Journal of Gastroenterology* 79(11):831–834, November 1984.

BAUERFEIND, P., CILLUFFO, T., FIMMEL, C.J., EMDE, C., VON RITTER, C., KOHLER, W., GUGLER, R., GASSER, T., BLUM, A.L. Does smoking interfere with the effect of histamine H2-receptor antagonists on intragastric acidity in man? *Gut* 28(5): 549–556, May 1987.

BIANCHI PORRO, G., PARENTE, F. Recent developments in peptic ulcer treatment. *Scandinavian Journal of Gastroenterology* 2 (Supplement 146):159–165, 1988.

BIANCHI PORRO, G., PETRILLO, M., GROSSI, E., LAZZARONI, M., ELASHOFF, J.D., GROSSMAN, M.I. Smoking and duodenal ulcer. (Letter.) *Gastroenterology* 79(1):180–181, July 1980.

BIANCHI PORRO, G., PRADA, A., LAZZARONI, M., PETRILLO, M., BENOWITZ, N.L. Smoking and gastric inhibition by H2 antagonists. (Letter.) *Lancet* 1(8324):584, March 12, 1983.

BIANCHI PORRO, G., PRADA, A., PETRILLO, M., LAZZARONI, M. Women and duodenal ulcer. (Letter.) *British Medical Journal* 283(6285):235, July 18, 1981.

BIANCHI PORRO, G., PRADA, A., PETRILLO, M., LAZZARONI, M., ACHORD, J.L. Gastric acid secretion, smoke, and duodenal ulcer healing. (Letter.) *Gastroenterology* 82(2):394–395, February 1982.

BILBREY, G.L., WEIX, J., KAPLAN, G.D. Value of single photon absorptiometry in osteoporosis screening. *Clinical Nuclear Medicine* 13(1):7–12, January 1988.

BOLIN, T.D., DAVIS, A.E., DUNCOMBE, V.M., BILLINGTON, B. Role of maintenance sucralfate in prevention of duodenal ulcer recurrence. *American Journal of Medicine* 83(3B): 91–94, September 28, 1987.

BORSCH, G. Roxatidine acetate in the long term maintenance of gastric ulcers. *Drugs* 35(Supplement 3): 134–138, 1988.

BOSTON, D.W. Smokers' wrinkles. (Letter.) *Journal of the American Medical Association* 226(7):788, November 12, 1973.

BRAND, D.L., ROUFAIL, W.M., THOMSON, A.B.R., TAPPER, E.J. Misoprostol, a synthetic PGE$_1$ analog, in the treatment of duodenal ulcers. *Digestive Diseases and Sciences* 30(Supplement 11):147S–158S, November 1985.

BRUNNER, G. Roxatidine acetate in the long term maintenance of duodenal ulcers. *Drugs* 35(Supplement 3):102–105, 1988.

BYNUM, T.E., KOCH G. G. Sucralfate tablets 1 g twice a day for the prevention of duodenal ulcer recurrence. *American Journal of Medicine* 86(6A):127–132, June 9, 1989.

CAMPBELL, A.J. Femoral neck fractures in elderly women: A prospective study. *Age and Ageing* 5:102–109, 1976.

CAULEY, J.A., GUTAI, J.P., SANDLER, R.B., LAPORTE, R.E., KULLER, L.H., SASHIN, D. The relationship of endogenous estrogen to bone density and bone area in normal postmenopausal women. *American Journal of Epidemiology* 124(5):752–761, 1986.

CERULLI, M.A., CLOUD, M.L., OFFEN, W.W., CHERNISH, S.M., MATSUMOTO, C. Nizatidine as maintenance therapy of duodenal ulcer disease in remission. *Scandinavian Journal of Gastroenterology* (Supplement 136):79–83, 1987.

CLASSEN, M., BETHGE, H., BRUNNER, G., DIRR, B., FROTZ, H., GABOR, M., GAIL, H., GRABNER, R., HAGENMULLER, F., HEINKEL, K., KAESS, H., KERSTAN, E., KUNTZEN, O., MAIER, K., MEIDERER, S., REICHEL, W., REISSIGL, H., SCHWAMBERGER, K., SEIFERT, E., THALER, H., WEISS, W., WORDEHOFF, D., WOTZKA, R. Effect of sucralfate on peptic ulcer recurrence: A controlled double-blind multicenter study. *Scandinavian Journal of Gastroenterology* (Supplement 83):61–68, 1983.

CONSENSUS CONFERENCE. Osteoporosis. *Journal of the American Medical Association* 252(6):799–802, August 10, 1984.

COOPER, C., BARKER, D.J.P., WICKHAM, C. Physical activity, muscle strength, and calcium intake in fracture of the proximal femur in Britain. *British Medical Journal* 297:1443–1446, December 3, 1988.

CRAWFORD, F.E., BACK, D.J., L'E ORME, M., BRECKENRIDGE, A.M. Oral contraceptive steroid plasma concentrations in smokers and non-smokers. *British Medical Journal* 282:1829–1830, June 6, 1981.

CUMMINGS, S.R., BLACK, D. Should perimenopausal women be screened for osteoporosis? *Annals of Internal Medicine* 104:817–823, 1986.

CUMMINGS, S.R., KELSEY, J.L., NEVITT, M.C., O'DOWD, K.J. Epidemiology of osteoporosis and osteoporotic fractures. *Epidemiologic Reviews* 7:178–208, 1985.

DANIELL, H.W. Smoker's wrinkles. A study in the epidemiology of "crow's feet." *Annals of Internal Medicine* 75:873–880, 1971.

DANIELL, H.W. Smokers' wrinkles. (Letter.) *Journal of the American Medical Association* 226(7):788–789, November 12, 1973.

DANIELL, H.W. Osteoporosis of the slender smoker. *Archives of Internal Medicine* 136:298–304, March 1976.

DANIELL, H.W. Anti-estrogenic effect of cigarette smoke. (Letter.) *New England Journal of Medicine* 316(21):1342, May 21, 1987.

DAVIDSON, B.J., RIGGS, B.L., WAHNER, H.W., JUDD, H.L. Endogenous cortisol and sex steroids in patients with osteoporotic spinal fractures. *Obstetrics and Gynecology* 61(3):275–288, March 1983.

DEAKIN, M., RAMAGE, J.K., WILLIAMS, J.G. Smoking, gastric secretion and inhibition by cimetidine. *Biomedicine and Pharmacotherapy* 42(2):89–92, 1988.

DOLL, R., JONES, F.A., PYGOTT, F. Effect of smoking on the production and maintenance of gastric and duodenal ulcers. *Lancet* 1:657–662, March 29, 1958.

EHSANULLAH, R.S., PAGE, M.C., TILDESLEY, G., WOOD, J.R. Prevention of gastroduodenal damage induced by non-steroidal anti-inflammatory drugs: Controlled trial of ranitidine. *British Medical Journal* 297(6655):1017–1021, October 22, 1988.

ETTINGER, B., GENANT, H.K., CANN, C.E. Long-term estrogen replacement therapy prevents bone loss and fractures. *Annals of Internal Medicine* 102:319–324, 1985.

EULER, A.R., POPIELA, T., TYTGAT, G.N., KULIG, J., LOOKABAUGH, J.L., PHAN, T.D., KITT, M.M. A multiclinic trial evaluating arbaprostil (15(R)-15-methyl prostaglandin E2) as a therapeutic agent for gastric ulcer. *Gastroenterology* 96(4):967–971, April 1989.

FARLEY, A., LÉVESQUE, D., PARÉ, P., THOMSON, A.B.R., SHERBANIUK, R., ARCHAMBAULT, A., MAHONEY, K. A comparative trial of ranitidine 300 mg at night with ranitidine 150 mg twice daily in the treatment of duodenal and gastric ulcer. *American Journal of Gastroenterology* 80(9):665–668, 1985.

FARMER, M.E., HARRIS, T., MADANS, J.H., WALLACE, R.B., CORNONI-HUNTLEY, J., WHITE, L.R. Anthropometric indicators and hip fracture. The NHANES I epidemiologic followup study. *Journal of the American Geriatrics Society* 37:9–16, 1989.

FELSON, D.T., KIEL, D.P., ANDERSON, J.J., KANNEL, W.B. Alcohol consumption and hip fractures: The Framingham Study. *American Journal of Epidemiology* 128(5):1102–1110, 1988.

FRIEDMAN, A.J., RAVNIKAR, V.A., BARBIERI, R.L. Serum steroid hormone profiles in postmenopausal smokers and nonsmokers. *Fertility and Sterility* 47(3):398–401, March 1987.

GALLAGHER, J.C., MELTON, L.J., RIGGS, B.L., BERGSTRATH, E. Epidemiology of fractures of the proximal femur in Rochester, Minnesota. *Clinical Orthopaedics and Related Research* 150:163–171, July–August 1980.

GARRAWAY, W.M., STAUFFER, R.N., KURLAND, L.T., O'FALLON, W.M. Limb fractures in a defined population. II. Orthopedic treatment and utilization of health care. *Mayo Clinic Proceedings* 54:708–713, 1979.

GIBINSKI, K., NOWAK, A., GABRYELEWICZ, A., SZALAJ, W., HASIK, J., KLINCEWICZ, H., BUTRUK, E., KOSECKI, P., POKORA, J., RADWAN, P. Ranitidine in the maintenance therapy of gastro-duodenal ulcer disease: Polish open multicentre study. *Hepatogastroenterology* 31(4):180–182, August 1984.

GRAFFNER, H., LINDELL, G. Increased ulcer relapse rate after PCV in smokers. *World Journal of Surgery* 12(2):277–281, April 1988.

GRAHAM, D.Y. *Campylobacter pylori* and duodenal ulcer disease. *Gastroenterology* 96:615–625, 1989.

GRIFFIN, M.R., RAY, W.A., SCHAFFNER, W. Nonsteroidal anti-inflammatory drug use and death from peptic ulcer in elderly persons. *Annals of Internal Medicine* 109(5):359–363, September 1, 1988.

GUGLER, R., ROHNER, H.-G., KRATOCHVIL, P., BRANDSTATTER, G., SCHMITZ, H. Effect of smoking on duodenal ulcer healing with cimetidine and oxmetidine. *Gut* 23(10):866–871, October 1982.

HALLERBACK, B., SOLHAUG, J.-H., CARLING, L., GLISE, H., HALLGREN, T., KAGEVI, I., SVEDBERG, L.-E., WAHLBY, L. Recurrent ulcer after treatment with cimetidine or sucralfate. *Scandinavian Journal of Gastroenterology* 22(7):791–797, 1987.

HAUPT, B.J., GRAVES, E.H. *Detailed Diagnoses and Surgical Procedures for Patients Discharged from Short-Stay Hospital: United States, 1979.* US DHHS Publication No. 82-1274-1, 1982.

HEMENWAY, D., COLDITZ, G.A., WILLETT, W.C., STAMPFER, M.J., SPEIZER, F.E. Fractures and lifestyle: Effect of cigarette smoking, alcohol intake, and relative weight on the risk of hip and forearm fractures in middle-aged women. *American Journal of Public Health* 78(12):1554–1558, December 1988.

HERRMANN, R.P., PIPER, D.W. Factors influencing the healing rate of chronic gastric ulcer. *American Journal of Digestive Diseases* 18(1):1–6, January 1973.

HETZEL, D.J., HANSKY, P.J., SHEARMAN, D.J., KORMAN, M.G., HECKER, R., TAGGART, G.J., JACKSON, R., GABB, B.W. Cimetidine treatment of duodenal ulceration: Short term clinical trial and maintenance study. *Gastroenterology* 74(2, Part 2):389–392, February 1978.

HEUMAN, R., LARSSON, J., NORRBY, S. Perforated duodenal ulcer—Long term results following simple closure. *Acta Chirurgica Scandinavica* 149(1):77–81, 1983.

HIGGINS, M.W., KJELSBERG, M. Characteristics of smokers and nonsmokers in Tecumseh, Michigan. II. The distribution of selected physical measurements and physiologic variables and the prevalence of certain diseases in smokers and nonsmokers. *American Journal of Epidemiology* 86(1):60–77, 1967.

HODNETT, R.M., GONZALEZ, F., LEE, W.C., NANCE, F.C., DEBOISBLANC, R. The need for definitive therapy in the management of perforated gastric ulcers. Review of 202 cases. *Annals of Surgery* 209(1):36–39, January 1989.

HOLBROOK, T.L., BARRETT-CONNOR, E., WINGARD, D.L. Dietary calcium and risk of hip fracture: 14-year prospective population study. *Lancet* 2:1046–1049, November 5, 1988.

HOLLO, I., GERGELY, I., BOROSS, M. Influence of heavy smoking upon the bone mineral content of the radius of the aged and effect of tobacco smoke on the sensitivity to calcitonin of rats. *Aktuel Gerontologie* 9:365–368, 1979.

HULL, D.H., BEALE, P.J. Cigarette smoking and duodenal ulcer. *Gut* 26:1333–1337, 1985.

HUTCHINSON, T.A., POLANSKY, S.M., FEINSTEIN, A.R. Post-menopausal oestrogens protect against fractures of hip and distal radius. A case-control study. *Lancet* 2:705–709, October 6, 1979.

IPPEN, M., IPPEN, H. Approaches to a prophylaxis of skin aging. *Journal of the Society of Cosmetic Chemists* 16:305–308, 1965.

JENSEN, G.F. Osteoporosis of the slender smoker revisited by epidemiologic approach. *European Journal of Clinical Investigation* 16:239–242, 1986.

JENSEN, J., CHRISTIANSEN, C., RØDBRO, P. Cigarette smoking, serum estrogens, and bone loss during hormone-replacement therapy early after menopause. *New England Journal of Medicine* 313(16):973–975, 1985.

JENSEN, J.S., BAGGER, J. Long-term social prognosis after hip fractures. *Acta Orthopaedica Scandinavica* 53:97–101, 1982.

JENSEN, J.S., TØNDEVOLD, E. Mortality after hip fractures. *Acta Orthopaedica Scandinavica* 50:161–167, 1979.

JOHNELL, O., NILSSON, B.E. Life-style and bone mineral mass in perimenopausal women. *Calcified Tissue International* 36:354–356, 1984.

KELLOW, J.E., BARR, G.D., COWEN, A.E., WARD, M., WOOD, L., PIPER, D.W. Comparison of ranitidine and cimetidine in the treatment of chronic gastric ulcer. *Digestion* 27(2):105–110, June 1983.

KIEL, D.P., FELSON, D.T., ANDERSON, J.J., WILSON, P.W.F., MOSKOWITZ, M.A. Hip fracture and the use of estrogens in postmenopausal women. The Framingham Study. *New England Journal of Medicine* 317(19):1169–1174, November 5, 1987.

KIKENDALL, J.W., EVAUL, J., JOHNSON, L.F. Effect of cigarette smoking on gastrointesinal physiology and non-neoplastic digestive disease. *Journal of Clinical Gastroenterology* 6(1):65–78, February 1984.

KLEMP, P., STABERG, B., THOMSEN, K. Skin circulation in regular smokers. *Ugeskr Laeger* 144(22):1604–1606, May 31, 1982.

KLIGMAN, A.M. Early destructive effect of sunlight on human skin. *Journal of the American Medical Association* 210(13):2377–2380, December 29, 1969.

KNOX, J.M., COCKERELL, E.G., FREEMAN, R.G. Etiological factors and premature aging. *Journal of the American Medical Association* 179(8):630–636, February 24, 1962.

KOELZ, H.R., HALTER, F. Sucralfate and ranitidine in the treatment of acute duodenal ulcer: Healing and relapse. *American Journal of Medicine* 86(6A):98–103, June 9, 1989.

KORMAN, M.G., HANSKY, J., EAVES, E.R., SCHMIDT, G.T. Influence of cigarette smoking on healing and relapse in duodenal ulcer disease. *Gastroenterology* 85:871–874, 1983.

KORMAN, M.G., HANSKY, J., MERRETT, A.C., SCHMIDT, G.T. Ranitidine in duodenal ulcer. Incidence of healing and effect of smoking. *Digestive Diseases and Sciences* 27(8):712–715, August 1982.

KORMAN, M.G., HETZEL, D.J., HANSKY, J., SHEARMAN, D.J.C., EAVES, E.R., SCHMIDT, G.T., HECKER, R., FITCH, R. Oxmetidine or cimetidine in duodenal ulcer: Healing rate and effect of smoking. *Gastroenterology* 82:1104, 1982.

KORMAN, M.G., SHAW, R.G., HANSKY, J., SCHMIDT, G.T., STERN, A.I. Influence of smoking on healing rate of duodenal ulcer in response to cimetidine or high-dose antacid. *Gastroenterology* 80(6):1451–1453, June 1981.

KREIGER, N., HILDITCH, S. Cigarette smoking and estrogen-dependent diseases. (Letter.) *American Journal of Epidemiology* 123(1):200, 1986.

KREIGER, N., KELSEY, J.L., HOLFORD, T.R., O'CONNOR, T. An epidemiologic study of hip fracture in postmenopausal women. *American Journal of Epidemiology* 116(1):141–148, 1982.

KURATA, J.H., ELASHOFF, J.D., HAILE, B.M., HONDA, G.D. A reappraisal of time trends in ulcer disease: Factors related to changes in ulcer hospitalization and mortality rates. *American Journal of Public Health* 73(9):1066–1072, 1983.

KURATA, J.H., ELASHOFF, J.D., NOGAWA, A.N., HAILE, B.M. Sex and smoking differences in duodenal ulcer mortality. *American Journal of Public Health* 76(6):700–702, June 1986.

LAM, S.-K. Implications of sucralfate-induced ulcer healing and relapse. *American Journal of Medicine* 86 (6A):122–126, June 9, 1989.

LAM, S.-K., HUI, W.M., LAU, W.Y., BRANICKI, F.J. Sucralfate overcomes adverse effect of cigarette smoking on duodenal ulcer healing and prolongs subsequent remission. *Gastroenterology* 92(5):1193–1201, May 1987.

LAM, S.-K., LAM, K.C., LAI, C.L., YEUNG, C.K., YAM, L.Y., WONG, W.S. Treatment of duodenal ulcer with antacid and sulpiride. A double-blind controlled study. *Gastroenterology* 76(2):315–322, February 1979.

LAM, S.-K., LAU, W.-Y., CHOI, T.-K., LAI, C.-L., LOK, A.S.F., HUI, W.-M., NG, M.M.T., CHOI, S.K.Y. Prostaglandin E_1 (misoprostol) overcomes the adverse effect of chronic cigarette smoking on duodenal ulcer healing. *Digestive Diseases and Sciences* 31(2):68S–74S, February 1986.

LAU, E., DONNAN, S., BARKER, D.J.P., COOPER, C. Physical activity and calcium intake in fracture of the proximal femur in Hong Kong. *British Medical Journal* 297:1441–1443, December 3, 1988.

LAURITSEN, K., DANISH OMEPRAZOLE STUDY GROUP. Relapse of gastric ulcers after healing with omeprazole and cimetidine. A double-blind follow-up study. *Scandinavian Journal of Gastroenterology* 24(5):557–560, June 1989.

LAURITSEN, K., HAVELUND, T., LAURSEN, L.S., BYTZER, P., KJAERGAARD, J., RASK-MADSEN, J. Enprostil and ranitidine in prevention of duodenal ulcer relapse: One-year double blind comparative trial. *British Medical Journal* 294(6577):932–934, April 11, 1987.

LEE, F.I., SAMLOFF, I.M., HARDMAN, M. Comparison of tri-potassium di-citrato bismuthate tablets with ranitidine in healing and relapse of duodenal ulcers. *Lancet* 1(8441):1299–1302, June 1985.

LEWINNEK, G.E., KELSEY, J., WHITE, A.A. III, KREIGER, N.J. The significance and a comparative analysis of the epidemiology of hip fractures. *Clinical Orthopaedics and Related Research* 152:35–43, October 1980.

LINDERGÅRD, B. Bone mineral content measured by photon absorptiometry—A methodological study carried out on normal individuals. *Scandinavian Journal of Urology and Nephrology* 59(Supplement):1–37, 1981.

LINDQUIST, O. Influence of the menopause on ischaemic heart disease and its risk factors and on bone mineral content. *Acta Obstetricia et Gynecologica Scandinavica* 110(Supplement):1–32, 1982.

LINDQUIST, O., BENGTSSON, C. The effect of smoking on menopausal age. *Maturitas* 1:171–173, 1979.

LINDQUIST, O., BENGTSSON, C., HANSSON, T., ROOS, B. Bone mineral content in relation to age and menopause in middle-aged women. *Scandinavian Journal of Clinical Laboratory Investigation* 41:215–223, 1981.

MACMAHON, B., TRICHOPOULOS, D., COLE, P., BROWN, J. Cigarette smoking and urinary estrogens. *New England Journal of Medicine* 307(17):1062–1065, October 21, 1982.

MARKS, I.N., GIRDWOOD, A.H., NEWTON, K.A., O'KEEFE, S.J., MAROTTA, F., LUCKE, W. A maintenance regimen of sucralfate 2 g at night for reduced relapse rate in duodenal ulcer disease. A one-year follow-up study. *American Journal of Medicine* 86(6A):136–140, June 9, 1989.

MARKS, I.N., GIRDWOOD, A.H., WRIGHT, J.P., NEWTON, K.A., GILINSKY, N.H., KALVARIA, I., BURNS, D.G., O'KEEFE, S.J., TOBIAS, R., LUCKE, W. Nocturnal dosage regimen of sucralfate in maintenance treatment of gastric ulcer. *American Journal of Medicine* 83(3B):95–98, September 28, 1987.

MARKS, I.N., WRIGHT, J.P., DENYER, M., GARISCH, J.A.M., LUCKE, W. Comparison of sucralfate with cimetidine in the short-term treatment of chronic peptic ulcers. *South African Medical Journal* 57(15):567–572, April 12, 1980.

MARKS, I.N., WRIGHT, J.P., GIRDWOOD, A.H., GILINSKY, N.H., LUCKE, W. Maintenance therapy with sucralfate reduces rate of gastric ulcer recurrence. *American Journal of Medicine* 79(Supplement 2C):32–35, August 30, 1985.

MARKS, R. *Common Facial Dermatoses.* Bristol: John Wright and Sons, 1976.

MARTIN, F. Sucralfate suspension 1 g four times per day in the short-term treatment of active duodenal ulcer. *American Journal of Medicine* 86(6A):104–107, June 9, 1989.

MASSARRAT, S., EISENMANN, A. Factors affecting the healing rate of duodenal and pyloric ulcers with low-dose antacid treatment. *Gut* 22:97–102, 1981.

MASSARRAT, S., MÜLLER, H.G., SCHMITZ-MOORMANN, P. Risk factors for healing of duodenal ulcer under antacid treatment: Do ulcer patients need individual treatment? *Gut* 29(3):291–297, March 1988.

MAZESS, R.B. On aging bone loss. *Clinical Orthopaedics and Related Research* 165:239–252, May 1982.

MCCULLOUGH, A.J., GRAHAM, D.Y., KNUFF, T.E., LANZA, F.L., LEVENSON, H.L., LYON, D.T., MUNSELL, W.P., PEROZZA, J., ROUFAIL, W.M., SINAR, D.R., ET AL. Suppression of nocturnal acid secretion with famotidine accelerates gastric ulcer healing. *Gastroenterology* 97(4):860–866, October 1989.

MCDERMOTT, M.T., WITTE, M.C. Bone mineral content in smokers. *Southern Medical Journal* 81(4):477–480, April 1988.

MCNAIR, P., CHRISTENSEN, M.S., MADSBAD, S., CHRISTIANSEN, C., BINDER, C., TRANSBOL, I. Bone loss in patients with diabetes mellitus: Effects of smoking. *Mineral and Electrolyte Metabolism* 3:94–97, 1980.

MELLSTRÖM, D., RUNDGREN, Å., JAGENBURG, R., STEEN, B., SVANBORG, A. Tobacco smoking, ageing and health among the elderly: A longitudinal population study of 70-year-old men and an age cohort comparison. *Age and Ageing* 11:45–58, 1982.

MELTON, L.J. III, RIGGS, B.L. Epidemiology of age-related fractures. In: Avioli (ed.) *The Osteoporosis Syndrome: Detection, Prevention and Treatment.* New York: Grune and Stratton, 1983, pp. 45–72.

MICHNOVICZ, J.J., HERSHCOPF, R.J., NAGANUMA, H., BRADLOW, H.L., FISHMAN, J. Increased 2-hydroxylation of estradiol as a possible mechanism for the anti-estrogenic effect of cigarette smoking. *New England Journal of Medicine* 315(21):1305–1309, November 20, 1986.

MILLER, C.W. Survival and ambulation following hip fracture. *Journal of Bone and Joint Surgery* 60A:930–934, 1978.

MODEL, D. Smoker's face: An underrated clinical sign? *British Medical Journal* 291:1760–1762, December 21–28, 1985.

MUELLER-LISSNER, S.A. Bile reflux is increased in cigarette smokers. *Gastroenterology* 90(5):1205–1209, May 1986.

NAGY, G.S. Evaluation of carbenoxolone sodium in the treatment of duodenal ulcer. *Gastroenterology* 74(1):7–10, January 1978.

NASIRY, R.W., MCINTOSH, J.H., BYTH, K., PIPER, D.W. Prognosis of chronic duodenal ulcer: A prospective study of the effects of demographic and environmental factors and ulcer healing. *Gut* 28:533–540, 1987.

NICHOLSON, P.A. A multicenter international controlled comparison of two dosage regimens of misoprostol and cimetidine on the treatment of duodenal ulcer in out-patients. *Digestive Diseases and Sciences* 30(Supplement 11):171S–177S, November 1985.

OWEN, R.A., MELTON, L.J. III, JOHNSON, K.A., ILSTRUP, D.M., RIGGS, B.L. Incidence of Colles' fracture in a North American community. *American Journal of Public Health* 72(6):605–607, June 1982.

PAAKKONEN, M., AUKEE, S., JANATUINEN, E., LAHTINEN, J., LAXEN, F., OLSEN, M., PIKKARAINEN, P., POIKOLAINEN, E. Sucralfate as maintenance treatment for the prevention of duodenal ulcer recurrence. *American Journal of Medicine* 86(6A): 133–135, June 9, 1989.

PAGANINI-HILL, A., ROSS, R.K., GERKINS, V.R., HENDERSON, B.E., ARTHUR, M., MACK, T.M. Menopausal estrogen therapy and hip fractures. *Annals of Internal Medicine* 95:28–31, 1981.

PARENTE, F., LAZZARONI, M., SANGALETTI, O., BARONI, S., BIANCHI PORRO, G. Cigarette smoking, gastric acid secretion, and serum pepsinogen I concentrations in duodenal ulcer patients. *Gut* 26(12):1327–1332, December 1985.

PETERSON, W.L., STURDEVANT, R.A.L., FRANKL, H.D., RICHARDSON, C.T., ISENBERG, J.I., ELASHOFF, J.D., SONES, J.Q., GROSS, R.A., MCCALLUM, R.W., FORDTRAN, J.S. Healing of duodenal ulcer with an antacid regimen. *New England Journal of Medicine* 297(7):341–345, August 18, 1977.

PICARD, D., STE-MARIE, L.G., COUTU, D., CARRIER, L., CHARTRAND, R., LEPAGE, R., FUGÈRE, P., D'AMOUR, P. Premenopausal bone mineral content relates to height, weight and calcium intake during early adulthood. *Bone and Mineral* 4:299–309, 1988.

PIPER, D.W., MCINTOSH, J.H., HUDSON, H.M. Factors relevant to the prognosis of chronic duodenal ulcer. *Digestion* 31(17):9–16, January 1985.

QUIMBY, G.F., BONNICE, C.A., BURSTEIN, S.H., EASTWOOD, G.L. Active smoking depresses prostaglandin synthesis in human gastric mucosa. *Annals of Internal Medicine* 104(5):616–619, May 1986.

REUS, W.F., ROBSON, M.C., ZACHARY, L., HEGGERS, J.P. Acute effects of tobacco smoking on blood flow in the cutaneous micro-circulation. *British Journal of Plastic Surgery* 37:213–215, 1984.

RICHARDSON, D. Effects of tobacco smoke inhalation on capillary blood flow in human skin. *Archives of Environmental Health* 42(1):19–25, January–February 1987.

RICHELSON, L.S., WAHNER, H.W., MELTON, L.J. III, RIGGS, B.L. Relative contributions of aging and estrogen deficiency to postmenopausal bone loss. *New England Journal of Medicine* 311(20):1273–1275, 1984.

RIIS, B., THOMSEN, K., CHRISTIANSEN, C. Does calcium supplementation prevent postmenopausal bone loss? A double-blind, controlled clinical study. *New England Journal of Medicine* 316(4):173–177, January 22, 1987.

ROBERT, M.E., LEUNG F.W., GUTH, P.H. Nicotine and smoking do not decrease basal gastric mucosal blood flow in anesthetized rats. *Digestive Diseases and Sciences* 31(5):530–534, May 1986.

ROOK, A., WILKINSON, D.S., EBLING, F.J.G. (eds.) *Textbook of Dermatology*, Volume 2. Third Edition. London: Blackwell Scientific Publications, 1979.

ROSS, A.H., SMITH, M.A., ANDERSON, J.R., SMALL, W.P. Late mortality after surgery for peptic ulcer. *New England Journal of Medicine* 307(9):519–522, 1982.

RUNDGREN, Å., MELLSTRÖM, D. The effect of tobacco smoking on the bone mineral content of the ageing skeleton. *Mechanisms of Ageing and Development* 28:273–277, 1984.

RYDNING, A., AADLAND, E., BERSTAD, A., ODEGAARD, B. Prophylactic effect of dietary fibre in duodenal ulcer disease. *Lancet* 2(8301):736–739, October 2, 1982.

SEEMAN, E., MELTON, L.J. III, O'FALLON, W.M., RIGGS, B.L. Risk factors for spinal osteoporosis in men. *American Journal of Medicine* 75:977–983, December 1983.

SHELLEY, W.B., WOOD, M.G. Unilateral wrinkles. Manifestation of unilateral elastic tissue defect. *Archives of Dermatology* 110:775–778, November 1974.

SLEMENDA, C.W., HUI, S.L., LONGCOPE, C., JOHNSTON, C.C. JR. Sex steroids and bone mass. A study of changes about the time of menopause. *Journal of Clinical Investigation* 80:1261–1269, November 1987.

SLEMENDA, C.W., HUI, S.L., LONGCOPE, C., JOHNSTON, C.C. JR. Cigarette smoking, obesity, and bone mass. *Journal of Bone and Mineral Research* 4(5):737–741, October 1989.

SMEDLEY, F., HICKISH, T., TAUBE, M., YALE, C., LEACH, R., WASTELL, C. Perforated duodenal ulcer and cigarette smoking. *Journal of the Royal Society of Medicine* 81(2):92–94, February 1988.

SONNENBERG, A. Smoking and mortality from peptic ulcer in the United Kingdom. *Gut* 27(11):1369–1372, November 1986.

SONNENBERG, A., MUELLER-LISSNER, S.A., VOGEL, E., SCHMID, P., GONVERS, J.J., PETER, P., STROHMEYER, G., BLUM, A.L. Predictors of duodenal ulcer healing and relapse. *Gastroenterology* 81(6):1061–1067, December 1981.

SONTAG, S., GRAHAM, D.Y., BELSITO, A., WEISS, J., FARLEY, A., GRUNT, R., COHEN, N., KINNEAR, D., DAVIS, W., ARCHAMBAULT, A., ACHORD, J., THAYER, W., GILLIES, R., SIDOROV, J., SABESIN, S.M., DYCK, W., FLESHLER, B., CLEATOR, I., WENGER, J., OPEKUN, A. JR. Cimetidine, cigarette smoking, and recurrence of duodenal ulcer. *New England Journal of Medicine* 311(11):689–693, September 13, 1984.

SOWERS, M.F., WALLACE, R.B., LEMKE, J.H. Correlates of forearm bone mass among women during maximal bone mineralization. *Preventive Medicine* 14:585–596, 1985.

SPARROW, D., BEAUSOLEIL, N.I., GARVEY, A.J., ROSNER, B., SILBERT, J.E. The influence of cigarette smoking and age on bone loss in men. *Archives of Environmental Health* 37(4):246–249, July–August 1982.

STEVENSON, J.C., LEES, B., DEVENPORT, M., CUST, M.P., GANGER, K.F. Determinants of bone density in normal women: Risk factors for future osteoporosis? *British Medical Journal* 298:924–928, April 8, 1989.

SUOMINEN, H., HEIKKINEN, E., VAINIO, P., LAHTINEN, T. Mineral density of calcaneus in men at different ages: A population study with special reference to life-style factors. *Age and Ageing* 13:273–281, 1984.

TATSUTA, M., IISHI, H., OKUDA, S. Effects of cigarette smoking on the location, healing and recurrence of gastric ulcers. *Hepato-gastroenterology* 5(34):223–228, October 1987.

THOMAS, T.G., STEVENS, R.S. Social effects of fractures of the neck of the femur. *British Medical Journal* 3:456–458, 1974.

U.S. DEPARTMENT OF HEALTH AND HUMAN SERVICES. *Reducing the Health Consequences of Smoking: 25 Years of Progress. A Report of the Surgeon General.* U.S. Department of Health and Human Services, Public Health Service, Centers for Disease Control, Center for Chronic Disease Prevention and Health Promotion, Office on Smoking and Health. DHHS Publication No. (CDC) 89-8411, 1989.

U.S. DEPARTMENT OF HEALTH, EDUCATION, AND WELFARE. *The Health Consequences of Smoking. A Report of the Surgeon General: 1971.* U.S. Department of Health, Education, and Welfare, Public Health Service, Health Services and Mental Health Administration. DHEW Publication No. (HSM) 71-7513, 1971.

U.S. DEPARTMENT OF HEALTH, EDUCATION, AND WELFARE. *The Health Consequences of Smoking. A Report of the Surgeon General: 1972.* U.S. Department of Health, Education, and Welfare, Public Health Service, Health Services and Mental Health Administration. DHEW Publication No. (HSM) 72-7516, 1972.

U.S. DEPARTMENT OF HEALTH, EDUCATION, AND WELFARE. *Smoking and Health. A Report of the Surgeon General.* U.S. Department of Health, Education, and Welfare, Public Health Service, Office of the Assistant Secretary for Health, Office on Smoking and Health. DHEW Publication No. (PHS) 79-50066, 1979.

U.S. PUBLIC HEALTH SERVICE. *Smoking and Health. Report of the Advisory Committee to the Surgeon General of the Public Health Service.* U.S. Department of Health, Education, and Welfare, Public Health Service, Center for Disease Control. PHS Publication No. 1103, 1964.

VAN DEVENTER, G.M., SCHNEIDMAN, D., WALSH, J.H. Sucralfate and cimetidine as single agents and in combination for treatment of active duodenal ulcers. A double-blind, placebo-controlled trial. *American Journal of Medicine* 79(Supplement 2C):39–44, August 30, 1985.

VANTRAPPEN, G., JANSSENS, J., POPIELA, T., KULIG, J., TYTGAT, G.N., HUIBREGTSE, K., LAMBERT, R., PAUCHARD, J.P., ROBERT, A. Effect of 15(R)-15-methyl prostaglandin E_2 (arbaprostil) on the healing of duodenal ulcer: A double-blind multicenter study. *Gastroenterology* 83(2):357–363, August 1982.

WEISS, N.S., URE, C.L., BALLARD, J.H., WILLIAMS, A.R., DALING, J.R. Decreased risk of fractures of the hip and lower forearm with postmenopausal use of estrogen. *New England Journal of Medicine* 303(21):1195–1198, 1980.

WEISS, W. Smokers' wrinkles. (Letter.) *Journal of the American Medical Association* 226(7):788, November 12, 1973.

WHITFIELD, P.F., HOBSLEY, M. Maximal gastric secretion in smokers and nonsmokers with duodenal ulcer. *British Journal of Surgery* 72(12):955–957, December 1985.

WILLIAMS, A.R., WEISS, N.S., URE, C.L., BALLARD, J., DALING, J.R. Effect of weight, smoking, and estrogen use on the risk of hip and forearm fractures in postmenopausal women. *Obstetrics and Gynecology* 60(6):695–999, December 1982.

WILLOUGHBY, J.M.T., ESSIGMAN, W.K., WEBER, J.C.P., PINERUA, R.F. Smoking and peptic ulcer in rheumatoid arthritis. *Clinical and Experimental Rheumatology* 4(1):31–35, January–March 1986.

WRIGHT, J.P., MARKS, I.N., MEE, A.S., GIRDWOOD, A.H., BORNMAN, P.C., GILINSKY, N.H., TOBIAS, P., LUCKE, W. Ranitidine in the treatment of gastric ulceration. *South African Medical Journal* 61(5):155–158, January 1982.

WYSHAK, G. Hip fracture in elderly women and reproductive history. *Journal of Gerontology* 36(4):424–427, 1981.

YEOMANS, N.D., ELLIOTT, S.L., EDWARDS, J., BUCHANAN, R., STURROCK, D., SMALLWOOD, R. Gastroduodenal damage during therapy with nonsteroidal anti-inflammatory drugs: Prevalence in arthritis clinic patients and effect of smoking. (Abstract.) *Gastroenterology* 94(5, Part 2):A510, May 1988.

YOUNG, G.P., ST. JOHN, D.J.B. Smoking and ulcer healing. (Letter.) *Gastroenterology* 82(1):163, January 1982.

CHAPTER 10
SMOKING CESSATION AND BODY WEIGHT CHANGE

CONTENTS

Introduction 473
Amount of Weight Gain After Smoking Cessation and Likelihood of Gaining
  Weight 473
Causes of Postcessation Weight Gain 483
  Food Intake 484
  Physical Activity 486
  Energy Expenditure 487
Relationship Between Overweight and Adverse Medical and Psychosocial
  Outcomes 490
Change in Weight-Related Health Risks After Smoking Cessation 497
Strategies to Control Postcessation Weight Gain 500
  Behavioral Methods for Reducing Postcessation Weight Gain 500
  Pharmacologic Methods for Reducing Postcessation Weight Gain 502
Conclusions 505
References 507

INTRODUCTION

Cigarette smoking is associated with decreased body weight, and many smokers report that a major reason they smoke is to reduce body weight (Grunberg 1986; Klesges et al. 1989; US DHHS 1988a). However, as documented in this Chapter, the weight gain associated with smoking cessation is generally small and poses a minimal health risk.

This Chapter is organized into six sections. Drawing from prospective investigations meeting specific criteria, the first section of this Chapter determines average weight gain following smoking cessation compared with continued smoking, assesses the percentage of continuing smokers and quitters gaining weight, and calculates the risk of gaining weight after smoking cessation versus continued smoking. The next section of this Chapter discusses the mechanisms responsible for weight gain after smoking cessation. The available literature is reviewed on dietary, activity, and metabolic changes after smoking cessation. The third section reviews the relationship between body weight and adverse medical and psychosocial outcomes. The fourth section examines whether weight-related health effects accompany weight gain in ex-smokers. The fifth section presents potential treatments for reducing postcessation weight gain, including pharmacologic (e.g., nicotine polacrilex gum, phenylpropanolamine, and d-fenfluramine) and nonpharmacologic approaches. The sixth section presents conclusions regarding smoking cessation and body weight change.

AMOUNT OF WEIGHT GAIN AFTER SMOKING CESSATION AND LIKELIHOOD OF GAINING WEIGHT

To evaluate postcessation weight gain and to determine the likelihood or relative risk of gaining weight after smoking cessation, longitudinal investigations after 1970 of postcessation weight gain were examined. Only studies that included a control group of continuing smokers were evaluated. Requirements for studies in this review included a minimum followup period of 1 month and at least 10 smokers who quit. Studies were excluded if a weight loss component or severe caloric restriction was part of the intervention or if an agent known to affect body weight (e.g., nicotine polacrilex gum) was used; however, placebo conditions within drug trials were considered. A few studies were excluded for methodologic or interpretive reasons, such as relapsed subjects included in data analysis along with quit subjects or whenever a weight change could not be calculated. Table 1 summarizes the 15 studies that fulfilled these inclusionary and exclusionary criteria.

The following information is included for each study listed in Table 1: the study reference, the followup or period of abstinence, the mean weight gain among individuals who quit smoking, the mean weight gain of subjects who did not quit smoking, the percentage of subjects quitting smoking who gained weight from baseline to the followup period, the percentage of nonabstinent subjects who gained weight during the same period, and the relative risk of gaining any weight after smoking cessation versus continued smoking. Adjusted averages of weight gain are provided to summarize across all studies. These adjusted averages control for differing sample sizes and assign

TABLE 1.—Summary of prospective studies on smoking and body weight

Reference	Sample size	Number of quitters	Quit period	Mean weight gain (lb) Quitters	Mean weight gain (lb) Continuing smokers	% quitters who gain weight	% continuing smokers who gain weight	Relative risk of gaining weight
Bossé, Garvey, Costa (1980)	705	237	5 yr	6.35	2.01	—	—	—
Cambien et al. (1981)	475	41	2 yr	7.5	2.2	—	—	—
Coates and Li (1983)	335	13	1 yr	5.15	0.04	76.9	46.3	1.66
Comstock and Stone (1972)	290	46	5 yr	11.2	2.4	87.0	60.7	1.43
Friedman and Siegelaub (1980)	9,539	2,738	18 mo (median)	3.18	0.9	—	—	—
Gritz, Carr, Marcus (1988)	554	61	1 yr	6.1	0.3	—	—	—
Hickey and Mulcahy (1973)	88	60	2 yr	1.6	0.9	—	—	—
Kramer (1982)	134	59	1 yr	—	—	78.0	56.0	1.39
Lund-Larsen and Tretli (1982)	6,580	1,047	3 yr	6.94	0.44	—	—	—
Noppa and Bengtsson (1980)	526	72	6 yr	7.7	2.4	80.6	61.7	1.31

TABLE 1.—Continued

Reference	Sample size	Number of quitters	Quit period	Mean weight gain (lb) Quitters	Mean weight gain (lb) Continuing smokers	% quitters who gain weight	% continuing smokers who gain weight	Relative risk of gaining weight
Puddey et al. (1985)	28	14	1.5 mo	3.97	0.44	—	—	—
Rabkin (1984b)	107	35	3 mo	4.4	0.7	—	—	—
Rodin (1987)	42	24	1.5 mo	3.18	0.30	58.3	33.3	1.75
Seltzer (1974)	318	104	5 yr	7.9	3.5	—	—	—
Tuomilehto et al. (1986)	496	155	5 yr	6.02	1.57	—	—	—
Total sample size=20,217; Average sample size=1,348; Number of studies reported=15			Median followup period=2 yr	Average weight gain among quitters=4.6; N=4,647	Average weight gain among continuing smokers=0.8; N=15,046	Average % of quitters who gain weight=79%; Number of studies reporting=5; N=214	Average % of continuing smokers who gain weight=56%; Number of studies reporting=5; N=1,113	Average relative risk of gaining weight=1.45; Number of studies reporting=5; N=1,327

NOTE: Averages are weighted for differing sample sizes.

more weight to large versus small samples. Table 2 provides more detailed information (e.g., 95-percent confidence intervals for weight gain and relative risk) regarding each of these investigations.

As indicated in Tables 1 and 2, the average sample size of these investigations was 1,348 (range=28–9,539). The followup period ranged from 1 month to 5 years, with a median followup period of 2 years. Consistent with previous reviews of the smoking and body weight literature (Klesges et al. 1989; US DHHS 1988a), the adjusted average weight gain among smokers who quit was approximately 5 pounds (mean=4.6; range=1.6–11.2 pounds). The weight gain among smokers who quit was considerably greater than the adjusted average gain of 0.8 pounds observed among subjects who continued to smoke (range=0 to +3.5 pounds). Thus, although variability of weight gain is quite marked (Tables 1 and 2), smoking cessation produces approximately a 4-pound greater weight gain than that associated with continued smoking.

A commonly reported, but erroneous, estimate regarding postcessation weight gain is that one-third of smokers gain weight after smoking cessation, one-third maintain body weight, and one-third lose weight after cessation (US DHEW 1977). In the five investigations providing detailed information regarding changes in body weight, the actual percentage of quitters gaining weight appears to be much greater than previously estimated. Considering the results of all five studies and adjusting for sample size, 79 percent of those who quit smoking experienced a weight gain (range=58–87 percent). Over the same followup period, an adjusted average of 56 percent of continuing smokers experienced an increase in body weight (range=33–62 percent) and, as presented above, the average amount of weight gain was less among continuing smokers.

Data allowing computation of a relative risk estimate of weight gain after smoking cessation were available from five investigations. This relative risk estimate compares the likelihood of weight gain in quitters versus continuing smokers. That is, a higher relative risk ratio indicates that the percentage of quitters who gained weight was higher compared with that of corresponding continuing smokers. Overall, the risk of weight gain after cessation was 45 percent greater for quitters (mean=1.45, range=1.31–1.75) than for continuing smokers. This increased risk of weight gain was consistent across differing followup periods, appearing as early as 6 weeks (Rodin 1987; relative risk (RR)=1.75) and lasting up to 6 years after smoking cessation (Noppa and Bengtsson 1980; RR=1.31). Additionally, one investigation found the relative risk of gaining more than 2 pounds after smoking cessation to be 1.38 (Bossé, Garvey, Costa 1980). In another investigation, the risk of gaining more than 10 pounds was 88 percent higher for quitters than for continuing smokers (RR=1.88) (Friedman and Siegelaub 1980).

Although the risk of gaining more than 10 pounds appears to be almost 90 percent greater among quitters than continuing smokers (Friedman and Siegelaub 1980), actual occurrence of 10-pound weight gains was relatively low (20.3 vs. 10.8 percent among quitters and continuing smokers, respectively). Friedman and Siegelaub (1980), with a large sample of quitters (N=2,738) and continuing smokers (N=6,801), presented the percentages of those gaining 20 pounds or more over a median 18-month followup. Among males, 3.7 percent of those who quit smoking gained more than 20 pounds compared with 0.9 percent of those who continued to smoke. Among females, 3.1

TABLE 2.—Details of prospective studies in which change in weight relative to continuing smokers was reported

Reference	Sample	Quit period	Average gain ±SD (lb)	95% CI for average gain (lb)	Results
Bossé, Garvey, Costa (1980)	705 males aged 24–81[a]	≤5 yr	Quitters: 6.35±12.15	(4.80–7.90)	Gained ≥2 lb Gained ≤2 lb or lost Quit 64.1% (152) 35.9% (85) Continued 46.4% (217) 53.6% (251)
			Continuing smokers: 2.01±9.61	(1.14–2.88)	Relative risk of gaining more than 2 lb=1.38 95% CI (1.21–1.58)
Cambien et al. (1981)	475 male Parisians aged 25–35 in control condition of randomized trial	≤2 yr	Quitters: 7.5		
			Continuing smokers and nonsmokers: 2.2		
Coates and Li (1983)	335 asbestos-exposed males, average age 42	1 yr	Quitters: 5.15±7.53	(1.06–9.24)	Gained No change or lost Quit 76.9% (10) 23.1% (3) Continued 46.3% (149) 53.7% (173)
			Continuing smokers: 0.35±7.53	(−0.47–1.17)	Relative risk of gaining any weight=1.66 95% CI (1.21–2.29) Quitters Continuing smokers Lost ≥5 lb 15.4% (2) 19.9% (64) Lost 1–4 lb 7.7% (1) 33.8% (109) Gained 0–4 lb 30.8% (4) 23.0% (74) Gained ≥5 lb 46.1% (6) 23.3% (75)

TABLE 2.—Continued

Reference	Sample	Quit period	Average gain ±SD (lb)	95% CI for average gain (lb)	Results

Comstock and Stone (1972)	290 males, aged 40–59	≤5 yr	Quitters: 11.2
			
			Continuing smokers: 2.4
					Gained
					  Quit 87.0% (40)
					  Continued 60.7% (148)
					
					Relative risk of gaining any weight=1.43
					95% CI (1.23–1.67)
						No change or lost
						  13.0% (6)
						  39.3% (96)

Friedman and Siegelaub (1980)	9,539 participants aged 20–70 in health screening in California	18 mo (median)	Quitters: 3.18
			  Males: 4.1
			  Females: 3.5
			
			Continuing smokers: 0.9
			  Males: 0.9
			  Females: 0.9
					Gained >10 lb
					  Quit 20.3% (557)
					  Continued 10.8% (734)
					
					Relative risk of gaining >10 lb=1.88
					95% CI (1.70–2.08)
						Gained <10 lb or lost
						  79.7% (2,181)
						  89.2% (6,067)

Males

	Quitters	Continuing smokers
Gained <10 lb	77.6% (930)	88.6% (2550)
Gained >10 lb	18.7% (224)	10.5% (302)
Gained >20 lb	3.7% (44)	0.9% (26)

Females

	Quitters	Continuing smokers
Gained <10 lb	81.2% (1251)	89.6% (3517)
Gained >10 lb	15.7% (242)	8.8% (344)
Gained >20 lb	3.1% (47)	1.6% (62)

TABLE 2.—Continued

Reference	Sample	Quit period	Average gain ±SD (lb)	95% CI for average gain (lb)	Results
Gritz, Carr, Marcus (1988)	554 self-quitters, average age 41.4 yr	1 yr	Quitters: 6.1 Continuing smokers: 0.3		
Hickey and Mulcahy (1973)	88 male smokers surviving first MI, average age 50.2 yr	2 yr	Quitters: 1.6 Continuing smokers: 0.9		

Kramer (1982)	134 participants from a commercial cessation program	≥1 yr			Gained
					  Quit 78.0% (46)
					  Continued 56.0% (42)
					No change or lost
					  22.0% (13)
					  44.0% (33)
					Relative risk of gaining weight=1.39
					95% CI (1.09–1.77)

Lund-Larsen and Tretli (1982)	6,580 Norwegians from a CV screening, aged 20–49	≤3 yr	Quitters: 6.94
			  Males: 7.94
			  Females: 5.95
			
			Continuing smokers: 0.44
			  Males: 0.88
			  Females: 0		

TABLE 2.—Continued

Reference	Sample	Quit period	Average gain ±SD (lb)	95% CI for average gain (lb)	Results

Noppa and Bengtsson (1980)	526 Swedish women, aged 38–60[a]	≤ 6 yr	Quitters: 7.7±10.8
			
			Continuing smokers: 2.4±11.5
				(5.2–10.2)
				
				(1.3–3.5)
					Gained
					  Quit 80.6% (58) No change or lost
					  Continued 61.7% (280) 19.4% (14)
					                                      38.3% (174)
					
					Relative risk of gaining any weight=1.31
					95% CI (1.14–1.49)
					
					                Quitters Continuing smokers
					Lost ≥22 lb 0.0% (0) 2.4% (11)
					Lost 11–22 lb 4.2% (3) 5.5% (25)
					Lost 0–11 lb 15.3% (11) 30.4% (138)
					Gained 0–11 lb 45.8% (33) 44.5% (202)
					Gained 11–22 lb 22.2% (16) 13.7% (62)
					Gained ≥ 22 lb 12.5% (9) 3.5% (16)

Puddey et al. (1985)	14 quitters and 14 matched smoking controls, aged 24–63	6 wk	Quitters: 3.97 Continuing smokers: 0.44		

TABLE 2.—Continued

Reference	Sample	Quit period	Average gain ±SD (lb)	95% CI for average gain (lb)	Results
Rabkin (1984b)	107 participants of cessation program, average age 40	≤3 mo	Quitters: 4.4±3.9 Males: 5.9±4.1 Females: 3.3±3.0 Continuing smokers: 0.7±3.7 Males: 2.2±3.4 Females: −0.4±3.0	(3.1–5.7) (3.8–8.1) (2.0–4.6) (−0.2–1.5) (0.9–3.5) (−1.3–0.4)	

Rodin (1987)	42 participants of smoking cessation program, average age 44	8 wk	Quitters: 3.18
			
			Continuing smokers: 0.30
					Gained
					  Quit 58.3% (14)
					  Continued 33.3% (6)
					Relative risk of gaining any weight=1.75
					95% CI (0.84–3.65)

Seltzer (1974)	318 white male veterans from Boston, aged 25–64	≤5 yr	Quitters: 7.9
			
			Continuing smokers: 3.5
					No change or lost
					  41.7% (10)
					  66.7% (12)

TABLE 2.—Continued

Reference	Sample	Quit period	Average gain ±SD (lb)	95% CI for average gain (lb)	Results

Tuomilehto et al. (1986)	496 participants in CV prevention trial in Finland, aged 25–59	≤5 yr	Quitters:
			  Males: 8.16
			  Females: −0.37
			
			Continuing smokers:
			  Males: 2.27
			  Females: −2.56		

NOTE: SD=standard deviation; CI=confidence interval; MI=myocardial infarction; CV=cardiovascular.
[a]Younger subjects gained more weight.

percent of those who quit smoking gained more than 20 pounds compared with 1.6 percent of those who continued to smoke.

In summary, while approximately four-fifths of smokers who quit will gain weight after cessation, average weight gain is approximately 4 pounds greater than that expected among continuing smokers. The risk of weight gain after cessation is 45 percent greater than the risk associated with continued smoking, although individual weight gains of 20 pounds or more are rare.

Although weight gain is common after cessation, little is known concerning the types of individuals at risk for substantial increases in body weight. Researchers have concluded that women, moderate smokers, and older smokers have the greatest weight control effect from smoking (US DHHS 1988a), although the tremendous variability in body weight changes after cessation has yet to be explained. That is, while the average weight gain after smoking cessation is approximately 5 pounds, individual responses range from weight loss to a weight gain exceeding 20 pounds. Studies are needed that focus carefully on individuals at risk of excessive weight gain after smoking cessation and the differences between these individuals and those who do not gain weight.

Additionally, investigators hypothesize that the relationship between smoking and body weight is attenuated by other health behaviors (Marti et al. 1989). Although the effects of smoking to reduce body weight are acknowledged, individuals who smoke are more likely than nonsmokers to have unhealthy lifestyles associated with increased body weight (e.g., lower levels of physical activity and higher dietary intakes) (Klesges, Eck et al. 1990; Chapter 11).

CAUSES OF POSTCESSATION WEIGHT GAIN

Cross-sectional and longitudinal studies clearly indicate the inverse relationship between smoking and body weight in humans and between nicotine and body weight in animals (Grunberg 1986; Klesges et al. 1989; US DHHS 1988a; Winders and Grunberg 1989). However, no study has included a simultaneous evaluation of the long-term changes in all of the variables that may account for this relationship, including food intake, physical activity, and energy expenditure. Of the currently published investigations, the longest followup period evaluating all three aspects of the energy balance equation has been 8 weeks (Stamford et al. 1986). A recent study evaluated food intake and physical activity changes over a 26-week followup but did not include metabolic measures (Hall et al. 1989). Short-term evaluations do not allow for an adequate determination of predictors of weight gain. This review focuses on those studies that have directly evaluated either food intake, physical activity, and/or metabolic rate as a function of smoking cessation, nicotine administration, or nicotine deprivation. The available data on changes in the energy balance equation that result from smoking cessation are summarized below.

Food Intake

Most short-term evaluations (e.g., 3 days or less) found that food intake, particularly the consumption of sweet foods and simple carbohydrates, increases after smoking cessation. For example in a 1-day experiment, Grunberg (1982a) reported that smokers who were allowed to smoke ate fewer sweet foods, but consumed similar amounts of non-sweet foods, compared with nonsmokers and smokers not allowed to smoke. This between-subjects laboratory study was short term and did not measure body weight changes. In another short-term study, Hatsukami and colleagues (1984) hospitalized 27 smokers for 7 days. After a 3-day baseline, 20 of the subjects were deprived of smoking for 4 days while the remaining 7 served as a control group. During this 4-day abstinence, caloric intake increased significantly in the abstinence group and was accompanied by a 1.76-pound increase in weight compared with baseline. Recently, Duffy and Hall (1988) assessed smokers who differed in degree of eating disinhibition, defined as eating that occurs in situations in which self-control behaviors are disrupted (e.g., binge eating). Smokers who were allowed to smoke before eating ice cream did not show food consumption differences as a function of level of disinhibition. However, results for smokers who had abstained from smoking for 24 hours showed a different pattern. Abstaining smokers who scored high on eating disinhibition ate more than three times (273.6 g) as much ice cream as those who scored low (86.4 g) on eating disinhibition. The results from this investigation indicate that dietary changes following smoking cessation may vary as a function of dieting history, use of cigarettes to curb appetite, and other weight history variables.

Some prospective investigations have qualitatively asked participants who quit smoking if they believed that their dietary intake had changed. These studies also reported that food intake increases after cessation. For example, Manley and Boland (1983) examined the side effects experienced by 94 subjects quitting smoking and whether these side effects varied as a function of relapse. On a withdrawal rating system, those who quit smoking rated themselves as furthest from "optimal" at followup on general appetite and overeating. On a separate rating scale, abstainers also gave higher ratings than relapsers at followup on "eating more." In a study of 53 self-quitters, Black and coworkers (1988) found that of those reporting that they ate more, average weight gain was 6.9 pounds. In contrast, of those reporting that they ate the same or less, average weight gain was 1.4 pounds.

Unfortunately, there are few prospective human investigations that have attempted to quantify carefully food intake changes over time among subjects after quitting smoking. These studies generally indicate that food intake increases after cessation; however, results vary greatly across investigations. Of eight studies to date, two reported clear increases in food consumption after cessation (Leischow and Stitzer 1989; Stamford et al. 1986), four provided qualified support for increased food consumption after cessation (Hall et al. 1989; Klesges et al., in press; Perkins, Epstein, Pastor 1990; Rodin 1987), and two reported no changes in food intake after cessation (Dallosso and James 1984; DiLorenzo et al. 1988).

In what may be the most comprehensive evaluation to date of change in energy balance, Stamford and colleagues (1986) analyzed changes in food intake, physical activity, and resting metabolic rate in 13 sedentary females who quit smoking for 48 days. Mean daily food intake increased by 227 kcal and explained 69 percent of the variance in changes in weight (4.85 pounds). No changes in physical activity or resting metabolic rate were observed.

To evaluate dietary changes after cessation, Leischow and Stitzer (1989) assigned subjects, in an inpatient setting, to either smoke-ad-libidum (N=6) or quit-smoking (N=9) conditions for at least 14 days after a 4-day baseline period. Results revealed a significant difference in weight gain (p<0.05) between smokers and those who quit smoking (2.0 vs. 4.7 pounds, respectively). The weight gain in those who quit smoking was associated with a significant increase in food intake over time compared with continuing smokers.

Four investigations have provided qualified support for dietary changes after cessation. Perkins, Epstein, and Pastor (1990) evaluated caloric intake, resting energy expenditure (REE), and physical activity in seven female smokers for 3 weeks, which included normal smoking (week 1), smoking cessation (week 2), and resumption of smoking (week 3). Total caloric intake did not increase during the week of cessation. However, once smokers resumed smoking during week 3, caloric intake decreased significantly. Caloric intake from alcohol, however, rose from 219 kcal per day in the first week to 432 kcal per day during the week of abstinence. When subjects resumed smoking during the third week, alcohol intake dropped to 129 kcal per day. During the cessation week, REE did not decrease compared with baseline. However, a significant increase in REE was observed when subjects resumed smoking compared with the week of abstinence (p<0.001). No changes in physical activity were observed.

Rodin (1987) evaluated changes in food intake and physical activity in 24 subjects who quit smoking and 18 smokers who failed to quit smoking. Subjects who quit smoking gained an average of 3.2 pounds over the 8-week study. Consistent with the literature concerning animals as subjects and some studies using humans (Grunberg 1986; Winders and Grunberg 1989), smokers who gained weight after stopping smoking increased their carbohydrate consumption, particularly sugar. This increase was accompanied by decreased protein consumption. However, these subjects did not increase their total food intake nor did they decrease their levels of physical activity. Levels of physical activity generally increased.

Hall and coworkers (1989) assessed changes in food intake and physical activity among 95 subjects who enrolled in a stop-smoking program. In contrast to all other investigations reviewed in this Section, Hall and coworkers (1989) evaluated long-term changes in food intake and physical activity (for a 6-month followup). Caloric intake increased significantly in one group and marginally in another group during the first 8 weeks of abstinence. Both sugar and total fat increases were noted in the group that significantly increased energy intake. Total dietary intake increased approximately 200 kcal per day over the 8-week period. In assessing 6-month changes, Hall and coworkers (1989) reported a gender difference in caloric intake with time. Among men who quit, mean daily caloric intake decreased by almost 1,000 kcal from a mean of 3,014 kcal during week 1 to 2,035 kcal at week 26. Among women, caloric intake remained stable (mean=1,841 kcal at week 1; mean=1,867 kcal at week 26). However, weight continued to increase for both groups. From the 12-week to the 6-month followup, men increased their weight 3.56 pounds (8.65 pounds total), and women increased their weight by 4.53 pounds (10.34 pounds total). No changes in physical activity were observed. Weight continued to increase despite no changes from baseline in dietary intake and physical activity in female ex-smokers and despite decreases in dietary intake and no physical activity changes in male ex-smokers.

Klesges and coworkers (in press) reported gender differences in response to smoking cessation. In this study, the food intake and physical activity of 68 smokers and nonsmokers were evaluated during a 2-week period. At the end of the first week, the smokers were paid to quit smoking, and 36 percent were successful at remaining abstinent for the entire week (confirmed by carbon monoxide (CO) readings). Nonsmokers continued to monitor their food intake and physical activity. At the end of the second week, subjects were allowed to return to smoking. In this investigation, female smokers who quit smoking increased their body weight in comparison with nonsmokers. Smokers who quit increased their consumption of mono- and polyunsaturated fats and decreased their intake of fiber. In contrast, males who quit smoking did not change either their weight or dietary intake compared with males in the other groups. No changes in physical activity were detected in any of the groups.

Dallosso and James (1984) reported on 10 subjects who quit smoking and were observed for 6 weeks after they participated in a stop-smoking clinic. Resting metabolic rate dropped by 4 percent in smokers who quit, a drop which was significant only when the data were expressed as per kilogram of body weight. The average food intake increased by 6.5 percent, but this difference was not statistically significant.

DiLorenzo and colleagues (1988) evaluated changes in body weight and caloric consumption in 16 subjects who quit smoking for 5 weeks compared with 11 subjects who continued to smoke and 16 nonsmokers studied over the same time period. Subjects who quit smoking gained an average of 5 pounds over the 5 weeks; the smoking and nonsmoking control groups did not change body weight significantly ($p<0.0001$). This weight gain was not associated with changes in dietary intake.

Physical Activity

In contrast to the findings on dietary intake and smoking cessation, the available data indicate that change in physical activity does not play a role in either differences in body weight between smokers and nonsmokers or the weight gain associated with smoking cessation. The small number of prospective investigations has generally reported unchanged physical activity after smoking cessation (Hall et al. 1989; Hatsukami et al. 1984; Klesges et al., in press; Perkins, Epstein, Pastor 1990; Stamford et al. 1986), and those that found a change in activity reported an increase in physical activity after smoking cessation (Leischow and Stitzer 1989; Rodin 1987). The literature consistently indicates that reduced physical activity after cessation cannot account for postcessation weight gain.

Energy Expenditure

An important and often overlooked variable in energy imbalance leading to weight gain is REE. Approximately 75 percent of total energy expenditure is in the form of metabolism (Ravussin et al. 1982). Ample indirect evidence supports the hypothesis of increased energy expenditure in smokers. That is, given that smokers do not have higher levels of physical activity compared with nonsmokers, the only known mechanism remaining to explain the energy imbalance is some aspect of metabolism (Blair, Jacobs, Powell 1985); smokers' dietary intakes may be the same or higher than those of nonsmokers (Picone et al. 1982; Stamford, Matter, Fell, Sady, Cresanta et al. 1984; Stamford, Matter, Fell, Sady, Papanek et al. 1984); smokers maintain lower body weights than do nonsmokers (Klesges et al. 1989; US DHHS 1988a); and weight gain has been reported in individuals quitting smoking without any dietary and physical activity changes (DiLorenzo et al. 1988; Hall et al. 1989). Additionally, several reports document nicotine-induced reductions in body weight in laboratory animals without a concomitant reduction in food intake (Grunberg, Bowen, Morse 1984; Schechter and Cook 1976; Wellman et al. 1986). However, those few studies that have evaluated metabolic changes in response to smoking cessation among humans have produced inconclusive and equivocal results.

Eight studies have reported either acute changes in REE following smoking or nicotine administration or have reported decreases in REE after smoking cessation. An early study (Glauser et al. 1970) reported decreases in oxygen consumption for seven male subjects who quit smoking for 1 month. Food intake and physical activity were not monitored. Reanalysis of these data (Klesges et al. 1989) revealed that the changes in metabolic rate reported by Glauser and coworkers (1970) were significant only with improper methods of statistical analysis. In the only study that utilized an indirect calorimetry respiration chamber, Hofstetter and coworkers (1986) reported a 10-percent difference in total energy expenditure during a 24-hour period of smoking compared with a 24-hour period of abstinence among eight smokers. However, this difference in energy expenditure disappeared after 24 hours. No changes were observed in mean basal (sleeping) metabolic rate. Diet was held constant.

Perkins and colleagues have conducted a series of studies evaluating the effects of nicotine, in the form of nicotine nasal spray, on changes in REE. In a study of nicotine administration in 18 male smokers, Perkins and colleagues (Perkins, Epstein, Stiller, Marks et al. 1989) reported REE changes that were 6 percent above baseline after nicotine administration, which was significantly greater than the 3-percent increase after placebo administration. Another investigation (Perkins et al. 1989a) sought to determine if nicotine-induced increases in metabolic rate observed at rest were also present during physical activity. Ten male smokers were administered nicotine and were then compared with 10 male smokers who were administered placebo. Metabolic rates increased both at rest and during light exercise. Although the percent change in REE due to nicotine was equivalent both at rest and during activity, the excess energy expenditure (in kilocalories) attributable to nicotine, was more than twice as great during exercise. A third study using nicotine nasal spray assessed the combined effects of nicotine and consumption of a meal on REE (Perkins, Epstein, Stiller, Sexton et al.

1989). Eight male smokers were assessed using a repeated measures design. These individuals were given a caloric load (vs. water) and nicotine (vs. placebo). Both the caloric load and nicotine increased REE significantly. However, no interaction between these factors emerged, and the effects were slightly less than additive when combined. Nicotine alone increased REE by 4.95 kcal per hour, food alone increased metabolic rate by 14.30 kcal per hour, but nicotine plus food increased metabolic rate by 17.00 kcal per hour. Finally, in a study of the effects of changes in energy balance as a function of smoking cessation, Perkins, Epstein, and Pastor (1990) evaluated REE in seven female smokers across 3 weeks: normal smoking (week 1), smoking cessation (week 2), and resumption of smoking (week 3). REE did not drop during the week of abstinence compared with baseline. However, a significant increase in REE was observed when subjects resumed smoking compared with the week that they were abstinent.

The effects of smoking and coffee consumption on REE were recently evaluated by Klesges, Brown, and colleagues (1990). Of 45 regular cigarette smokers and coffee drinkers, 15 were randomly assigned to smoke 2 cigarettes, 15 were assigned to drink two standardized cups of coffee, and 15 were assigned to smoke cigarettes and drink coffee. All three groups had acute increases in REE with a similar pattern of response in each group.

In the largest study to date of all-day changes in metabolic rate, Klesges, Coday, and coworkers (1990) evaluated changes in REE among 39 individuals over a 10-hour period using multiple assessments of REE. Of the 30 smokers, 20 were assigned randomly to continuous, regular smoking and 10 were assigned to a no-smoking group. A nonsmoking control group of nine subjects was also evaluated over the same time period. The increase in REE among nonsmokers was not significant. In marked contrast, smokers who did not smoke decreased REE over the course of the day. Additionally, there were two distinct patterns of results among smokers who smoked over time. Of the 20 smokers, 14 (70 percent) markedly increased their REE over time, but 6 smokers (30 percent) decreased REE over time (similar to the pattern of smokers who did not smoke). Closer inspection of the minute-by-minute metabolic changes of those subjects who increased metabolic rate indicated an acute metabolic increase followed by a return to baseline early in the day, or an acute metabolic increase followed by a reduction, but to a level higher than baseline later in the day. In contrast, subjects who had a mean decrease in REE also had an acute metabolic increase followed by a drop below baseline early in the day, or an acute metabolic increase followed by a return to baseline later in the day. Subjects who responded with decreases in REE smoked more (as measured by expired CO) than those who responded with a cumulative increase in energy expenditure. These results are consistent with recent observations of a U-shaped relationship between daily cigarette consumption and body weight, with moderate smokers weighing less than nonsmokers but heavy smokers approximating the body weights of nonsmokers (Albanes et al. 1987).

Four studies found no relationship between smoking and metabolic rate. Burse and coworkers (1982) did not observe chronic changes in resting metabolism in a sample of three smokers who quit for 3 weeks. However, the small sample size in this investigation limits interpretation of the results. Although Robinson and York (1986) reported an elevated metabolic response to food intake (i.e., thermic effect of food), chronic REE did not change as a function of smoking and total energy expenditure after a meal during the cessation period. Stamford and colleagues (1986) did not find changes in oxygen consumption in 13 subjects who quit smoking for 48 days. These investigators did find marked food intake changes that accounted for 69 percent of the variance of postcessation weight gain. In a study of the chronic effects of smoking status on REE, Perkins and coworkers (1989b) assessed 20 male smokers and 10 male nonsmokers after overnight abstinence from food and caffeine in both groups and after overnight abstinence from smoking in the smoking group. No differences in REE were observed.

Two recent studies evaluating the acute effects of cigarette smoking on REE have provided equivocal findings. In a sample of five occasional and five regular smokers (Warwick, Chapple, Thomson 1987), REE did not increase after smoking, even during the first 15 to 30 minutes after smoking. Additionally, the thermic effect of food was slightly, but not significantly, lower with smoking than without smoking. Dallosso and James (1984) evaluated short- and long-term metabolic changes associated with smoking. The thermogenic (metabolic) response for 1 hour after smoking 1 cigarette was not significant, although an acute increase was observed during the first 30 minutes. However, variability of responses was marked, ranging from a 4.5-percent decrease in metabolic rate to a 9.0-percent increase. No consistent long-term changes in metabolic rate were observed. Rather, the metabolic rate of four smokers clearly decreased after cessation; the rate stayed the same in two smokers and increased in two others.

The literature generally indicates that both dietary and metabolic changes are responsible for weight gain after smoking cessation, but these changes probably occur through complex mechanisms. Physical activity does not appear to be related to postcessation weight gain. Although the pattern generally indicates that both dietary and metabolic factors are involved, there is inconsistency both within and between studies indicating tremendous individual differences in subjects' dietary and metabolic changes after smoking cessation.

Investigators need to try to determine carefully the potential moderator variables of dietary and metabolic changes after smoking cessation. Factors such as gender, age, race, weight history, and concerns about postcessation weight gain may all play a role in predicting dietary changes after cessation. Some individuals, for example, may respond to smoking cessation by dramatically increasing their dietary intake (Duffy and Hall 1988), whereas others may impose dietary restrictions in an attempt to avoid postcessation weight gain (Klesges et al., in press).

There also appears to be tremendous individual variation in the metabolic response to smoking and smoking cessation. Overall, evaluations of short-term, acute responses to smoking generally report increases in metabolic rate as a function of nicotine administration and smoking (Hofstetter et al. 1986; Perkins et al. 1989a; Klesges, Brown et al. 1990), although long-term (overnight or longer) studies generally do not indicate changes in metabolic rate as a function of smoking cessation (Stamford et al. 1986). However, some investigators have reported that the acute effects of smoking have not produced a change in REE (Warwick, Chapple, Thomson 1987).

Research needs to focus on a number of potential moderators of smoking and metabolic rate. Levels of plasma nicotine vary greatly even for the same level of cigarette consumption and for the same nicotine content of cigarettes (US DHHS 1988a). The relationship between nicotine, as well as other constituents of tobacco smoke, and metabolic rate needs to be evaluated carefully. It is also possible that heavier, chronic smokers may habituate to the effects of nicotine over time (US DHHS 1988a) and their metabolic responses may become blunted (Klesges, Coday et al. 1990). Other important moderators, such as years smoked, gender, and relative weight, should also be carefully evaluated in future investigations.

RELATIONSHIP BETWEEN OVERWEIGHT AND ADVERSE MEDICAL AND PSYCHOSOCIAL OUTCOMES

Obesity refers to excess body fat, whereas overweight refers to excess body weight relative to height compared with gender-specific norms (Powers 1980). Obesity and overweight are highly correlated across the population, although some individuals are overweight but not obese (e.g., bodybuilders), and others are obese but not overweight (e.g., a normal weight "couch potato") (Grunberg 1982b). In the context of this Chapter, the relevant data are those that are related to health risks. The most commonly used methods to measure or estimate body fat in studies of health consequences of body size are measures of height and weight in comparison with gender-specific norms (which actually determine overweight) and measurement of subcutaneous fat by skinfold thickness at one or more sites (which determines obesity). Therefore, the data cited in this Chapter are sometimes based on estimates of obesity and sometimes based on estimates of overweight; both terms appear in the text. Normative values for these anthropometric measures have generally been derived in one of two ways: either by averaging the values found in populations of healthy persons or by tabulating values reported to be associated with greatest longevity in population-based studies. Inclusion of data based on these various standard measures provides the most complete information available. Although the volume of research related to obesity and health risk precludes comprehensive review here, a summary of this literature is a useful starting point for examining the health risks of weight gain following smoking cessation.

Large amounts of epidemiologic and clinical data clearly indicate a positive association between excess body weight and medical risk. Cross-sectional, longitudinal, ecologic, and case–control studies indicate that there is a graded relationship between weight and various diseases and disease risk factors. Positive associations have been reported between body weight and glucose intolerance and type II diabetes (Kannell, Gordon, Castelli 1979; Rimm et al. 1972; West and Kalbfleisch 1971; Negri et al. 1988; Hadden and Harris 1987); elevated blood pressure and hypertension (MacMahon et al. 1987; Chiang, Perlman, Epstein 1969; MacMahon et al. 1984; Blackburn and Prineas 1983; Pan et al. 1986); elevated total blood cholesterol and lowered high-density lipoprotein cholesterol (HDL-C) (Jooste et al. 1988; Garrison et al. 1980; Nanas et al. 1987); gout (Larsson, Bjorntorp, Tibblin 1981); kidney stones (Larsson, Bjorntorp, Tibblin 1981); gall bladder disease (Rimm et al. 1972); cardiovascular disease (CVD) (Rabkin, Mathewson, Hsu 1977; Noppa et al. 1980; Garrison and Castelli 1985);

cancers of the endometrium and colon (Garfinkel 1985; Graham et al. 1988; Verreault et al. 1989); arthritis (Anderson and Felson 1988; Felson 1988); and varicose veins. Obese women are more likely than lean women to experience menstrual abnormalities (Hartz et al. 1979) and complications in pregnancy (Abrams and Parker 1988). Obese individuals require more medical care (Tsai, Lucas, Bernacki 1988), experience more complications during and following surgical procedures (Schwartz 1955), and report greater limitations in performing tasks of everyday living (Stewart, Brook, Kane 1980).

The strength and consistency of the data and the understanding of causal mechanisms underlying obesity–disease associations vary from end-point to end-point. Nevertheless, there is little doubt that obesity represents an important health risk that may reduce both the quality and duration of life. The overall evidence linking overweight to disease has led to recommendations from numerous health organizations for individuals in the general population to control their weight as a means of preventing future illness (National Institutes of Health Consensus Development Conference Statement 1985; Subcommittee on Nonpharmacological Therapy of the 1984 Joint National Committee on Detection, Evaluation, and Treatment of High Blood Pressure 1986; US DHHS 1988b).

Despite convincing data linking obesity to ill health, several issues in the area remain controversial. A key issue that is particularly germane to smoking cessation-induced weight gain is the extent to which modest degrees of overweight represent a health hazard. The most commonly recognized standards for acceptable body weights are those developed by the life insurance industry based on followup studies of policy holders conducted in 1959 and 1979 (Metropolitan Life Insurance Company 1960; Society of Actuaries and Association of Life Insurance Medical Directors of America 1980).

Each of these studies evaluated the mortality of approximately 4,000,000 life insurance policy holders. "Ideal" weight standards that were developed from these studies and widely used in subsequent research represent the gender- and height-specific weights associated with lowest mortality. Overall, a J-shaped relationship is observed between weight and mortality. Lowest premature mortality is associated with body weights that are about 10 percent below the population average. Excess premature mortality is associated with extremely low weights (i.e., body weights more than 10 percent below the standards), and premature mortality increases incrementally for increasing weights above the standard. In the range of weights that encompasses the vast majority of the population (i.e., relative weights of 1.0 to 1.3), the relationship between weight and mortality was approximately linear with each 1-percent increase in weight associated with about a 1-percent increase in premature mortality. Above relative weights of about 1.3, the curve rises even more steeply so that premature mortality may double at relative weights of 1.5 or more (Manson et al. 1987).

The overall relationship between weight and mortality has been confirmed in several other large scale prospective studies. For example, the American Cancer Society followup study of 750,000 men and women from the general U.S. population provides confirmatory data with specific detail on various causes of death (Lew and Garfinkel 1979). Table 3 presents mortality ratios for this study group by weight status for selected causes. Table 4 presents mortality ratios by weight and smoking status. Most of the deaths associated with leanness occur among smokers, and although the shape of the weight-mortality curves are similar among smokers and never smokers, smokers have nearly twice the mortality rate compared with never smokers over much of the weight distribution. A recent 10-year followup study of 1,700,000 Norwegians confirms these findings in a non-U.S. population with regard to the shape of the weight mortality association and the causes of death at both ends of the distribution (Waaler 1988).

The reported relationship with age further complicates the relationship between body weight and health (Andres et al. 1985). For example, the strongest relationship between body weight and premature mortality holds for younger age groups (i.e., under 40 years of age). In older adults, the relationship between weight and mortality is weak over much of the weight distribution, and in the oldest groups studied (i.e., over 60 years of age), mortality appears inversely related to weight. Indeed, many prospective studies of middle-aged adults have observed little or no prognostic significance of body weight for either total premature mortality or major disease endpoints except at the extremes of the body weight distribution. These findings have led some researchers to argue that concerns about weight and overall health for most individuals have been exaggerated (Keys 1981; Barrett-Connor 1985). In contrast, other investigators have noted that cigarette smoking has not been statistically controlled in many of these analyses, and in addition, pathophysiologic effects of obesity, such as hypertension and hyperglycemia, have been inappropriately adjusted (Manson et al. 1987). Therefore, the health risks of obesity may have been underestimated.

Another issue to consider in the relationship between body weight and health is that all forms of overweight may not pose the same health risks. In particular, health risk may depend on weight status at different times in an individual's life. A study by Abraham, Collins, and Nordsieck (1971), for example, studied 1,087 white males for whom height and weight data were available at ages 9 to 13 and after a period of approximately 40 years. By cross-classifying respondents by childhood and adult weight status, these researchers found that individuals who were at the low end of the weight distribution as children, but who gained weight to reach the high end of the weight distribution as adults, were at significantly higher risk of hypertensive vascular disease and cardiovascular renal disease than were individuals who had high weights both as children and as adults. Similarly, in a report based on the Normative Aging Study, Borkan and colleagues (1986) found age by weight gain interactions, relating weight gain to health risk. Weight gain had a stronger positive association with change in fasting glucose levels for older men compared with younger men; however, weight gain was more strongly related to change in uric acid (positive) and forced vital capacity (negative) in younger men (Borkan et al. 1986).

The importance of timing issues in the relationship between body weight and disease is also apparent in weight cycling. Weight cycling refers to gaining and losing weight repeatedly over time. Such weight fluctuations might occur in individuals who repeatedly diet but are unable to maintain weight losses. Weight cycling might be caused by recurrent illnesses or major fluctuations in lifestyle. Such fluctuations might conceivably also occur among smokers who quit but relapse to smoking on multiple occasions. Several recent reports suggest that weight cycling may be associated with

TABLE 3.—Mortality ratios for all ages combined in relation to the death rate of those 90–109% of average weight

Cause of death	7th rev ICD	Gender	<80	80–89	90–109	110–119	120–129	130–139	≥140
Total deaths		Male	1.25	1.05	1.00	1.15	1.27	1.46	1.87
		Female	1.19	0.96	1.00	1.17	1.29	1.46	1.89
CHD	420	Male	0.88	0.90	1.00	1.23	1.32	1.55	1.95
		Female	1.01	0.89	1.00	1.23	1.39	1.54	2.07
Cancer, all sites	140–205	Male	1.33	1.13	1.00	1.02	1.09	1.14	1.33
		Female	0.96	0.92	1.00	1.10	1.19	1.23	1.55
Diabetes	260	Male	0.88	0.84	1.00	1.65	2.56	3.51	5.19
		Female	0.65	0.61	1.00	1.92	3.34	3.78	7.90
Digestive diseases	540–542 570–578	Male	1.39	1.28	1.00	1.45	1.88	2.89	3.99
	584–586	Female	1.58	0.92	1.00	1.66	1.61	2.19	2.29
Cerebrovascular diseases	330–334	Male	1.21	1.09	1.00	1.15	1.17	1.54	2.27
		Female	1.33	0.98	1.00	1.09	1.16	1.40	1.52

NOTE: CHD=coronary heart disease.
[a] Calculated by dividing a person's actual weight by the corresponding average weight for the appropriate sex-inch of height-5-yr age group, multiplied by 100.
SOURCE: Lew and Garfinkel (1979).

TABLE 4.—Mortality ratios for all ages combined according to smoking status in relation to those 90–109% of average age

Cause of death	Gender	Smoking status	<80	80–89	90–109	110–119	120–129	130–139	≥140
All causes of death	Male	Never smoked	0.88	0.75	0.75	0.91	0.98	1.16	1.69
		≥20 cig/day	1.68	1.40	1.34	1.53	1.76	2.00	2.21
		Other	1.22	1.01	0.93	1.04	1.15	1.29	1.66
	Female	Never smoked	1.10	0.88	0.93	1.08	1.20	1.37	1.74
		≥20 cig/day	1.98	1.59	1.64	1.82	2.22	2.30	2.73
		Other	1.53	1.13	1.12	1.40	1.42	1.62	2.04
Coronary artery disease (ICD 420)	Male	Never smoked	0.72	0.66	0.76	0.96	1.04	1.24	1.73
		≥20 cig/day	1.06	1.13	1.33	1.66	1.81	2.11	2.11
		Other	0.91	0.90	0.93	1.12	1.19	1.37	1.84
	Female	Never smoked	0.93	0.82	0.92	1.10	1.29	1.39	1.86
		≥20 cig/day	1.51	1.70	2.12	2.20	3.48	3.79	4.74
		Other	1.54	1.14	1.18	1.88	1.44	2.01	2.33
Cancer, all sites (ICD 140–205)	Male	Never smoked	0.60	0.60	0.66	0.69	0.79	0.90	0.76
		≥20 cig/day	2.07	1.71	1.43	1.46	1.55	1.71	2.00
		Other	1.20	1.03	1.90	0.89	1.05	0.87	1.22
	Female	Never smoked	0.85	0.85	0.96	1.06	1.16	1.19	1.50
		≥20 cig/day	1.49	1.36	1.34	1.50	1.34	1.70	1.49
		Other	1.11	0.98	1.03	1.06	1.16	1.11	1.60

[a] See Table 3 for definition.
SOURCE: Lew and Garfinkel (1979).

elevated premature mortality compared with maintaining a more stable weight over time. In a study by Hamm, Shekelle, and Stamler (1989), for example, CVD and cancer mortality and total mortality were compared among individuals who reported either having gained significant weight (N=133), having remained at the same weight (N=178), or both having gained and lost significant weight (N=98). Both gainers and cyclers had significantly elevated total mortality experience, relative risks of 1.5 and 1.4, respectively, compared with individuals whose weights remained constant. Three recently published abstracts (Lissner et al. 1989; Lissner, Collins et al. 1988; Lissner, Odell et al. 1988) have reported even greater health risks of weight cycling. Using prospective data from the Multiple Risk Factor Intervention Trial (MRFIT) (Lissner, Collins et al. 1988), two prospective studies from Göteborg, Sweden (Lissner et al. 1987), and the Framingham Study (Lissner, Odell et al. 1988), weight cycling was defined as the variability of weights recorded at repeat examinations. Controlling for a variety of possible confounding variables, weight cycling was independently predictive of total premature mortality and CVD mortality. In the analyses based on MRFIT, premature mortality among men with the most variable weights was 36 to 89 percent higher than among men with the most stable weights.

An additional issue to consider in the relationship between body weight and health is the distribution of body fat. Individuals differ in the location of stored adipose tissue. Research data show that individuals who store greater amounts of body fat in the abdominal region rather than in the hips or limbs have elevated cardiovascular risk factors (Gillum 1987; Selby, Friedman, Quesenberry 1989), CVD, and diabetes rates (Freedman and Rimm 1989; Lapidus and Bengtsson 1988) as well as reproductive system cancers among women (Bjorntorp 1988).

Usually measured by the ratio of abdominal circumference to hip circumference or the ratio of trunk versus peripheral skinfolds, a central body fat distribution is positively correlated with absolute body weight. However, in several studies, the centrality of fat distribution has proven to be a much stronger predictor of disease than body weight. A landmark study in this area was conducted by Larsson and colleagues (1984) who reported on 13 years of followup for 792 Swedish men aged 54 years at the time of first observation. Outcome measures were stroke, ischemic heart disease, and all-cause mortality. None of these health outcomes was significantly related to measures of adiposity (body mass index weight/height^2, the sum of several skinfold measurements, and body circumferences). However, the ratio of waist to hip circumference (WHR) was significantly and positively related to all three measures of illness and death. The relevance of this finding for ex-smokers, as discussed below, is that smoking is positively related to WHR and that smoking cessation is associated with a reduced WHR (Shimokata, Muller, Andres 1989).

Compared with pathophysiologic health risks, social and psychological pathologies associated with overweight are not as well established. This situation may reflect the relative absence of research in this area, but it may also indicate the absence of a strong relationship. Obesity is strongly disapproved of and discriminated against in this society (Allon 1973; Grunberg 1982b; Wadden and Stunkard 1985). Overweight individuals are falsely stereotyped as having a variety of undesirable characteristics, including self-indulgence, laziness, lack of self-control, and lack of intelligence.

The perception in this culture of obesity as unattractive has been documented in various populations. For example Richardson (1971), in a study of 10- and 11-year-olds' perception of the likableness of children with a variety of handicaps, found that obese children were judged less attractive than were children with amputations and facial disfigurement or children confined to wheelchairs. Similar biased impressions have been documented among adults and among physicians and medical students (Allon 1973; Maddox and Liederman 1969). Canning and Mayer (1966) found that the prevalence of obese students in college was less than the prevalence of obese students in high school despite no difference in academic performance in high school or in college application rates. A survey of employers indicates that many profess not to hire obese individuals (Roe and Eickwort 1976), and at least one survey of business executives suggests an inverse association between obesity and salary (*Industry Week* 1974). In a survey of college students, Kallen and Doughty (1984) found lower rates of reported dating in overweight subjects, although no less satisfaction with intimate relationships.

Although it is obvious that many overweight individuals are dissatisfied with their personal appearance, desire to lose weight, and frequently make efforts to lose weight (Wadden et al. 1989; Polivy, Garner, Garfinkel 1986; Adams 1980; Guggenheim, Poznanski, Kaufmann 1973; Dwyer, Feldman, Mayer 1975; Dwyer and Mayer 1970; Stewart and Brook 1983; Jeffery et al. 1984), evidence for severe psychological or social impairment in all but the most severe cases of obesity is generally lacking. Moore, Stunkard, and Srole (1962), reporting data from the Midtown Manhattan Study, found higher scores on three measures of psychological disability in the obese compared with the nonobese.

Data from the Rand Health Study and a Dutch population-based study indicated that obese individuals report that their weight imposes some restrictions on their everyday activities and causes them more pain and worry compared with the nonobese (Stewart, Brook, Kane 1980; Stewart and Brook 1983; Seidell et al. 1986). However, Stewart and Brook (1983) also reported that obese persons are less depressed than normal-weight persons, a finding corroborated in a study of British citizens by Crisp and McGuiness (1976). These mixed and inconsistent findings from studies of obese adults also have characterized studies of obese children (Wadden et al. 1989; Wadden et al. 1984). In extremely obese individuals presenting themselves for treatment (i.e., those 75 percent or more overweight), higher levels of psychological disturbance have been reported (Halmi et al. 1980; Atkinson and Ringuette 1967). Even here, it has been questioned whether such pathology is greater than that observed in normal-weight individuals presenting for medical or surgical procedures (Wise and Fernandez 1979; Swenson, Pearson, Osborne 1973). It has been suggested that unwarranted concerns about weight gain may contribute to eating disorders such as anorexia and bulimia (Wooley and Wooley 1984). Data supporting this idea, however, are largely anecdotal (Wadden and Stunkard 1985).

Prospective studies on the effects of weight gain on psychosocial functioning have not yet been reported. Studies of psychological changes accompanying weight loss generally show positive effects, even when weight loss is modest and not well maintained (Wing et al. 1984). Therefore, consistent with intuition, many people feel better about themselves when they lose weight. However, the extrapolation of these findings to weight gain lacks empirical support.

In summary, although adverse psychological and social consequences of overweight have been much discussed in both lay and professional circles, such effects have not been well documented. Moreover, to the extent that associations have been reported, the direction of causation is unclear. More research in this area is warranted, particularly because the available research is not extensive and much of it is methodologically weak. At this time, data suggest that only the most extreme forms of obesity, the upper 1 or 2 percent of the weight distribution in this domain, pose significant hazards. However, it is important to emphasize that these conclusions reflect the lack of evidence for serious psychosocial problems resulting from modest weight gains. Nevertheless, many persons want to lose weight, many persons seek ways to lose weight, and many persons feel better about themselves when they lose weight.

CHANGE IN WEIGHT-RELATED HEALTH RISKS AFTER SMOKING CESSATION

As documented earlier in this Chapter, smoking cessation is associated with weight gain. An important question is the extent to which this weight gain might lead to elevations in blood pressure, cholesterol, glucose intolerance, or other factors that would offset the benefits of smoking cessation discussed in detail throughout this Report.

Relatively few studies have specifically examined the effect of smoking cessation on weight-related health risks. Seven studies were reviewed for this Report. Gordon and coworkers (1975) reported changes over an 18-year period in weight and related risk characteristics among individuals in the Framingham Study. At entry into the study, 61 percent of men and 40 percent of women smoked cigarettes; at the 18-year followup, 37 percent of men and 31 percent of women continued to smoke. Analyses of changes were restricted to men because of the small numbers of women who quit smoking in this sample. Male quitters were similar to those who continued to smoke in baseline characteristics except that the former group contained more diabetics. The authors interpret this finding as suggesting that ill health is an incentive to stop smoking.

Short-term effects of smoking cessation, defined as the change between the last examination at which smoking was reported and the first examination at which nonsmoking was reported (2-year intervals), included a weight gain of 3.8 pounds, an increase in systolic blood pressure of 1.6 mm Hg, and an increase in serum cholesterol of 0.2 mg/dL. Continuing smokers had an average weight gain of 0.3 pound, increased systolic blood pressure of 0.7 mm Hg, and decreased serum cholesterol of 0.2 mg/dL. For the same time period, nonsmokers had an average weight gain of 0.5 pound, increased systolic blood pressure of 0.7 mm Hg, and increased serum cholesterol of 0.3 mg/dL. Differences among groups in blood pressure and cholesterol changes were not statistically significant. Long-term changes associated with smoking cessation were evaluated by comparing changes between the fourth and the tenth examination, a period of 12 years, among continuing smokers, nonsmokers, and individuals smoking at entry but not smoking from the fourth to the tenth examination. Trends in weight, blood pressure, serum cholesterol, and blood glucose did not differ significantly among these three groups.

Schoenenberger (1982) reported the relationship between smoking cessation and changes in body weight, blood pressure, and serum cholesterol over 3 years among men in the special intervention group in MRFIT. All men in the study were at high risk for heart disease and were being counseled throughout the study in smoking cessation and dietary changes to effect cholesterol reduction. When necessary, the men were also treated pharmacologically for elevated blood pressure. Results indicated significantly less weight loss in quitters (–0.6 pounds, i.e., a gain of 0.6 pounds) compared with nonsmokers and continuing smokers (5.7 and 3.6 pounds, respectively), no differences in blood pressure change (–9.6, –8.7, and –9.4 mm Hg, respectively, for systolic blood pressure among men not on medication), and greater reductions in serum cholesterol among quitters (–13.4 mg/dL) than in the other two groups (–10.0 and –8.1 mg/dL). The latter effect was interpreted as possibly reflecting a higher level of generalized motivation to reduce risk in the quitting group.

In a 5-year followup study of 2,283 persons with mild hypertension in eastern Finland, Tuomilehto and colleagues (1986) found that 26 percent of men and 35 percent of women who smoked at the time of the initial examination had quit. Among men, smoking cessation was associated with a 7.9-pound weight gain compared with 0.2-pound and 2.2-pound weight gains among nonsmokers and continuing smokers, respectively. Among women, weight loss after smoking cessation averaged 0.7 pound compared with gains of 0.1 pound and 2.2 pounds among nonsmokers and continuing smokers, respectively. Smoking cessation was not associated with a significant increase in blood pressure or serum cholesterol compared with continuing smokers or nonsmokers. Mean arterial pressure fell by 5.0 and 13.1 mm Hg in male and female quitters, respectively, compared with decreases of 6.9 and 8.7 mm Hg among nonsmokers and of 7.0 and 9.6 mm Hg among continuing smokers. Serum cholesterol fell between 0.63 and 0.66 mmol/L across the various subgroups.

Two papers relating smoking cessation to weight-related risks have been published based on data from the Normative Aging Study. The first report examined change over 5 years among 214 continuing smokers and 104 quitters (Garvey, Bossé, Seltzer 1974). An average weight gain of 4.2 pounds, which was accompanied by a 3.6 mm Hg increase in diastolic blood pressure, was observed among quitters compared with continuing smokers. The second report examined the relationship between smoking and body fat distribution, both cross-sectionally and longitudinally between examination visits scheduled 2 years apart (Shimokata, Muller, Andres 1989). Central body fat distribution, which poses increased health risks, as assessed by WHR was positively associated with smoking. Moreover, among smokers, daily cigarette consumption was positively associated with central adiposity. Smoking cessation was associated with increased body weight. However, despite the weight gain, the change in WHR among ex-smokers was small and, in fact, decreased slightly because hip circumference increased. Therefore, based on WHR data only, smoking rather than smoking cessation may pose a weight-related health risk.

Stamford and coworkers (1986) studied the short-term effects of smoking cessation on lipoprotein fractions. Among 13 women who successfully quit smoking for a period of 48 days, these investigators observed a weight increase of 4.9 pounds. This weight change was accompanied by a nonsignificant increase in total cholesterol of 9 mg/dL and a significant increase in HDL-C of 7 mg/dL. Over the subsequent year, these favorable HDL-C changes were maintained in three individuals continuing to abstain from smoking, but were lost in nine individuals who returned to smoking.

One randomized trial of smoking cessation and weight-related health risks was located for this review. Rabkin (1984a) randomized 107 smokers to smoking cessation and 33 to continued smoking in a comparative study of smoking cessation strategies. A battery of physiologic measures was obtained at baseline and repeated 2 to 3 months following randomization. No differences were found in cessation rates among the different quitting strategies. Physiologic changes observed in the smoking cessation group as a whole (i.e., all those randomized) included a significant increase in weight (1.8 pounds) and skinfold thickness (6.6 mm) compared with the control group (0.4 pound and −7.0 mm), but no significant change in lipid profiles, fasting glucose, or blood pressure. Only 35 subjects in the cessation groups were successful in quitting smoking. Successful quitters gained significant amounts of weight compared with individuals who did not quit (4.4 vs. 0.7 pounds, respectively). Successful quitters also experienced significant increases in HDL-C compared with nonquitters (4.2 vs. 0.1 mg/dL). Changes in other weight-related risk factors did not differ among groups.

The studies reviewed above are consistent in their findings. Individuals who quit smoking and gain weight appear to experience relatively small changes in health-related risk factors such as blood pressure, serum cholesterol, and blood glucose. Moreover, some of the potentially adverse effects of weight gain on health risks are mitigated by changes in lipid profiles and in body fat distribution in a direction predictive of improved health outcomes. It seems likely that only those smokers who have large weight gains after smoking cessation would experience important changes in weight-related risk factors.

The characteristics of individuals most likely to gain harmfully large amounts of weight after smoking cessation merit additional investigation. Bossé, Garvey, and Costa (1980) have reported relevant findings from the Normative Aging Study. Over a 5-year period these investigators found that factors most predictive of weight gain among recent quitters were younger age, leanness of body build, and greater amounts of smoking. The latter finding is confirmed by other studies (Blitzer, Rimm, Giefer 1977; Gordon et al. 1975). There are no data available on specific predictors of excessive weight gain among ex-smokers. Research on predictors of weight gain suggest that those persons most likely to gain weight after smoking cessation may be those who can best afford it because they are relatively lean. They also may be those who need smoking cessation most because they smoke the most.

Quantitatively estimating the extent of health risk associated with weight gain after smoking cessation is a complex process. The health risks of obesity vary with age, the temporal patterning of weight changes, type of obesity, and other risk factors. Moreover, smoking cessation itself appears to have independent effects on some weight-related risk factors that may actually be beneficial.

It has been estimated that the health risks posed by regular smoking double overall mortality rates compared with never smoking (US DHHS 1989). Moreover, as detailed elsewhere in this Report, there are clear health benefits associated with smoking cessation. The amount of excess body weight that would have to occur to offset the benefits of smoking cessation would have to be considerable. Yet, average weight gains after smoking cessation are only about 5 pounds, bringing most individuals to a weight level similar to that of their nonsmoking peers. As discussed in this Chapter, the proportion of ex-smokers who are likely to gain large amounts of weight (e.g., more than 20 pounds) is small. Therefore, although some individuals may experience these large weight gains, the number of individuals likely to gain enough weight to offset the benefits of smoking cessation is negligible. Also, the likelihood of adverse psychosocial consequences because of small weight gain seems remote for most people. Although further research in this area is warranted, there is little reason to expect weight gain to pose a substantive medical or psychosocial hazard to the vast majority of smokers who are quitting. For those persons who do gain excessive amounts of weight after smoking cessation, the health benefits of cessation still exist, and weight control programs rather than smoking relapse should be implemented. In conclusion, the clear reduction in health risks that results from smoking cessation overshadows any health risks that may result from smoking cessation-induced body weight gain.

STRATEGIES TO CONTROL POSTCESSATION WEIGHT GAIN

Because weight gain after smoking cessation commonly occurs and because many people, particularly young women, report smoking to control weight gain (Klesges and Klesges 1988; US DHHS 1990), strategies that successfully moderate postcessation weight gain may encourage weight-conscious smokers to attempt cessation and may facilitate the efforts of successful quitters to remain abstinent. Only a few controlled investigations have examined interventions for reducing weight gain after smoking cessation. Currently existing behavioral and pharmacologic interventions are summarized below.

Behavioral Methods for Reducing Postcessation Weight Gain

Smoking cessation programs that include a weight control component have not successfully increased smoking cessation. In one study, 79 women were randomly assigned to a 7-week smoking cessation program either with or without weight control information (Mermelstein 1987). At posttreatment and at followup, there were no significant differences in smoking cessation rates between the two groups. Participants in both groups gained weight during treatment; however, the weight increase for the smoking-cessation-plus-weight-control group was significantly less than the increase for the smoking-cessation-only group (1.4 vs. 2.4 pounds).

Several weight control strategies, as adjuncts to smoking cessation, were evaluated by Grinstead (1981). Forty-five subjects were randomly assigned to a 4-week smoking aversion program with one of three weight control interventions. No differences in smoking cessation rates were observed, and there were no weight change differences among the groups. Subjects in all groups gained weight during treatment.

In another smoking cessation study, Bowen, Spring, and Fox (submitted for publication) randomly assigned 31 participants to either a high- or low-carbohydrate diet. Subjects in the high-carbohydrate group were given specific dietary advice encouraging the use of carbohydrates; they were also given tryptophan as a dietary supplement. In the low-carbohydrate group, dietary advice focused on consumption of foods low in carbohydrates. Each group attended four 2-hour meetings per week. Sessions for both groups stressed information about the effects of tobacco, self-management strategies, rapid smoking, and relapse prevention techniques.

The rationale for this treatment approach is based on a 1982 report that smoking cessation is accompanied by an increase in preference for sweet-tasting high carbohydrate foods (Grunberg 1982a). Grunberg (1986) suggested that carbohydrates act through serotonergic mechanisms to attenuate withdrawal. Tryptophan is thought to increase the production of serotonin in the brain. At the end of treatment, 13 of 16 subjects (81 percent) in the high-carbohydrate group were abstinent (confirmed by CO assessments) compared with 9 of 15 subjects (60 percent) in the low-carbohydrate group. This difference was in the hypothesized direction but was not statistically significant. Also consistent with the hypothesis, nonabstainers in the high-carbohydrate group were smoking significantly fewer cigarettes than nonabstainers in the low-carbohydrate group. In both groups subjects gained weight after quitting smoking. No significant differences were observed between experimental groups in the number of subjects who gained weight or in the average amount of weight gain per subject.

Of the three investigations that have evaluated the impact of a weight-control program on weight gain and cessation (Bowen, Spring, Fox, submitted for publication; Grinstead 1981; Mermelstein 1987), none were successful in preventing weight gain and only one (Mermelstein 1987) reported a significant between-groups difference in the amount of weight gain. None of the smoking-plus-weight-control programs were clearly successful in significantly enhancing cessation rates.

At least three investigations have indicated that individuals can stop smoking without significant weight gain. However, these studies have been limited to subjects typically at high risk of CVD who participated in multicomponent CVD risk factor reduction trials. In a study involving MRFIT participants at the upper 10 to 15 percent on a measure of CVD risk, Schoenenberger (1982) reported that continuing smokers had lost an average of 4.6 pounds at a 3-year followup, but that those who quit smoking had gained less than 1 pound. All subjects participated in several treatments that focused on stopping smoking and improving diet. In a 6-year followup of these participants, quitters had gained 4.7 pounds compared with a 1.3-pound weight loss among nonquitters overall (Gerace et al., in press). However, weight gained after cessation varied as a function of baseline daily cigarette consumption. For those who had smoked 1 to 19 cigarettes per day, quitters averaged a 0.5-pound weight gain compared with a 2.4-pound weight loss among continuing smokers. For those who had smoked 20 to 39 cigarettes per day, quitters averaged a 4.6-pound weight gain compared with a 1.4-pound weight loss among continuing smokers. For those who had smoked more than 40 cigarettes per day, quitters averaged a 7.2-pound weight gain compared with a 1.0-pound weight loss among continuing smokers. Thus, weight gain after smoking cessation was positively related to daily cigarette consumption before quitting (Gerace et al., in press).

Hickey and Mulcahy (1973) reported on 124 male smokers who survived a myocardial infarction and participated in a lifestyle modification program. At 2-year followup, these investigators found an average weight gain of 1.6 pounds (change not significant) among the 60 individuals (48 percent) who quit smoking. Those individuals who continued to smoke averaged a small, but nonsignificant weight loss (0.8 pound). In a study of CVD risk factor assessment in Paris, Ducimetière and colleagues (1978) randomly assigned 271 smokers to either a cessation-plus-diet advice group or a smoking cessation-only group. The two groups did not differ in weight at pretest, but at 2-year followup, subjects in the cessation-plus-diet group had significantly lower weights than subjects in the cessation-only group. However, the two groups did not differ in smoking cessation, and the large degree of attrition in the cessation-plus-diet group must be noted when evaluating treatment outcome.

Thus, it appears that for individuals at high risk for CVD participating in intensive, multicomponent risk factor trials, smoking cessation can occur without significant increases in body weight. Future research needs to focus on whether similar results can be obtained with the typical smoker in a more cost-effective intervention.

Pharmacologic Methods for Reducing Postcessation Weight Gain

Three pharmacologic approaches have been evaluated as potential treatments for reducing postcessation weight gain: nicotine polacrilex gum, d-fenfluramine, and phenylpropanolamine (PPA). The available information on pharmacologic interventions for reducing postcessation weight gain is summarized below.

There is substantial evidence that nicotine is the agent in tobacco that causes changes in body weight (US DHHS 1988a). Therefore, the most obvious pharmacologic approach that may prove useful in reducing postcessation weight gain is nicotine replacement. The least hazardous vehicle currently available to deliver nicotine is nicotine polacrilex gum. As literature documenting the use of the gum to aid in quitting smoking has grown (Schwartz 1987; US DHHS 1988a), several correlational studies have reported that use of the gum reduces postcessation weight gain (Emont and Cummings 1987; Fagerström 1987; Hajek, Jackson, Belcher 1988), although this effect is not observed uniformly (Hjalmarson 1984; Tonnesen et al. 1988). In one study, Fagerström (1987) conducted a followup of 28 patients who were still abstinent at 6-month posttreatment after attending a smoking cessation clinic. These subjects received 2 mg of nicotine gum. Subjects were divided at the median (263) number of pieces of gum chewed. Six months after treatment, less frequent gum users had gained an average of 6.8 pounds, whereas the body weight of more frequent gum users had increased by 2.0 pounds. Fagerström (1987) hypothesized that higher nicotine polacrilex gum use was necessary to produce blood nicotine levels approaching the effective dosages achieved by smoking.

Emont and Cummings (1987) also found that nicotine polacrilex gum use reduced postcessation weight gain and that this effect was related to the amount of gum chewed. These investigators studied 104 participants of a 2.5-week stop-smoking clinic. Of the subjects who were either abstinent at 1 month or had smoked fewer than 5 cigarettes in the month since treatment, 20 had used nicotine polacrilex gum in their attempts to quit. Use of nicotine polacrilex gum in general was not significantly related to weight gain. However, when number of pieces of gum chewed per day was considered, there was a significant inverse correlation ($r=-0.37$) between nicotine polacrilex gum use and increase in body weight. When broken down by initial daily cigarette consumption, the relationship between nicotine polacrilex gum use and weight gain held only for individuals who had smoked more than 26 cigarettes per day. Neither the Fagerström (1987) nor the Emont and Cummings (1987) studies biochemically verified smoking status or measured blood nicotine levels.

In the only controlled investigation of this kind, Gross, Stitzer, and Maldonado (1989) examined the relationship between nicotine polacrilex gum use and body weight. Subjects were randomly assigned in a double-blind study either to a nicotine polacrilex gum or a placebo condition. Smoking and nicotine polacrilex gum use were verified with CO, thiocyanate, and cotinine measurements. Of the original 127 subjects, 40 completed the 10-week abstinence trial. In this period, abstinent subjects in the placebo group gained an average of 7.8 pounds, 4.0 pounds more than the abstinent nicotine polacrilex gum users. There was also evidence for a nicotine dose effect on weight gain. Users of fewer than 6.5 pieces of gum per day gained 5.0 pounds over the 10 weeks, whereas more frequent nicotine polacrilex gum users gained 1.5 pounds. Gross, Stitzer, and Maldonado (1989) present strong support for nicotine polacrilex gum's suppression of postcessation weight gain in this rigorous study. Once nicotine polacrilex gum use was discontinued, weight gain in both active gum and placebo conditions was comparable (6.8 vs. 8.7 pounds at 6-month followup). Thus, in this study, nicotine replacement delayed rather than prevented postcessation weight gain.

A recent controlled study (Spring et al., in press) evaluated the effects of d-fenfluramine on postcessation changes in food intake and weight gain. D-fenfluramine, which releases and blocks re-uptake of serotonin, is a prescription drug that has anorectic qualities without stimulating the central nervous system (CNS). For this study, 31 overweight female smokers were placed either on placebo or 30 mg d-fenfluramine per day in a double-blind assignment. Subjects then quit smoking and were observed for 4 weeks. Although the numbers of subjects remaining abstinent were small (five in the placebo group and eight in the d-fenfluramine group), significant differences in food intake between the two groups were observed over time. By 48 hours after discontinuing smoking, placebo-treated subjects consumed approximately 300 cal more per day than during the baseline measurement period. This increase resulted largely from increased consumption of carbohydrate-rich meal and snack foods. The difference in weight gain between the two groups was significant, with the placebo-treated subjects gaining an average of 3.5 pounds and the d-fenfluramine-treated subjects losing an average of 1.8 pounds. No significant differences in smoking cessation were observed, although statistical power to detect a difference was low.

A recently completed, placebo-controlled investigation evaluated the effects of phenylpropanolamine (PPA), which is an over-the-counter sympathomimetic agent that has weak CNS effects and more pronounced peripheral effects, on weight gain associated with smoking cessation (Klesges, Klesges et al. 1990). It is used both as an anorectic agent and as a decongestant. Subjects were 57 adult female cigarette smokers who were randomly assigned, in a double-blind procedure, to either gum with PPA, (25 mg tid), placebo gum, or no gum. After a baseline assessment, subjects were paid to quit smoking for 2 weeks. Smoking cessation was verified by weekly as well as by random (spot), CO assessments. Of the 57 subjects enrolled in the study, 41 (72 percent) were successful in quitting smoking. Of subjects receiving PPA, 94 percent quit smoking, whereas 63 percent of the two control groups quit smoking. Of those subjects remaining continuously abstinent over the 2 weeks, dietary intake decreased 630 kcal on average in the PPA group, whereas intake in the other two groups remained unchanged. Decreases in intake of all major nutrients (carbohydrate, fat, and protein) were observed in the PPA group. Abstinent subjects receiving PPA gained significantly less weight (mean change=0.09 pounds) compared with either the placebo gum group (mean change=1.59 pounds) or the no gum group (mean change=1.94 pounds).

To summarize this Section, additional minor weight control modifications to smoking cessation programs do not generally yield beneficial effects in terms of reducing postcessation weight gain or increasing cessation rates. However, aggressive weight control programs, perhaps offered after individuals have quit smoking (Wittsten 1988), may be able to produce smoking cessation without unwanted weight gain. Nicotine polacrilex gum, d-fenfluramine, and PPA all have promise as adjuncts for reducing postcessation weight gain, but research to date is extremely preliminary.

Focus needs to be on more effective behavioral methods for reducing unwanted postcessation weight gain and on combination therapies that include behavioral and pharmacologic strategies. High priority must be given to the development and evaluation of effective programs that can be offered in a cost-effective manner. Given the probable role of metabolic rate on postcessation weight gain, weight programs may need to focus on reduction of dietary intake rather than dietary maintenance. Additionally, aggressive weight management programs may not be necessary, or even wanted, for many subjects who quit smoking (Gritz, Klesges, Meyers 1989). Future investigations need to determine, of those who quit smoking, the individuals best suited for weight management programs without compromising smoking cessation.

Studies on the effects of nicotine polacrilex gum, d-fenfluramine, and PPA on postcessation weight gain yield some cautious optimism. However, longer followup periods and larger, more heterogeneous samples must be utilized in future investigations. It also appears, at least with nicotine polacrilex gum (Gross, Stitzer, Maldonado 1989), that weight gain can occur rapidly after gum use is discontinued. This delayed weight gain, and its possible role on post-drug relapse, needs to be investigated. Future research also needs to focus on specifying the influence of moderator variables, such as initial daily cigarette consumption, age, gender, and level of drug use on the effectiveness of these pharmacologic agents in preventing weight gain. Finally, the relative efficacy of these agents needs to be evaluated, and comparisons between pharmacologic and behavioral approaches to postcessation weight gain should be considered.

CONCLUSIONS

1. Average weight gain after smoking cessation is only about 5 pounds (2.3 kg). This weight gain poses a minimal health risk.

2. Approximately 80 percent of smokers who quit gain weight after cessation, but only about 3.5 percent of those who quit smoking gain more than 20 pounds.

3. Increases in food intake and decreases in resting energy expenditure are largely responsible for postcessation weight gain.

References

ABRAHAM, S., COLLINS, G., NORDSIECK, M. Relationship of childhood weight status to morbidity in adults. *HSMHA Health Reports* 86(3):273–284, March 1971.
ABRAMS, B., PARKER, J. Overweight and pregnancy complications. *International Journal of Obesity* 12(4):293–303, 1988.
ADAMS, G.R. Social psychology of beauty: Effects of age, height, and weight on self-reported personality traits and social behavior. *Journal of Social Psychology* 112:287–293, 1980.
ALBANES, D.M., JONES, Y., MICOZZI, M.S., MATTSON, M.E. Associations between smoking and body weight in the US population: Analysis of NHANES II. *American Journal of Public Health* 77(4):439–444, April 1987.
ALLON, N. The stigma of overweight in everyday life. In: Bray, G.A. (ed.) *Obesity in Perspective.* Volume II. Washington, DC: U.S. Government Printing Office, DHEW Publication No. (NIH) 75-708, 1973, pp. 83–102.
ANDERSON, J.J., FELSON, D.T. Factors associated with osteoarthritis of the knee in the first National Health and Nutrition Examination Survey (NHANES I): Evidence for an association with overweight, race, and physical demands of work. *American Journal of Epidemiology* 128(1):179–189, July 1988.
ANDRES, R., ELAHI, D., TOBIN, J.D., MULLER, D.C., BRANT, L. Impact of age on weight goals. *Annals of Internal Medicine* 103(6, Part 2):1030–1033, December 1985.
ATKINSON, R.M., RINGUETTE, E.L. A survey of biographical and psychological features in extraordinary fatness. *Psychosomatic Medicine* 29:121–133, March–April 1967.
BARRETT-CONNOR, E.L. Obesity, atherosclerosis, and coronary artery disease. *Annals of Internal Medicine* 103(6, Part 2):1010–1019, December 1985.
BJORNTORP, P. The associations between obesity, adipose tissue distribution and disease. *Acta Medica Scandinavica Supplement* 723:121–134, 1988.
BLACK, P.M., GIOVINO, G.A., OSSIP-KLEIN, D.J., LURIER, A., MEGAHED, N., DEBOLE, N., VALENZUELA, L., LEONE, M.A., STIGGINS, J. Smoking, weight gain, and relapse: Preliminary findings from a self-help population. Poster presented at the meeting of the Association for the Advancement of Behavior Therapy, New York, 1988.
BLACKBURN, H., PRINEAS, R. Diet and hypertension: Anthropology, epidemiology, and public health implications. *Progress in Biochemical Pharmacology* 19:31–79, 1983.
BLAIR, S.N., JACOBS, D.R., POWELL, K.E. Relationships between exercise or physical activity on other health behaviors. *Public Health Reports* 100:172–180, March–April 1985.
BLITZER, P.H., RIMM, A.A., GIEFER, E.E. The effect of cessation of smoking on body weight in 57,032 women: Cross-sectional and longitudinal analyses. *Journal of Chronic Diseases* 30(7):415–429, July 1977.
BORKAN, G.A., SPARROW, D., WISNIEWSKI, C., VOKONAS, P.S. Body weight and coronary disease risk: Patterns of risk factor change associated with long-term weight change. The Normative Aging Study. *American Journal of Epidemiology* 124(3):410–419, September 1986.
BOSSÉ, R., GARVEY, A., COSTA, P.T. Predictors of weight change following smoking cessation. *International Journal of the Addictions* 15(7):969–991, 1980.
BOWEN, D.J., SPRING, B., FOX, E. Dietary advice and smoking cessation. Submitted for publication.
BURSE, R.L., GOLDMAN, R.F., DANFORTH, E., HORTON, E.S., SIMS, E.A.H. *Effects of Cigarette Smoking on Body Weight, Energy Expenditure, Appetite, and Endocrine Function.* U.S. Army Medical Research and Development Command, Fort Detrick, Frederick, Maryland. Report No. M25/82, NTIS No. AD-A114 213/2, 1982.

CAMBIEN, F., RICHARD, J.-L., DUCIMETIERE, P., WARNET, J.M., KAHN, J. The Paris Cardiovascular Risk Factor Prevention Trial: Effects of two years of intervention in a population of young men. *Journal of Epidemiology and Community Health* 35:91–97, 1981.

CANNING, H., MAYER, J. Obesity—Its possible effect on college acceptance. *New England Journal of Medicine* 275(21):1172–1174, November 29, 1966.

CHIANG, B.N., PERLMAN, L.V., EPSTEIN, F.H. Overweight and hypertension: A review. *Circulation* 39(3):403–421, March 1969.

COATES, T.J., LI, V.C. Does smoking cessation lead to weight gain? The experience of asbestos-exposed shipyard workers. *American Journal of Public Health* 73(11):1303–1304, November 1983.

COMSTOCK, G.W., STONE, R.W. Changes in body weight and subcutaneous fatness related to smoking habits. *Archives of Environmental Health* 24(4):271–276, April 1972.

CRISP, A.H., MCGUINESS, B. Jolly fat: Relation between obesity and psychoneurosis in general population. *British Medical Journal* 1(6000):7–9, January 3, 1976.

DALLOSSO, H.M., JAMES, W.P.Y. The role of smoking in the regulation of energy balance. *International Journal of Obesity* 8(4):365–375, 1984.

DILORENZO, T.M., SHER, K., WALITZER, K., FARHA, J., POWERS, R. The effects of smoking cessation on food craving. Poster presented at the meeting of the Association for the Advancement of Behavior Therapy, New York, 1988.

DUCIMETIÈRE, P., KRITSIKIS, S., RICHARD, J.L., PEQUIGNOT, G. Changes in body weight of middle-aged smokers after modification of their tobacco consumption. *Epidemic and Public Health Review* 26(2):193–198, 1978.

DUFFY, J., HALL, S.M. Smoking abstinence, eating style, and food intake. *Journal of Consulting and Clinical Psychology* 56(3):417–421, June 1988.

DWYER, J.T., FELDMAN, J.J., MAYER, J. The social psychology of dieting. In: Hafen, B.Q. (ed.) *Overweight and Obesity: Causes, Fallacies, Treatment.* Provo, Utah: Brigham Young University Press, 1975, pp. 112–130.

DWYER, J.T., MAYER, J. Potential dieters: Who are they? *Journal of the American Dietetic Association* 56(6):510–514, June 1970.

EMONT, S.L., CUMMINGS, K.M. Weight gain following smoking cessation: A possible role for nicotine replacement in weight management. *Addictive Behaviors* 12(2):151–155, 1987.

FAGERSTRÖM, K.O. Reducing the weight gain after stopping smoking. *Addictive Behaviors* 12(1):91–93, 1987.

FELSON, D.T. Epidemiology of hip and knee osteoarthritis. *Epidemiological Reviews* 10:1–28, 1988.

FREEDMAN, D.S., RIMM, A.A. The relation of body fat distribution, as assessed by six girth measurements, to diabetes mellitus in women. *American Journal of Public Health* 79(6):715–720, June 1989.

FRIEDMAN, G.D., SIEGELAUB, A.B. Changes after quitting smoking. *Circulation* 61(4):716–723, April 1980.

GARFINKEL, L. Overweight and cancer. *Annals of Internal Medicine* 103(6, Part 2):1034–1036, December 1985.

GARRISON, R.J., CASTELLI, W.P. Weight and thirty-year mortality of men in the Framingham Study. *Annals of Internal Medicine* 103(6, Part 2):1006–1009, December 1985.

GARRISON, R.J., WILSON, P.W., CASTELLI, W.P., FEINLEIB, M., KANNEL, W.B., MCNAMARA, P.M. Obesity and lipoprotein cholesterol in the Framingham offspring study. *Metabolism* 29(11):1053–1060, October 1980.

GARVEY, A.J., BOSSÉ, R., SELTZER, C.C. Smoking, weight change, and age. A longitudinal analysis. *Archives of Environmental Health* 28(6):327–329, June 1974.

GERACE, T.A., HOLLIS, J., OCKENE, J.K., SVENDSEN, K. Cigarette smoking intervention in the Multiple Risk Factor Intervention Trial: Results and relationships to other outcomes.

Chapter 5—Relationship of smoking cessation to diastolic blood pressure, body weight, and plasma lipids. *Preventive Medicine*, in press.

GILLUM, R.F. The association of body fat distribution with hypertension, hypertensive heart disease, coronary heart disease, diabetes and cardiovascular risk factors in men and women aged 18–79 years. *Journal of Chronic Diseases* 40(5):421–428, 1987.

GLAUSER, S.C., GLAUSER, E.M., REIDENBERG, M.M., RUSY, B.F., TALLARIDA, R.J. Metabolic changes associated with the cessation of cigarette smoking. *Archives of Environmental Health* 20(3):377–381, March 1970.

GORDON, T., KANNEL, W.B., DAWBER, T.R., MCGEE, D. Changes associated with quitting cigarette smoking: The Framingham Study. *American Heart Journal* 90(3):322–328, September 1975.

GRAHAM, S., MARSHALL, J., HAUGHEY, B., MITTELMAN, A., SWANSON, M., ZIELEZNY, M., BYERS, T., WILKINSON, G., WEST, D. Dietary epidemiology of cancer of the colon in western New York. *American Journal of Epidemiology* 128(23):490–503, September 1988.

GRINSTEAD, O.A. *Preventing Weight Gain Following Smoking Cessation: A Comparison of Behavioral Treatment Approaches.* Doctoral Dissertation. University of California Los Angeles, University of Microfilms International, Thesis No. 82-06024, 1981, 174 pp.

GRITZ, E.R., CARR, C.R., MARCUS, A.C. Unaided smoking cessation: Great American Smokeout and New Year's Day Quitters. *Psychosocial Oncology* 6(3/4): 217–234, 1988.

GRITZ, E.R., KLESGES, R.C., MEYERS, A.W. The smoking and body weight relationship: Implications for intervention and postcessation weight control. *Annals of Behavioral Medicine* 11(4):144–153, 1989.

GROSS, J., STITZER, M.L., MALDONADO, J. Nicotine replacement: Effects of postcessation weight gain. *Journal of Consulting and Clinical Psychology* 57(1):87–92, February 1989.

GRUNBERG, N.E. The effects of nicotine and cigarette smoking on food consumption and taste preferences. *Addictive Behaviors* 7(4):317–331, 1982a.

GRUNBERG, N.E. Obesity: Etiology, hazards, and treatment. In: Gatchel, R.J., Baum, A., Singer, J.E. (eds.) *Handbook of Psychology and Health, Volume I. Clinical Psychology and Behavioral Medicine: Overlapping Disciplines.* Hillsdale, New Jersey: Lawrence Erlbaum Press, 1982b, pp. 103–120.

GRUNBERG, N.E. Behavioral and biological factors in the relationship between tobacco use and body weight. In: Katkin, E.S., Manuck, S.B. (eds.) *Advances in Behavioral Medicine.* Volume 2. Greenwich, Connecticut: JAI Press, 1986, pp. 97–129.

GRUNBERG, N.E., BOWEN, D.J., MORSE, D.E. Effects of nicotine on body weight and food consumption in rats. *Psychopharmacology* 83(1):93–98, April 1984.

GUGGENHEIM, K., POZNANSKI, R., KAUFMANN, N.A. Body build and self-perception in 13 and 14-year-old Israel children and their relationship to obesity. *Israel Journal of Medical Sciences* 9(2):120–128, February 1973.

HADDEN, W.C., HARRIS, M.I. Prevalence of diagnosed diabetes, undiagnosed diabetes, and impaired glucose tolerance in adults 20–74 years of age. *Vital and Health Statistics* Series 11, (237):1–55, February 1987.

HAJEK, P., JACKSON, P., BELCHER, M. Long-term use of nicotine chewing gum. Occurrence, determinants, and effect on weight gain. *Journal of the American Medical Association* 260(11):1593–1596, September 16, 1988.

HALL, S.M., MCGEE, R., TUNSTALL, C., DUFFY, J., BENOWITZ, N. Changes in food intake and activity after quitting smoking. *Journal of Consulting and Clinical Psychology* 57(1):81–86, February 1989.

HALMI, K.A., LONG, M., STUNKARD, A.J., MASON, E. Psychiatric diagnosis of morbidly obese gastric bypass patients. *American Journal of Psychiatry* 137(4):470–472, April 1980.

HAMM, P., SHEKELLE, R.B., STAMLER, J. Large fluctuations in body weight during young adulthood and twenty-five-year risk of coronary death in men. *American Journal of Epidemiology* 129(2):312–318, February 1989.

HARTZ, A.J., BARBORIAK, P.N., WONG, A., KATAYAMA, K.P., RIMM, A.A. The association of obesity with infertility and related menstrual abnormalities in women. *International Journal of Obesity* 3(1):57–73, 1979.

HATSUKAMI, D.K., HUGHES, J.R., PICKENS, R.W., SVIKIS, D. Tobacco withdrawal symptoms: An experimental analysis. *Psychopharmacology* 84(2):231–236, October 1984.

HICKEY, N., MULCAHY, R. Effect of cessation of smoking on body weight after myocardial infarction. *American Journal of Clinical Nutrition* 26(4):385–386, April 1973.

HJALMARSON, A.I.M. Effect of nicotine chewing gum in smoking cessation: A randomized, placebo-controlled, double-blind study. *Journal of the American Medical Association* 252(20):2835–2838, November 1984.

HOFSTETTER, A., SCHUTZ, Y., JEQUIER, E., WAHREN, J. Increased 24-hour energy expenditure in cigarette smokers. *New England Journal of Medicine* 314(2):79–82, January 1986.

INDUSTRY WEEK. Fatter execs get slimmer paychecks. *Industry Week* 180:21, 24, January 14, 1974.

JEFFERY, R.W., FOLSOM, A.R., LUEPKER, R.V., JACOBS, D.R. JR., GILLUM, R.F., TAYLOR, H.L., BLACKBURN, H. Prevalence of overweight and weight loss behavior in a metropolitan adult population: The Minnesota Heart Survey experience. *American Journal of Public Health* 74(4):349–352, April 1984.

JOOSTE, P.L., STEENKAMP, H.J., BENADE, A.J., ROSSOUW, J.E. Prevalence of overweight and obesity and its relation to coronary heart disease in the CORIS study. *South African Medical Journal* 74(3):101–104, August 6, 1988.

KALLEN, D.J., DOUGHTY, A. The relationship of weight, the self perception of weight and self esteem with courtship behavior. In: Kallen, D.J., Sussman, M.B. (eds.) *Obesity and the Family.* New York: The Haworth Press, Inc. 1984, pp. 93–114.

KANNEL, W.B., GORDON, T., CASTELLI, W.P. Obesity, lipids, and glucose intolerance. The Framingham Study. *American Journal of Clinical Nutrition* 32(6):1238–1245, June 1979.

KEYS, A. Overweight, obesity, coronary heart disease, and mortality. In: Selby, N., White, P.L. (eds.) *Nutrition in the 1980s: Constraints on Our Knowledge. Proceedings of the Western Hemishpere Nutrition Congress VI Held in Los Angeles, California, August 10–14, 1980.* New York: Alan R. Liss, Inc., 1981, pp. 31–46.

KLESGES, R.C., CODAY, M., PASCALE, R., MEYERS, A., WINDERS, S., HULTQUIST, C., KLESGES, L.M. The cumulative effects of cigarette smoking on resting energy expenditure. *Proceedings of the Society of Behavioral Medicine*, Chicago, Illinois, 1990.

KLESGES, R.C., ECK, L.H., CLARK, E., MEYERS, A.W., HANSON, C.L. The effects of smoking cessation and gender on dietary intake, physical activity, and weight gain. *International Journal of Eating Disorders*, 9:435–446, 1990.

KLESGES, R.C., ECK, L.H., ISBELL, T., FULLITON, W., HANSON, C.L. The effects of smoking status on the dietary intake, physical activity, and body fat of adult men. *American Journal of Clinical Nutrition* 51:784–789, 1990.

KLESGES, R.C., KLESGES, L.M. Cigarette smoking as a dieting strategy in a university population. *International Journal of Eating Disorders* 7:413–419, 1988.

KLESGES, R.C., KLESGES, L.M., MEYERS, A.W., KLEM, M.L., ISBELL, T. The effects of phenylpropanolamine on dietary intake, physical activity, and body weight after smoking cessation. *Clinical Pharmacology and Therapeutics* 47(6):747–754, 1990.

KLESGES, R.C., MEYERS, A.W., KLESGES, L.M., LA VASQUE, M.E. Smoking, body weight, and their effects on smoking behavior: A comprehensive review of the literature. *Psychological Bulletin* 106(2):204–230, September 1989.

KRAMER, J.F. A one-year follow-up of participants in a smoke stoppers program. *Patient Counselling and Health Education* 4(2):89–94, 1982.

LAPIDUS, L., BENGTSSON, C. Regional obesity as a health hazard in women—A prospective study. *Acta Medica Scandinavica Supplement* 723:53–59, 1988.

LARSSON, B., BJORNTORP, P., TIBBLIN, G. The health consequences of moderate obesity. *International Journal of Obesity* 5(2):97–116, 1981.

LARSSON, B., SVARDSUDD, K., WELIN, L., WILHELMSEN, L., BJORNTORP, P., TIBBLIN, G. Abdominal adipose tissue distribution, obesity, and risk of cardiovascular disease and death: 13 year follow up of participants in the study of men born in 1913. *British Medical Journal* 288(6428):1401–1404, May 12, 1984.

LEISCHOW, S.J., STITZER, M.L. Smoking cessation and weight gain. *Proceedings of the Society of Behavioral Medicine Ninth Annual Scientific Sessions*, 172 [Abstract], 1989.

LEW, E.A., GARFINKEL, L. Variations in mortality by weight among 750,000 men and women. *Journal of Chronic Diseases* 32(8):563–576, 1979.

LISSNER, L., BENGTSSON, C., LAPIDUS, L., LARSSON, B., BENGTSSON, B., BROWNELL, K. Body weight variability and mortality in the Göteborg prospective studies of men and women. In: Bjorntorp, P., Rossner, S. (eds.) *Proceedings of the First European Congress of Obesity, June 1987*. London: Libbey, 1989, pp. 55–60.

LISSNER, L., COLLINS, G., BLAIR, S.N., BROWNELL, K.D. Weight fluctuation and mortality in the MRFIT population. Abstract presented at the Society for Epidemiologic Research, June 15–17, Vancouver, British Columbia, Canada, 1988.

LISSNER, L., ODELL, P., D'AGOSTINO, R., STOKES, J., KREGER, B., BELANGER, A., BROWNELL, K. Health implications of weight cycling in the Framingham population. Abstract presented at the Society for Epidemiologic Research, June 15–17, Vancouver, British Columbia, Canada, 1988.

LUND-LARSEN, P.G., TRETLI, S. Changes in smoking habits and body weight after a three-year period: The cardiovascular disease study in Finnmark. *Journal of Chronic Diseases* 35(10):773–780, 1982.

MACMAHON, S., CUTLER, J., BRITTAIN, E., HIGGINS, M. Obesity and hypertension: Epidemiological and clinical issues. *European Heart Journal* 8(Supplement B):57–70, May 1987.

MACMAHON, S.W., BLACKET, R.B., MACDONALD, G.J., HALL, W. Obesity, alcohol consumption and blood pressure in Australian men and women: The National Heart Foundation of Australia Risk Factor Prevalence study. *Journal of Hypertension* 2(1):85–91, February 1984.

MADDOX, G.L., LIEDERMAN, V. Overweight as a social disability with medical implications. *Journal of Medical Education* 44(3):214–220, March 1969.

MANLEY, R.S., BOLAND, F.J. Side-effects and weight gain following a smoking cessation program. *Addictive Behaviors* 8(4):375–380, 1983.

MANSON, J.E., STAMPFER, M.J., HENNEKENS, C.H., WILLETT, W.C. Body weight and longevity: A reassessment. *Journal of the American Medical Association* 257(3):353–358, January 16, 1987.

MARTI, B., TUOMILEHTO, J., KORHONEN, H.J., KARTOVAARA, L., VARTIAINEN, E., PIETINEN, P., PUSKA, P. Smoking and leanness: Evidence for change in Finland. *British Medical Journal* 298(6683):1287–1290, May 13, 1989.

MERMELSTEIN, R. Preventing weight gain following smoking cessation. Poster presented at the meeting of the Society of Behavioral Medicine Eighth Annual Scientific Session, Washington, DC, March 1987.

METROPOLITAN LIFE INSURANCE COMPANY. Overweight: Its prevention and significance. Statistical bulletin, 1960.

MOORE, M.E., STUNKARD, A., SROLE, L. Obesity, social class and mental illness. *Journal of the American Medical Association* 181(11):962–966, September 15, 1962.

NANAS, S., PAN, W.H., STAMLER, J., LIU, K., DYER, A., STAMLER, R., SCHOENBERGER, J.A., SHEKELLE, R.B. The role of relative weight in the positive association between age and serum cholesterol in men and women. *Journal of Chronic Diseases* 40(9):887–892, 1987.

NATIONAL INSTITUTES OF HEALTH CONSENSUS DEVELOPMENT CONFERENCE STATEMENT. Health implications of obesity. *Annals of Internal Medicine* 103(6, Part 2):1073–1077, December 1985.

NEGRI, E., PAGANO, R., DECARLI, A., LA VECCHIA, C. Body weight and the prevalence of chronic diseases. *Journal of Epidemiology and Community Health* 42(1):24–29, March 1988.

NOPPA, H., BENGTSSON, C. Obesity in relation to smoking: A population study of women in Göteberg, Sweden. *Preventive Medicine* 9(4):534–543, July 1980.

NOPPA, H., BENGTSSON, C., WEDEL, H., WILHELMSEN, L. Obesity in relation to morbidity and mortality from cardiovascular disease. *American Journal of Epidemiology* 111(6):682–692, June 1980.

PAN, W.H., NANAS, S., DYER, A., LIU, K., MCDONALD, A., SCHOENBERGER, J.A., SHEKELLE, R.B., STAMLER, R., STAMLER, J. The role of weight in the positive association between age and blood pressure. *American Journal of Epidemiology* 124(4):612–623, October 1986.

PERKINS, K.A., EPSTEIN, L.H., MARKS, B.L., STILLER, R.L., JACOB, R.G. The effect of nicotine on energy expenditure during light physical activity. *New England Journal of Medicine* 320(14):898–903, April 6, 1989a.

PERKINS, K.A., EPSTEIN, L.H., MARKS, B.L., STILLER, R.L., JACOB, R.G. Resting metabolic rate in male nonsmokers versus recently abstinent smokers. *Proceedings of the Society of Behavioral Medicine Ninth Annual Scientific Sessions*, 169 [Abstract], 1989b.

PERKINS, K.A., EPSTEIN, L.H., PASTOR, S. Changes in energy balance following smoking cessation and resumption of smoking in women. *Journal of Consulting and Clinical Psychology* 58(1):121–125, 1990.

PERKINS, K.A., EPSTEIN, L.H., STILLER, R.L., MARKS, B.L., JACOB, R.G. Acute effects of nicotine on resting metabolic rate in cigarette smokers. *American Journal of Clinical Nutrition* 50(3):545–550, September 1989.

PERKINS, K.A., EPSTEIN, L.H., STILLER, R.L., SEXTON, J., JACOB, R.G., DEBSKI, T. The combined effects of nicotine and consumption of a meal on metabolic rate. Poster presented at the meeting of the Society of Behavioral Medicine, San Francisco, California, 1989.

PICONE, T.A., ALLEN, L.H., SCHRAMM, M.M., OLSEN, P.N. Pregnancy outcome in North American women. I. Effects of diet, cigarette smoking, and psychological stress on maternal weight gain. *American Journal of Clinical Nutrition* 36(6):1205–1213, December 1982.

POLIVY, J., GARNER, D.M., GARFINKEL, P.E. Causes and consequences of the current preference for thin female physiques. In: Herman, C.P., Zanna, M.P., Higgins, E.T. (eds.) *Physical Appearance, Stigma, and Social Behavior: The Ontario Symposium, Volume 3.* Hillsdale, New Jersey: Lawrence Erlbaum Associates, Publishers, 1986, pp. 89–112.

POWERS, P.S. *Obesity, the Regulation of Weight.* Baltimore: Williams and Wilkins, 1980.

PUDDEY, I.B., VANDONGEN, R., BEILIN, L.J., ENGLISH, D.R., UKICH, A.W. The effect of stopping smoking on blood pressure—A controlled trial. *Journal of Chronic Diseases* 38(6):483–493, 1985.

RABKIN, S.W. Effect of cigarette smoking cessation on risk factors for coronary atherosclerosis: A control clinical trial. *Atherosclerosis* 53(2):173–184, November 1984a.

RABKIN, S.W. Relationship between weight change and the reduction or cessation of cigarette smoking. *International Journal of Obesity* 8(6):665–673, 1984b.

RABKIN, S.W., MATHEWSON, F.A., HSU, P.H. Relation of body weight to development of ischemic heart disease in a cohort of young North American men after a 26 year observation period: The Manitoba Study. *American Journal of Cardiology* 39(3):452–458, March 1977.

RICHARDSON, S.A. Research report: Handicap, appearance and stigma. *Social Science and Medicine* 5(6):621–628, December 1971.

RIMM, A.A., WERNER, L.H., BERNSTEIN, R., VAN YSERLOO, B. Disease and obesity in 73,532 women. *Obesity and Bariatric Medicine* 1(4):77–84, November–December 1972.

ROBINSON, S., YORK, D.A. The effect of cigarette smoking on the thermic response to feeding. *International Journal of Obesity* 10(5):407–417, 1986.

RODIN, J. Weight change following smoking cessation: The role of food intake and exercise. *Addictive Behaviors* 12:303–317, 1987.

ROE, D.A., EICKWORT, K.R. Relationship between obesity and associated health factors with unemployment among low income women. *Journal of the American Medical Women's Association* 31(5):193–194, May 1976.

SCHECHTER, M.D., COOK, P.G. Nicotine-induced weight loss in rats without an effect on appetite. *European Journal of Pharmacology* 38(1):63–69, July 1976.

SCHOENENBERGER, J.C. Smoking change in relation to changes in blood pressure, weight, and cholesterol. *Preventive Medicine* 11:441–453, 1982.

SCHWARTZ, H. Problems of obesity in anesthesia. *New York State Journal of Medicine* 55:3277–81, November 15, 1955.

SCHWARTZ, J.L. Review and Evaluation of Smoking Cessation Methods: The United States and Canada, 1978–1985. U.S. Department of Health and Human Services, National Cancer Institute, Division of Cancer Prevention. NIH Publication No. 87-2940, 1987.

SEIDELL, J.C., BAKX, K.C., DEURENBERG, P., BUREMA, J., HAUTVAST, J.G.A.J., HUYGEN, F.J.A. The relation between overweight and subjective health according to age, social class, slimming behavior and smoking habits in Dutch adults. *American Journal of Public Health* 76(12):1410–1415, December 1986.

SELBY, J.V., FRIEDMAN, G.D., QUESENBERRY, C.P. JR. Precursors of essential hypertension. The role of body fat distribution pattern. *American Journal of Epidemiology* 129(1):43–53, January 1989.

SELTZER, C.C. Effect of smoking on blood pressure. *American Heart Journal* 87(5):558–564, May 1974.

SHIMOKATA, H., MULLER, D.C., ANDRES, R. Studies in the distribution of body fat. III. Effects of cigarette smoking. *Journal of the American Medical Association* 261(8):1169–1173, February 24, 1989.

SOCIETY OF ACTUARIES AND ASSOCIATION OF LIFE INSURANCE MEDICAL DIRECTORS OF AMERICA. Build Study, 1979. Philadelphia: Recording and Statistical Corporation, 1980.

SPRING, B., WURTMAN, J., GLEASON, R., WURTMAN, R., KESSLER, K. Weight gain and withdrawal symptoms after smoking cessation: A preventive intervention using d-fenfluramine. *Health Psychology*, in press.

STAMFORD, B.A., MATTER, S., FELL, R.D., PAPANEK, P. Effects of smoking cessation. *American Journal of Clinical Nutrition* 43(4):486–494, April 1986.

STAMFORD, B.A., MATTER, S., FELL, R.D., SADY, S., CRESANTA, M.K., PAPANEK, P. Cigarette smoking, physical activity, and alcohol consumption: Relationship to blood lipids and lipoproteins in premenopausal females. *Metabolism* 33(7):585–590, July 1984.

STAMFORD, B.A., MATTER, S., FELL, R.D., SADY, S., PAPANEK, P., CRESANTA, M. Cigarette smoking, exercise, and high density lipoprotein cholesterol. *Atherosclerosis* 52(1):73–83, July 1984.

STEWART, A.L., BROOK, R.H. Effects of being overweight. *American Journal of Public Health* 73(2):171–178, February 1983.

STEWART, A.L., BROOK, R.H., KANE, R.L. Conceptualization and measurement of health habits for adults in the health insurance study: Volume II, Overweight. *Rand Report* (R-2374/2-HEW), July 1980.

SUBCOMMITTEE ON NONPHARMACOLOGICAL THERAPY OF THE 1984 JOINT NATIONAL COMMITTEE ON DETECTION, EVALUATION, AND TREATMENT OF HIGH BLOOD PRESSURE. Nonpharmacological approaches to the control of high blood pressure. *Hypertension* 8(5):444–467, May 1986.

SWENSON, W.M., PEARSON, J.S., OSBORNE, D. *An MMPI Source Book: Basic Item, Scale, and Pattern Data on 50,000 Medical Patients* Minneapolis: University of Minnesota Press, 1973.

TONNESEN, P., FRYD, V., HANSEN, M., HELSTED, J., GUNNERSEN, A.B., FORCHAMMER, H., STOCKNER, M. Effect of nicotine chewing gum in combination with group counseling on the cessation of smoking. *New England Journal of Medicine* 318(1):15–18, January 7, 1988.

TSAI, S.P., LUCAS, L.J., BERNACKI, E.J. Obesity and morbidity prevalence in a working population. *Journal of Occupational Medicine* 30(7):589–591, July 1988.

TUOMILEHTO, J., NISSINEN, A., PUSKA, P., SALONEN, J.T., JALKANEN, L. Long-term effects of cessation of smoking on body weight, blood pressure and serum cholesterol in the middle-aged population with high blood pressure. *Addictive Behaviors* 11:1–9, 1986.

U.S. DEPARTMENT OF HEALTH AND HUMAN SERVICES. *The Health Consequences of Smoking: Nicotine Addiction. A Report of the Surgeon General, 1988.* U.S. Department of Health and Human Services, Public Health Service, Centers for Disease Control, Center for Health Promotion and Education, Office on Smoking and Health. DHHS Publication No. (CDC) 88-8406, 1988a.

U.S. DEPARTMENT OF HEALTH AND HUMAN SERVICES. *The Surgeon General's Report on Nutrition and Health, 1988.* U.S. Department of Health and Human Services, Public Health Service. DHHS (PHS) Publication No. 88-50211, 1988b.

U.S. DEPARTMENT OF HEALTH AND HUMAN SERVICES. *Reducing the Health Consequences of Smoking: 25 Years of Progress. A Report of the Surgeon General.* U.S. Department of Health and Human Services, Public Health Service, Centers for Disease Control, Center for Chronic Disease Prevention and Health Promotion, Office on Smoking and Health. DHHS Publication No. (CDC) 89-8411, 1989.

U.S. DEPARTMENT OF HEALTH AND HUMAN SERVICES. *Tobacco Use in 1986. Methods and Basic Tabulations from Adult Use of Tobacco Survey.* Public Health Service, Centers for Disease Control, Center for Chronic Disease Prevention and Health Promotion, Office on Smoking and Health. DHHS Publication No. (OM) 90-2004, 1990.

U.S. DEPARTMENT OF HEALTH, EDUCATION, AND WELFARE. *The Smoking Digest: Progress Report on a Nation Kicking the Habit.* U.S. Department of Health, Education, and Welfare, Public Health Service, National Institutes of Health, Office of Cancer Communications, National Cancer Institute, The Smoking Digest, October 1977, p. 127.

VERREAULT, R., BRISSON, J., DESCHENES, L., NAUD, F. Body weight and prognostic indicators in breast cancer: Modifying effect of estrogen receptors. *American Journal of Epidemiology* 129(2):260–268, February 1989.

WAALER, H.T. Hazard of obesity—The Norwegian experience. *Acta Medica Scandinavica Supplement* 723:17–21, 1988.

WADDEN, T.A., FOSTER, G.D., BROWNELL, K.D., FINLEY, E. Self-concept in obese and normal-weight children. *Journal of Consulting and Clinical Psychology* 52(6):1104–1105, December 1984.

WADDEN, T.A., FOSTER, G.D., STUNKARD, A.J., LINOWITZ, J.R. Dissatisfaction with weight and figure in obese girls: Discontent but not depression. *International Journal of Obesity* 13(1):89–97, February 1989.

WADDEN, T.A., STUNKARD, A.J. Social and psychological consequences of obesity. *Annals of Internal Medicine* 103(6, Part 2):1062–1067, December 1985.

WARWICK, P.M., CHAPPLE, R.S., THOMSON, E.S. The effect of smoking two cigarettes on resting metabolic rate with and without food. *International Journal of Obesity* 11(3):229–237, 1987.

WELLMAN, P.J., MARMON, M.M., REICH, S., RUDDLE, J. Effects of nicotine on body weight, food intake and brown adipose tissue thermogenesis. *Pharmacology Biochemistry and Behavior* 24(6):1605–1609, June 1986.

WEST, K.M., KALBFLEISCH, J.M. Influence of nutritional factors on prevalence of diabetes. *Diabetes* 20(2):99–108, February 1971.

WINDERS, S., BROWN, K., KLESGES, R.C., HAYES, A., MEYERS, A.W. The effects of smoking and coffee consumption on resting energy expenditure. *Proceedings of the Society of Behavioral Medicine*, Chicago, Illinois, 1990.

WINDERS, S.E., GRUNBERG, N.E. Nicotine, tobacco smoke, and body weight: A review of the animal literature. *Annals of Behavioral Medicine* 11(4):125–133, 1989.

WING, R.R., EPSTEIN, L.H., MARCUS, M.D., KUPFER, D.J. Mood changes in behavioral weight loss programs. *Journal of Psychosomatic Research* 28(3):189–196, 1984.

WISE, T., FERNANDEZ, F. Psychological profiles of candidates seeking surgical correction for obesity. *Obesity and Bariatric Medicine* 8(3):83–86, May–June 1979.

WITTSTEN, A.B. Weight control program reinforces smoking cessation [news]. *American Journal of Public Health* 78(9):1240–1241, September 1988.

WOOLEY, S.C., WOOLEY, O.W. Should obesity be treated at all? In: Stunkard, A.J., Stellar, E. (eds.) *Eating and Its Disorders*. Research Publications: Association for Research in Nervous and Mental Disease, Volume 62. New York: Raven Press, 1984, pp. 185–192.

CHAPTER 11
PSYCHOLOGICAL AND BEHAVIORAL CONSEQUENCES AND CORRELATES OF SMOKING CESSATION

CONTENTS

Introduction ... 521
Short-Term Effects of Smoking Cessation: Nicotine Withdrawal ... 521
   Brief Review of Previous Work ... 521
   Craving as a Withdrawal Symptom ... 523
   Changes in Alcohol and Caffeine Use ... 524
   Withdrawal Relief Versus Enhancement Models of the Effects of Smoking on Performance ... 525
   Variability in Withdrawal ... 526
   Timecourse of Withdrawal ... 529
   Withdrawal as a Cause of Relapse ... 530
   Summary ... 531

Long-Term Psychological and Behavioral Consequences and Correlates of Smoking Cessation ... 532
   Introduction ... 532
   Mood, Anxiety, Perceived Stress, and Psychological Well-Being ... 533
      Research Results ... 534
   Self-Efficacy and Locus of Control ... 541
      Self-Efficacy ... 541
      Locus of Control ... 542
   Coping and Self-Management Skills ... 543
   Social Support and Interpersonal Interactions ... 545
   Summary ... 546

Health Practices of Former Smokers ... 546
   Introduction ... 546
   Physical Activity ... 551
   Dietary Practices ... 554
   Use of Other Substances ... 555
      Other Tobacco Products ... 555
      Alcohol ... 556
   Studies of Multiple Health Habits ... 559
   Summary ... 561

Participation of Former Smokers in Health-Screening Programs ... 561

Summary ... 565

Conclusions ... 565

References ... 567

INTRODUCTION

Former smokers often describe quitting smoking as a turning point in their lives. For many individuals, cessation leads to an improved sense of well-being and often serves as a catalyst for other positive health-related lifestyle changes (Finnegan and Suler 1985; Knudsen et al. 1984; Suedfeld and Best 1977). These improvements in psychosocial functioning and health-related lifestyle behaviors may contribute to and reinforce continued abstinence. However, some smokers may hesitate to try to quit because they fear negative changes in mood and well-being (Gritz 1980; Hall 1984; Tamerin 1972). In addition, relapsers often attribute their return to smoking to unwanted changes in mood or to a strong desire for a cigarette (Baer 1985; Chapman, Smith, Layden 1971; Marlatt and Gordon 1980; Russell 1970; Shiffman 1982).

This Chapter reviews findings on short-term withdrawal effects and the longer term psychological and behavioral effects related to abstinence from smoking. Short-term withdrawal effects are described in the 1988 Report of the Surgeon General on nicotine addiction (US DHHS 1988). The first Section of this Chapter updates this review by examining recent studies in six areas: craving as a withdrawal symptom, changes in alcohol and caffeine use, withdrawal relief versus enhancement models of the effects of abstinence on performance, variability in withdrawal, timecourse of withdrawal, and nicotine withdrawal as a cause of relapse. The second Section reviews longer term changes, such as changes in the use of alcohol, illicit drugs, and other tobacco products as well as increases in other health-related practices and preventive health behaviors, including participation in cardiovascular and cancer screening. A major portion of this Section reviews the relationship of long-term abstinence to psychological factors such as mood, coping with stress, self-efficacy, and locus of control. Because the long-term psychological and behavioral effects of smoking abstinence have never been summarized, this Section will include a more indepth review of studies than will be provided in the Section on short-term effects.

Providing smokers with information on transient adverse withdrawal effects and the distinction between these and the longer term psychological and behavioral benefits of abstinence may allay fears and help remove barriers to quitting or to maintaining abstinence. This information may also help to develop more effective programs that help the smoker plan and cope with the effects of cigarette abstinence. For example, education about the signs and symptoms of withdrawal from tranquilizers appears to help long-term users stop using tranquilizers (Lader and Higgitt 1986).

SHORT-TERM EFFECTS OF SMOKING CESSATION: NICOTINE WITHDRAWAL

Brief Review of Previous Work

Over the last decade, several reviews have been published on nicotine withdrawal (Hatsukami, Hughes, Pickens 1985; Henningfield 1984; Hughes, Higgins, Hatsukami 1990; Murray and Lawrence 1984; Shiffman 1979; US DHHS 1988; West 1984). Perhaps the most widely-accepted description of nicotine withdrawal is that which appears in the *Diagnostic and Statistical Manual of Mental Disorders* (DSM-III-R, American Psychiatric Association 1987) (Table 1). In addition to the signs and symptoms listed in DSM-III-R, depression, disrupted sleep, impatience, and perhaps increased pleasantness of sweets are common and valid indicators of nicotine withdrawal (Hughes, Higgins, Hatsukami 1990). However, an especially important effect not included in DSM-III-R is impaired performance, particularly on vigilance and rapid information processing tasks (Snyder, Davis, Henningfield 1989; Wesnes and Warburton 1983). Other consequences of withdrawal, which may not be clinically evident, include slowing of the electroencephalogram, changes in rapid eye movement during sleep, decreased levels of catecholamines, decreased thyroid function, increased levels of medications, decreased orthostatis, and increased skin temperature (American Psychiatric Association 1987; Hughes, Higgins, Hatsukami 1990).

TABLE 1.—Diagnostic categorization and criteria for nicotine withdrawal— nicotine-induced organic mental disorder

The essential feature of this disorder is a characteristic withdrawal syndrome due to the abrupt cessation of or reduction in the use of nicotine-containing substances (e.g., cigarettes, cigars, pipes, chewing tobacco, or nicotine gum) and that has been at least moderate in duration and amount.

Among many heavy cigarette smokers, changes in mood and performance that are related to withdrawal can be detected within 2 hr after the last tobacco use. The sense of craving appears to reach a peak within the first 24 hr after cessation of tobacco use and gradually declines thereafter over a few days to several weeks. In any given case it is difficult to distinguish a withdrawal effect from the emergence of psychological traits that are suppressed, controlled, or altered by the effects of nicotine or from a behavioral reaction (e.g., frustration) to the loss of a reinforcer.

Mild symptoms of withdrawal may occur after switching to low-tar (nicotine) cigarettes and after stopping the use of smokeless (chewing) tobacco or nicotine polacrilex gum.

Diagnostic criteria for nicotine withdrawal:

A. Daily use of nicotine for at least several weeks.

B. Abrupt cessation of nicotine use or reduction in the amount of nicotine used followed within 24 hr by at least four of the following signs:

(1) craving for nicotine

(2) irritability, frustration, or anger

(3) anxiety

(4) difficulty concentrating

(5) restlessness

(6) decreased heart rate

(7) increased appetite or weight gain

SOURCE: Condensed from the American Psychiatric Association (1987).

The signs and symptoms of nicotine withdrawal are observable; they are often of clinically significant magnitude and occur in self-quitters as well as those who attend smoking cessation clinics (Hughes, Higgins, Hatsukami 1990). Most withdrawal symptoms are opposite to those produced by administration of nicotine, occur for a specified period of time, and with continued abstinence, return to levels similar to those experienced by a smoker. Relief of withdrawal by use of nicotine polacrilex gum, occurrence of withdrawal upon cessation of nicotine polacrilex gum, and occurrence of withdrawal upon switching to low-nicotine cigarettes indicate that a lack of nicotine is responsible for most withdrawal effects (Hughes, Higgins Hatsukami 1990; West 1984).

Craving as a Withdrawal Symptom

Recent articles have attempted to clarify the role of craving in cigarette smoking (Kozlowski and Wilkinson 1987a; West and Kranzler 1990; West and Schneider 1987). The term "craving" has been used loosely and interchangeably by both smokers and investigators to indicate a strong desire or urge to smoke. The problems associated with this terminology and the advantages to using the term "strong desire" have been outlined (Hughes 1986a; Kozlowski and Wilkinson 1987a; Kozlowski and Wilkinson 1987b; Marlatt 1987; Rankin 1987; Shiffman 1987; Stockwell 1987; West 1987; West and Schneider 1987; Kozlowski, Mann et al. 1989). Although an increased desire for a cigarette is a common consequence of abstinence, part of the craving may result from the desire to relieve other withdrawal symptoms by having a cigarette. For example, a review by West and Schneider (1987) demonstrated that withdrawal effects, such as irritability and restlessness, are positively associated with craving. They noted that drugs such as clonidine may alleviate craving because these agents reduce the other symptoms. Thus, craving might be alleviated by reducing other withdrawal symptoms (Kozlowski and Wilkinson 1987a).

An urge to smoke may be due to several factors, such as response to environmental stimuli associated with cigarette smoking or deprivation, onset of withdrawal symptoms, and protracted withdrawal. That such effects are physiologically, behaviorally, or cognitively mediated has been debated widely (Kozlowski and Wilkinson 1987a, b; West and Kranzler 1990; West and Schneider 1987).

The desire to smoke as indicative of nicotine withdrawal has been a subject of some controversy for five reasons. First, the referent for the terms craving and desire is unclear. In 1955, the World Health Organization (WHO) stated, "a term such as 'craving' with its everyday connotations should not be used in the scientific literature . . . if confusion is to be avoided" (WHO 1955, p. 63). On the other hand, craving for a cigarette is the most commonly reported postcessation symptom (Hughes, Higgins, Hatsukami 1990); and therefore, it is difficult to ignore these self-reports.

Second, craving readily occurs even when smokers are not trying to abstain (Hughes, Higgins, Hatsukami 1990; Hughes and Hatsukami 1986). However, many other withdrawal symptoms, such as irritability, are also experienced by smokers (Hughes, Higgins, Hatsukami 1990).

Third, several factors other than abstinence, such as sensory cues associated with smoking (Rose 1988), the "behavior" of smoking (Hajek et al. 1989), and expectancy (Hughes et al. 1989; Gottlieb et al. 1987), can influence craving. However, these factors can also affect other withdrawal symptoms (Francis and Nelson 1984). In addition, demonstrating that a symptom is influenced by a nonabstinence variable does not mean that the symptom cannot be induced by abstinence; it simply suggests nonspecificity; that is, abstinence is only one of many causes.

Fourth, nicotine polacrilex gum does not predictably reduce the desire for a cigarette (Hughes 1986b; West 1984; West and Schneider 1987). However, one possibility is that more cigarette-like (i.e., more bolus-like) routes of administration of nicotine, such as aerosols, nasal sprays, and vapors, would decrease desire to smoke (Pomerleau et al. 1988).

Fifth, managing craving may be critical to cessation of smoking. Recent prospective studies have indicated that postcessation self-reports of craving are predictive of later relapse (Gritz, Carr, Marcus 1990; West, Hajek, Belcher 1989; Killen et al. 1990). Also, the ubiquity of smoking cues and the availability of cigarettes may make craving especially prevalent and difficult to resist.

Recent research contradicts the commonly held notion that the desire for cigarettes is less than that for prototypic drugs of abuse (Kozlowski, Wilkinson et al. 1989). Persons presenting for treatment of alcohol and drug problems compared the strongest urge they had for cigarettes with their strongest urge for the alcohol or drug for which they were seeking treatment. Among alcohol-dependent persons, 50 percent reported that their strongest urges for cigarettes were greater than their strongest alcohol urges, 32 percent reported that the strongest urges were about the same for both cigarettes and alcohol, and 18 percent reported that their strongest urges for alcohol were greater than for cigarettes. Among drug-dependent persons, 25 percent said their strongest urges were for cigarettes, 27 percent said their strongest urges were about the same, and 48 percent said their strongest urges were for their drug of choice.

In the treatment of drug dependencies, such as alcohol, use of the term craving has been historically associated with theories of loss of control (Ludwig and Wikler 1974). Typically, tobacco researchers are not implying loss of control over smoking when they use the term craving (Kozlowski and Wilkinson 1987a). Smokers may or may not be implying loss of control when they use the term.

In summary, although the desire to smoke may have a more complex origin than other withdrawal symptoms, it is a predictable and important withdrawal effect. The occurrence of craving after cessation has several implications. It suggests that nicotine delivered in a cigarette-like system may be the best method to relieve the desire to smoke because the delivery would mimic some of the sensory cues associated with smoking (Rose 1988; Hajek et al. 1989). Also, it suggests that for smokers who wish to avoid medication, behavioral strategies could be used to combat even pharmacologically mediated desires to smoke.

Changes in Alcohol and Caffeine Use

Initial short-term changes in alcohol and caffeine intake upon smoking abstinence are of increasing interest. It is unclear that smoking cessation impedes abstinence or prompts relapse back to drinking among those with alcohol dependence (Kozlowski, Ferrence, Corbit 1990). Such changes in alcohol and caffeine use were not reviewed extensively in the 1988 Surgeon General's Report on nicotine addiction (US DHHS

1988). Long-term effects of abstinence on alcohol intake are reviewed later in this Chapter.

Two prospective studies found that among smokers trying to stop smoking permanently, alcohol use significantly decreased, by about 75 percent per drink per day in one study, during the first week after abstinence (Hughes and Hatsukami 1986; Puddey et al. 1985). A third study reported that subjects who had a larger decrease in the number of cigarettes smoked postcessation had a larger decrease in alcohol use (Olbrisch and Oades-Souther 1986). However, a recent study suggested the opposite; that is, alcohol use increased among females who stopped smoking temporarily for 1 week for the duration of an experiment (Perkins, Epstein, Pastor 1990). This discrepancy across experiments may be due to gender or motivational differences in the populations. In the latter case, an increase in alcohol consumption may occur when smokers in an experiment do not try to control their alcohol intake during temporary smoking abstinence; however, when smokers are trying to stop permanently they may decrease alcohol use voluntarily as an aid to smoking cessation.

Abstinence does not appear to change short-term caffeine intake (Benowitz, Hall, Modin 1989; Hughes and Hatsukami 1986; Hughes 1990; Hughes et al. 1990; Kozlowski 1976; Puddey et al. 1985; Rodin 1987). Smoking increases the elimination of caffeine, probably through non-nicotine-related mechanisms (Benowitz 1988); thus, when smokers stop, their rates of elimination of caffeine decrease (Benowitz, Hall, Modin 1989; Brown et al. 1988). With no change in caffeine intake, blood levels of caffeine increase 2.5-fold (Brown et al. 1988). Because several of the symptoms of caffeine intoxication are similar to those of nicotine withdrawal (e.g., anxiety, restlessness, and irritability), it has been suggested that these increased levels of caffeine may mimic or potentiate symptoms attributed to tobacco withdrawal (Sachs and Benowitz 1990).

Withdrawal Relief Versus Enhancement Models of the Effects of Smoking on Performance

The effects of abstinence on performance were reviewed in the Surgeon General's Report on nicotine addiction (US DHHS 1988). This review and others (Hughes, Higgins, Hatsukami 1990) have concluded that abstinence impairs performance on attention tasks, especially those labeled as rapid information processing, selective attention, sustained attention, or vigilance tasks. This impairment may persist for at least 7 to 10 days (Snyder, Davis, Henningfield 1989) and is reversed by nicotine replacement (Snyder and Henningfield 1989). However, it is not clear that abstinence impairs learning, memory, performance on more complex tasks, problem solving, or reaction time.

In the prototypic procedure for studying the effects of smoking on performance, smokers abstain overnight; performance is then measured before and after smoking a cigarette. A possible result would be that performance on a vigilance task was better after smoking than before smoking. Some researchers might interpret this difference as an indication that smoking enhances performance (Wesnes, Warburton, Matz 1983). However, another interpretation is that the presmoking performance level was poor because of tobacco withdrawal and that the improvement in performance occurred because smoking relieves tobacco withdrawal (Schachter 1979; Silverstein 1982). This latter interpretation assumes that overnight deprivation induces withdrawal; although this assumption has not been tested directly, withdrawal effects can occur after only 12 hours of deprivation (Hughes, Higgins, Hatsukami 1990).

Ideally, studying smokers before initiation would allow comparison of this baseline with before and after a smoking episode. As this is impractical, one solution has been to add a control group of nonsmokers (Hughes, Higgins, Hatsukami 1990). For example, smokers performed better after smoking and the same as nonsmokers in several studies of errors on a vigilance task (Taylor and Blezard 1979; Hughes, Keenan, Yellin 1989; Lyon et al. 1975; Heimstra et al. 1980; Tong et al. 1977; Tarriere and Hartmann 1983; Keenan, Hatsukami, Anton 1989) and a tracking task (Lyon et al. 1975) (Figure 1, upper panel). The effect was attributed to relief of withdrawal.

One study provided evidence for enhancement of performance from smoking independent of reversing withdrawal. Wesnes and Warburton (1978) reported a pattern consistent with enhancement when errors on vigilance tasks were studied (Figure 1, lower panel).

Other indirect evidence can be used to test the withdrawal relief versus enhancement models. Two studies reported enhancement of tracking or motor skills when smokers were not deprived (Parrott and Winder 1989; Hindmarch, Kerr, Sherwood 1990; Larson, Finnegan, Haag 1950; Pomerleau and Pomerleau 1986). Several studies have examined the effect of cigarette smoking or nicotine administration on the performance of nonsmokers (Dunne, MacDonald, Hartley 1986; Hindmarch, Kerr, Sherwood 1990; Wesnes, Warburton, Matz 1983; Wesnes and Revell 1984; West and Jarvis 1986; Wesnes and Warburton 1984). In two studies, the improvement in nonsmokers was similar to that of deprived smokers (Wesnes, Warburton, Matz 1983; Wesnes and Revell 1984). One study reported performance to be similar between deprived smokers and nonsmokers (Warburton 1990). Finally, nicotine appears to improve the performance of animals not previously exposed to nicotine (Clarke 1987; Emley and Hutchinson 1984).

In summary, the results of studies to assess if smoking increases performance through withdrawal relief or by direct enhancement appear contradictory. One possible explanation of this discrepancy is that smoking may increase performance through both withdrawal relief and direct enhancement. The specific mechanism that is operative may vary not only among smokers but also within smokers across situations.

Variability in Withdrawal

Whereas the necessary and sufficient condition to establish dependence is repeated exposure to the drug, other factors may exacerbate nicotine withdrawal symptoms. Although several investigators have commented on the variability of postcessation symptoms, it is unclear that this variability is greater than with other drug withdrawal syndromes (Hughes, Higgins, Hatsukami 1990; US DHHS 1988). The results of retrospective and postcessation studies on self-reported withdrawal symptoms (e.g., hunger, restlessness, or inability to concentrate) among smokers who have a greater

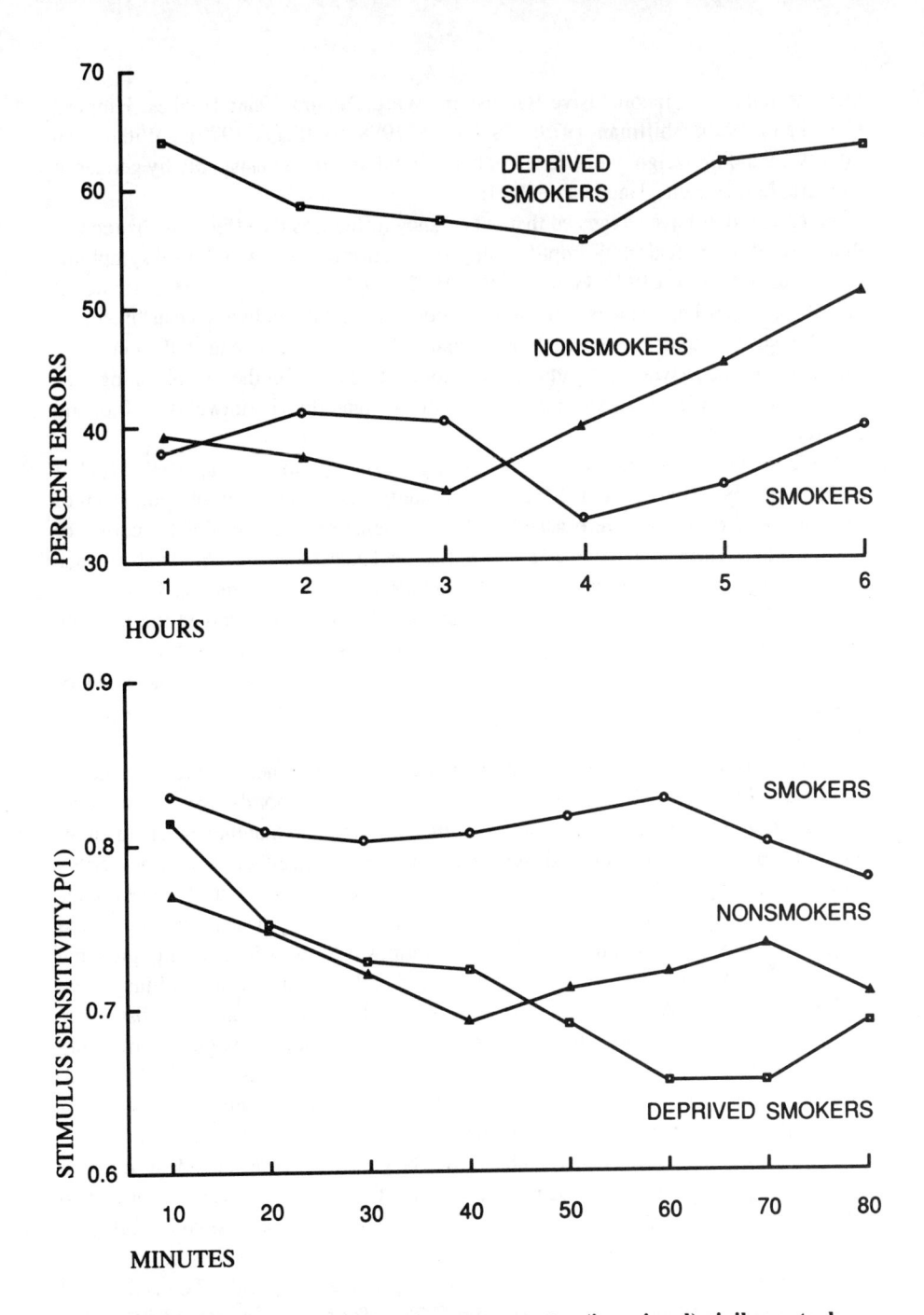

FIGURE 1.—*Upper panel:* **Performance on a meter (i.e., visual) vigilance task**
SOURCE: Heimstra et al. 1980.

Lower panel: **Performance on the continuous clock task, a visual vigilance task**

NOTE: Increased stimulus sensitivity refers to fewer errors.

SOURCE: Wesnes and Warburton (1978).

nicotine intake are inconclusive (Goldstein, Ward, Niaura 1988; Hughes, Higgins, Hatsukami 1990; Shiffman 1979; US DHHS 1988; Williams 1979). Withdrawal effects, including weight gain, have not been found to differ consistently by gender or age (Hughes, Higgins, Hatsukami 1990).

Several studies have suggested that expectancy influences the effects of abstinence; that is, some individuals may amplify, deny, or misattribute their withdrawal symptoms (Barefoot and Girodo 1972; Gottlieb et al. 1987; Hughes and Krahn 1985; Hughes et al. 1989). According to the misattribution model, at times the individual can "mistake" withdrawal symptoms for other possible events. For example, in one study a labeling mistake was made when individuals were told that a placebo they were taking was alleged to have side effects similar to the effects of cigarette withdrawal (Barefoot and Girodo 1972).

Three direct tests of expectancy have been published (Gottlieb et al. 1987; Hughes and Krahn 1985; Hughes et al. 1989). In one study, subjects in a double-blind trial of nicotine polacrilex gum were asked if they thought they had received nicotine or placebo gum. Those who believed they had received placebo gum had more abstinence discomfort than those who could not differentiate what they had received; this latter group had more discomfort than those who thought they had received the nicotine polacrilex gum (Hughes and Krahn 1985). Because this study used post hoc ratings, it is unclear that the belief in which gum had been received modified the level of abstinence effects, or that the level of abstinence effects modified the belief of which gum had been received.

Two experimental trials have manipulated instructions and thereby directly tested if expectancy influences abstinence effects. The first study randomly assigned smokers to a 2x2 design of contrasting instructions; subjects were told that they received either nicotine polacrilex gum or placebo gum, and actually received either nicotine polacrilex gum or placebo gum (Gottlieb et al. 1987). Most of the measures of abstinence effects were unchanged by instructions or by actual drugs. The physical symptoms and stimulation scores on the Shiffman-Jarvik Withdrawal Scale were less only on some days in the group told they were receiving nicotine than in the group told they were receiving placebo. A second study used a similar design and found that abstinence symptoms were fewer among those who received nicotine polacrilex gum than among those who received placebo gum, but found no effect of instructions (Hughes et al. 1989). In summary, the seemingly valid proposition that abstinence effects are influenced by expectancy has not been completely supported by empirical tests.

Abstinence effects have been hypothesized to be greater in more dependent smokers. However, the scales for dependence used to test this hypothesis vary according to whether they are quantifying physical dependence (withdrawal), behavioral dependence (desire for tobacco or tendency to relapse), or dependence on tobacco or on the nicotine in tobacco (Hughes 1984). The Fagerström Tolerance Scale (TQ) is the most widely used dependence scale (Fagerström 1978). TQ consists mostly of items that refer to behavioral dependence on tobacco. The total TQ score predicted total abstinence discomfort in one study (Fagerström 1980) and weight gain in another study (Tønnesen et al. 1988). However, two detailed studies failed to indicate that TQ predicted weight gain (Emont and Cummings 1987) or self-reported withdrawal symptoms.

The Reasons for Smoking Scale has two scales relevant to the dependence construct—the addiction scale and the negative affect scale (Ikard, Green, Horn 1969). Neither of these has been shown to predict weight gain (Bossé, Garvey, Costa 1980), self-reported withdrawal (Hughes and Hatsukami 1986), or relief by nicotine polacrilex gum (Hughes and Hatsukami 1986).

Russell's Smoking Motivation Questionnaire has a subscale for dependence (Russell, Peto, Patel 1974). In one study, the scale predicted total abstinence discomfort and irritability but did not predict restlessness, depression, hunger, or inability to concentrate (West and Russell 1985).

Another measure somewhat related to dependence includes the severity of abstinence discomfort in the past, which appears to predict self-reported abstinence (Hughes and Hatsukami 1986). Other generic scales, such as the MacAndrews Scale for Addiction (MacAndrew 1979) and Eysenk Personality Questionnaire (Eysenk and Eysenk 1975), do not predict abstinence discomfort and weight gain (Bossé, Garvey, Costa 1980). Although one study found that self-reported smoking for stimulation predicted abstinence effects (Niaura et al. 1989), an earlier study had found no such relationship (West and Russell 1985).

In summary, the evidence that any dependence scale predicts abstinence effects is quite limited. Further tests that use scales that more specifically determine physical versus behavioral dependence and dependence on nicotine versus tobacco may provide more informative data.

Timecourse of Withdrawal

Several recent studies produced concordant results on the timecourse of nicotine withdrawal. Most signs and symptoms of nicotine withdrawal are readily detected within 24 hours (Hughes, Higgins, Hatsukami 1990). Previous studies have suggested that abstinence effects can occur even sooner, for example, within 2 hours (US DHHS 1988). These studies have measured effects during smoking and 2 to 6 hours postsmoking; it was noted that 2 to 6 hours after smoking, self-ratings of performance were worse than during smoking. Several investigators have interpreted the scores during smoking as representing baseline and the postsmoking scores as representing withdrawal. However, as discussed earlier, an alternate interpretation is possible: the scores 2 to 6 hours postsmoking represent baseline scores and the scores during smoking represent the acute effects of smoking (Hughes et al. 1990).

The results of several prospective studies indicate that the signs and symptoms of nicotine withdrawal peak in the first 1 to 2 days following cessation (Cummings et al. 1985; Hughes and Hatsukami 1986; West et al. 1984; Shiffman and Jarvik 1976; Schneider, Jarvik, Forsythe 1984) and last about 1 month (Gritz, Carr, Marcus 1990; Cummings et al. 1985; Gross and Stitzer 1989; Hughes 1990; Hughes et al. 1990; Lawrence, Amoedi, Murray 1982; West, Hajek, Belcher 1987). For each of 10 weeks, Gross and Stitzer (1989) recorded symptoms of quitters and found a peak during the first week and a return to baseline 3 to 4 weeks postcessation. Snyder, Davis, and

Henningfield (1989) tracked performance on several tasks over 10 days. Impairment in performance peaked at 1 to 2 days, and performance on most tasks returned to baseline during the 10 days; however, performance on some tasks was still impaired after 10 days. A study by Cummings and colleagues (1985) included 33 subjects who kept a daily record of 8 withdrawal symptoms. At 21 days, few subjects were reporting withdrawal symptoms, with the exception of an occasional desire for a cigarette. A fourth study (Hughes 1990) provided a less-detailed timecourse but included groups of never smokers, ex-smokers, and continuing smokers. The withdrawal scores of abstinent smokers at 1 month were equivalent to their baseline scores and to those of never smokers and continuing smokers (Hughes 1990). Although the average withdrawal symptom score returned to baseline at 1 month, 45 percent of subjects reported symptoms still above precessation levels at 1-month followup (Hughes 1990). Further followup of these subjects indicated that their withdrawal scores had returned to baseline or below baseline by 6 months postcessation. Craving, hunger, and weight gain are exceptions to the 1-month duration; they may continue at least through the first 6-months after cessation (Gritz, Carr, Marcus 1990; Hughes 1990; Hughes et al. 1990; West, Hajek, Belcher 1987).

With cessation of other drugs, a prolonged withdrawal syndrome has been postulated (Martin and Jasinski 1969). There is no evidence of a prolonged nicotine withdrawal syndrome. In fact, scores on withdrawal scales appear to decrease below precessation levels at followup (Figure 2); that is, positive mood changes occur after long-term abstinence from smoking (Chapter 11, see section on long-term psychological and behavioral consequences and correlates of smoking cessation) (Gritz, Carr, Marcus 1990; Gross and Stitzer 1989; Hughes 1990; Hughes et al. 1990).

Withdrawal as a Cause of Relapse

Seven recent studies have examined nicotine withdrawal as a predictor of relapse, that is, whether smokers with severe withdrawal are more likely to relapse. Five studies found that some withdrawal symptoms predicted relapse at some points in time (Gritz, Carr, Marcus 1990; West, Hajek, Belcher 1990; Hughes 1990; Killen et al. 1990; Swan et al. 1988). The two studies that did not indicate such a relationship examined the ability of withdrawal to predict abstinence at very early followup (Hughes and Hatsukami 1986) or very late followup (Hughes et al. 1990). In the five positive studies, mood changes, such as depression and anxiety, were the more common predictors. However, both across and within the studies, there was no consistent or clear grouping of symptoms predicting withdrawal at specific points in time. One common finding was that the number of symptoms appeared to be a predictor (Gritz, Carr, Marcus 1990; Hughes 1990). For subgroups of smokers, such as more dependent smokers, withdrawal may be an especially important factor in relapse, but this relationship has not been demonstrated.

Postcessation weight gain has often been hypothesized to be a major cause of relapse, especially among women (Hall, Ginsberg, Jones 1986). Contrary to several *a priori* hypotheses, three prospective studies have found that more weight gain predicted less relapse (Duffy and Hall 1990; Hall, Ginsberg, Jones 1986; Hughes et al. 1990). There

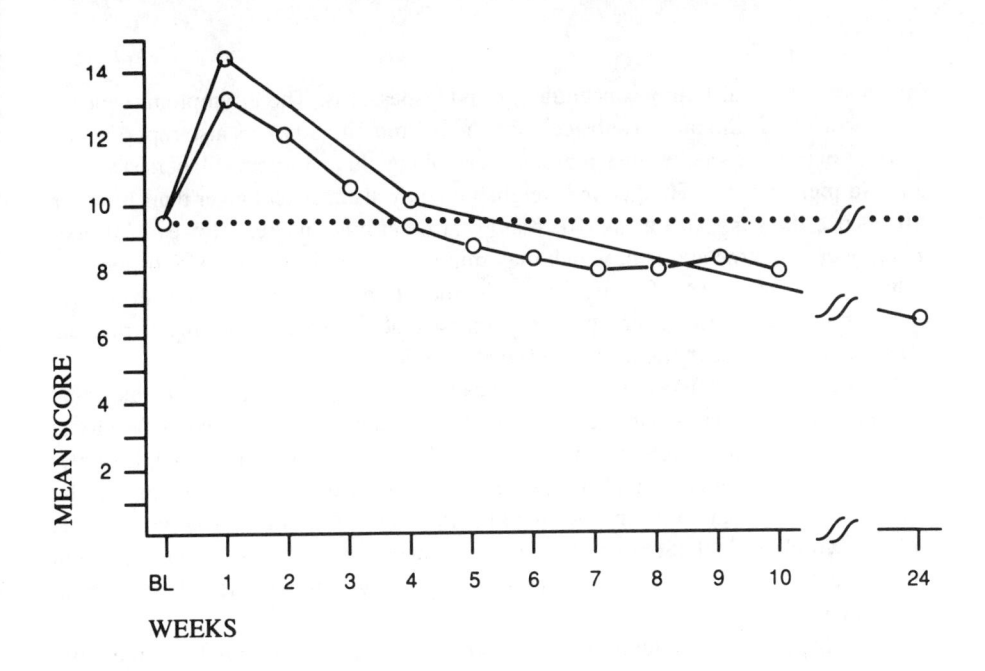

FIGURE 2.—Self-reported withdrawal discomfort among abstinent smokers
SOURCE: Gross and Stitzer 1989; Hughes (1990).

was no gender difference in this prediction in any of the three studies. This finding is further supported by a study in which women who reported eating more in the first 4 days of cessation were more likely to be abstinent at 6-month followup (Guilford 1966). One explanation for the weight gain–relapse finding is that food deprivation increases the reinforcing effects of drugs (Carroll and Meisch 1984). Cessation of smoking may decrease metabolic rate (Perkins, Epstein, Pastor 1990); if this is true, to avoid weight gain, smokers may deprive themselves of food and thereby increase the reinforcing effects of cigarettes smoked during periods of relapse.

In summary, this recent evidence shows that smokers with more severe withdrawal symptoms are more likely to relapse. However, these results should not be misinterpreted. First, prediction is not equivalent to causality; withdrawal symptoms may predict relapse, not because they cause relapse, but because they are associated with some other variable, such as degree of dependence. Second, those symptoms that predict the occurrence of relapse and the timing of relapse—very early (<2 days), early (2–10 days), or later (10–30 days)—vary across studies. Third, although studies have shown that withdrawal is an early predictor of relapse, these studies have not shown that withdrawal predicts eventual outcome (i.e., long-term abstinence).

Summary

Strong evidence indicates that smokers who stop smoking experience a nicotine withdrawal syndrome that includes the short-term consequences of anxiety, irritability, frustration, anger, difficulty concentrating, and restlessness. These symptoms generally occur within 24 hours and subside after about 1 month. Smokers also report strong cravings or urges to smoke when they are not smoking; this symptom will persist among some former smokers. Hunger and weight gain may also persist longer than 1 month. Abstinence does not appear to affect short-term caffeine intake. However, it does increase caffeine metabolism, which may mimic or potentiate symptoms of nicotine withdrawal. There are conflicting data on the short-term effects of smoking abstinence on alcohol intake. However, the data suggest that smokers attempting permanent smoking abstinence experience decreased alcohol intake.

Research on the effects of smoking abstinence on performance indicates that abstinence impairs performance on attention tasks. This impairment may persist for at least 7 to 10 days and is relieved by nicotine replacement. Other more complex types of tasks as well as memory and learning have not been clearly shown to be impaired by abstinence. The relation of improvement in attention tasks with nicotine may be due either to withdrawal relief or to performance enhancement; findings are consistent with both models. However, evidence more strongly suggests withdrawal relief from receiving nicotine.

Variability in tobacco withdrawal symptoms resembles that observed for other drug withdrawal syndromes. Several studies have suggested that expectancy influences withdrawal effects. However, this has not been completely supported by empirical tests. Although abstinence effects have been hypothesized to be greater in more dependent smokers, the evidence is conflicting. Recent data indicate that smokers with more severe withdrawal symptoms are more likely to relapse. However, no symptoms or groups of symptoms consistently predict relapse at any given point in time.

LONG-TERM PSYCHOLOGICAL AND BEHAVIORAL CONSEQUENCES AND CORRELATES OF SMOKING CESSATION

Introduction

Most long-term studies of self-quitters or smokers taking part in treatment programs only include data on smoking behavior or smoking status (Adesso 1979; Gordon and Cleary 1986; Orleans and Shipley 1982; Shipley, Rosen, Williams 1982); followup measures of psychological and behavioral consequences are rarely included. Thus, although former smokers represent a large and growing segment of the U.S. population (Volume Appendix), the long-term psychological and behavioral consequences of smoking cessation have not been well studied.

Very few studies of former smokers have employed prospective or longitudinal designs; rather, most have used retrospective or cross-sectional designs. In the typical retrospective study, subjects are asked whether after quitting or during their experience of trying to quit, they were more or less nervous, irritable, depressed, sedentary, or health conscious than before quitting. While relevant to the experience of a person abstaining from tobacco, retrospective studies potentially suffer from several limitations, including the absence of information about baseline group similarities or differences and the problem of recall bias. (See Chapter 2 for a discussion of methodologic problems.) Successful former smokers may minimize or fail to recall their difficulties or exaggerate their prowess (Heinold et al. 1982); recidivists may exaggerate withdrawal problems to justify their relapse (Graham and Gibson 1971). Cross-sectional studies do not permit the establishment of comparability at baseline. Conclusions from the data are therefore limited, often identifying the correlates of cessation rather than the consequences. Both consequences and correlates of cessation will be discussed in this Section.

Most prospective studies of smoking cessation sequelae have been conducted with smokers participating in formal treatment programs rather than with smokers quitting on their own (Hughes, Higgins, Hatsukami 1990). Treatment participants may differ in several ways from self-quitters. In a recent review of findings concerning short-term withdrawal effects, Hughes, Higgins, and Hatsukami (1990) noted that self-quitters had fewer and less severe withdrawal symptoms than treated quitters; they noted, as did Schachter (1982), that clinic populations may include a higher proportion of hardcore, highly dependent smokers. On the other hand, treated quitters may learn new coping skills such as relaxation, self-reward, or exercise and gain additional support for their initial quitting efforts. Therefore, their short-term postquitting experiences may not be representative of the 90 percent of former smokers who quit on their own (US DHHS 1988; Fiore et al. 1990). Thus, in drawing conclusions from studies of participants in treatment programs, it is important to be aware of the possible differences between these two populations of abstainers.

Mood, Anxiety, Perceived Stress, and Psychological Well-Being

Tobacco use has often been described as a maladaptive response to, or a way to cope with, life stress and a way to regulate negative affect (Tomkins 1966; Billings and Moos 1981; Ockene et al. 1981; Orleans 1985; Abrams et al. 1987). Smokers often believe that smoking helps them cope with stress and anxiety (Ikard, Green, Horn 1969). Thus, in addition to the stress of separation from cigarettes (Tamerin 1972), abstaining from cigarettes potentially could make the smoker feel less able to cope with stress (Abrams et al. 1987; Marlatt and Gordon 1985) and thereby constitute a biologically based source of stress (Grunberg and Baum 1985). If the quitter feels unable to cope with stress without cigarettes, perceived stress may increase, and self-efficacy may decrease, resulting in heightened anxiety and an overall negative shift in well-being. Alternatively, Cohen and Lichtenstein (in press) have hypothesized that for smokers who want to quit smoking, continued smoking may prove more stressful than cessation, and quitting smoking may result in a more positive self-appraisal and heightened feelings of self-esteem and personal competence. Similarly, other researchers have proposed that smoking may cause negative self-evaluations and feelings of guilt and helplessness among smokers who want to quit, so that quitting would result in an overall long-term improvement in mood, self-image, and self-esteem (Frerichs et al. 1981; Knudsen et al. 1984; Schwartz and Dubitzky 1968).

Possible long-term changes in anxiety levels after quitting might also reflect quitting-related changes in physiologic stress reactivity (Abrams et al. 1987). To the extent that smoking contributes to excess physiologic stress reactivity and more ready arousal to anxiety (Emmons et al. 1986; Williams, Hudson, Redd 1982; US DHHS 1988), cessation might lead to stable reductions in general anxiety.

Several models have been proposed to understand the possible long-term consequences of smoking cessation for depression or dysphoria (Frerichs et al. 1981; Hughes 1988; Hughes, Higgins, Hatsukami 1990; Tamerin 1972). Studies of withdrawal effects have found depressed mood or dysphoria to be a common, transient withdrawal effect, partly reflecting multiple pharmacologic effects of nicotine abstinence (Backon 1983; Hughes, Higgins, Hatsukami 1990; US DHHS 1988). Covey, Glassman, and Stetner (in press) found that smokers with a history of major depression had more severe symptoms of depression 2 weeks after a behavioral treatment for smoking than those without such a history. However, some theorists have proposed that for smokers who want to quit, quitting could result in improved mood, well-being, and self-esteem (Frerichs et al. 1981).

Research Results

Five cross-sectional studies have compared former smokers with continuing smokers or relapsers on measures of mood, affect, anxiety, and psychological well-being (Abrams et al. 1987; Giannetti, Reynolds, Rihn 1985; Orleans et al. 1983; Pederson and Lefcoe 1976; Pomerleau, Adkins, Pertschuk 1978). Of these five studies, three found no differences between these groups, and two found differences demonstrating more healthy outcomes for former smokers. Pederson and Lefcoe (1976) compared 46 former smokers, mostly self-quitters who had not smoked cigarettes for 1 year or longer, with 46 current smokers volunteering for treatment. These researchers found no differences on Jackson Personality Inventory scales that included measures of anxiety and self-esteem. Likewise, Pomerleau, Adkins, and Pertschuk (1978) used the Symptom Checklist (SCL-56) as a 2-year followup measure of dysphoria among 60 smoking cessation treatment participants and found no differences between quitters and continued smokers. Mean duration of smoking abstinence was not reported. Giannetti, Reynolds, and Rihn (1985) compared 47 former smokers who had been abstinent for at least 6 months with 35 current smokers hospitalized for cardiovascular disease and found no differences in "habits of nervous tension."

In the only study to employ multiple self-report, physiologic, and observer measures, Abrams and colleagues (1987) found no significant differences between 22 former smokers (mean abstinence approximately 2 years) and 22 relapsers on the State-Trait Anxiety Inventory, but did find that former smokers reported significantly less anxiety and had significantly lower heart rates in response to simulated smoking-related stressors. In a study of worksite health screen participants, Orleans and colleagues (1983) compared 525 long-term former smokers who had been abstinent for more than 12 months (mean abstinence = approximately 9 years) with 856 current smokers and found that the long-term former smokers had significantly better age- and sex-adjusted scores on the Health and Nutrition Examination Survey (HANES) General Well-Being Index, including its anxiety and depression subscales, and on the Framingham measures of anger symptoms and anger internalization. However, there were no differences on these measures between current smokers and recent ex-smokers, those who had been abstinent for less than 12 months.

Prospective longitudinal studies of smokers who become former smokers or remain continuing smokers are needed to establish whether any differences between former and current smokers existed prior to quitting, especially since baseline or "prequitting" measures of psychological well-being and self-esteem have been found to predict success in quitting smoking (Hall et al. 1983; Ockene et al. 1982; Schwartz and Dubitzky 1968; Straits 1970; West et al. 1977). The few prospective studies (Table 2) that have been conducted have either documented no significant change in psychological factors from baseline among former smokers, or no difference in the magnitude of change for former and continuing smokers, or have indicated improvements for former smokers. None of these studies demonstrated long-term negative psychological changes for former smokers.

Two of the prospective studies found no significant changes in a variety of mood and psychological measures from a prequitting baseline to long-term followup among former smokers and no significant differences between quitters and continuing smokers in the magnitude of such change. Pertschuk and coworkers (1979) asked 24 participants in a nonaversive cognitive-behavioral treatment to complete pretreatment and 2-month followup ratings of psychological functioning. These researchers found no significant changes in stress, affect, symptoms of psychological distress, or utilization of psychiatric treatment as indicated by need for psychotropic medication or mental health services. Changes from baseline to followup were not evaluated separately for quitters and nonquitters, but these groups did not differ on 4-month followup ratings. Emmons and associates (1986) studied the effects of smoking cessation on cardiovascular reactivity to stress among quit-smoking clinic participants and found no significant changes from baseline to a 6-month followup among 16 abstainers or 8 relapsers. However, this study noted that an average weight gain of 5 pounds among abstainers may have masked improvements in reactivity scores. Because weight was related to baseline and followup cardiovascular measures, it is possible that in each of these studies, treatment assisted quitters in avoiding persistent unwanted side effects.

Two studies of nicotine withdrawal effects that extended measurement beyond 4 weeks of abstinence have yielded no evidence for a withdrawal syndrome beyond 4 to 5 weeks (Hughes, Gust, Pechacek 1987; Gross and Stitzer 1989). These studies, reviewed in detail by Hughes, Higgins, and Hatsukami (1990), found that adverse postquitting changes in levels of anxiety, restlessness, impatience, irritability, and dysphoria peaked during the first 2 weeks after quitting, returned to baseline or below-baseline levels by 4 weeks, and remained at those levels at 10- to 26-week followups.

Gross and Stitzer (1989) studied 40 smokers who quit after a 3-session cessation class and maintained biochemically validated smoking abstinence for 10 weeks while using nicotine polacrilex gum or a placebo. Subjects completed weekly ratings of withdrawal symptoms, including symptoms of psychological distress such as irritability, anxiety, and impatience. Weekly followup ratings were adjusted for baseline ratings and baseline smoking rate. For the 20 placebo subjects, mean ratings for irritability, anxiety, and impatience increased from baseline to the first postquit week, returned to baseline

TABLE 2.—Prospective studies of quitting-related changes in mood, anxiety, stress reactivity, perceived stress, self-image, and psychological well-being

Reference	Sample size	Type of study	Findings	Strengths or limitations
Pertschuk et al. (1979)	24 smoking cessation clinic participants	Stress, affect, psychological distress, and utilization of psychiatric treatment were assessed at the start of treatment and 2 mo posttreatment	No significant pre- to posttreatment change in self-reported anxiety, depression, anger, irritability, appetite loss, insomnia, hopelessness, difficulty concentrating, apathy, use of psychotropic medication	Although posttreatment scores did not differentiate abstainers (N=16) and recidivists (N=8), these groups were not compared on pre- to posttreatment changes
Emmons et al. (1986)	24 smoking cessation clinic participants	Cardiovascular reactivity (SBP, DBP, HR) in response to cognitive and physical stressors were assessed 1 wk prior to treatment and 6 mo after treatment	No significant pre- to posttreatment change for abstainers (N=16) in mean SBP, DBP, or HR, and no difference in amount of change between abstainers and recidivists (N=8)	Only abstainers had a significant weight increase during the following period; this may account for lack of reduction in cardiovascular reactivity
Gross and Stitzer (1989)	40 abstainers using nicotine polacrilex gum or a placebo following a 3-session treatment	A 15-item withdrawal symptom measure was completed weekly for 10 postquit weeks	For placebo subjects, rated symptoms of psychological distress (irritability, anxiety, impatience) increased from baseline to first postquit week, returned to baseline by week 4, then declined below baseline initially, stabilizing after 5 wk; scores for active gum users declined below baseline initially, stabilizing after 3 wk at below-baseline levels	Self-reported abstinence biologically confirmed and baseline scores and baseline smoking rate used as covariates, but no control for repeated measurement

TABLE 2.—Continued

Reference	Sample size	Type of study	Findings	Strengths or limitations
Hughes, Gust, Pechacek (1987)	315 smokers followed for 6 mo after a contact treatment with physician advice and active nicotine polacrilex or placebo gum	At 1–2 wk, 1 mo, and 6 mo, subjects rated 5 withdrawal symptoms relevant to mood and psychological functioning (anger, anxiety, difficulty concentrating, impatience, restlessness)	Among abstinent subjects, these ratings peaked at 1–2 wk postquitting, returned to baseline by 1 mo, and declined further to below-baseline at 6 mo	Below-baseline 6-mo ratings among nonquitters suggest a drift in measures due to a repeated testing effect
Hall et al. (1983)	35 participants in a cessation clinic for smokers with chronic cardiopulmonary disease	POMS was administered before and 6 mo after treatment	A measure of total mood disturbance (anger/irritability + tension + anxiety + fatigue + confusion + depression/dejection − vigor) at 6 mo was significantly negatively correlated with smoking reduction; parallel significant relations were noted for the scales anger/irritability and tension/anxiety	Analyses controlled for pretreatment measures
Orleans et al. (1983)	72 ex-smokers (N=7 mo abstinent) who had quit during the year following a worksite health screen (49 at companies with health promotion programs, 23 at control companies)	HANES well-being, anxiety, and depression scales and the Framingham anger symptom scales were administered at a baseline health screen and 1-yr followup	Significant baseline to 1-yr improvements in the HANES well-being and depression scales were observed for new ex-smokers at treatment sites only; no changes in Framingham anger measures were observed	Analyses controlled for age, sex, baseline values, and duration of abstinence; comparisons with never smokers, long-term former smokers, or recidivists at treatment sites were not conducted

TABLE 2.—Continued

Reference	Sample size	Type of study	Findings	Strengths or limitations
Prochaska et al. (in press)	63 smokers quitting on their own rated their self-change processes semiannually for 2.5 yr	Self-reevaluation scale items assessed changes in self-image related to smoking	T-scores declined progressively for smokers going from action to maintenance stages	Analyses assessed stage-based patterns of change; comparisons with smokers who did not progress were not reported
Cohen and Lichtenstein (in press)	150 smokers planning to quit on their own	Smoking status and perceived stress were assessed at baseline, 1, 3, and 6 mo	Smokers who never quit (N=57) and those who quit and relapsed (N=81) maintained baseline stress levels over the 6-mo followup; smokers who quit and remained abstinent (N=12) showed a significant decrease in perceived stress from baseline to followup	Causality is unclear—stress may have contributed to the failure to quit smoking and failure to quit may have raised perceived stress

NOTE: SBP= systolic blood pressure; DBP= diastolic blood pressure; HR= heart rate; POMS=Profile of Mood States; HANES=Health and Nutrition Examination Survey.

levels by week four, then continued to decline, stabilizing at below-baseline levels by week six. There were significant interactions between use of the gum and the weeks during which it was used for each of these symptoms, with nicotine polacrilex gum significantly suppressing postcessation ratings only during the first 4 to 5 weeks after quitting. The authors concluded that several of the most disturbing aspects of the tobacco withdrawal syndrome appear to resolve within 4 to 5 weeks after quitting (Gross and Stitzer 1989). Although findings suggest positive changes over baseline for these recent quitters, below-baseline 6- to 10-week scores may reflect the effects of the initial treatment or a repeated-testing effect.

In a similar study of the effects of nicotine polacrilex gum on tobacco withdrawal, Hughes, Gust, and Pechacek (1987) studied 315 smokers for 6 months after a minimal contact treatment involving brief physician counseling, instruction in nicotine polacrilex gum use, and prescription of nicotine polacrilex gum or a placebo. At a pretreatment baseline, and again at 1- to 2-week, 1-month, and 6-month followups, subjects rated six withdrawal symptoms related to mood and psychological functioning including anger, anxiety, difficulty concentrating, impatience, and restlessness in addition to four others—craving, hunger, insomnia, and physical symptoms. For 75 subjects abstinent at 6 months, of whom 57 used nicotine polacrilex gum and 18 used a placebo, ratings for anger, anxiety, difficulty concentrating, restlessness, and impatience peaked at the 1- to 2-week followup, returned to baseline at 1 month, then dipped to below-baseline levels at 6 months. Subjects receiving nicotine polacrilex gum compared with those using placebo reported smaller increases from baseline to 1- to 2-week and 1-month ratings for most withdrawal symptoms, but nicotine polacrilex gum effects were not explored at the 6-month followup because too few subjects continued using the gum. However, 6-month ratings were lower on many symptoms even among 240 nonquitters, suggesting a drift in ratings due to a testing effect. In fact, the only symptom change from baseline, which differentiated quitters and nonquitters at 6 months, was that quitters had a greater increase in hunger than did nonquitters ($p<0.001$).

Hughes, Gust, and Pechacek (1987) concluded that, with the possible exception of hunger and craving or an urge to smoke, there was no evidence for prolonged withdrawal reactions lasting 6 months or more. (See Chapter 11 for discussion of hunger and weight effects.) However, these researchers also noted that results based on a select group of smokers who enrolled in a study and the absence of control groups of long-term former smokers and continuing smokers not trying to quit limit the generalizations that can be made about the symptoms of long-term abstainers.

Two other prospective studies comparing quitters and nonquitters have documented 6-month improvements in mood and well-being among former smokers who had participated in cessation treatments. Hall and associates (1983) administered the Profile of Mood States to 35 smokers with cardiopulmonary disease both before and 6 months after, 1 of 2 different 6-session quitting treatments. Controlling for baseline scores, they found that total mood disturbance, including anger/irritability, tension/anxiety, fatigue, confusion, and depression/dejection, was negatively correlated with smoking reduction ($p<0.02$). That is, smokers achieving the greatest smoking reduction showed the greatest improvements in overall mood. The same held true for the separate factors of anger/irritability (p<0.05) and tension/anxiety (p<0.05). Treatment differences were not explored.

Orleans and colleagues (1983) studied a group of 72 smokers who had quit in the previous year (mean abstinence, 7 months), and compared the changes in mood and well-being occurring among 49 quitters at 4 worksites where a range of employee health promotion programs had been offered including smoking cessation, exercise, weight control, and stress management, with those occurring among 23 quitters at 4 no-treatment control worksites. The investigators controlled for age, sex, baseline values, and months since quitting. Significant improvements in HANES well-being, anxiety, and depression scores were observed only among former smokers at treatment companies, but not among those at control companies (p<0.01). These results suggest that treatment may have potentiated positive changes among new quitters. However, never smokers, long-term former smokers, continuing smokers, or recidivists at treatment companies were not compared.

Two studies have documented long-term, quitting-related improvements in psychosocial outcomes among self-quitters. Prochaska and associates (in press) assessed the processes that smokers undergo during different stages of smoking behavior change in a 2.5-year longitudinal study of self-change among 63 self-quitters. These researchers found significant decreases from baseline in smoking-related negative self-evaluations (e.g., "My dependency on cigarettes makes me feel disappointment in myself") from a prequitting baseline for 9 subjects who progressed from the contemplation stage to the action stage and then to maintenance, and for 54 subjects who progressed from action to maintenance. Formal comparisons with subjects who did not progress in their stage of change were not reported. (See Chapter 2 for a discussion of stages of change.)

Cohen and Lichtenstein (in press) found significant long-term reductions in perceived stress in a prospective study of 150 unaided quitters. They administered the Perceived Stress Scale (Cohen, Kamarck, Mermelstein 1983) prior to quitting and again at 1, 3, and 6 months after the quit date. This scale measures the degree to which individuals perceive the stresses in their lives to exceed their abilities to cope (range=0–16). For the 12 subjects who quit and remained continuously abstinent, perceived stress decreased significantly from a prequitting mean of 5.7 to a 6-month followup mean of 2.9. Among 57 continuing smokers, perceived stress levels increased slightly from 6.1 prior to quitting to 6.3 at 6 months. Likewise, for the 81 smokers who quit but relapsed, perceived stress levels increased slightly from a prequitting mean of 5.8 to a 6-month mean of 6.1. There were no significant differences between quitters, continuing smokers, and relapsers in prequitting perceived stress levels. The investigators suggest that among smokers who want to stop smoking, quitting may have a beneficial influence on perceived stress, self-esteem, and general self-efficacy (a belief that one has the ability to perform a specific behavior such as smoking cessation) (Bandura 1982), and failing to quit may have opposite effects. However, these researchers also noted that a causal explanation cannot be clearly invoked: It is possible both that perceived stress contributed to the failure to quit smoking (Marlatt 1985a; Shiffman 1982) and that failure to quit contributed to stress.

More prospective studies are needed to clarify the long-term postwithdrawal psychological consequences of smoking abstinence suggested by the research reviewed for this Report. Studies designed specifically to assess long-term abstinence effects will require longer followup, larger samples of unselected quitters, and control groups of smokers who are not trying to quit. When possible and appropriate, self-report and physiologic and observer ratings of emotional and psychological changes should be included (Abrams et al. 1987; Hughes, Higgins, Hatsukami 1990) with measures of health-related quality of life (Kaplan 1988).

Self-Efficacy and Locus of Control

Self-Efficacy

Self-efficacy has been shown to be a strong mediator of smoking behavior change and to predict short- and long-term quitting outcomes (Condiotte and Lichtenstein 1981; Coelho 1984; McIntyre, Lichtenstein, Mermelstein 1983). As defined by Bandura (1982), self-efficacy refers to one's perceived ability to perform a specific behavior, such as resist temptations to smoke under specific circumstances; that is, self-efficacy is a response to a stressful event rather than a global sense of personal competence. As such, self-efficacy related to smoking cessation is likely to influence both the decision to engage in a quit attempt and perseverance in coping after quitting (Coelho 1984; Marlatt 1985b).

The self-efficacy measures employed in smoking cessation research have concerned only expectations for smoking behavior control. However, several researchers have proposed that successful smoking cessation might itself result in feelings of increased general self-mastery and self-confidence. That is, generalized self-efficacy may be a consequence of smoking cessation (Cohen and Lichtenstein, in press; Marlatt 1985b,c; Prochaska et al., in press). No studies have yet examined prequitting to postquitting changes in generalized self-efficacy.

However, the relationship between cessation and self-efficacy around smoking control has been studied. Cross-sectional studies among smokers wanting to quit have found that successful quitters score significantly higher on measures of self-efficacy than either those who tried to quit and failed (Abrams et al. 1987; Barrios and Niehaus 1985; Prochaska et al. 1982) or continuing smokers (Katz and Singh 1986). These differences may reflect that successful quitters generally have higher efficacy scores to begin with (Fleisher et al., in press; Mothersill, McDowell, Rosser 1988; Ockene et al. 1982; Prochaska et al. 1985) or that one's expectations that smoking can be resisted would rise significantly as a function of actual success in doing so.

Prospective longitudinal studies, with followup periods ranging from several weeks to 2.5 years postquitting, lend support to the hypothesis that increases in self-efficacy concerning smoking control are related to smoking cessation both for untreated self-quitters (Prochaska et al., in press) and for smokers enrolled in treatment programs (Coelho 1984; Killen, Maccoby, Taylor 1984; Nicki, Remington, MacDonald 1984; Schwartz and Dubitzky 1968). Coelho (1984) reported that smoking control self-efficacy scores increased significantly from a mean of 77.1 at the time of enrolling in treatment to a mean of 127.4 at 3 months posttreatment for 18 subjects who had quit smoking. (Abstinence was defined as continuous nonsmoking since a quit date, but mean duration of abstinence was not reported.) Conversely, pretreatment and posttreatment means for 48 nonquitters were unchanged from 78.1 to 75.1, respectively.

Two studies examined the effects of different types of smoking intervention treatments on self-efficacy ratings. Killen, Maccoby, and Taylor (1984) found no differences in the amount of positive change in self-efficacy among abstainers of 4 weeks or longer who took part in different treatments that included nicotine polacrilex gum, nonsmoking skill training, or combined nicotine polacrilex gum and skill training. Nicki, Remington, and MacDonald (1984) followed 53 subjects for 1 year after treatment and found significantly greater increases in smoking control self-efficacy among quitters and nonquitters randomized to a behavioral smoking intervention treatment designed explicitly to enhance smoking control self-efficacy than among those randomized to a standard control treatment ($p<0.05$). The mean duration of abstinence for quitters was not reported.

Locus of Control

Measures of locus of control reflect the extent to which an individual believes that he or she has control over personal happenings and circumstances. Measures of a generalized locus of control reflect either expectations that one has internal (i.e., personal) control over the reinforcements for one's behavior, indicating an internal locus of control, rather than believing that these reinforcements are determined by fate, luck, or other forces beyond control (Rotter 1966), which reflects a more external locus of control. Measures of health locus of control reflect beliefs that important health outcomes can be controlled through behavior rather than by being at the mercy of luck, fate, or powerful others (Wallston, Wallston, DeVellis 1978). It is possible that former smokers would shift toward a more positive or more internal control orientation in reaction to their successful quitting. Anecdotal evidence suggests that when smokers quit smoking they feel both more competent and more in control of their lives and that they experience pride in their perceived "strength of will" (Knudsen et al. 1984).

Cross-sectional studies have demonstrated that former smokers, both self-quitters and treated quitters, exhibit significantly more internal control orientations than either those who tried to quit and failed (Rosenbaum and Argon 1979) or continued to smoke and did not attempt cessation (Mlott and Mlott 1974; Orleans et al. 1983; Rosenbaum and Argon 1979). However, prequitting measures of generalized (Ockene et al. 1982) and health-specific (Horwitz, Hindi-Alexander, Wagner 1985) locus of control also differentiate these groups.

Locus of control may be related to the duration of abstinence. Orleans and associates (1983) found no significant differences between 1,343 current smokers and 856 short-term ex-smokers (abstinent for <3 months) in a baseline measure of perceived personal control over preventable illness. However, 89 medium-term former smokers (abstinent 3–12 months) and 525 long-term former smokers (abstinent for >12 months) scored significantly higher on personal control than current smokers ($p<0.01$). A followup conducted 1 year later showed a significant ($p<0.01$) increase toward internal control among 72 smokers who had quit since baseline (mean abstinence, 7 months).

Conversely, Orleans and colleagues (1983) found a significant shift toward more external health locus of control of similar magnitude among 30 individuals who had been former smokers at baseline, but who had relapsed by the 1-year followup. A similar pattern was reported by Horwitz, Hindi-Alexander, and Wagner (1985) who followed 219 participants in a single-session hypnosis treatment over a 1-year period. These researchers found a significant shift ($p<0.001$) toward a more external orientation among 79 smokers who had tried to quit but failed, with the mean falling from 27.6 pretreatment to 24.2 at the 1-year followup. The investigators suggested that generalized expectancies for control over one's health might be diminished by failure and by the "abstinence violation effect" (i.e., when individuals take a cigarette or relapse, they may feel guilty or depressed or believe that they are lacking in will power and may decide they are not maintaining control over smoking) (Marlatt 1985b). However, Horwitz, Hindi-Alexander, and Wagner (1985) found no significant pretreatment to followup shift toward an internal health locus of control among 56 continuously abstinent quitters who had quit with hypnosis. This lack of change toward an internal health locus of control may in part reflect that treatment using hypnosis does not engender strong personal, internal attributions for success.

Two studies suggest that treatment factors can influence shifts in locus of control. Orleans and associates (1983) divided 72 recent former smokers into 2 groups: 49 at 4 worksite companies where a comprehensive employee health promotion program had been introduced and 23 at 4 no-treatment control companies. The significant overall shift toward an internal health locus of control was accounted for wholly by the former smokers at treatment companies. It is possible that the intervening health promotion program emphasizing personal control over health, well-being, and preventable illness potentiated or hastened this shift. Blittner, Goldberg, and Merbaum (1978) randomly assigned 54 smokers seeking treatment to 1 of 3 conditions: a stimulus control treatment coupled with bogus feedback of superior self-control abilities, a stimulus control treatment alone, or a wait list control. A statistically significant pretreatment to posttreatment increase in internal orientation was observed only for the subjects who received feedback to enhance their expectations of inner control ability. This group also achieved the greatest 14-month smoking reductions ($p<0.001$).

Thus, most of the available data suggest that smoking cessation is related to an increase in a more internal locus of control orientation; no data indicate a shift toward an external locus of control for abstainers. There is some support to suggest that treatment method may have a differential effect on an increase in internal locus of control orientation.

Coping and Self-Management Skills

The relation of abstinence from cigarettes to a generalized improvement in the extent and use of coping and self-management skills has not been studied. To the extent that stopping smoking results in an individual's acquiring or strengthening generally applicable stress-coping and temptation-coping skills, long-term benefits of abstinence might be expected to include the generalized use of such skills. However, no studies have assessed whether increases in generalized stress-coping skills occur as a consequence of cessation. Longitudinal studies have not included prequitting and postquitting measures of generic coping strategies. A brief review of the relation of coping to smoking cessation and maintenance of abstinence may help to provide direction for this line of needed research.

Shiffman and Wills (1985) have developed a conceptual framework of coping that distinguishes stress-coping skills, that is, skills used to cope with general life stressors, and temptation-coping skills, or skills relevant for coping with a situation in which there is a specific temptation for substance use or an urge to smoke. Folkman and Lazarus (1988) defined stress-coping as constantly changing cognitive and behavioral efforts to manage specific external and internal demands that are appraised as taxing or exceeding the resources of the person to maintain an appropriate balance between environmental demands and resources available to the individual to meet those demands. Temptation coping can be separated into what smokers do when faced with the immediate temptation to smoke and anticipatory coping or the strategies smokers use to maintain commitment to abstinence and prevent temptation (Shiffman and Wills 1985).

To the extent that smoking constitutes a maladaptive response for coping with stress and negative affects such as anxiety, depression, anger, frustration, loneliness, or boredom (Abrams et al. 1987; Marlatt 1985b,c; Ockene et al. 1981), the former smoker must find alternative strategies for coping. The use of healthy all-purpose coping strategies such as self-reinforcement, assertive behavior, social support, relaxation, and exercise has proven important to success in maintaining abstinence in some studies (Ashenberg, Morgan, Fisher 1984; Grunberg and Bowen 1985; Marlatt 1985c; Shiffman 1982).

However, two large worksite studies demonstrated no differences between current and former smokers in the self-reported use of healthy and unhealthy techniques for coping with stress (Blair et al. 1980; Orleans et al. 1983). In support of the importance of coping skills, Katz and Singh (1986) found that 77 former smokers who had abstained for 6 months or more (mean 6.7 years) had significantly higher scores on the Rosenbaum Self-Control Schedule (a self-report measure of individual differences in applying self-control or coping methods) than 52 smokers recruited for a quit-smoking treatment. "Self-cured" and treated former smokers did not differ on this measure. The investigators concluded that former smokers may have succeeded because they possessed better self-coping skills initially. The same interpretation could be applied to the study by Abrams and associates (1987) in which 22 former smokers (mean abstinence 22 months) exhibited better observer-rated skills to resist the temptation to smoke than did 22 recidivists in simulations involving interpersonal smoking triggers. Shiffman (1982) found that former smokers who reported using cognitive and behavioral strategies to cope with smoking temptations were less likely to relapse. These few studies support the conclusion that use of skills to cope with stress and with temptations or urges to smoke seem to be more prevalent among former smokers compared with current smokers.

Social Support and Interpersonal Interactions

Research has not addressed how smoking cessation influences the level of general or quitting-relevant social support available to the quitter or how cessation affects the quality of the individual's interpersonal interactions. Research on social support processes has focused on examining baseline or posttreatment measures of social support as predictors of quitting success (Graham and Gibson 1971; Lichtenstein, Glasgow, Abrams 1986; Mermelstein et al. 1986; Ockene et al. 1982; US DHHS 1989). Several studies have demonstrated that successful quitters had significantly fewer smokers in their social networks at baseline than did continuing smokers (Eisinger 1971; Graham and Gibson 1971; Ockene et al. 1982). Others have demonstrated that the quitter's success stimulated quitting by others, especially spouses (Suedfeld and Best 1977).

A few studies are relevant to the investigation of cessation effects on social support. A large-scale, cross-sectional and longitudinal worksite study (Orleans et al. 1983) found no differences among current smokers, former smokers, and never smokers at baseline in satisfaction with personal relationships and interpersonal communication or in satisfaction with coworker relationships. However, at 1-year followup, 72 baseline smokers who had quit (mean abstinence, 7 months) showed a significant decline from baseline in satisfaction with coworker relationships ($p<0.01$) and scored significantly lower in satisfaction with personal relationships ($p<0.05$) than a group of 30 baseline former smokers who had relapsed since baseline. Whether new former smokers were in no-treatment control companies or in treatment companies where they benefitted from multiple health promotion programming, designed in part to boost coworker support, did not affect changes in satisfaction with interpersonal relationships. These negative changes in interpersonal relationships are difficult to interpret because former smokers in this study also demonstrated decreases in anxiety and depression and improvements in coping strategies compared with baseline. One possibility is that new former smokers may be less tolerant of smokers in their environment. Further study is needed to replicate and explain this isolated finding.

In contrast, Prochaska and colleagues (in press) monitored a group of 63 self-quitters who progressed through the stages of smoking behavior change to maintain abstinence over 2.5 years (mean duration of abstinence was not reported) (Chapter 2). They found that their use of helping relationships continued to increase with time. Similarly, Horwitz, Hindi-Alexander, and Wagner (1985) found that 56 successful quitters reported significantly greater social support from spouses and friends 1 year after a single-session hypnosis treatment than they did at baseline. No changes in reported level of support were noted for 84 continuing smokers, but even 79 recidivists reported significant increases in spouse support over baseline. Notwithstanding hypnotic suggestions that "other peoples' smoke will not bother you," successful quitters reported significantly ($p<0.05$) more often expressing objections to others smoking around them (mean=2.38) than either recidivists (mean=0.75) or continuing smokers (mean=0.50) at the 1-year followup. Likewise, more former smokers requested nonsmoking areas in restaurants (53 percent) and public transport (32 percent) than did recidivists (12 percent and 12 percent, respectively) or continuing smokers (8 percent and 6 percent, respectively). This practice may have helped to minimize social pressures to smoke commonly precipitating relapse (Marlatt and Gordon 1985), and helped to assure support for maintenance. It is also possible that these practices simply resulted from, rather than contributed to, smoking abstinence.

The results of these studies, although somewhat conflicting, suggest that former smokers played an active role in structuring the improved support they reported as a way of maintaining abstinence. However, given the limited information, no conclusions regarding the effect of smoking cessation on social interactions can be made at present.

Summary

Research findings provide no evidence for any long-term negative psychological effects beyond hunger and craving. However, the available findings suggest that there are some postwithdrawal psychological benefits that may increase with duration of abstinence.

HEALTH PRACTICES OF FORMER SMOKERS

Introduction

Several studies have found that both good health practices and poor health practices cluster (Belloc and Breslow 1972; Tapp and Goldenthal 1982; Verbrugge 1982; Marsden, Bray, Herbold 1988). Self-defined former smokers appear more likely than current smokers to engage in regular exercise and to practice other recommended health behaviors. In general, smokers who quit and who subsequently or concurrently change other health behaviors may represent a more distinct health-conscious group. Castro and coworkers (1989) have suggested that cigarette smokers exhibit less healthy lifestyles along cognitive, behavioral, and motivational dimensions. As the authors noted, addictive behaviors seldom occur in isolation but are instead embedded within complex behavioral chains or lifestyles. Conversely, the data presented in this Section suggest that when individuals stop smoking, other beneficial health practices also may emerge. Given the nature of the available data, it is not possible to determine whether these other beneficial health behaviors reflect the characteristics of a distinct health-conscious subgroup of smokers, emerge as part of the smokers' efforts to maintain abstinence (e.g., increased exercise), represent a response to adverse withdrawal symptoms (e.g., changes in dietary practices), or are direct effects of quitting.

This Section reviews data on former smokers' physical activity and dietary practices and use of other substances such as alcohol and other forms of tobacco, and former smokers' profiles with regard to multiple health-enhancing behaviors. Changes in former smokers' physical activity and dietary practices, as they relate to postcessation weight changes, are also reviewed in Chapter 10.

The studies reviewed in Chapter 10 are longitudinal investigations in which former and continuing smokers are compared. This Section focuses on cross-sectional data from two nationwide surveys, the National Health Interview Survey (NHIS) conducted by the National Center for Health Statistics (Kovar and Poe 1985; Schoenborn and Benson 1988) and the Behavioral Risk Factor Surveillance System (BRFSS) coordinated by the Centers for Disease Control and conducted by State health departments (Remington et al. 1988). Both surveys provide large data sets on health behaviors in the noninstitutionalized adult population. The limitations of drawing conclusions from cross-sectional data apply here (Chapter 2).

For its yearly interviews, NHIS uses a multistage probability scheme sampling technique developed in collaboration with the Bureau of the Census and employs personnel trained for the decennial census. BRFSS uses a multistage cluster technique of random digit dialing to select households for its yearly telephone survey. Both randomly select a respondent from a list of residents identified when a household is chosen.

A core set of questions each year is used in NHIS, then additional questions are added in supplements to the core survey in keeping with each year's chosen focus. In 1985, the NHIS special topic was health promotion, with variables such as physical activity, dietary practices, sleep, weight, alcohol use, and smoking that were similar to those used in the pioneering Alameda County study. The health promotion portion of the interview was completed by an estimated 90 percent of eligible respondents (Schoenborn and Benson 1988). In 1987, the special topic was cancer, with questions on diet, smoking, smokeless tobacco use, alcohol use, vitamin and mineral consumption, knowledge about cancer risks, cancer screening and preventive care, and family history of cancer. The cancer-related portion of the interview was completed by approximately 86 percent of eligible respondents (Schoenborn and Boyd 1989). In both NHIS surveys, a former smoker self-reported as having smoked at least 100 cigarettes and not smoking at the time of the survey. Mean duration of abstinence was not reported (Schoenborn and Benson 1988; Schoenborn and Boyd 1989).

In 1987, BRFSS covered blood pressure, physical activity, weight and dieting, diet, alcohol use, preventive practices, seatbelt use, stress, pregnancy status, use of oral contraceptives, and use of smokeless tobacco and cigarettes. The median cooperation rate (the ratio of completed interviews to the sum of completed interviews and refusals) among the participating States was 84 percent (Remington et al. 1988). Similar to NHIS, BRFSS defined a former smoker as an individual who had smoked at least 100 cigarettes in his or her lifetime and was not smoking at the time of the survey. (Mean abstinence of former smokers cannot be calculated. However, 64 and 54 percent of men and women, respectively, were abstinent from cigarettes for more than 5 years.)

Although these three surveys are similar, the published data available from them differ in several respects. Data from the 1985 NHIS, presented in Table 3, are age-adjusted (Schoenborn and Benson 1988). Data from the 1987 NHIS, presented in Table 4, are simple proportions with no variables controlled (Schoenborn and Boyd 1989). Data from the 1987 BRFSS were analyzed to assess the relationships between cigarette smoking and lifestyle and preventive practices (Table 5) and to examine the same relationships with respect to the duration of cigarette abstinence (Table 6). The odds ratios, presented in Tables 5 and 6, are controlled for age, ethnicity, and level of education.

TABLE 3.—Summary of data from 1985 NHIS, behaviors of never, former, and current smokers aged 20 and older

Behavior	Never smokers %	Former smokers %	Current smokers %
MEN			
Alcohol consumption			
Heavier drinker[a]	7.9	12.7	18.9
≥5 drinks[b]	13.8	21.2	28.7
Weight/diet/exercise			
Never eats breakfast	18.9	22.3	33.3
Snacks daily	39.3	40.4	38.5
Less physically active[c]	13.2	14.6	18.8
Sedentary[d]	46.6	47.7	57.2
Overweight[e]	28.1	30.0	21.2
Other			
Sleeps ≤6 hr	21.5	22.5	24.9
WOMEN			
Alcohol consumption			
Heavier drinker[a]	1.1	3.7	6.1
≥5 drinks[b]	2.2	5.0	8.5
Weight/diet/exercise			
Never eats breakfast	17.7	19.8	37.6
Snacks daily	37.6	41.5	35.3
Less physically active[c]	19.9	23.3	24.9
Sedentary[d]	61.1	58.5	64.3
Overweight[e]	24.9	23.0	17.9
Other			
Sleeps ≤6 hr	20.4	19.9	24.4

NOTE: All percentages are age adjusted; NHIS=National Health Interview Survey.
[a]Measure developed by the National Institute on Alcohol Abuse and Alcoholism. Categories based on ounces of ethanol consumed during the past 2 wk; heavier drinker is defined as having an average of 1.0 oz (2 drinks) or more/day.
[b]Five drinks or more on 10 days or more in the past year.
[c]Based on perceived level of physical activity relative to others.
[d]Energy expenditure on leisure activity of 0 to 1.4 kcal kg/day.
[e]Twenty percent or more above desirable weight based on 1983 Metropolitan Life Insurance Company standards, according to self-report of weight.
SOURCE: Schoenborn and Benson (1988).

TABLE 4.—Summary of data from 1987 NHIS behaviors of never, former, and current smokers aged 18 and older

Behavior	Never smokers %	Former smokers %	Current smokers %
MEN			
Alcohol consumption			
Drinks beer ≥5/wk	6.4	12.6[a,b]	17.1[c]
Drinks ≥3 beers/episode	36.3	30.5[a,b]	52.1[c]
Drinks wine ≥5/wk	1.2	3.1[a,b]	1.7[c]
Drinks ≥3 glasses wine/episode	12.9	11.6[a,b]	20.2[c]
Drinks liquor ≥5/wk	1.7	4.8[a,b]	4.1[c]
≥3 drinks/episode	30.4	25.8[a,b]	45.1[c]
Dietary practices			
3 meals/day on weekdays	48.6	50.9[a,b]	32.8[c]
3 meals/day on weekends	44.3	44.0[b]	35.0[c]
Avoids snacks weekdays	24.5	30.5[a,b]	26.5[c]
Avoids snacks weekends	21.0	25.9[a,b]	23.6[c]
Has changed diet for health	35.0	44.8[a,b]	26.4[c]
≥20% above desirable weight	24.9	34.2[a,b]	23.8[c]
Preventive care			
Digital rectal exam (ever)	59.5	66.8[a,b]	59.4
Blood stool test (ever)	38.6	44.9[a,b]	33.9[c]
Proctoscopic exam (ever)	24.0	27.7[a,b]	21.0[c]
WOMEN			
Alcohol consumption			
Drinks beer ≥5/wk	0.9	2.3[a,b]	4.0[c]
Drinks ≥3 beers/episode	17.1	17.2[b]	32.7[c]
Drinks wine ≥5/wk	1.3	4.3[a,b]	1.9[c]
Drinks ≥3 glasses wine/episode	7.0	10.9[a,b]	17.8[c]
Drinks liquor ≥5/wk	0.7	2.7[a]	2.7[c]
≥3 drinks/episode	13.7	14.1[b]	32.0[c]
Dietary practices			
3 meals/day on weekdays	50.1	49.5[b]	29.5[c]
3 meals/day on weekends	44.2	41.8[a,b]	29.4[c]
Avoids snacks weekdays	26.6	26.9	26.8
Avoids snacks weekends	23.6	24.4[a,d]	23.6
Has changed diet for health	38.7	49.0[a,b]	34.5[c]
≥20% above desirable weight	24.3	24.8[b]	20.3[c]
Preventive care			
Digital rectal exam (ever)	56.8	67.4[a,b]	60.6[c]
Blood stool test (ever)	37.9	46.2[a,b]	35.7[c]
Proctoscopic exam (ever)	20.8	27.2[a,b]	21.1
Pap smear (within year)	39.2	43.5[a,b]	40.7[c]
Breast self-exam (within yr)	34.8	40.3[a,b]	34.0
Breast exam (monthly)	51.5	52.2	52.1
Mammogram (ever)	38.5	46.7[a,b]	35.1[c]

NOTE: NHIS=National Health Interview Survey.
[a] Former smokers differ from never (p≤0.5).
[b] Former smokers differ from current (p≤0.5).
[c] Current differ from never (p≤0.5).
[d] This is (a) but not (b) because of sample size despite same point estimate.
SOURCE: Schoenborn and Boyd (1989).

TABLE 5.—Summary of data from 1987 BRFSS, behaviors of former smokers and current smokers aged 18 and older

Behavior	Former smokers relative to never smokers	Current smokers relative to never smokers	Former smokers relative to current smokers
MEN			
Alcohol consumption			
Any alcohol/mo	1.75[a]	2.11[a]	0.82[a]
≥5 drinks/episode	1.67[a]	2.64[a]	0.63[a]
≥60 drinks/mo	1.75[a]	3.03[a]	0.58[a]
Drinking and driving	1.44[a]	1.99[a]	0.71[a]
Weight/diet/exercise			
Obese (BMI)[c]	1.05	0.62[a]	1.68[a]
Obese (Met. Life)[d]	1.06	0.64[a]	1.63[a]
Trying to lose pounds	1.22[a]	0.63[a]	1.92[a]
More exercise	0.98	0.82[a]	1.17[b]
Eating fewer kcal	0.85[b]	0.82[b]	1.04
Physical activity	1.10[b]	0.69[a]	1.57[a]
Sedentary	0.91[b]	1.44[a]	0.64[a]
Preventive care			
Cholesterol test	1.27[a]	0.94	1.34[a]
Flu shot past month	1.09	0.87[b]	1.26[a]
Other			
Use ST	1.74[a]	0.84[b]	2.09[a]
Use seatbelt	0.92[b]	0.58[a]	1.60[a]
WOMEN			
Alcohol consumption			
Any alcohol/mo	2.07[a]	2.34[a]	0.87[a]
≥5 drinks/episode	1.86[a]	3.35[a]	0.55[a]
≥60 drinks/mo	2.88[a]	5.45[a]	0.52[a]
Drinking and driving	1.87[a]	2.92[a]	0.65[a]
Weight/diet/exercise			
Obese (BMI)[c]	0.98	0.63[a]	1.59[a]
Obese (Met. Life)[d]	0.96	0.65[a]	1.52[a]
Trying to lose pounds	1.19[a]	0.75[a]	1.60[a]
More exercise	1.07	0.72[a]	1.48[a]
Eating fewer kcal	0.97	0.96	0.99
Physical activity	1.17[a]	0.81[a]	1.45[a]
Sedentary	0.86[a]	1.24[a]	0.69[a]
Preventive care			
Cholesterol test	1.15[a]	1.11[a]	1.05
Flu shot past month	0.95	0.91[b]	1.05

TABLE 5.—Continued

	Adjusted odds ratios		
Behavior	Former smokers relative to never smokers	Current smokers relative to never smokers	Former smokers relative to current smokers
Other			
Use ST	0.73	0.46[a]	1.53
Use seatbelt	1.03	0.62[a]	1.63[a]

NOTE: BRFSS=Behavioral Risk Factor Surveillance System; ST=smokeless tobacco.
[a] $p<0.01$.
[b] $0.01<p<0.05$.
[c] BMI=body mass index.
[d] Met. Life=Metropolitan Life height and weight tables.
SOURCE: Samet and Wiggins, unpublished analyses of the 1987 BRFSS.

Physical Activity

Evidence from the 1985 NHIS, the 1987 BRFSS, and other cross-sectional studies suggests that smokers are less likely than nonsmokers to make regular exercise part of their lives (Goldbourt and Medalie 1975; Schoenborn and Benson 1988; Martin and Dubbert 1982). These differences may be the consequence of cessation and result partly from changes in physiologic function, such as lung function, that make exercise more pleasurable or tolerable for former smokers compared with current smokers (Castro et al. 1989). They also may reflect the former smokers' efforts to maintain abstinence. Blair and colleagues (1980) found mixed results in their studies of workers in a South Carolina company. Among men living within a 0.5 mile of work, current smokers were less likely than never smokers to walk to work. Among women, former smokers were more likely than either never smokers or current smokers to walk to work. (Mean duration of abstinence for former smokers was not reported.) There were no significant differences between smoking categories in other measures of physical activity, such as time spent sitting, use of stairs versus elevator, level of leisure time versus physical activity, and participation in a company exercise program. However, many measures for former smokers were between those of current smokers and never smokers.

The 1985 NHIS used 2 measures of physical activity, the perception of being less physically active than others and a more rigorous definition of sedentary behavior based on subjects' reports of participation in 23 leisure activities during the preceding 2 weeks (Schoenborn and Benson 1988). The perception of being less physically active was significantly more common among current smokers than former smokers and never smokers (Table 3). When separated by sex, these differences appear to be greater for men than for women. Men who were former smokers were significantly less likely to report being sedentary than current smokers and not significantly different from never smokers. Among women, former smokers were significantly less likely than current smokers and never smokers to be sedentary.

In two studies among Navy personnel, Conway and Cronan (1988a,b) studied the relationship among smoking, exercise, and physical fitness. The first study (Conway and Cronan 1988a) included 3,045 Navy personnel randomly selected from a group who volunteered to participate in an evaluation of physical fitness and health. Both

TABLE 6.—Summary of data from 1987 BRFSS, behaviors of former smokers aged 18 and older by duration of abstinence

	Adjusted odds ratios by duration of abstinence		
Behavior	13–24 mo relative to 1–12-mo quitters	25–60 mo relative to 1–12-mo quitters	≥61 mo relative to 1–12-mo quitters
MEN			
Alcohol consumption			
Any alcohol/mo	1.01	1.02	1.09
≥5 drinks/episode	1.03	1.05	0.95
≥60 drinks/mo	1.00	1.26	1.09
Drinking and driving	1.27	1.14	1.17
Weight/diet/exercise			
Obese (BMI)[b]	1.51[a]	1.46[a]	1.43[a]
Obese (Met. Life)[c]	1.45[a]	1.38[a]	1.39[a]
Trying to lose pounds	1.02	1.18	1.08
More exercise	0.85	1.06	0.86
Eating fewer kcal	0.92	1.46	1.37
Physical activity	0.98	1.13	1.25[a]
Sedentary	1.02	0.88	0.80[a]
Preventive care			
Cholesterol test	0.94	1.03	0.98
Flu shot past month	0.88	0.96	0.95
Other			
Use ST	0.64[a]	0.97	0.74[a]
Use seatbelt	1.02	1.09	1.22[a]
WOMEN			
Alcohol consumption			
Any alcohol/mo	1.02	1.28[a]	1.22[a]
≥5 drinks/episode	0.97	1.03	0.83
≥60 drinks/mo	1.30	1.03	1.15
Drinking and driving	1.55	0.60	0.72
Weight/diet/exercise			
Obese (BMI)[b]	1.28	1.31[a]	1.42[a]
Obese (Met. Life)[c]	1.07	1.16	1.30[a]
Trying to lose pounds	1.17	1.15	1.04
More exercise	0.97	1.10	0.98
Eating fewer kcal	1.10	1.01	0.90
Physical activity	1.05	1.06	1.11
Sedentary	0.95	0.95	0.90
Preventive care			
Cholesterol test	0.89	1.05	0.88
Flu shot past month	1.26	0.97	1.04

TABLE 6.—Continued

	Adjusted odds ratios by duration of abstinence		
Behavior	13–24 mo relative to 1–12-mo quitters	25–60 mo relative to 1–12-mo quitters	≥61 mo relative to 1–12-mo quitters
Other			
Use ST	0.49	0.27	1.07
Use seatbelt	1.28[a]	1.14	1.24[a]

NOTE: BRFSS=Behavioral Risk Factor Surveillance System; ST=smokeless tobacco.
[a]Significantly different from 1–12-mo quitters (p<0.05). There were no significant differences among the three categories of cessation >1 yr.
[b]BMI=body mass index.
[c]Met. Life=Metropolitan Life height and weight index.
SOURCE: Samet and Wiggins, unpublished analyses of the 1987 BRFSS.

never smokers and former smokers engaged in significantly more exercise sessions per week than did current smokers. Current smokers exercised for significantly less time per session and had significantly lower overall physical fitness scores compared with never smokers or former smokers. In a second study, the same authors examined the association between physical fitness and smoking among 1,357 Navy men (Conway and Cronan 1988b). Again, current smokers had poorer levels of physical fitness with lower scores than former smokers or never smokers on tests of cardiorespiratory and muscular endurance. Overall, never smokers performed better than former smokers and current smokers. In both studies, participants were young, with an average age of 26 years (study 1) and 28 years (study 2), suggesting that both decrements associated with smoking and improvements associated with quitting can appear at an early age.

A cross-sectional study of 781 runners found that as mileage increased, the percentage of self-defined former smokers also increased (Macera, Pate, Davis 1989). These investigators suggested that high-mileage runners seemed to quit smoking at a higher rate than low-mileage runners. Although the sample size was probably too small to show significant differences and the data were cross-sectional, the results support both empirical and anecdotal data about the relationship between abstinence from smoking and increased participation in exercise. Gordon and Polen (1987) studied 1,061 men and women who participated in smoking cessation clinics at Kaiser Permanente medical facilities from 1980 to 1983. Men and women who had increased their exercise after program participation were more likely to be abstinent from smoking 7 to 12 months later. These studies suggest that increasing exercise may be part of a former smoker's efforts to remain abstinent, a direct consequence of cessation, or both. The study by Gordon and Polen (1987) lends support to the first hypothesis.

The 1987 BRFSS allows a comparison among current smokers, never smokers, and former smokers on a range of health practices (Table 5). Two measures of physical activity were used. One asked a very general question about any physical activity in the past month, including nonaerobic activities, such as gardening, as well as major aerobic activities. The second identified sedentary lifestyle as the lowest category on a complex scale of life activities. On both measures, men and women who had quit smoking were more active than never smokers, who were in turn more active than current smokers. Among men, those who had been smoke-free for more than 5 years were significantly more active and less sedentary than new quitters, those who had been abstinent less than 1 year. This difference was not significant among women.

Prospective investigations of changes in physical activity after smoking cessation have indicated either no change or an increase in activity (Chapter 10). An additional prospective study focusing on exercise specifically, rather than weight changes, also found increased exercise among quitters. In a 1-year study of a large worksite population, Orleans and associates (1983) found that 72 recent ex-smokers (mean abstinence, 7 months) significantly increased their self-rated levels of activity compared with 347 continuing smokers ($p<0.01$) and that the ex-smokers achieved significant increases ($p<0.01$) from a prequitting baseline in the frequency of activities involving moderate exertion, such as walking or climbing stairs. Gordon and Cleary (1986) analyzed data from the 1979–1980 National Survey of Personal Health Practices and Consequences and found a more limited positive relationship. Aerobic exercise increased for women who tried to quit smoking but was not related to successful quitting in the last year among women or to any change in smoking behavior among men.

More studies are needed to clarify the effects of smoking abstinence on the level of physical activity. The relationship between increased physical activity and smoking abstinence may be a consequence of cessation, may reflect more successful quitting among smokers who have a higher level of prequitting physical activity, may be evidence that former smokers use exercise as a strategy to avoid smoking, or as a way to deal with the possible adverse effects of weight gain, or may be due to some combination of these possibilities. The cross-sectional nature of the data available do not permit a conclusion with regard to these alternatives.

Dietary Practices

Cross-sectional data from NHIS, BRFSS, and other studies present a mixed picture of the dietary practices of smokers, former smokers, and never smokers. Schoenborn and Benson (1988), reporting on the 1985 NHIS, found that current smokers are more likely to skip breakfast than never or former smokers (Table 3). This finding is consistent with the 1987 NHIS data showing that both former and never smokers are more likely than current smokers to eat no more than or no less than three meals a day (Schoenborn and Boyd 1989) (Table 4). As shown in Table 4, whether former smokers are more likely, less likely, or equally likely to eat three meals than are never smokers depends on gender and whether the day is a weekday or weekend day. Two NHIS surveys present contradictory results on snacking. The age-adjusted 1985 study indicated that among women, former smokers are the most likely to snack, but that there was no significant difference among men (Table 3). Raw percentages in the 1987 NHIS data show that among men, former smokers avoid snacks more than either never or current smokers, but that among women, there is essentially no difference (Table 4).

BRFSS data (Table 5) indicate that former smokers are the most likely group to be "trying to lose weight," although no more likely than never smokers to be obese.

Similarly, the 1987 NHIS data show that former smokers of both sexes are the most likely to report that they have changed their diet for the sake of their health (Table 3). In these same NHIS data, not controlled for age, men who are former smokers are more obese than never smokers, although women who are former smokers and never smokers are equally likely to be obese. Among the 10,000 Israeli men in Goldbourt and Medalie's 1975 study of Government employees, former smokers (duration of abstinence not noted) consumed fewer calories and were more likely to be on some sort of special diet for weight loss, diabetes, heart disease, hypertension, or ulcers. Former smokers surveyed for all three of these data sets may have initiated special diets or quit smoking following the diagnosis of illness. However, the Israeli data demonstrate that among those individuals who had experienced heart attacks or peptic ulcers, former smokers were more likely to report themselves compliant with their diets than current smokers (Goldbourt and Medalie 1975).

Former smokers often report retrospectively that they increased food consumption when they quit smoking (Carmody et al. 1986). The first part of this Chapter and a review by Hughes, Higgins, and Hatsukami (1990) indicate that increased hunger and appetite are common smoking withdrawal reactions, often extending beyond the initial 4-week withdrawal period. However, most longitudinal studies of changes in dietary practices after quitting have examined only short-term changes (Chapter 10). The majority of these studies have found evidence for increased dietary intake, especially of sweet foods and simple carbohydrates, after quitting. In a prospective study Orleans and coworkers (1983) found approximately a 6-pound weight gain at 1-year followup over baseline for 72 former smokers who had been abstinent from cigarettes for an average of 7 months. These researchers also found evidence for significant ($p<0.01$) improvements in overall nutritional practices for former smokers.

Better dietary behavior among former smokers when compared with current smokers may reflect changes made by former smokers in their efforts to remain abstinent, a response to their concerns regarding possible weight gain, or an overall desire to be healthy that is motivated by smoking cessation. Adequate data are not available to permit an assessment of these alternative hypotheses.

Use of Other Substances

Other Tobacco Products

In data from the United Kingdom, the cessation of cigarette smoking has been linked to the increased use of other smoked tobacco products, including pipes and cigars, by men (Jarvis 1984). These researchers noted that many of the alleged gender differences in cigarette smoking cessation rates are due to the adoption of pipe and cigar use by men. Comparable analyses have been performed on data from the 1987 NHIS Cancer Epidemiology and Control Supplement (Schoenborn and Boyd 1989) (Volume Appendix). When former cigarette smokers who used any other forms of tobacco were reclassified as smokers, the difference in cessation rates between men and women decreased.

Data from the 1987 NHIS indicate that the overall prevalence of the use of smokeless tobacco products and cigars or pipes is low; the prevalence of use ranges from 3.0 to 5.2 percent for men and from 0 to 0.5 percent for women; former cigarette smokers are more likely than never cigarette smokers to be current smokers of pipes or cigars (Table 7). Because the prevalence of pipe or cigar smoking increases as a function of age, it is important to use age adjustments in future investigations of the relationship between cigarette cessation and pipe or cigar smoking.

Alcohol

Smokers are more likely than nonsmokers to drink alcohol and use other drugs (Istvan and Matarazzo 1984; US DHHS 1988). Cross-sectional data from the 1983 NHIS (Kovar and Poe 1985) show a strong association between smoking status and daily alcohol intake (Figures 3 and 4); former smokers tend to be heavier drinkers than are never smokers, and daily alcohol intake increases with heavier smoking (Kozlowski and Ferrence 1990). The drinking and smoking scales differ for men and women to compensate for the relative rarity among women of very heavy drinking and heavy smoking; at the same levels per day as men, fewer drinks per day are required for women than for men to be placed in the "heavy drinking" category.

In the 1987 NHIS, alcohol consumption was divided into beer, wine, and liquor consumption. Published data report on the proportion of respondents consuming "5 or more drinks per week" and "3 or more drinks on days you drank" for each category. These data are generally consistent with the 1983 (Figures 3 and 4) and the 1985 age-adjusted NHIS data (Table 2) and with the age-, education-, and ethnicity-adjusted data from the 1987 BRFSS (Table 5) in showing lower alcohol consumption among former than among current smokers but higher than among never smokers. These data regarding alcohol consumption of former smokers are also consistent with data presented previously in this Chapter on the short-term effects of smoking abstinence on alcohol consumption (Hughes and Hatsukami 1986; Olbrisch and Oades-Souther 1986; Puddey et al. 1985).

In the 1987 BRFSS survey, two measures of alcohol were used: the amount consumed and whether drinking and driving occurred together (Tables 5 and 6). Men and women who had quit smoking drank significantly more than never smokers and were significantly more likely to drink and drive. However, former smokers drank significantly less than current smokers and were significantly less likely to drink and drive.

The intermediate position of former smokers seen in the 1987 BRFSS and the 1985 NHIS is paralleled in the 1987 NHIS by the percentage of both sexes who drink five beers or more per week, the percentage of women who drink three glasses or more of wine when they drink wine, and the percentage of men who drink three drinks or more when they drink liquor (Table 4). In the 1987 NHIS, male former smokers are significantly less likely than either comparison group to have three beers or more when they drink beer or three glasses or more of wine when they drink wine. Although a very small percentage of adults drink wine or liquor five times or more per week, men who are former smokers are more likely than current or never smokers to drink this often. Female former smokers are more likely than current or never smokers to drink wine

TABLE 7.—Percent distribution of persons aged 18 and older by tobacco product and use status, according to gender and cigarette smoking status, United States, 1987

Tobacco product and use status	Both genders				Men				Women			
	Total	Never smokers	Former smokers	Current smokers	Total	Never smokers	Former smokers	Current smokers	Total	Never smokers	Former smokers	Current smokers
Total	100.0	100.0	100.0	100.0	100.0	100.0	100.0	100.0	100.0	100.0	100.0	100.0
Chewing tobacco												
Never	93.8	96.7	89.8	92.0	87.6	92.5	83.5	85.3	99.3	99.3	99.2	99.2
Former	4.2	1.8	7.3	5.8	8.4	4.1	11.9	10.6	0.4	0.3	0.6	0.6
Current	2.0	1.5	2.9	2.2	4.0	3.4	4.6	4.1	0.3	0.4	0.2[a]	0.2[a]
Snuff												
Never	95.9	93.3	94.3	94.8	92.3	94.6	90.9	90.5	99.2	99.0	99.2	99.4
Former	2.4	1.1	3.8	3.5	4.7	2.4	6.1	6.4	0.4	0.3	0.5	0.5
Current	1.7	1.6	1.9	1.6	3.0	3.0	3.0	3.1	0.5	0.7	0.3[a]	0.1[a]
Pipe												
Never	91.1	97.4	79.3	89.7	81.5	93.9	85.9	80.5	99.7	100.0	99.2	99.5
Former	7.3	1.7	18.5	7.9	15.2	4.4	30.4	15.1	0.3	0.0[a]	0.8	0.4
Current	1.6	0.8	2.2	2.3	3.3	2.2	3.7	4.4	0.0[a]	—[a]	0.0[a]	0.2[a]
Cigars												
Never	91.1	97.0	80.5	89.7	81.7	92.5	87.8	80.8	99.6	99.8	99.4	99.2
Former	6.4	1.8	16.3	6.2	13.1	4.4	26.9	11.5	0.3	0.1[a]	0.6	0.6
Current	2.5	1.2	3.2	4.1	5.2	3.1	5.3	7.8	0.1[a]	0.0[a]	0.0[a]	0.1[a]

[a]Data do not meet standard of reliability or precision (more than 30% relative standard error in numerator of percentage or rate).

SOURCE: National Health Interview Survey (1987); Schoenborn and Boyd (1989).

MALES

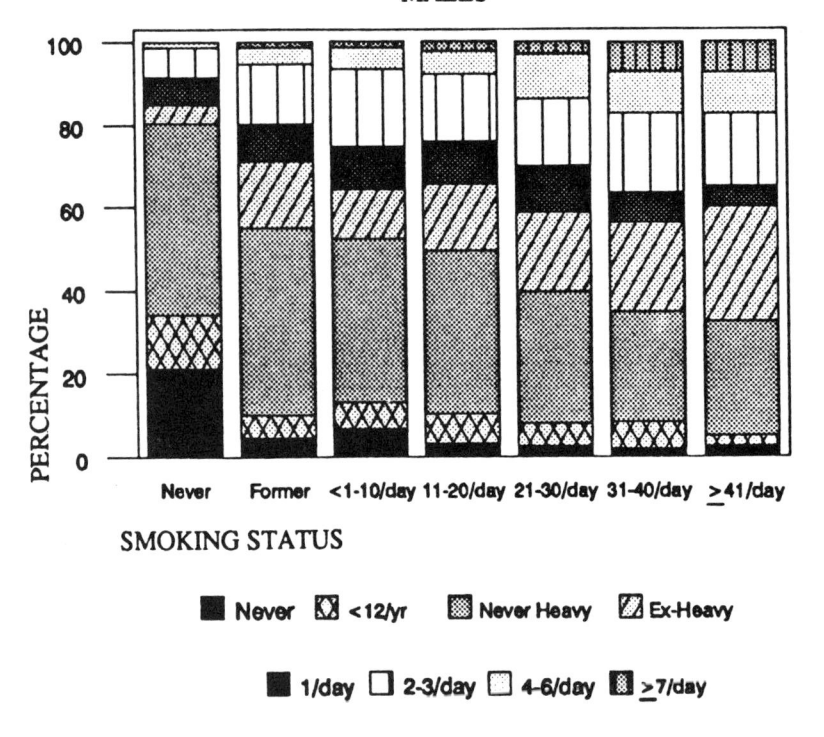

FIGURE 3.—Drinking relative to smoking status for men, 1983 NHIS (Kovar and Poe 1985)

NOTE: Samples for each category are, from never smoker to heaviest smoker, 1,397, 874, 295, 653, 263, 190, 57. NHIS=National Health Interview Survey.

SOURCE: Kozlowski and Ferrence (1990).

five times or more per week; they are as likely as current smokers to drink liquor this often. However, this represents a very small proportion of women. Female former smokers are less likely than current smokers and no more likely than never smokers to drink three beers or more when they drink beer or to have three drinks or more when they drink liquor.

These cross-sectional data are consistent with other cross-sectional data that demonstrate a relationship between alcohol use and smoking status (Istvan and Matarazzo 1984). However, the contribution of tobacco cessation to alcohol and drug use by individuals with alcohol and drug problems is unknown (Sobell et al. 1990). The majority of smokers consume approximately 1 pack per day, and most smokers do not have serious alcohol problems. The most significant effects might be seen in those few individuals who both smoke very heavily, more than 40 cigarettes per day, and use drugs or alcohol heavily (Kozlowski and Ferrence 1990). Bobo (1989) and Miller, Hedrik, and Taylor (1983) reported data that indicate that smoking cessation does not

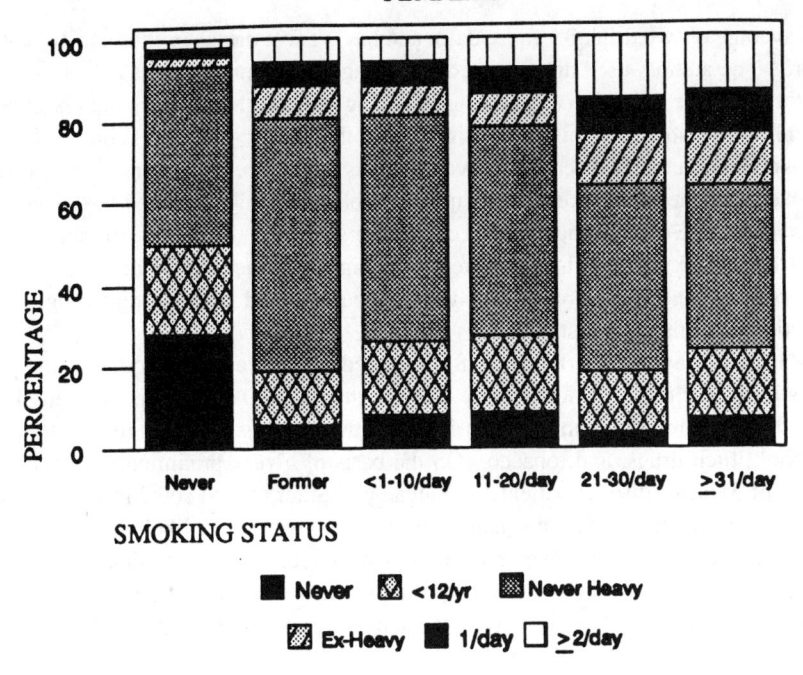

FIGURE 4.—Drinking relative to smoking status for women, 1983 NHIS (Kovar and Poe 1985)

NOTE: Samples for each category are, from never smoker to heaviest smoker, 2,661, 789, 505, 786, 205, 176. NHIS=National Health Interview Survey.

SOURCE: Kozlowski and Ferrence (1990).

impair the course of treatment for alcohol problems and may be associated with better outcomes.

Studies of Multiple Health Habits

It is of interest to examine not only single behaviors, such as diet or exercise, in relation to smoking cessation, but also combinations of behaviors. Use of alcohol and other substances, use of other tobacco products, coffee consumption, physical activity, and diet have been the health behaviors studied most widely in conjunction with smoking and smoking cessation.

Schoenborn and Benson (1988) reported on the following eight unhealthy behaviors surveyed in the 1985 NHIS: sleeping 6 hours or less, skipping breakfast, snacking daily, being less physically active than other persons of the same age, being sedentary in terms of leisure-time sports activities, being significantly overweight (10 percent or more based on the 1983 Metropolitan Life Insurance Company standards), drinking heavily (an average of two drinks or more/day), and having five drinks or more on 10 days or more. The authors used age-adjusted percentages to eliminate age as a confounding factor. With the exception of snacking and being overweight, current smokers engaged in unhealthy habits at significantly higher rates than never smokers (Table 2). Former smokers more closely resembled never smokers than current smokers. Fewer former smokers and never smokers than current smokers slept 6 hours or less, never ate breakfast, were less physically active, or were sedentary. However, former smokers tended to snack daily and be overweight in slightly higher percentages than current smokers, which is concordant with the previously noted findings regarding dietary practices and smoking abstinence.

Marsden, Bray, and Herbold (1988) examined substance use and other health practices in a large cross-sectional study of more than 17,000 military personnel. These researchers found the number of positive health practices inversely related to use of alcohol, illicit drugs, and tobacco. On the basis of a very preliminary retrospective study of 35 heart disease patients, Finnegan and Suler (1985) concluded that former smokers (mean duration of abstinence, unspecified) were more likely to maintain diet and exercise changes. Former smokers may have represented a particularly adherent subgroup of patients, but the authors postulated that success in maintaining diet and exercise changes may have been influenced by the psychological effects of attempting cessation.

Maron and colleagues (1986) examined seatbelt use in a sample of high school students and found modest but significant negative effects of smoking, frequency of getting drunk, and illicit drug use (cocaine and marijuana), and positive effects of "heart-healthy nutrition" and physical activity on seatbelt use. In a study of 874 community college students, Castro and associates (1989) found that moderate-to-heavy smokers had exhibited more unhealthy behaviors than nonsmokers. As in some of the other cross-sectional studies reported here, these investigators did not distinguish former smokers from never smokers.

Among males, former smokers interviewed as part of the 1987 BRFSS (which examined multiple health behaviors) were more likely than current smokers but less likely than never smokers to use seatbelts. However, among females, never smokers and former smokers were equally likely to use seatbelts, and both were significantly more likely to use seatbelts than current smokers (Table 3). Long-time quitters were more likely than new quitters (<1 year) to use their seatbelts, although this association was small and significant only for men who had been abstinent from smoking cigarettes for 5 years or more and for women abstinent for 1 to 2 years and for 5 years or more (Table 5).

Among Multiple Risk Factor Intervention Trial (MRFIT) participants, Schoenenberger (1982) found that smokers who had quit between baseline and a 3-year followup survey made successful changes across a number of dimensions. Former smokers were more likely to avoid gaining weight, to lower their serum cholesterol, and, if hypertensive, to lower their blood pressure. Supporting the conclusions of Schoenenberger (1982) regarding MRFIT participants, Tuomilehto and associates (1986) studied a random sample of 2,119 Finnish subjects at 2 points in time and found that both men and women who had quit smoking between baseline and the 5-year followup reduced their fat intake, increased their physical activity, and made more attempts to reduce body weight than did current smokers. Baseline differences suggested that these quitters (duration of abstinence not specified) may have been more health conscious at the outset.

Orleans and colleagues (1983) performed a prospective analysis of health behavior changes experienced by 72 employees quitting smoking between baseline and year one. As part of the "Live for Life" program they included baseline health behavior values, age, and sex as covariates. Their findings indicated an overall positive shift in healthy lifestyle with improvements in subjective health status, emotions, and well-being. New ex-smokers (average abstinence, 7 months) showed improvements over baseline in resting pulse, perceived personal control over preventable illness, knowledge of health risks, overall nutrition practices, regular moderate exercise, and seatbelt use. The only negative changes were body mass and weight changes associated with slightly less than a mean 6-pound weight gain, which took place along with an improvement in overall nutrition, and declines in job satisfaction measured by satisfaction with growth opportunities and personal relationships on the job.

Summary

In the absence of more systematic longitudinal research, data from cross-sectional and longitudinal studies suggest that abstinence from smoking is related to improvements in other positive lifestyle behaviors contributing to overall good health. These behaviors may be used by the former smoker to prevent relapse (e.g., exercise), to cope with adverse withdrawal symptoms (e.g., increased food intake as a response to increased appetite), or as part of a commitment to a healthier lifestyle. Exercise may help new quitters to remain abstinent and to avoid or minimize weight gain. The data from the MRFIT (Schoenenberger 1982) and other large data bases (Friedman et al. 1979) confirm that former smokers often take active steps to lower their disease risks. These studies should alleviate concerns that smoking cessation may result in unhealthy lifestyle shifts through unwanted symptom substitution.

Given the strong association between smoking and other kinds of substance use, it is important to know if smoking cessation impairs the ability to stop other drug use. The limited evidence suggests that this is not the case (Bobo 1989; Miller, Hedrik, Taylor 1983). How multiple drug use and multiple drug withdrawal may interact with cigarette smoking and its cessation is an area requiring study.

PARTICIPATION OF FORMER SMOKERS IN HEALTH-SCREENING PROGRAMS

The literature presented earlier in this Chapter suggests that former smokers are more likely than current smokers to engage in a variety of health-enhancing behaviors, such as regular physical activity. Another area in which improvement may occur for individuals who stop smoking is participation in, or benefits from, health-screening programs. Participation in programs of health screening by those who are presumably healthy and asymptomatic is a health-enhancing or health-protective behavior, much like wearing seatbelts or performing regular exercise. This participation is to be distinguished from health screening sought for diagnostic purposes. Calnan and Rutter (1986) cautioned, however, that there are important conceptual differences between behaviors such as not smoking or regular flossing and utilization of screening. In the first case, the emphasis is on the individual performing the recommended action. In the second, the individual makes a decision to use the service, but a professional performs the procedure. Smokers exhibit a decreased propensity to use preventive services in contrast to nonsmokers. The data suggest that former smokers occupy an intermediate position between current and never smokers in their seeking of health screening.

Data from the large Johnson and Johnson "Live for Life" worksite trial discussed earlier showed that current smokers were less willing than former or never smokers to complete health risk assessments (Shipley et al. 1988). A survey of randomly selected nonrespondents to the "Live for Life" health screening found that significantly more nonrespondents reported ever having smoked cigarettes and significantly more female nonrespondents currently smoked (Settergren et al. 1983). Additional support for the position that smokers may have lower response rates to health risk appraisals is provided by Seltzer, Bossé, and Garvey (1974), who found current smokers significantly less likely than never smokers to respond to a health questionnaire.

One source of data about the health-screening practices of former smokers consists of results from a 1988 nationwide randomized survey of American Association of Retired Persons (AARP) members aged 50 and older to assess differences among current smokers, former smokers (abstinent for 1 week or longer with a mean duration of 19.3 years), and never smokers (Rimer et al. 1990). In addition to the usual quitting-related variables, respondents were asked about their use of health services, including routine cardiovascular and cancer screening. Questionnaires were received from 3,129 persons, a 54-percent response rate. In this older population for whom health screening is especially important, the never, current, and former smokers differed significantly on utilization of screening (Table 8). The results suggest that smoking may act as a deterrent to appropriate use of screening services for older smokers and possibly for younger smokers as well, or that there is a general unhealthy approach taken by smokers. That former smokers were more likely to avail themselves of preventive checks and services than current smokers suggests that former smokers may have a more preventive health orientation than current smokers, may participate in screening as an approach to maintain abstinence, or may be concerned about the effects of smoking on their health. As with exercise and other health promotion practices, the data are retrospective; therefore, it cannot be determined if the former smokers were always different from current smokers in their health screening habits or if they changed as a result of cessation.

The results of the AARP survey suggest that with time former smokers may resemble never smokers in their use of screening services. Maintaining health was the primary reason for quitting among former smokers who responded to the AARP survey; perhaps the subset of smokers who quit was more health conscious at the outset. Or having quit, former smokers may be more willing to take a proactive stand to maintain their health. It is also possible that having admitted vulnerability to the harms of smoking and

TABLE 8.—Physician visits and medical tests within the past year among AARP members aged 50 and older, by smoking status

	Current smokers (N=339) 11%	Former smokers (N=1489) 47%	Never smokers (N=1316) 42%	Overall (N=3147) 100%	p-value[a]
Physician visit (≥1)	77	88	86	86	<0.001
Complete physical or checkup	50	60	60	59	<0.001
Blood pressure check	79	90	87	87	<0.001
Electrocardiogram	41	52	45	48	<0.001
Stool blood test	28	38	36	36	<0.001
Digital rectal examination	23	34	30	31	<0.001
Mammogram (women only)	24	41	36	36	<0.014
Pap smear (women only)	33	43	39	40	<0.006

NOTE: All rates are age adjusted.   AARP=American Association of Retired Persons.
[a] Current smokers vs. former or never smokers.
SOURCE: Rimer et al. (1990).

experiencing the benefits of quitting, former smokers are more amenable to adopting other health-enhancing behaviors. This would be consistent with the tenets of the Health Belief Model (Janz and Becker 1984) and with preliminary findings about the increased value of health expressed by self-defined former smokers (Tipton and Riebsame 1987).

In two measures of disease prevention assessed in the 1987 BRFSS data, male former smokers appeared to be more health conscious than current smokers and at least as much as never smokers (Table 5). These individuals are significantly more likely than never smokers to have had their cholesterol tested in the past year; never smokers, in turn, are more likely than current smokers to have had this test. Although former smokers were slightly more likely than never smokers to have had a flu shot in the past month, this difference was not statistically significant. Both former smokers and never smokers were significantly more likely to have had the shot than were current smokers. Female former smokers were more likely to have had their cholesterol tested than were never smokers, but were not significantly different from current smokers. Women in all three smoking categories were similar, indicating no statistically significant differences in their probability of having received a flu shot in the past month. Among former smokers, length of time since cessation did not predict any differences in either of these behaviors among men or women.

The 1987 NHIS data show higher rates of preventive care among former smokers than among never or current smokers (Table 4). Women who had quit were significantly more likely to report ever having had a digital rectal exam, a stool blood test, and a proctoscopic exam. Women who had stopped smoking were also significantly more likely to have had a Pap smear or a breast examination within the past year and to ever have had a mammogram. However, women did not differ by smoking status in their practice of monthly breast self-examination. These data did not control for age and may reflect the greater number of former smokers in the higher risk ages, in addition to the unavoidable problems inherent in cross-sectional data such as not being able to determine the order of smoking cessation and preventive care.

A study of participation among 600 female members of a health maintenance organization showed that female smokers were less likely than former smokers or never smokers to complete a health risk assessment or to obtain mammograms (Rimer et al. 1988, 1989). When residents of a large retirement community were surveyed about their health habits, Chao and colleagues (1987) found differential use of several screening tests, including blood pressure, fecal occult blood tests, mammograms, and Pap tests among current smokers, former smokers, and never smokers, with former smokers having the highest rates of screening. Macrae and colleagues (1984) studied 581 individuals who completed health questionnaires before being offered fecal occult blood tests. These researchers found that whereas smokers were not less likely to decline the initial offer, they were significantly less likely to comply, that is, to follow through with the test. These same investigators suggested that smokers may have been more susceptible to interpersonal pressure publicly, but later succumbed to a strategy of defensive avoidance. Although Macrae and associates (1984) did not distinguish the screening behavior of never smokers and former smokers, other studies reported here suggest that these groups would have been similar.

The suggestion that former smokers are more oriented to prevention and early detection is also consistent with Verbrugge's (1982) conclusions that smokers have poorer health, increased risks due to smoking, and are more oriented to remedial as opposed to preventive health actions. As smokers move toward maintenance of nonsmoking, they appear to value their health more highly (Tipton and Riebsame 1987; Horwitz, Hindi-Alexander, Wagner 1985). This finding is consistent with the greater utilization of screening found among AARP former smokers (Rimer et al. 1990). These findings undoubtedly are affected by the relationship between socioeconomic status (SES) and preventive care utilization. That is, lower SES is associated with less use of preventive services (Dutton 1986). To the extent that they are represented disproportionately among those of lower SES, current smokers will be at risk for underuse of age-appropriate prevention and early detection services.

The literature about the health screening practices of former smokers is suggestive but inconclusive. It appears that former smokers are more likely than current smokers, but perhaps less likely than never smokers, to seek regular cardiovascular and cancer screening.

SUMMARY

The data suggest that as the duration of abstinence lengthens, former smokers begin to resemble never smokers in their utilization of health screening and their participation in a variety of health-enhancing behaviors, such as physical activity. However, it is not clear if former smokers are different from current smokers at the outset, if the method of cessation affects these outcomes, or if the reason for quitting affects subsequent health practices. There is reason to believe that former smokers, especially those who quit while they are healthy, come to value their health more and take health-enhancing action as an extension of this valuing (Tipton and Riebsame 1987). These conclusions are consistent with the Health Belief Model (Janz and Becker 1984) and the Protection Motivation Theory (Prentice-Dunn and Rogers 1986). Longitudinal, prospective studies would make an important contribution to understanding these issues.

Increased participation in screening and other health-enhancing behaviors also may result from enhanced self-esteem and an increased sense of self-control. Ockene and colleagues (1988) concluded that successful behavior change is likely to promote a perception of general self-efficacy. The perception of oneself as capable may generalize to other areas of one's life. Kronenfeld and associates (1988) stressed that it may be difficult for most people to change multiple habits simultaneously. Having gained a sense of mastery from stopping smoking, former smokers may attempt to improve other health practices. However, some studies suggest that former smokers seem to undertake a number of health-enhancing steps proximally, if not simultaneously (Schoenenberger 1982; Friedman et al. 1979; Gerace et al., in press). For example, quitters in MRFIT (baseline smokers who were biochemically verified ex-smokers at the sixth annual visit) reported a greater decrease in their number of alcoholic drinks per day and sucrose consumption than nonquitters (Gerace et al., in press).

CONCLUSIONS

1. Short-term consequences of smoking cessation include anxiety, irritability, frustration, anger, difficulty concentrating, increased appetite, and urges to smoke. With the possible exception of urges to smoke and increased appetite, these effects soon disappear.
2. Smokers who abstain from smoking show short-term impairment of performance on a variety of simple attention tasks, which improves with nicotine administration. Memory, learning, and the performance of more complex tasks have not been clearly shown to be impaired. Whether the self-reported improvement in attention tasks upon nicotine administration is due entirely to relief of withdrawal effects or is also due in part to enhancement of performance above the norm is unclear.
3. In comparison with current smokers, former smokers have a greater perceived ability to achieve and maintain smoking abstinence (self-efficacy) and a greater perceived control over personal circumstances (locus of control).
4. Former smokers, compared with current smokers, practice more health-promoting and disease-preventing behaviors.

References

ABRAMS, D.B., MONTI, P.M., PINTO, R.P., ELDER, J.P., BROWN, R.A., JACOBUS, S.I. Psychosocial stress and coping in smokers who relapse or quit. *Health Psychology* 6(4):289–303, 1987.

ADESSO, V.J. Some correlates between cigarette smoking and alcohol use. *Addictive Behaviors* 4:269–273, 1979.

AMERICAN PSYCHIATRIC ASSOCIATION. *Diagnostic and Statistical Manual of Mental Disorders,* Third Edition, revised. Washington, D.C.: American Psychiatric Association, 1987, pp. 165–168.

ASHENBERG, Z.S., MORGAN, G.D., FISHER, E.B. Psychological stress and smoking recidivism: A prospective assessment. Paper presented at the SBM Fifth Annual Conference, Philadelphia, Pennsylvania, 1984.

BACKON, J. Prostaglandins, depression and not smoking. (Letter.) *American Journal of Psychiatry* 140(5):645, May 1983.

BAER, J.S. Patterns of relapse after cessation of smoking. Unpublished doctoral dissertation, University of Oregon, Eugene, 1985.

BANDURA, A. Self-efficacy mechanism in human agency. *American Psychologist* 37(2):122–147, February 1982.

BAREFOOT, J.C., GIRODO, M. The misattribution of smoking cessation symptoms. *Canadian Journal of Behavioral Science* 4(4):358–363, 1972.

BARRIOS, F.X., NIEHAUS, J.C. The influence of smoker status, smoking history, sex, and situational variables on smokers' self-efficacy. *Addictive Behaviors* 10:425–429, 1985.

BELLOC, N.B., BRESLOW, L. Relationship of physical health status and health practices. *Preventive Medicine* 1:409–421, 1972.

BENOWITZ, N.L. Pharmacologic aspects of cigarette smoking and nicotine addiction. *New England Journal of Medicine* 319(20):1318–1330, November 17, 1988.

BENOWITZ, N.L., HALL, S.M., MODIN, G. Persistent increase in caffeine concentrations in people who stop smoking. *British Medical Journal* 298:1075–1076, April 22, 1989.

BILLINGS, A.G., MOOS, R.H. The role of coping responses and social resources in attenuating the stress of life events. *Journal of Behavioral Medicine* 4:139–146, 1981.

BLAIR, A., BLAIR, S.N., HOWE, H.G., PATE, R.R., ROSENBERG, M., PARKER, G.M., PICKLE, L.W. Physical, psychological, and sociodemographic differences among smokers, ex-smokers, and nonsmokers in a working population. *Preventive Medicine* 9:747–759, 1980.

BLITTNER, M., GOLDBERG, J., MERBAUM, M. Cognitive self-control factors in the reduction of smoking behavior. *Behavior Therapy* 9:553–561, 1978.

BOBO, J.K. Nicotine dependence and alcoholism epidemiology and treatment. *Journal of Psychoactive Drugs* 21(3):323–329, July–September 1989.

BOSSÉ, R., GARVEY, A.J., COSTA, P.T. Predictors of weight change following smoking cessation. *International Journal of the Addictions* 15:969–991, 1980.

BROWN, C.R., JACOB, P. III, WILSON, M., BENOWITZ, N.L. Changes in rate and pattern of caffeine metabolism after cigarette abstinence. *Clinical Pharmacology and Therapeutics* 43(5):488–491, May 1988.

CALNAN, M., RUTTER, D.R. Preventive health practices and their relationship with sociodemographic characteristics. *Health Education Research* 1(4):247–253, 1986.

CARMODY, T.P., BRISCHETTO, C.S., PIERCE, D.K., MATARAZZO, J.D., CONNOR, W.E. A prospective five-year follow-up of smokers who quit on their own. *Health Education Research* 1(2):101–109, 1986.

CARROLL, M.E., MEISCH, R.A. Increased drug-reinforced behavior due to food deprivation. In: Thompson, T., Dews, P.B., Barrett, J.E. (eds.) *Advances in Behavioral Pharmacology,* Volume 4. New York: Academic Press, 1984, pp. 47–88.

CASTRO, F.G., NEWCOMB, M.D., MCCREARY, C., BAEZCONDE-GARBANATI, L. Cigarette smokers do more than just smoke cigarettes. *Health Psychology* 8(1):107–129, 1989.

CHAO, A., PAGANINI-HILL, A., ROSS, R.K., HENDERSON, B.E. Use of preventive care by the elderly. *Preventive Medicine* 16:710–722, 1987.

CHAPMAN, R.F., SMITH, J.W., LAYDEN, T.A. Elimination of cigarette smoking by punishment and self-management training. *Behavioral Research and Therapy* 9:255–264, 1971.

CLARKE, P.B.S. Nicotine and smoking: A perspective from animal studies. *Psychopharmacology* 92:135–143, 1987.

COELHO, R.J. Self-efficacy and cessation of smoking. *Psychological Reports* 54:309–310, 1984.

COHEN, S., KAMARCK, T., MERMELSTEIN, R. A global measure of perceived stress. *Journal of Health and Social Behavior* 24:385–396, December 1983.

COHEN, S., LICHTENSTEIN, E. Perceived stress, quitting smoking, and smoking relapse. *Health Psychology*, in press.

CONDIOTTE, M.M., LICHTENSTEIN, E. Self-efficacy and relapse in smoking cessation programs. *Journal of Consulting and Clinical Psychology* 49(5):648–658, October 1981.

CONWAY, T.L., CRONAN, T.A. Smoking, exercise, and physical fitness. Paper presented at the 1988 Annual Convention of the American Psychological Association, Atlanta, Georgia, August 1988a.

CONWAY, T.L., CRONAN, T.A. Smoking and physical fitness among navy shipboard men. *Military Medicine* 153(11):589–594, November 1988b.

COVEY, L.S., GLASSMAN, A.H., STETNER, F. Depression and depressive symptoms in smoking cessation. *Comprehensive Psychiatry*, in press.

CUMMINGS, K.M., GIOVINO, G., JAÈN, C.R., EMRICH, L.J. Reports of smoking withdrawal symptoms over a 21 day period of abstinence. *Addictive Behaviors* 10(4):373–381, 1985.

DUFFY, J., HALL, S.M. *Weight control and maintaining nonsmoking: Two incompatible goals?* Paper presented at the annual convention of the American Psychological Association, Boston, 1990.

DUNNE, M.P., MACDONALD, D., HARTLEY, L.R. The effects of nicotine upon memory and problem solving performance. *Physiology and Behavior* 37(6):849–854, 1986.

DUTTON, D. Financial, organizational and professional factors affecting health care utilization. *Social Science and Medicine* 23(7):721–735, 1986.

EISINGER, R.A. Psychosocial predictors of smoking recidivism. *Journal of Health and Social Behavior* 12:355–362, December 1971.

EMLEY, G.S., HUTCHINSON, R.R. Behavioral effects of nicotine. In: Thompson, T., Dews, P.B., Barrett, J.E. (eds.) *Advances in Behavioral Pharmacology*, Volume 4. New York: Academic Press, 1984, pp. 105–129.

EMMONS, K.M., WEIDNER, G., FOSTER, W.M., COLLINS, R.L. The effect of smoking cessation on cardiovascular reactivity to stress. Paper presented at the 20th Annual Meeting of the Association for Advancement of Behavior Therapy, Chicago, Illinois, 1986.

EMONT, S.L., CUMMINGS, K.M. Weight gain following smoking cessation: A possible role for nicotine replacement in weight management. *Addictive Behaviors* 12:151–155, 1987.

EYSENK, J.H., EYSENK, S.B.G. *Manual of the Eysenk Personality Questionnaire*. London: Hodder and Stoughton, 1975.

FAGERSTRÖM, K.-O. Measuring degree of physical dependence to tobacco smoking with reference to individualization of treatment. *Addictive Behaviors* 3:235–241, 1978.

FAGERSTRÖM, K.-O. Physical dependence on nicotine as a determinant of success in smoking cessation. *World Smoking and Health* 5:22–23, 1980.

FINNEGAN, D.L., SULER, J.R. Psychological factors associated with maintenance of improved health behaviors in postcoronary patients. *Journal of Psychology* 119(1):87-94, January 1985.

FIORE, M.C., NOVOTNY, T.E., PIERCE, J.P., GIOVINO, G.A., HATZIANDREU, E.J., NEWCOMB, P.A., SURAWICZ, T.S., DAVIS, R.M. Methods used to quit smoking in the United States. Do cessation programs help? *Journal of the American Medical Association* 263(20):2760-2765, May 23/30, 1990.

FLEISHER, L., KEINTZ, M., RIMER, B., UTT, M., WORKMAN, S., ENGSTROM, P.F. Process evaluation of a minimal-contact smoking cessation program in an urban nutritional assistance (WIC) program. In: Engstrom, P.F., Rimer, B., Mortenson, L.E. (eds.) *Advances in Cancer Control.* New York: Alan R. Liss, Inc., in press.

FOLKMAN, S., LAZARUS, R.S. Coping as a mediator of emotion. *Journal of Personality and Social Psychology* 54(3):466-475, 1988.

FRANCIS, D.A., NELSON, A.A. JR. Effect of patient recognition of tranquilizers on their use in alcohol detoxification. *American Journal of Hospital Pharmacy* 41:488-492, March 1984.

FRERICHS, R.R., ANESHENSEL, C.S., CLARK, V.A., YOKOPENIC, P. Smoking and depression: A community survey. *American Journal of Public Health* 71(6):637-640, June 1981.

FRIEDMAN, G.D., SIEGELAUB, A.B., DALES, L.G., SELTZER, C.C. Characteristics predictive of coronary heart disease in ex-smokers before they stopped smoking: Comparison with persistent smokers and nonsmokers. *Journal of Chronic Diseases* 32:175-190, 1979.

GERACE, T.A., HOLLIS, J., OCKENE, J.K., SVENDSEN, K. Cigarette smoking intervention in the Multiple Risk Factor Intervention Trial: Results and relationships to other outcomes. 5. Relationship of smoking cessation to diastolic blood pressure, body weight, and plasma lipids. *Preventive Medicine*, in press.

GIANNETTI, V.J., REYNOLDS, J., RIHN, T. Factors which differentiate smokers from ex-smokers among cardiovascular patients: A discriminant analysis. *Social Science and Medicine* 20(3):241-245, 1985.

GOLDBOURT, U., MEDALIE, J.H. Characteristics of smokers, nonsmokers and ex-smokers among 10,000 adult males in Israel. I. Distribution of selected sociodemographic and behavioral variables and the prevalence of disease. *Israel Journal of Medical Science* 11(11):1079-1101, November 1975.

GOLDSTEIN, M.G., WARD, K., NIAURA, R. Nicotine gum, tobacco dependence and withdrawal. Paper presented at the annual meeting of the American Psychiatric Association, Montreal, Canada, May 1988.

GORDON, N.P., CLEARY, P.D. Smoking cessation in a national probability sample cohort 1979-1980: Health attitudes, practices, and smoking behavior associated with quit attempts and behavior change at one year. *Smoking and Behavior Policy.* Cambridge, Massachusetts: Harvard University, October 1986.

GORDON, N.P., POLEN, M.R. Predicting success for men and women smokers in stop smoking programs. Paper presented at the 115th Annual Meeting of the American Public Health Association, New Orleans, Louisiana, October 20, 1987.

GOTTLIEB, A.M., KILLEN, J.D., MARLATT, G.A., TAYLOR, C.B. Psychological and pharmacological influences in cigarette smoking withdrawal: Effects of nicotine gum and expectancy on smoking withdrawal symptoms and relapse. *Journal of Consulting and Clinical Psychology* 55(4):606-608, 1987.

GRAHAM, S., GIBSON, R.W. Cessation of patterned behavior: Withdrawal from smoking. *Social Science and Medicine* 5:319-337, 1971.

GRITZ, E.R. Smoking behavior and tobacco abuse. In: Mello, N.K. (ed.) *Advances in Substance Abuse*, Volume 1. Greenwich, Connecticut: JAI Press, Inc., 1980, pp. 91-158.

GRITZ, E.R., CARR, C.R., MARCUS, A.C. The tobacco withdrawal syndrome in unaided quitters. Unpublished manuscript, 1990.

GROSS, J., STITZER, M.L. Nicotine replacement: Ten-week effects on tobacco withdrawal symptoms. *Psychopharmacology* 98:334–341, 1989.

GRUNBERG, N.E., BAUM, A. Biological commonalities of stress and substance abuse. In: Shiffman, S., Wills, T.A. (eds.) *Coping and Substance Use.* New York: Academic Press, 1985, pp. 25–61.

GRUNBERG, N.E., BOWEN, D.J. Coping with the sequelae of smoking cessation. *Journal of Cardiopulmonary Rehabilitation* 5(6):285–289, June 1985.

GUILFORD J.S. *Factors Related to Successful Abstinence From Smoking.* Pittsburgh, Pennsylvania: American Institute for Research, July 1966.

HAJEK, P., JARVIS, M.J., BELCHER, M., SUTHERLAND, G., FEYERABEND, C. Effect of smoke-free cigarettes on 24 h cigarette withdrawal: A double-blind placebo-controlled study. *Psychopharmacology* 97:99–102, 1989.

HALL, S.M. The abstinence phobias: Links between substance abuse and anxiety. *International Journal of the Addictions* 19(6):613–631, 1984.

HALL, S.M., BACHMAN, J., HENDERSON, J.B., BARSTOW, R., JONES, R.T. Smoking cessation in patients with cardiopulmonary disease: An initial study. *Addictive Behaviors* 8:33–42, 1983.

HALL, S.M., GINSBERG, D., JONES, R.T. Smoking cessation and weight gain. *Journal of Consulting and Clinical Psychology* 54:342–346, 1986.

HATSUKAMI, D.K., HUGHES, J.R., PICKENS, R.W. Characterization of tobacco withdrawal: Physiological and subjective effects. In: Grabowski, J., Hall, S. (eds.) *Pharmacological Adjuncts in Smoking Cessation*, NIDA Research Monograph 53. DHHS Publication No. (ADM) 85-1333, 1985, pp. 56–67.

HEIMSTRA, N.W., FALLESEN, J.J., KINSLEY, S.A., WARNER, N.W. The effects of deprivation of cigarette smoking on psychomotor performance. *Ergonomics* 23(11):1047–1055, 1980.

HEINOLD, J.W., GARVEY, A.J., GOLDIE, C., BOSSÉ, R. Retrospective analysis in smoking cessation research. *Addictive Behaviors* 7:347–353, 1982.

HENNINGFIELD, J.E. Behavioral pharmacology of cigarette smoking. In: Thompson, T., Dews, P.B., Barrett, J.E. (eds.) *Advances in Behavioral Pharmacology*, Volume 4. New York: Academic Press, 1984, pp. 131–210.

HINDMARCH, I., KERR, J.S., SHERWOOD, N. Effects of nicotine gum on psychomotor performance in smokers and non-smokers. *Psychopharmacology* 100:535–541, 1990.

HORWITZ, M.B., HINDI-ALEXANDER, M., WAGNER, T.J. Psychosocial mediators of abstinence, relapse, and continued smoking: A one-year follow-up of a minimal intervention. *Addictive Behaviors* 10:29–39, 1985.

HUGHES, J.R. Identification of the dependent smoker: Validity and clinical utility. *Behavioral Medicine Abstracts* 5(4):202–204, Fall 1984.

HUGHES, J.R. Craving as a psychological construct. *British Journal of Addiction* 82:38–39, 1986a.

HUGHES, J.R. Problems of nicotine gum. In: Ockene, J.K. (ed.) *Pharmacologic Treatment of Tobacco Dependence: Proceedings of the World Congress, November 4–5, 1985.* Cambridge, Massachusetts: Institute for the Study of Smoking Behavior and Policy, 1986b, pp. 141–147.

HUGHES, J.R. Clonidine, depression, and smoking cessation. *Journal of the American Medical Association* 259(19):2901–2902, May 20, 1988.

HUGHES, J.R. Tobacco withdrawal in self-quitters. *American Review of Respiratory Disease*, 1990.

HUGHES, J.R., GULLIVER, S.B., AMORI, G., MIREAULT, G., FENWICK, J. Effect of instructions and nicotine on smoking cessation, withdrawal symptoms and self-administration of nicotine gum. *Psychopharmacology* 99:486–491, 1989.

HUGHES, J.R., GUST, S.W., PECHACEK, T.F. Prevalence of tobacco dependence and withdrawal. *American Journal of Psychiatry* 144(2):205–208, February 1987.

HUGHES, J.R., GUST, S.W., SKOOG, K., KEENAN, R., FENWICK, J.W. Symptoms of tobacco withdrawal: A replication and extension. *Archives of General Psychiatry*, 1990.

HUGHES, J.R., HATSUKAMI, D. Signs and symptoms of tobacco withdrawal. *Archives of General Psychiatry* 43(3):289–294, March 1986.

HUGHES, J.R., HIGGINS, S.T., HATSUKAMI, D. Effects of abstinence from tobacco: A critical review. In: Kozlowski, L.T., Annis, H., Cappell, H.D., Glaser, F., Goodstadt, M., Israel, Y., Kalant, H., Sellers, E.M., Vingilis, E. (eds.) *Research Advances in Alcohol and Drug Problems*, Volume 10. New York: Plenum Press, 1990, pp. 317–398.

HUGHES, J.R., KEENAN, R.M., YELLIN, A. Effect of tobacco withdrawal on sustained attention. *Addictive Behaviors* 14:577–580, 1989.

HUGHES, J.R., KRAHN, D. Blindness and the validity of the double-blind procedure. *Journal of Clinical Psychopharmacology* 5(3):138–142, 1985.

IKARD, F.F., GREEN, D.E., HORN, D. A scale to differentiate between types of smoking as related to the management of affect. *International Journal of the Addictions* 4(4):649–659, December 1969.

ISTVAN, J., MATARAZZO, J.D. Tobacco, alcohol, and caffeine use: A review of their interrelationships. *Psychological Bulletin* 95(2):301–326, 1984.

JANZ, N.K., BECKER, M.H. The health belief model: A decade later. *Health Education Quarterly* 11(1):1–47, Spring 1984.

JARVIS, M. Gender and smoking: Do women really find it harder to give up? *British Journal of Addiction* 79(4):383–387, December 1984.

KAPLAN, R.M. Health-related quality of life in cardiovascular disease. *Journal of Consulting and Clinical Psychology* 56(3):382–392, 1988.

KATZ, R.C., SINGH, N.N. Reflections on the ex-smoker: Some findings on successful quitters. *Journal of Behavioral Medicine* 9(2):191–202, 1986.

KEENAN, R.M., HATSUKAMI, D.K., ANTON, D.J. The effects of short-term smokeless tobacco deprivation on performance. *Psychopharmacology* 98:126-130, 1989.

KILLEN, J., TAYLOR, C., MACCOBY, N., YOUNG, J. Investigating predictors of smoking relapse: An analysis of biochemical and self-report measures of tobacco dependence. Unpublished manuscript, 1990.

KILLEN, J.D., MACCOBY, N., TAYLOR, C.B. Nicotine gum and self-regulation training in smoking relapse prevention. *Behavior Therapy* 15:234–248, 1984.

KNUDSEN, N., SCHULMAN, S., FOWLER, R., VAN DEN HOEK, J. Why bother with stop-smoking education for lung cancer patients? *Oncology Nursing Forum* 11(3):30–33, May–June 1984.

KOVAR, M.G., POE, G.S. The National Health Interview Survey design, 1973–84, and procedures, 1975–83. National Center for Health Statistics, Series 1, No. 18. DHHS Publication No. (PHS) 85-1320, 1985.

KOZLOWSKI, L.T. Effects of caffeine consumption on nicotine consumption. *Psychopharmacology* 47(2):165–168, 1976.

KOZLOWSKI, L.T., FERRENCE, R.G. Statistical control in research on alcohol and tobacco: An example from research on alcohol and mortality. *British Journal of Addiction* 85(2):271–278, February 1990.

KOZLOWSKI, L.T., FERRENCE, R.G., CORBIT, T. Tobacco use: A perspective for alcohol and drug researchers. *British Journal of Addiction* 85:245, 1990.

KOZLOWSKI, L.T., MANN, R.E., WILKINSON, D.A., POULOS, C.X. "Cravings" are ambiguous: Ask about urges or desires. *Addictive Behaviors* 14:443–445, 1989.

KOZLOWSKI, L.T., WILKINSON, D.A. Use and misuse of the concept of "craving" by alcohol, tobacco, and drug researchers. *British Journal of Addiction* 82(1):31–36, January 1987a.

KOZLOWSKI, L.T., WILKINSON, D.A. Comments on Kozlowski and Wilkinson's use and misuse of the concept of craving by alcohol, tobacco and drug researchers: A reply from the authors. *British Journal of Addiction* 82:489–492, 1987b.

KOZLOWSKI, L.T., WILKINSON, D.A., SKINNER, W., KENT, C., FRANKLIN, T., POPE, M.A. Comparing tobacco cigarette dependence with other drug dependencies: Greater or equal "difficulty quitting" and "urges to use," but less pleasure from cigarettes. *Journal of the American Medical Association* 261(6):898–901, February 10, 1989.

KRONENFELD, J.J., GOODYEAR, N., PATE, R., BLAIR, A., HOWE, H., PARKER, G., BLAIR, S.N. The interrelationship among preventive health habits. *Health Education Research* 3(3):317–323, 1988.

LADER, M.H., HIGGITT, A.C. Management of benzodiazepine dependence—Update 1986. *British Journal of Addiction* 81(1):7–10, February 1986.

LARSON, P.S., FINNEGAN, J.K., HAAG, H.B. Observations on the effect of cigarette smoking on the fusion frequency of flicker. *Journal of Clinical Investigation* 29:483–486, 1950.

LAWRENCE, P.S., AMOEDI, N., MURRAY, A. Withdrawal symptoms associated with smoking cessation. Paper presented at the Annual Convention of the Association for the Advancement of Behavior Therapy, Los Angeles, November 1982.

LICHTENSTEIN, E., GLASGOW, R.E., ABRAMS, D.B. Social support in smoking cessation: In search of effective interventions. *Behavior Therapy* 17:607–619, 1986.

LUDWIG, A.M., WIKLER, A. "Craving" and relapse to drink. *Journal of Studies on Alcohol* 35:108–130, 1974.

LYON, R.J., TONG, J.E., LEIGH, G., CLARE, G. The influence of alcohol and tobacco on the components of choice reaction time. *Journal of Studies on Alcohol* 36:587–596, 1975.

MACANDREW, C. On the possibility of the psychometric detection of persons who are prone to the abuse of alcohol and other substances. *Addictive Behaviors* 4(1):11–20, 1979.

MACERA, C.A., PATE, R.R., DAVIS, D.R. Runners' health habits, 1985—"The Alameda 7" revisited. *Public Health Reports* 104(4):341–349, July–August 1989.

MACRAE, F.A., HILL, D.J., ST. JOHN, D.J.B., AMBIKAPATHY, A., GARNER, J.F., BALLARAT GENERAL PRACTITIONER RESEARCH GROUP. Predicting colon cancer screening behavior from health beliefs. *Preventive Medicine* 13:115–126, 1984.

MARLATT, G.A. Relapse prevention: Theoretical rationale and overview of the model. In: Marlatt, G.A., Gordon, J.R. (eds.) *Relapse Prevention: Maintenance Strategies in the Treatment of Addictive Behaviors.* New York: Guilford Press, 1985a, pp. 3–67.

MARLATT, G.A. Cognitive factors in the relapse process. In: Marlatt, G.A., Gordon, J.R. (eds.) *Relapse Prevention: Maintenance Strategies in the Treatment of Addictive Behaviors.* New York: Guilford Press, 1985b, pp. 128–193.

MARLATT, G.A. Lifestyle modification. In: Marlatt, G.A., Gordon, J.R. (eds.) *Relapse Prevention: Maintenance Strategies in the Treatment of Addictive Behaviors.* New York: Guilford Press, 1985c, pp. 280–344.

MARLATT, G.A. Craving notes. *British Journal of Addiction* 82:42–43, 1987.

MARLATT, G.A., GORDON, J.R. Determinants of relapse: Implications for the maintenance of behavior change. In: Davidson, P.O., Davidson, S.M. (eds.) *Behavioral Medicine: Changing Health Lifestyles.* New York: Brunner/Mazel, Inc., 1980, pp. 410–452.

MARLATT, G.A., GORDON, J.R. (eds.) *Relapse Prevention: Maintenance Strategies in the Treatment of Addictive Behaviors.* New York: Guilford Press, 1985.

MARON, D.J., TELCH, M.J., KILLEN, J.D., VRANIZAN, K.M., SAYLOR, K.E., ROBINSON, T.N. Correlates of seat-belt use by adolescents: Implications for health promotion. *Preventive Medicine* 15:614–623, 1986.

MARSDEN, M.E., BRAY, R.M., HERBOLD, J.R. Substance use and health among U.S. military personnel: Findings from the 1985 worldwide survey. *Preventive Medicine* 17:366–376, 1988.

MARTIN, J.E., DUBBERT, P.M. Exercise applications and promotion in behavioral medicine: Current status and future directions. *Journal of Consulting and Clinical Psychology* 50(6):1004–1017, 1982.

MARTIN, W.R., JASINSKI, D.R. Physiological parameters of morphine dependence in man—Tolerance, early abstinence, protracted abstinence. *Journal of Psychiatric Research* 7:9–17, 1969.

MCINTYRE, K.O., LICHTENSTEIN, E., MERMELSTEIN, R.J. Self-efficacy and relapse in smoking cessation: A replication and extension. *Journal of Consulting and Clinical Psychology* 51(4):632–633, 1983.

MERMELSTEIN, R., COHEN, S., LICHTENSTEIN, E., BAER, J.S., KAMARCK, T. Social support and smoking cessation and maintenance. *Journal of Consulting and Clinical Psychology* 54(4):447–453, 1986.

MILLER, W.R., HEDRIK, K.E., TAYLOR, C.A. Addictive behaviors and life problems before and after behavioral treatment of problem drinkers. *Addictive Behaviors* 8(4):403–412, 1983.

MLOTT, S.R, MLOTT, Y.D. Dogmatism and locus of control in individuals who smoke, stopped smoking and never smoked. *Journal of Community Psychology* 3:53–57, 1974.

MOTHERSILL, K.J., MCDOWELL, I., ROSSER, W. Subject characteristics and long term post-program smoking cessation. *Addictive Behaviors* 13(1):29–36, 1988.

MURRAY, A.L., LAWRENCE, P.S. Sequelae to smoking cessation: A review. *Clinical Psychology Review* 4:143–157, 1984.

NATIONAL CENTER FOR HEALTH STATISTICS. Massey, J.T., Moore, T.F., Parsons, V.L., Tadros, W. *Design and Estimation for the National Health Interview Survey, 1985–94.* Series 2, No. 110, August 1989.

NIAURA, R., GOLDSTEIN, M.G., WARD, K.D., ABRAMS, D.B. Reasons for smoking and severity of residual nicotine withdrawal symptoms when using nicotine chewing gum. *British Journal of Addiction* 84:681–687, 1989.

NICKI, R.M., REMINGTON, R.E., MACDONALD, G.A. Self-efficacy, nicotine-fading/self-monitoring and cigarette-smoking behaviour. *Behavioral Research and Therapy* 22(5):477–485, 1984.

OCKENE, J.K., BENFARI, R.C., NUTTALL, R.L., HURWITZ, I., OCKENE, I.S. Relationship of psychosocial factors to smoking behavior change in an intervention program. *Preventive Medicine* 11:13–28, 1982.

OCKENE, J.K., NUTALL, R., BENFARI, R.C., HURWITZ, I., OCKENE, I.S. A psychosocial model of smoking cessation and maintenance of cessation. *Preventive Medicine* 10:623–638, 1981.

OCKENE, J.K., SORENSEN, G., KABAT-ZINN, J., OCKENE, I.S., DONNELLY, G. Benefits and costs of lifestyle change to reduce risk of chronic disease. *Preventive Medicine* 17:224–234, 1988.

OLBRISCH, M., OADES-SOUTHER, D. *Smoking Cessation and Changes in Food, Alcohol, and Caffeine Intake.* Paper presented at the annual convention of the American Psychological Association, Washington, D.C., 1986.

ORLEANS, C.T. Understanding and promoting smoking cessation: Overview and guidelines for physician intervention. *Annual Review of Medicine* 36:51–61, 1985.

ORLEANS, C.T., SHIPLEY, R.H. Assessment in smoking cessation research: Some practical guidelines. In: Keefe, F.J., Blumenthal, J.A. (eds.) *Assessment Strategies in Behavioral Medicine.* New York: Grune and Stratton, 1982.

ORLEANS, C.T., SHIPLEY, R.H., WILBUR, C., PISERCHIA, P., WHITEHURST, D. Wide-ranging improvements in employee health lifestyle and wellbeing accompanying smoking cessation in the Live For Life program. Paper presented at the Annual Meeting of the Society of Behavioral Medicine, Baltimore, Maryland, 1983.

PARROT, A.C., WINDER, G. Nicotine chewing gum (2 mg, 4 mg) and cigarette smoking: Comparative effects upon vigilance and heart rate. *Psychopharmacology* 97:257–261, 1989.

PEDERSON, L.L., LEFCOE, N.M. A psychological and behavioural comparison of ex-smokers and smokers. *Journal of Chronic Diseases* 29:431–434, 1976.

PERKINS, K.A., EPSTEIN, L.H., PASTOR, S. Changes in energy balance following smoking cessation and resumption of smoking in women. *Journal of Consulting and Clinical Psychology* 58:121–125, 1990.

PERTSCHUK, M.J., POMERLEAU, O.F., ADKINS, D., HIRSH, C. Smoking cessation: The psychological costs. *Addictive Behaviors* 4:345–348, 1979.

POMERLEAU, C.S., POMERLEAU, O.F. Performance anxiety, smoking and cardiovascular reactivity. *Psychosomatic Medicine* 48(3/4):300, March/April 1986.

POMERLEAU, O., ADKINS, D., PERTSCHUK, M. Predictors of outcome and recidivism in smoking cessation treatment. *Addictive Behaviors* 3:65–70, 1978.

POMERLEAU, O., POMERLEAU, C., FAGERSTRÖM, K.-O., HENNINGFIELD, J.E., HUGHES, J.R. *Nicotine Replacement. A Critical Evaluation.* New York: Alan R. Liss, Inc., 1988.

PRENTICE-DUNN, S., ROGERS, R.W. Protection Motivation Theory and preventive health: Beyond the Health Belief Model. *Health Education Research* 1(3):153–161, 1986.

PROCHASKA, J.O., CRIMI, P., LAPSANSKI, D., MARTEL, L., REID, P. Self-change processes, self-efficacy and self-concept in relapse and maintenance of cessation of smoking. *Psychological Reports* 51:983–990, 1982.

PROCHASKA, J.O., DICLEMENTE, C.C., VELICER, W.F., GINPIL, S., NORCROSS, J.C. Predicting change in smoking status for self-changers. *Addictive Behaviors* 10:395–406, 1985.

PROCHASKA, J.O., DICLEMENTE, C.C., VELICER, W.F., ROSSI, J.S., GUADAGNOLI, E. Patterns of change in smoking cessation: Between variable comparisons. *Multivariate Behavioral Research*, in press.

PUDDEY, I.B., VANDONGEN, R., BEILIN, L.J., ENGLISH, D.R., UKICH, A.W. The effect of stopping smoking on blood pressure—A controlled trial. *Journal of Chronic Diseases* 38(6):483–493, 1985.

RANKIN, H. Craving competition. *British Journal of Addiction* 76:1–2, 1987.

REMINGTON, P.L., SMITH, M.Y., WILLIAMSON, D.F., ANDA, R.F., GENTRY, E.M., HOGELIN, G.C. Design, characteristics, and usefulness of state-based behavioral risk factor surveillance: 1981–87. *Public Health Reports* 103(4):366–375, 1988.

RIMER, B.K., DAVIS, S.W., ENGSTROM, P.F., MYERS, R.E., ROSAN, J.R. Some reasons for compliance and noncompliance in a health maintenance organization breast cancer screening program. *Journal of Compliance in Health Care* 3(2):103–114, 1988.

RIMER, B.K., KEINTZ, M.K., KESSLER, H.B., ENGSTROM, P.F., ROSAN, J.R. Why women resist screening mammography: Patient-related barriers. *Radiology* 172:243–246, 1989.

RIMER, B.K., ORLEANS, C.T., KEINTZ, M.K., CRISTINZIO, S., FLEISHER, L. The older smoker: Status, challenges and opportunities for intervention. *Chest* 97(3):547–553, March 1990.

RODIN, J. Weight change following smoking cessation: The role of food intake and exercise. *Addictive Behaviors* 12:303–317, 1987.

ROSE, J.E. The role of upper airway stimulation in smoking. In: Pomerleau, O.F., Pomerleau, C., Fagerström, K.-O., Henningfield, J.E., Hughes, J.R. (eds.) *Nicotine Replacement in the Treatment of Smoking.* New York: Alan R. Liss, Inc., 1988, pp. 95–106.

ROSENBAUM, M., ARGON, S. Locus of control and success in self-initiated attempts to stop smoking. *Journal of Clinical Psychology* 35(4):870–872, October 1979.

ROTTER, J.B. Generalized expectancies for internal versus external control of reinforcement. *Psychological Monographs* 80(1), 1966.

RUSSELL, M.A.H. Effect of electric aversion on cigarette smoking. *British Medical Journal* 1:82–86, 1970.

RUSSELL, M.A.H., PETO, J., PATEL, U.A. The classification of smoking by factoral structure of motives. *Journal of the Royal Statistical Society* 137(Part 3):313–333, 1974.

SACHS, D.P.L., BENOWITZ, N.L. The nicotine withdrawal syndrome: Nicotine absence or caffeine excess? In: Harris, L.S. (ed.) *Problems of Drug Dependence,* NIDA Research Monograph Series, 1990.

SAMET, J.M., WIGGINS, C.L. Unpublished analyses of the 1987 Behavioral Risk Factor Surveillance System.

SCHACHTER, S. Regulation, withdrawal, and nicotine addiction. In: Krasnegor, N.A. (ed.) *Cigarette Smoking as a Dependence Process.* NIDA Research Monograph 23. U.S. Department of Health, Education, and Welfare, Public Health Service, Alcohol, Drug Abuse, and Mental Health Administration, National Institute on Drug Abuse. January 1979, pp. 123–133.

SCHACHTER, S. Recidivism and self-care of smoking and obesity. *American Psychologist* 37(4):436–444, April 1982.

SCHNEIDER, N.G., JARVIK, M.E., FORSYTHE, A.B. Nicotine vs. placebo gum in the alleviation of withdrawal during smoking cessation. *Addictive Behaviors* 9(2):149–156, 1984.

SCHOENBORN, C.A., BENSON, V. Relationships between smoking and other unhealthy habits: United States, 1985. *Vital and Health Statistics.* No. 154, U.S. Department of Health and Human Services, Public Health Service, DHHS Publication No. (PHS) 88-1250, May 27, 1988.

SCHOENBORN, C.A., BOYD, G.M. Smoking and other tobacco use: United States, 1987. *Vital and Health Statistics.* No. 169 (Series 10), U.S. Department of Health and Human Services, Public Health Service, DHHS Publication No. (PHS) 89-1597, September 1989, pp. 1–78.

SCHOENENBERGER, J.C. Smoking change in relation to changes in blood pressure, weight, and cholesterol. *Preventive Medicine* 11:441–453, 1982.

SCHWARTZ, J.L., DUBITZKY, M. Changes in anxiety, mood, and self-esteem resulting from an attempt to stop smoking. *American Journal of Psychiatry* 124(11):138–142, May 1968.

SELTZER, C.C., BOSSÉ, R., GARVEY, A.J. Mail survey response by smoking status. *American Journal of Epidemiology* 100(6):453–457, 1974.

SETTERGREN, S.K., WILBUR, C.S., HARTWELL, T.D., RASSWEILER, J.H. Comparison of respondents and nonrespondents to a worksite health screen. *Journal of Occupational Medicine* 25(6):475–480, June 1983.

SHIFFMAN, S. Relapse following smoking cessation: A situational analysis. *Journal of Consulting and Clinical Psychology* 50(1):71–86, 1982.

SHIFFMAN, S. Craving: Don't let us throw the baby out with the bathwater. *British Journal of Addiction* 82:37–38, 1987.

SHIFFMAN, S., WILLS, T.A. (eds.) *Coping and Substance Use.* Orlando, Florida: Academic Press, 1985.

SHIFFMAN, S.M. The tobacco withdrawal syndrome. In: Krasnegor, N.A. (ed.) *Cigarette Smoking as a Dependence Process*. NIDA Research Monograph 23, DHEW Publication No. (ADM) 79-800. January 1979, pp. 158–184.

SHIFFMAN, S.M., JARVIK, M.E. Smoking withdrawal symptoms in two weeks of abstinence. *Psychopharmacology* 50(1):35–39, 1976.

SHIPLEY, R.H., ORLEANS, C.T., WILBUR, C.S., PISERCHIA, P.V., MCFADDEN, D.W. Effect of the Johnson & Johnson Live for Life Program on employee smoking. *Preventive Medicine* 17:25–34, 1988.

SHIPLEY, R.H., ROSEN, T.J., WILLIAMS, C. Measurement of smoking: Surveys and some recommendations. *Addictive Behaviors* 7:299–302, 1982.

SILVERSTEIN, B. Cigarette smoking, nicotine addiction, and relaxation. *Journal of Personality and Social Psychology* 42(5):946–950, May 1982.

SNYDER, F.R., DAVIS, F.C., HENNINGFIELD, J.E. The tobacco withdrawal syndrome: Assessment on a computerized test battery. *Drug and Alcohol Dependence* 23:259–266, 1989.

SNYDER, F.R., HENNINGFIELD, J.E. Effects of nicotine administration following 12 h of tobacco deprivation: Assessment on computerized performance tasks. *Psychopharmacology* 97:17–22, 1989.

SOBELL, L.C., SOBELL, M.B., KOZLOWSKI, L.T., TONEATTO, T. Alcohol or tobacco research versus alcohol and tobacco research. *British Journal of Addiction* 85(2):263–269, February 1990.

STOCKWELL, T. Is there a better word than "craving?" *British Journal of Addiction* 82:44–45, 1987.

STRAITS, B.C. Social and psycho-physiological correlates of smoking withdrawal. *Social Science Quarterly* 51(1):80–96, 1970.

SUEDFELD, P., BEST, J.A. Satiation and sensory deprivation combined in smoking therapy: Some case studies and unexpected side-effects. *International Journal of the Addictions* 12(2/3):337–359, 1977.

SWAN, F., DENK, C., PARKER, S., CARMELLI, D., FURZE, C., ROSENMAN, R. Risk factors for late relapse in male and female ex-smokers. *Addictive Behaviors* 13:253–256, 1988.

TAMERIN, J.S. The psychodynamics of quitting smoking in a group. *American Journal of Psychiatry* 129(5):101–107, November 1972.

TAPP, J.T., GOLDENTHAL, P. A factor analytic study of health habits. *Preventive Medicine* 11:724–728, 1982.

TARRIERE, H.C., HARTMANN, F. Investigation into the effects of tobacco smoke on a visual vigilance task. *Pharmacology and Therapeutics* 21:208, 1983.

TAYLOR, D.H., BLEZARD, P.N. The effects of smoking and urinary pH on a detection task. *Quarterly Journal of Experimental Psychology* 31:635–640, 1979.

TIPTON, R.M., RIEBSAME, W.E. Beliefs about smoking and health: Their measurement and relationship to smoking behavior. *Addictive Behaviors* 12:217–223, 1987.

TOMKINS, S.S. Psychological model for smoking behavior. *American Journal of Public Health* 56(12):17–20, December 1966.

TONG, J.E., LEIGH, G., CAMPBELL, J., SMITH, D. Tobacco smoking, personality and sex factors in auditory vigilance performance. *British Journal of Psychology* 68:365–370, 1977.

TØNNESEN, P., FRYD, V., HANSEN, M., HELSTED, J., GUNNERSEN, A.B., FORCHAMMER, H., STOCKNER, M. Effect of nicotine chewing gum in combination with group counseling on the cessation of smoking. *New England Journal of Medicine* 318(1):15–18, 1988.

TUOMILEHTO, J., NISSINEN, A., PUSKA, P., SALONEN, J., JALKANEN, L. Long-term effects of cessation of smoking on body weight, blood pressure and serum cholesterol in the middle-aged population with high blood pressure. *Addictive Behaviors* 11:1–9, 1986.

U.S. DEPARTMENT OF HEALTH AND HUMAN SERVICES. *The Health Consequences of Smoking: Nicotine Addiction. A Report of the Surgeon General, 1988.* U.S. Department of Health and Human Services, Public Health Service, Centers for Disease Control, Center for Health Promotion and Education, Office on Smoking and Health. DHHS Publication No. (CDC) 88-8406, 1988.

U.S. DEPARTMENT OF HEALTH AND HUMAN SERVICES. *Reducing the Health Consequences of Smoking: 25 Years of Progress. A Report of the Surgeon General.* U.S. Department of Health and Human Services, Public Health Service, Centers for Disease Control, Center for Chronic Disease Prevention and Health Promotion, Office on Smoking and Health. DHHS Publication No. (CDC) 89-8411, 1989.

VERBRUGGE, L.M. Work satisfaction and physical health. *Journal of Community Health* 7(4):262–283, Summer 1982.

WALLSTON, K.A., WALLSTON, B.S., DEVELLIS, R. Development of the multidimensional health locus of control (MHLC) scales. *Health Education Monographs* 6(2):160–170, Spring 1978.

WARBURTON, D.M. Psychopharmacological aspects of nicotine. In: Wonnacott, S., Russell, M.A.H., Stolerman, I.P. (eds.) *Nicotine Psychopharmacology.* New York: Oxford University Press, 1990, pp. 76–111.

WESNES, K., REVELL, A. The separate and combined effects of scopolamine and nicotine on human information processing. *Psychopharmacology* 84:5–11, 1984.

WESNES, K., WARBURTON, D.M. The effects of cigarette smoking and nicotine tablets upon human attention. In: Thornton, R.E. (ed.) *Smoking Behaviour: Physiological and Psychological Influences.* London: Churchill Livingstone, 1978, pp. 131–147.

WESNES, K., WARBURTON, D.M. Smoking, nicotine and human performance. *Pharmacology and Therapeutics* 21:189–208, 1983.

WESNES, K., WARBURTON, D.M. Effects of scopolamine and nicotine on human rapid information processing performance. *Psychopharmacology* 82:147–150, 1984.

WESNES, K., WARBURTON, D.M., MATZ, B. Effects of nicotine on stimulus sensitivity and response bias in a visual vigilance task. *Neuropsychobiology* 9:41–44, 1983.

WEST, D.W., GRAHAM, S., SWANSON, M., WILKINSON, G. Five year follow-up of a smoking withdrawal clinic population. *American Journal of Public Health* 67(6):536–544, June 1977.

WEST, R. Use and misuse of craving. *British Journal of Addiction* 82:39–40, 1987.

WEST, R., SCHNEIDER, N. Craving for cigarettes. *British Journal of Addiction* 82(4):407–415, April 1987.

WEST, R.J. Psychology and pharmacology in cigarette withdrawal. *Journal of Psychosomatic Research* 28(5):379–386, 1984.

WEST, R.J., HAJEK, P., BELCHER, M. Time course of cigarette withdrawal symptoms during four weeks of treatment with nicotine gum. *Addictive Behaviors* 12:1–5, 1987.

WEST, R.J., HAJEK, P., BELCHER, M. Severity of withdrawal symptoms as a predictor of outcome of an attempt to quit smoking. *Psychological Medicine* 19(4):981–985, November 1989.

WEST, R.J., JARVIS, M.J. Effects of nicotine on finger tapping rate in non-smokers. *Pharmacology, Biochemistry and Behavior* 25:727–731, 1986.

WEST, R.J., JARVIS, M.J., RUSSELL, M.A.H., CARRUTHERS, M.E., FEYERABEND, C. Effect of nicotine replacement on the cigarette withdrawal syndrome. *British Journal of Addiction* 79:215–219, 1984.

WEST, R.J., KRANZLER, H.R. Craving for cigarettes and psychoactive drugs. In: Warburton, D. (ed.) *Comparative Drug Use*. Harwood Academic Publishers, 1990.

WEST, R.J., RUSSELL, M.A.H. Pre-abstinence smoke intake and smoking motivation as predictors of severity of cigarette withdrawal symptoms. *Psychopharmacology* 87:334–336, 1985.

WILLIAMS, D.G. Different cigarette-smoker classification factors and subjective state in acute abstinence. *Psychopharmacology* 64(2):231–235, August 8, 1979.

WILLIAMS, S.G., HUDSON, A., REDD, C. Cigarette smoking, manifest anxiety and somatic symptoms. *Addictive Behaviors* 7(4):427–428, 1982.

WORLD HEALTH ORGANIZATION. The craving for alcohol. Report of the WHO Expert Committee on Mental Health and on Alcohol. *Quarterly Journal of Studies on Alcohol* 16:33–66, 1955.

VOLUME APPENDIX
NATIONAL TRENDS IN SMOKING CESSATION

CONTENTS

Introduction 583
Sources of Data 583
  National Center for Health Statistics Surveys 583
  Office on Smoking and Health Surveys 584
Measures of Quitting Behavior 584
  Percentage of Former Smokers in the Entire Population 585
  Percentage of Ever Smokers Who Are Former Smokers ("Quit Ratio") 585
  The Smoking Continuum 585
  Other Measures 588
Trends in the Proportion of Ever Smokers Who Are Former Smokers
  ("Quit Ratio") 588
  Trends by Gender 588
  Trends by Race 593
  Trends by Age 593
  Trends by Level of Educational Attainment 595
Long-Term Abstinence and Relapse 595
  National Health and Nutrition Examination Survey Epidemiologic
  Followup Study 596
The Smoking Continuum 599
  Percentage of Ever Smokers Who Have Never Tried to Quit ... 599
  Percentage of Those Smoking at 12 Months Prior to a Survey Interview
  Who Quit for at Least 1 Day During Those 12 Months 606
  Percentage of Ever Smokers Who Had Been Abstinent for Less Than 1 Year . 606
  Percentage of Ever Smokers Who Had Been Abstinent for 1 to 4 Years 606
  Percentage of Ever Smokers Who Had Been Abstinent for at Least 5 Years ... 607
  Interpretation of Continuum Findings 607
Other Measures Related to Smoking Cessation 608
  Intention to Smoke in 5 Years 608
  Receipt of Advice to Quit From a Doctor 609
Conclusions 610
References 613

INTRODUCTION

This volume appendix discusses national trends in smoking cessation over the last 25 years, specifically updating and expanding descriptions of the national trends in quitting activity presented in previous Surgeon General's reports (US DHHS 1980, 1983, 1988, 1989a). This Section does not provide a detailed discussion of psychosocial, pharmacologic, and behavioral factors known to be related to cessation, because this information is available from other sources (US DHEW 1979; US DHHS 1980, 1988, 1989a).

Data are utilized from 5 national cross-sectional surveys on adult tobacco use that were performed by the Office on Smoking and Health (OSH) (formerly the National Clearinghouse for Smoking and Health) and the 12 National Health Interview Survey (NHIS) supplements and the National Health and Nutrition Examination Survey (NHANES) Epidemiologic Followup Study (NHEFS), both performed by the National Center for Health Statistics (NCHS). The surveys were conducted between 1965 and 1987. The national surveys and the measures of quitting activity are described below, followed by a discussion of the data. Information on smoking cessation during pregnancy is also included in Chapter 8.

Information on smoking behavior was obtained from these surveys by means of self-report (i.e., without biochemical validation). As discussed in Chapter 2, self-report is considered a valid measure of smoking status in cross-sectional surveys, although some underreporting of daily cigarette consumption likely occurs.

SOURCES OF DATA

National Center for Health Statistics Surveys

Survey data collected by NCHS and available for inclusion in this Report were derived from the 1965, 1966, 1970, 1974, 1976, 1977, 1978, 1979, 1980, 1983, 1985, and 1987 supplements to NHIS and the 1982 to 1984 NHEFS. Cigarette smoking status (current, former, and never) is assessed in the same manner in all surveys. The constructs assessed on the NHIS supplements vary from survey year to survey year. Variables assessed include attempts to quit smoking among current smokers, duration of abstinence among former smokers, and receipt of advice to quit from a doctor.

NHIS, a cross-sectional household interview survey, samples the civilian, noninstitutionalized population of the United States (NCHS 1958, 1985, 1989). Weighting procedures are used to provide national estimates. Sample sizes for the smoking supplements (ages 20+) vary from approximately 9,700 in 1980 to over 80,000 in 1966.

NHEFS was a followup study of persons enrolled in NHANES-I, which assessed lifetime patterns of cigarette smoking behavior among current and former smokers. Whereas NHANES-I participants were drawn from a national probability sample of the civilian, noninstitutionalized population, NHEFS participants included only those who underwent the medical examination in NHANES-I. Personal interviews with each participant or a proxy (for deceased NHANES-I participants) were completed for 12,200 of the 14,407 original examinees. Proxy interviews were conducted with 1,697 representatives of deceased NHANES-I examinees. The interval between NHANES-I and NHEFS was about 10 years (Madans et al. 1986; NCHS 1987).

Office on Smoking and Health Surveys

OSH has commissioned five national surveys of tobacco use among adults in this country, referred to as the Adult Use of Tobacco Surveys (AUTSs). The surveys ask detailed questions designed to assess the knowledge, attitudes, and practices of adults regarding all forms of tobacco use. These cross-sectional surveys were conducted in 1964, 1966, 1970, 1975, and 1986 (US DHEW 1969, 1973, 1976; US DHHS 1989b).

The similar or identical wording of several standard questions for all five surveys facilitates comparisons. Constructs assessed included tobacco use behavior, intentions regarding future smoking behavior among ever smokers, and receipt of a doctor's advice to quit smoking.

Some differences in the conduct and design of the studies occurred. The mode of interviewing changed with time. The 1964 survey obtained data solely from personal household interviews. Whereas personal household interviews were the major mode of data collection in the 1966 survey, telephone interviews and mailed questionnaires were also used to collect data from eligible household members not available when the interviewer was present in the house. The 1970 and 1975 surveys conducted telephone interviews when possible and personal household interviews in nontelephone households. The 1986 survey was conducted entirely by telephone. The 1964 and 1966 surveys drew samples only from the contiguous United States. Other AUTSs collected data from residents of all 50 States.

The actual number of respondents for each survey was 4,635 in 1964, 4,061 in 1966, 5,191 in 1970, 12,029 in 1975, and 13,031 in 1986 (US DHEW 1969, 1973, 1976; US DHHS 1989b). In each survey, weighting procedures were used to adjust for an oversampling of ever smokers in the original study population. Comparisons between the 1986 AUTS and the others will not be exact, because the 1986 AUTS weights to an estimate of the adult U.S. population, whereas the other surveys weight to their respective sample sizes.

MEASURES OF QUITTING BEHAVIOR

As documented in several previous Surgeon General's reports (US DHEW 1979; US DHHS 1988, 1989a) and discussed in Chapter 2 of this Report, smoking cessation is a multifactorial process for overcoming an addictive behavior. One model characterizes this process as having several stages—precontemplation, contemplation, action, and maintenance (Prochaska and DiClemente 1983; Chapter 2). People frequently cycle and recycle through the various stages (marked by frequent relapse episodes) on their way to becoming long-term ex-smokers (Prochaska and DiClemente 1983; Cohen et al. 1989). This analysis of national trends in smoking cessation will use several measures to describe the quitting process. The 1989 Surgeon General's Report (US DHHS 1989a) discusses three measures of quitting behavior. These interrelated parameters are discussed below.

Percentage of Former Smokers in the Entire Population

This measure of quitting behavior has been used to calculate the number of former smokers in the population. Based on data from the 1987 NHIS, for example, 23.6 percent of the 162.6 million civilian, noninstitutionalized adults 20 years of age and older were former cigarette smokers. There were, therefore, approximately 38.5 million former smokers 20 years old or older in the United States in 1987. The percentage of former smokers in the entire population is limited as a measure of quitting activity primarily because it does not take into account the percentage of the population that has ever smoked (and thus is "at risk" of quitting). It also does not differentiate between people who have been abstinent for a short period and people who have maintained abstinence for several years (US DHHS 1989a).

Percentage of Ever Smokers Who Are Former Smokers ("Quit Ratio")

By dividing the number of ever smokers into the number of former smokers, perspective is given to the magnitude of quitting in a population. The term "quit ratio" has been used to describe this measure (CDC 1986; Pierce, Aldrich et al. 1987; US DHHS 1988, 1989a; Fiore et al. 1989) and is the term used below; this measure has also been termed the "quit rate" (Kabat and Wynder 1987) or the "cessation rate" (Jarvis 1984). The term "ratio" is mostly used in sciences when the numerator and the denominator are two separate and distinct quantities (Elandt-Johnson 1975). "Quit ratio" is used here, even though the numerator is included in the denominator, because of its repeated use in the literature as well as in previous Surgeon General's reports. The percentage of ever smokers who have discontinued smoking indicates the prevalence of abstinence (Ossip-Klein et al. 1986).

In 1987, 23.6 percent of the population were former cigarette smokers and 29.1 percent of the population were current smokers. The quit ratio among ever smokers was 44.8 percent; that is, nearly one-half of all living adults who ever smoked cigarettes had quit. Quit ratios by gender and age were recently published for 36 States and the District of Columbia based on 1988 data from the Behavioral Risk Factor Surveillance System (Anda et al. 1990) (Table 1).

The measure is limited because it treats all former smokers equally, regardless of duration of abstinence. It also classifies current smokers who had never tried to stop smoking in the same manner as it does current smokers who had been abstinent for a long period of time and relapsed shortly before the time of the survey (US DHHS 1989a).

The Smoking Continuum

The 1989 Surgeon General's Report defined a 10-category smoking continuum based on data from the 1986 AUTS. This continuum expanded on the smoking status variable (current, former, and never) to incorporate the timing and duration of quit attempts (US DHHS 1989a). Respondents were asked whether they had ever made a serious attempt to quit, and if the response was affirmative, they were then asked about the timing of

TABLE 1.—Quit ratio[a] in selected States, by age group and gender—BRFSS, 1988

State	18–34 %	(±95% CI)[b]	35–49 %	(±95% CI)	50–64 %	(±95% CI)	≥65 %	(±95% CI)	Men %	(±95% CI)	Women %	(±95% CI)	Total %	(±95% CI)
Alabama	24.5	(7.0)	41.3	(7.3)	54.3	(8.3)	65.8	(10.1)	47.4	(5.6)	37.3	(5.9)	43.2	(4.1)
Arizona	45.5	(7.9)	54.2	(8.0)	61.2	(9.9)	67.9	(8.8)	60.1	(6.2)	49.8	(6.0)	55.4	(4.3)
California	40.1	(5.7)	54.3	(5.6)	64.3	(6.9)	65.6	(7.8)	56.9	(4.4)	49.3	(4.5)	53.7	(3.2)
Connecticut	38.6	(7.4)	49.0	(7.3)	60.7	(9.3)	74.9	(8.0)	55.1	(6.4)	50.4	(5.8)	52.8	(4.3)
District of Columbia	37.2	(8.8)	45.4	(9.9)	56.5	(11.6)	59.4	(12.5)	52.0	(8.0)	43.4	(7.3)	47.6	(5.5)
Florida	43.7	(7.4)	45.3	(7.2)	52.3	(7.7)	77.6	(5.7)	58.5	(4.8)	50.4	(5.2)	54.8	(3.5)
Georgia	39.5	(5.6)	40.3	(8.7)	53.1	(12.7)	70.2	(17.2)	44.2	(7.2)	46.6	(6.8)	45.3	(5.2)
Hawaii	33.7	(7.1)	45.0	(7.6)	61.5	(9.1)	70.9	(9.9)	49.6	(5.8)	44.3	(6.3)	47.3	(4.3)
Idaho	42.6	(7.1)	49.2	(6.9)	58.3	(8.3)	77.1	(6.2)	61.3	(5.5)	44.2	(5.5)	54.0	(3.9)
Illinois	35.1	(6.7)	42.6	(6.6)	53.6	(8.0)	64.1	(8.3)	48.9	(5.3)	42.4	(5.2)	45.8	(3.6)
Indiana	33.1	(5.5)	42.2	(5.8)	51.9	(6.7)	79.1	(5.9)	51.6	(4.4)	41.2	(4.6)	47.0	(3.2)
Iowa	30.0	(9.2)	59.5	(10.5)	55.4	(12.3)	71.1	(10.9)	60.3	(8.1)	39.1	(7.2)	50.7	(5.8)
Kentucky	22.6	(5.6)	33.6	(6.9)	48.2	(7.0)	63.6	(7.0)	42.6	(4.9)	31.1	(4.5)	37.8	(3.4)
Maine	38.3	(7.2)	50.4	(7.4)	65.3	(8.4)	72.7	(8.7)	60.5	(5.9)	44.5	(5.5)	53.2	(4.1)
Maryland	41.1	(9.0)	45.6	(8.3)	57.9	(9.9)	70.9	(9.3)	53.0	(7.3)	48.0	(6.5)	50.6	(5.0)
Massachusetts	35.2	(6.6)	50.8	(7.0)	59.8	(9.5)	75.5	(7.1)	56.2	(6.3)	47.6	(5.2)	51.9	(4.2)
Michigan	37.4	(7.0)	50.5	(7.3)	55.0	(10.3)	65.9	(13.4)	52.0	(6.4)	45.5	(5.8)	48.9	(4.5)
Minnesota	41.2	(4.4)	55.2	(4.3)	64.6	(5.4)	76.0	(5.0)	60.4	(3.4)	49.2	(3.8)	55.4	(2.5)
Missouri	35.8	(7.1)	42.9	(7.5)	57.5	(8.4)	79.2	(7.0)	54.7	(6.1)	43.5	(5.4)	49.6	(4.1)
Montana	45.7	(9.6)	58.8	(7.7)	58.8	(8.2)	79.0	(7.1)	62.0	(6.4)	54.1	(6.2)	58.6	(4.5)

TABLE 1.—Continued

State	18–34 %	(±95% CI)	35–49 %	(±95% CI)	50–64 %	(±95% CI)	≥65 %	(±95% CI)	Men %	(±95% CI)	Women %	(±95% CI)	Total %	(±95% CI)
Nebraska	39.6	(7.4)	57.6	(8.3)	57.6	(9.0)	74.5	(7.8)	59.0	(5.9)	47.2	(6.1)	54.0	(4.3)
New Hampshire	35.2	(7.0)	53.0	(7.4)	60.3	(9.9)	74.2	(9.2)	53.8	(6.1)	48.6	(6.0)	51.5	(4.6)
New Mexico	38.4	(8.7)	47.0	(9.2)	53.4	(9.8)	64.7	(11.7)	49.4	(7.3)	46.3	(7.0)	48.0	(5.2)
New York	29.8	(7.4)	42.7	(8.1)	66.3	(8.9)	80.3	(8.2)	54.2	(6.8)	46.8	(6.5)	50.5	(4.7)
North Carolina	37.0	(6.8)	47.5	(6.7)	47.9	(8.5)	72.3	(7.9)	50.4	(5.7)	43.4	(5.2)	47.3	(3.9)
North Dakota	38.7	(7.1)	50.9	(6.8)	62.2	(7.9)	73.3	(7.4)	58.3	(5.1)	45.5	(5.6)	53.1	(3.8)
Ohio	30.6	(6.5)	42.3	(7.6)	57.4	(9.0)	67.3	(8.4)	52.0	(6.2)	37.4	(5.7)	44.9	(4.2)
Oklahoma	37.1	(9.1)	43.6	(8.6)	55.9	(10.2)	62.9	(13.4)	53.4	(7.0)	39.6	(6.7)	47.5	(5.1)
Rhode Island	34.7	(6.4)	44.8	(6.8)	55.6	(8.5)	69.8	(7.2)	51.1	(5.6)	44.6	(5.1)	47.8	(3.8)
South Carolina	28.9	(5.8)	41.5	(6.6)	58.7	(7.6)	72.2	(8.8)	46.0	(5.1)	42.1	(5.4)	44.4	(3.8)
South Dakota	37.4	(9.2)	52.3	(8.6)	60.8	(9.2)	71.1	(8.7)	55.6	(5.8)	50.5	(6.7)	53.4	(4.3)
Tennessee	29.0	(4.8)	40.9	(5.7)	49.5	(6.8)	67.2	(7.9)	43.4	(4.5)	39.4	(4.1)	41.8	(3.2)
Texas	38.8	(8.6)	45.7	(8.4)	53.7	(10.5)	69.3	(12.5)	52.5	(6.7)	41.4	(6.8)	47.9	(4.8)
Utah	33.5	(7.5)	50.9	(8.1)	68.3	(11.3)	80.1	(9.2)	65.2	(5.8)	40.5	(8.6)	56.6	(5.0)
Washington	37.7	(7.3)	54.8	(7.5)	53.7	(8.7)	82.5	(7.9)	58.2	(5.8)	46.1	(5.8)	53.0	(4.2)
West Virginia	38.5	(7.1)	43.4	(6.5)	49.1	(7.2)	69.4	(7.2)	54.5	(5.2)	38.4	(5.0)	47.6	(3.7)
Wisconsin	35.0	(6.9)	52.0	(7.3)	62.2	(8.5)	76.0	(9.1)	63.8	(5.6)	46.3	(6.7)	56.5	(4.4)
Median prevalence	37.2		47.0		57.5		71.1		54.2		44.6		50.5	

NOTE: BRFSS=Behavioral Risk Factor Surveillance System.
[a] Defined as the percentage of ever smokers who were former smokers at the time of the survey.
[b] Confidence interval.
SOURCE: BRFSS 1988 (Anda et al. 1990)

their most recent quit attempt. This measure provides information on the recent quitting history of the population (Pierce, Giovino et al. 1989; US DHHS 1989a). The trend analyses presented below will use an eight-category continuum (Table 2) among ever smokers to incorporate data from the 1978, 1979, 1980, and 1987 NHISs. As opposed to the 1986 AUTS, the questions asked in these NHISs do not permit a dichotomous classification of current smokers who had never tried to quit according to interest in quitting.

In addition to a description of the overall smoking continuum, several segments of the continuum, or measures derived from the continuum, will be described separately. These measures include the following:

- The percentage of ever smokers who have never tried to quit;

- The percentage of people smoking at 12 months prior to a survey interview who had been abstinent for at least 1 day during those 12 months;

- The percentage of ever smokers who had stopped smoking for less than 1 year;

- The percentage of ever smokers who had stopped smoking for 1 to 4 years; and

- The percentage of ever smokers who had stopped smoking for at least 5 years.

Other Measures

Respondents to AUTSs were asked to estimate the possibility that they would be smoking 5 years after the survey. This question gives a measure of intention to smoke. Finally, respondents to several NHISs and to all OSH tobacco use surveys were asked if a physician had ever advised them to stop smoking.

TRENDS IN THE PROPORTION OF EVER SMOKERS WHO ARE FORMER SMOKERS ("QUIT RATIO")

Using data from NHISs for 1965 to 1987, trends in the proportion of ever cigarette smokers in the U.S. adult population who have stopped smoking cigarettes (quit ratio) are presented by gender and by race in Figures 1 and 2, respectively. Trends for the total adult population, as well as trends by age and by education, are shown in Table 3. These data, with the exception of the age-specific estimates, are age-adjusted to the 1985 population. In these analyses, the quit ratio was regressed on the calendar year of data collection. The R^2 statistic, supplied for each trend analysis, is a measure of the strength of the linear relationship. R^2 values may range from 0 (no linear trend) to 1.0 (a perfect positive or negative linear relationship).

Trends by Gender

As shown in Figure 1, the quit ratio for both genders has been increasing in an approximately linear fashion (R^2=0.94 for males and 0.97 for females) since 1965, and

TABLE 2.—Cigarette smoking continuum by year, percentage of ever cigarette smokers, NHISs, United States, 1978–87, adults aged 20 and older

Cigarette smoking continuum	1978	1979	1980	1987
1. Current smokers who had never tried to quit	25.9	26.1	25.4	18.9
2. Current smokers who had quit previously but not in past year	22.7	21.4	23.1	20.0
3. Current smokers who had quit for <7 days in past year	6.6	6.0	5.9	7.0
4. Current smokers who had quit for ≥7 days in past year	8.5	8.6	7.8	8.4
5. Former smokers who had quit within past 3 mo	1.3	1.6	1.4	1.8
6. Former smokers who had been abstinent for 3–12 mo	2.7	2.6	2.7	2.8
7. Former smokers who had been abstinent for 1–5 yr	9.0	10.0	9.5	10.4
8. Former smokers who had quit ≥5 yr earlier	23.3	23.6	24.1	30.7
Percentage of those smoking during the year prior to the survey who tried to quit during that year (Categories 3+4+5+6 divided by 1+2+3+4+5+6)	28.2	28.4	26.8	34.0
Percentage of those smoking during the year prior to the survey who quit during that year and were still abstinent at the time of the survey (Categories 5+6 divided by 1+2+3+4+5+6)	6.1	6.3	6.2	7.8

NOTE: NHIS=National Health Interview Survey.
SOURCE: NHISs 1978, 1979, 1980, 1987.

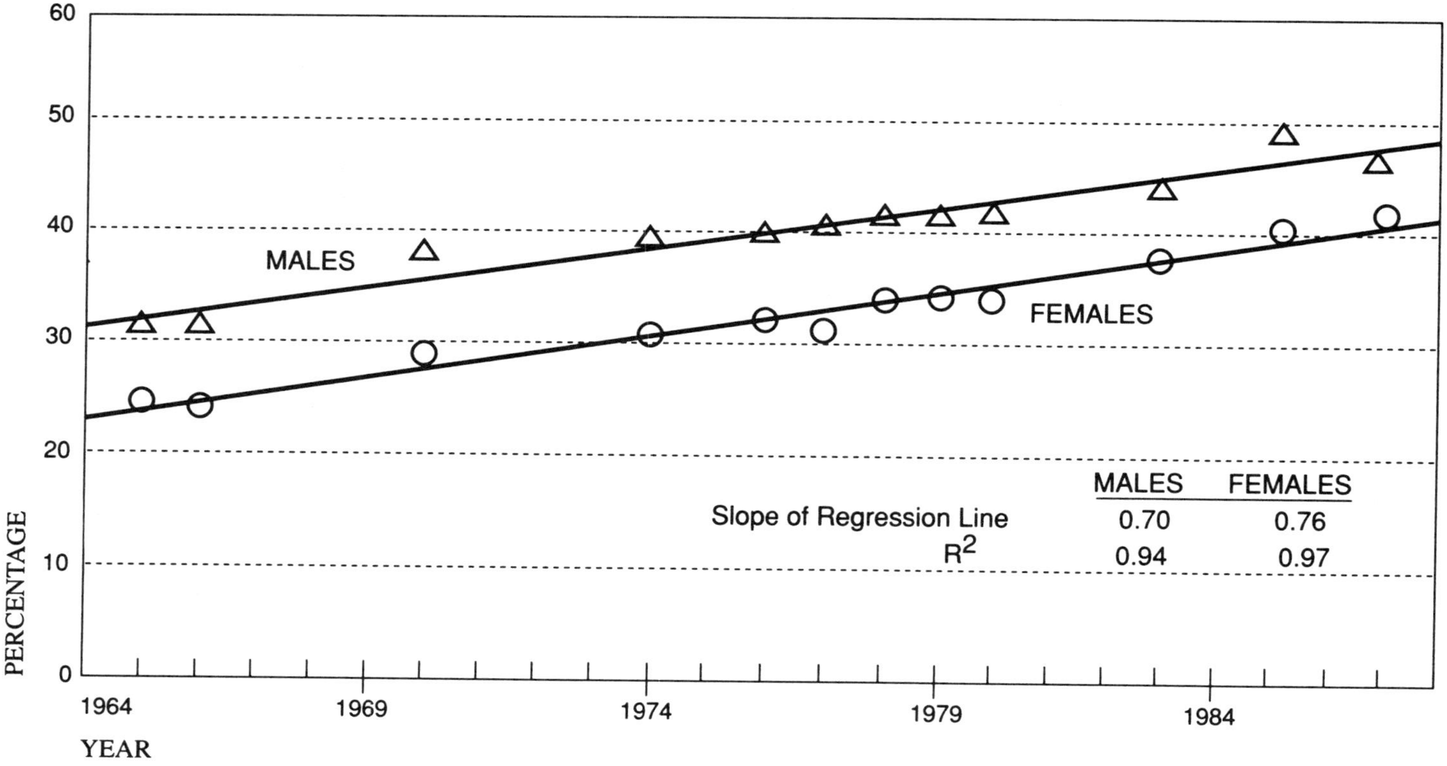

FIGURE 1.—Trends in the quit ratio, United States, 1965–87, by gender

NOTE: Quit ratio is the proportion of ever smokers who are former smokers. NHIS=National Health Intreview Survey; OSH=Office on Smoking and Health.

SOURCE: NHISs 1965, 1966, 1970, 1974, 1976, 1977, 1978, 1979, 1980, 1983, 1985, 1987: OSH, unpublished data.

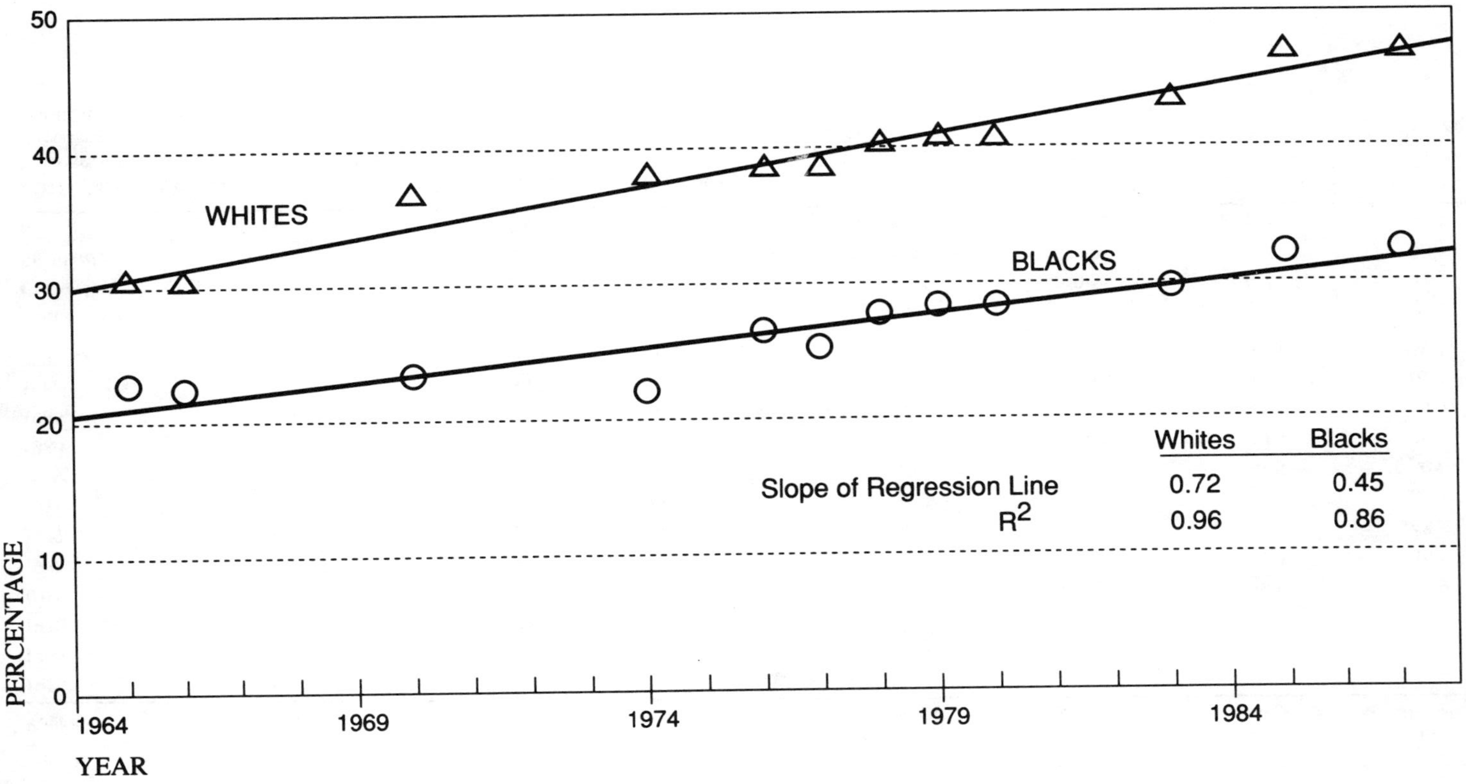

FIGURE 2.—Trends in the quit ratio, United States, 1965–87, by race

NOTE: NHIS=National Health Interview Survey; OSH=Office on Smoking and Health.
SOURCE: NHISs 1965, 1966, 1970, 1974, 1976, 1977, 1978, 1979, 1980, 1983, 1985, 1987; OSH, unpublished data.

TABLE 3.—Trends in quit ratio (%) (percentage of ever cigarette smokers who are former cigarette smokers), by age and by education, NHISs, United States, 1965–87, adults aged 20 and older

		Age (yr)				Educational level			
Year	Overall population	20–24	25–44	45–64	≥65	Less than high school graduate	High school graduate	Some college	College graduate
1965[a]	29.6	17.8	23.6	30.9	48.7	—	—	—	—
1966	29.5	17.0	23.4	30.9	50.5	33.3	28.0	28.7	39.7
1970	35.3	20.8	29.8	36.1	56.9	38.1	33.6	34.9	48.2
1974	36.3	20.9	29.3	39.7	57.8	38.0	35.2	36.6	47.9
1976	37.1	22.0	29.4	40.4	59.6	39.5	35.0	37.2	46.1
1977	36.8	22.9	29.6	39.5	58.7	38.3	34.0	36.8	48.6
1978	38.5	22.8	31.9	40.1	62.4	38.7	36.3	41.0	49.7
1979	39.0	22.6	31.8	42.4	61.7	40.8	36.7	37.5	50.6
1980	39.0	22.2	33.0	40.9	61.0	39.4	36.5	40.6	48.7
1983	41.8	21.4	34.3	46.4	64.7	42.1	38.7	41.2	54.9
1985	45.0	26.0	38.2	49.7	68.0	41.3	40.5	46.0	61.1
1987	44.8	23.8	37.2	49.2	69.2	44.3	41.1	45.5	59.1
Trend information (1965–87)									
Change[b]/yr	0.68	0.26	0.61	0.84	0.86	0.44	0.55	0.74	0.88
Standard error (±)	0.04	0.06	0.05	0.06	0.06	0.05	0.05	0.08	0.13
R^2	0.96	0.64	0.93	0.95	0.96	0.88	0.92	0.90	0.83

NOTE: The data stratified by education are age adjusted to the 1985 population. NHIS=National Health Interview Survey.
[a] For 1965, data stratified by education were unavailable.
[b] In percentage points.
SOURCE: NHISs 1965, 1966, 1970, 1974, 1976, 1977, 1978, 1979, 1980, 1983, 1985, 1987.

the rates of increase for both are also similar (0.70 percentage points/year for males and 0.76 percentage points/year for females). The quit ratio has been consistently higher for males than for females. Using data from the 1970 and 1975 AUTSs, Jarvis (1984) reclassified as current smokers males who gave up smoking cigarettes but who continued to smoke cigars and/or pipes. When the use of other forms of smoking tobacco was considered, the difference between males and females in the quit ratio (termed as the "cessation rate" by Jarvis) was reduced by more than two-thirds.

Data from the 1987 NHIS Cancer Epidemiology and Control supplement (Schoenborn and Boyd 1989) were analyzed to update the work of Jarvis (Table 4). The weighted percentage of ever cigarette smokers who were former cigarette smokers among males was 48.7 percent. The corresponding number among females was 40.1 percent. When former cigarette smokers who smoked cigars and/or pipes were reclassified as current smokers (without changing the denominator), the prevalence of cessation among ever smokers became 45 percent for males and 40 percent for females. Furthermore, when former cigarette smokers who used any other form of tobacco (cigars, pipes, snuff, and/or chewing tobacco) at the time of the survey were classified as current tobacco users, the figures became 42.1 percent for males and 39.9 percent for females (OSH, unpublished data). Thus, reclassification of former cigarette smokers who were smoking cigars and/or pipes as current smokers reduced the difference in the quit ratio between males and females from 8.6 to 5.0 percentage points. Former cigarette smokers who were using any other form of tobacco were reclassified as current tobacco users, and this reclassification further reduced the difference to 2.2 percentage points.

Trends by Race

Trends by race are presented in Figure 2. The quit ratio among both whites and blacks has been increasing steadily since 1965 (R^2=0.96 for whites and 0.86 for blacks). While the change per year since 1965 is higher for whites (0.72 percentage points/year) than it is for blacks (0.45 percentage points/year), the lines have been essentially parallel since 1974 (Fiore et al. 1989). Use of the 1987 NHIS data to reclassify as current smokers all former cigarette smokers who were smoking cigars or pipes reduced the quit ratio from 46.4 to 44.2 percent among whites and from 31.5 to 30.2 percent among blacks. Further reclassification, as current tobacco users, of former cigarette smokers who were using any other form of tobacco reduced the numbers to 42.5 percent for whites and 29.1 percent for blacks (OSH, unpublished data).

Trends by Age

Table 3 provides information on the quit ratio stratified by age. For all age categories, the quit ratio increased from 1965 to 1987. The rate of change was highest in the age categories of 45–64 years and 65 years and older. Reclassification of the 1987 data to account for cigar and pipe smoking and for any other tobacco use lowered the numbers from 23.8 percent to 23.4 and 22.2 percent, respectively, among the 20–24-year-olds; from 37.2 percent to 35.6 and 34.3 percent, respectively, among 25–44-year-olds; from

49.2 percent to 46.4 and 45.0 percent, respectively, among 45–64-year-olds; and from 69.2 percent to 66.2 percent and 62.8 percent, respectively, among those 65-years-old and older (Table 4) (OSH, unpublished data). A detailed analysis of trends in the quit ratio by age for the period 1974 through 1987 has been completed (Novotny et al., in press).

Differences in quit ratios between age groups may reflect actual differences in quitting activity by age—that is, older persons may be more prone to quit and maintain abstinence than younger smokers, perhaps because of the occurrence of smoking-related symptoms or illness. However, continuing smokers are less likely than former smokers to survive to old age (Chapter 3); this selective mortality will artifactually increase the quit ratio among older age groups.

TABLE 4.—Effect of adjusting for use of other tobacco products on quit ratio (percentage of ever cigarette smokers who are former cigarette smokers), 1987, NHIS, United States

	Quit ratio (%)		
	Unadjusted[a]	Adjusting for cigars/pipes[b]	Adjusting for cigars/pipes/snuff/chewing tobacco[c]
Gender			
Males	48.7	45.0	42.1
Females	40.1	40.0	39.9
Race			
Whites	46.4	44.2	42.5
Blacks	31.5	30.2	29.1
Age (yr)			
20–24	23.8	23.4	22.2
25–44	37.2	35.6	34.3
45–64	49.2	46.4	45.0
≥65	69.2	66.2	62.8
Education (yr)			
<12	39.7	38.1	35.2
12	40.9	39.2	37.8
13–15	46.9	44.9	43.5
≥16	61.4	57.3	56.6
Overall	44.8	42.8	41.1

NOTE: NHIS=National Health Interview Survey.
[a]The percentage of ever cigarette smokers who were former cigarette smokers at the time of the survey.
[b]As in footnote (a), but former cigarette smokers who were using cigars and/or pipes at the time of the survey reclassified as current smokers.
[c]As in footnote (a), but former cigarette smokers who were using either cigars, pipes, snuff, or chewing tobacco at the time of the survey reclassified as current tobacco users.
SOURCE: NHIS (1987).

Trends by Level of Educational Attainment

Table 3 shows the quit ratio among college graduates is consistently higher than the ratios among persons with less than high school graduation, high school graduation, or some college education. Also, the rate of increase per year rises as the educational level increases (0.44, 0.55, 0.74, and 0.88 percentage points/ year in persons with <12, 12, 13–15, and 16 or more years of education, respectively). From 1966 to 1977 the quit ratio among high school dropouts was higher than the ratios among the two middle education categories; the reason for this is unclear.

Reclassification of the 1987 NHIS former cigarette smokers based on the use of other tobacco products did not affect the magnitude of the relationships between education categories (Table 4). After reclassification, the quit ratio dropped from 39.7 percent to 38.1 and 35.2 percent in the less-than-high-school-graduation category, from 40.9 percent to 39.2 and 37.8 percent in the high-school-graduation category, from 46.9 percent to 44.9 and 43.5 percent in the some-college category, and from 61.4 percent to 57.3 and 56.6 percent in the college graduation category (OSH, unpublished data).

LONG-TERM ABSTINENCE AND RELAPSE

The prototypical pattern of relapse after cessation among group clinic participants was first published by Hunt, Barnett, and Branch (1971) and is cited in the 1988 Surgeon General's Report (US DHHS 1988). The relapse curve for smokers indicates that approximately 65 percent of all quitters relapsed within 3 months of quitting; another 10 percent relapsed from 3 to 6 months postcessation. About 3 percent more of the original sample of quitters relapsed from 6 to 12 months postcessation.

Because smokers who attend quit-smoking classes are likely to be different from smokers who attempt to quit on their own (Fiore et al. 1990), the probability of quitting success in one group may not apply to the other. Indeed, the results of a meta-analysis of 10 prospective studies of people attempting to quit without any assistance or using only self-help materials suggested that about 24 percent of those study participants who were continuously abstinent at the 6-month followup relapsed before the 1-year followup (Cohen et al. 1989); the corresponding percentage in the study of clinic attendees (Hunt, Barnett, Branch 1971) was 12 percent, as calculated using the percentages in the previous paragraph.

Few prospective studies of cessation have observed participants for longer than 1 year (Schwartz 1987; Glasgow and Lichtenstein 1987). Relapse data after 1 year of continuous abstinence are not presented in some of the intervention studies that include followup periods of more than 1 year (e.g., Lando and McGovern 1982; Lichtenstein and Rodrigues 1977; Ockene et al. 1982; West et al. 1977). In the Multiple Risk Factor Intervention Trial, 15 percent of the special-intervention group and 16 percent of the usual-care group who were abstinent from cigarettes at both the first- and second-year followup assessments reported recidivism during the third or fourth year of followup (Ockene et al. 1982).

Hammond and Garfinkel (1964) provided data from the Cancer Prevention Study I (CPS-I) on a cohort of 65,709 male former smokers (aged 30–89) who were reinterviewed after 2 years. Of those who had been abstinent for less than 1 year at baseline, 37.3 percent were smoking cigarettes again at followup. Of those who had been abstinent for at least 1 year but less than 2 years or for 2 years or more at baseline, 19.1 and 4.6 percent, respectively, were smoking cigarettes again at the 2-year followup interview.

In another report also based on CPS-I, Hammond and Garfinkel (1963) further subdivided the duration of abstinence at baseline for males aged 50 to 69. For those abstinent for 2 to 4 years, 5 to 9 years, and 10 years or more at baseline, 8.7, 4.1, and 2.2 percent, respectively, were smoking cigarettes at the 2-year followup interview.

Kirscht, Brock, and Hawthorne (1987) surveyed a probability sample of 3,073 Michigan adults in 1980. In 1982, completed followup questionnaires were obtained from 2,110 members (68.7 percent) of the original sample. In 1980, 23.0 percent of the entire sample were ex-smokers. Of those ex-smokers who had been abstinent for less than 6 months in 1980, 38.7 percent were smoking again when they completed the 1982 questionnaire. Among those ex-smokers who had been abstinent between 6 and 23 months in 1980, 29.5 percent were smoking in 1982. Among those abstinent between 24 and 119 months or for 120 months or more in 1980, 9.5 and 2.3 percent, respectively, reported that they were smoking again when the 1982 survey was conducted.

National Health and Nutrition Examination Survey Epidemiologic Followup Study

Data from NHEFS (NCHS 1987; Madans et al. 1986) were used to assess lifetime patterns of quitting in a sample of the adult population (OSH, unpublished data). Reconstructed cigarette smoking prevalence from NHEFS shows good agreement with self-reported smoking status recorded during the original NHANES-I interview (Machlin, Kleinman, Madans 1989).

The description of quitting and relapse discussed below is limited because only quit attempts of 12 months or more were assessed and the reclassification of former cigarette smokers who smoked cigars or pipes as current smokers is not always possible. Quit attempts that occurred before the age of 21 were not considered.

As shown by NHEFS data in Figure 3, of the 6,460 ever cigarette smokers, 55.2 percent had stopped smoking cigarettes for at least 1 year at some point before the NHEFS interview. Of these, 37.6 percent relapsed after at least 1 year of maintaining abstinence. Of those who relapsed, 43.0 percent quit again for at least 1 year. Among those who quit again for at least 1 year, 35.2 percent relapsed a second time. These data indicate that at least one-third of all ever smokers who quit for at least 1 year will eventually relapse.

The product–limit method (Lee 1980) was used to estimate the relapse rate after the first 1-year period of abstinence. As shown in Figure 4, most of the relapse after the first 1-year abstinence period occurred within a few years. About 28 percent of ever smokers who attained abstinence for at least 1 year relapsed within 5 years of quitting. Another 7 percent of the original sample of ever smokers who had quit for 1 year or more relapsed within the next 5 years. Thus, about one-third (35 percent) of former smokers who have maintained abstinence for at least 1 year may eventually relapse.

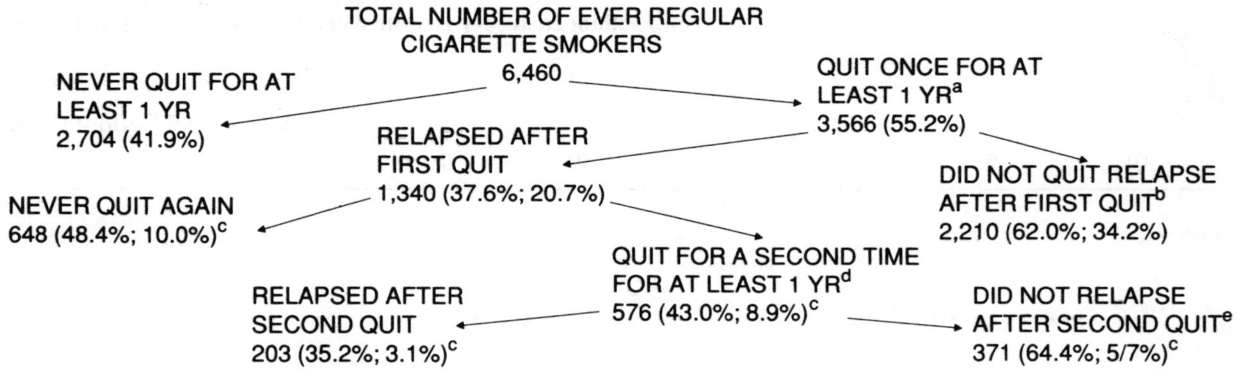

TOTAL NUMBER OF EVER REGULAR CIGARETTE SMOKERS
6,460

QUIT ONCE FOR AT LEAST 1 YR[a]
3,566 (55.2%)

→ DID NOT QUIT RELAPSE AFTER FIRST QUIT[b]
2,210 (62.0%; 34.2%)

→ RELAPSED AFTER FIRST QUIT
1,340 (37.6%; 20.7%)

QUIT FOR A SECOND TIME FOR AT LEAST 1 YR[d]
576 (43.0%; 8.9%)[c]

→ DID NOT RELAPSE AFTER SECOND QUIT[e]
371 (64.4%; 5.7%)[c]

NEVER QUIT FOR AT LEAST 1 YR
2,704 (41.9%)

NEVER QUIT AGAIN
648 (48.4%; 10.0%)[c]

RELAPSED AFTER SECOND QUIT
203 (35.2%; 3.1%)[c]

FIGURE 3.—Flow chart of quitting history, attempts lasting longer than 1 year, NHEFS

NOTE: NHEFS=National Health and Nutrition Examination Survey (NHANES-I) Epidemiologic Followup Study.

[a] Of the 6,640 ever regular cigarette smokers, 155 quit within the year preceding the NHEFS interview. Data on the first quit attempt were missing for 35 people (4 were current smokers, 6 were former smokers, and 25 were deceased at the time of the interview).

[b] Of the 3,566 people who quit for at least 1 year, data were not available on 16 (15 were former smokers and 1 was deceased at the time of the interview).

[c] The first number represents the percentage of the reference number one row above (e.g., 1,340 is 37.6% of 3,566); the second number represents the percentage of the total number of ever regular cigarette smokers in this sample (e.g., 1,340 is 20.7% of 6,460).

[d] Of the 1,340 people who relapsed after their first ≥1-yr period of abstinence, 74 quit within the year preceding the interview and 26 never returned to regular smoking. Data were not available on 16 others (11 were current smokers, 3 were former smokers, and 2 were deceased at the time of the interview).

[e] Of the 576 people who quit twice for at least 1 yr, data were not available for 2 (both were former smokers at interview).

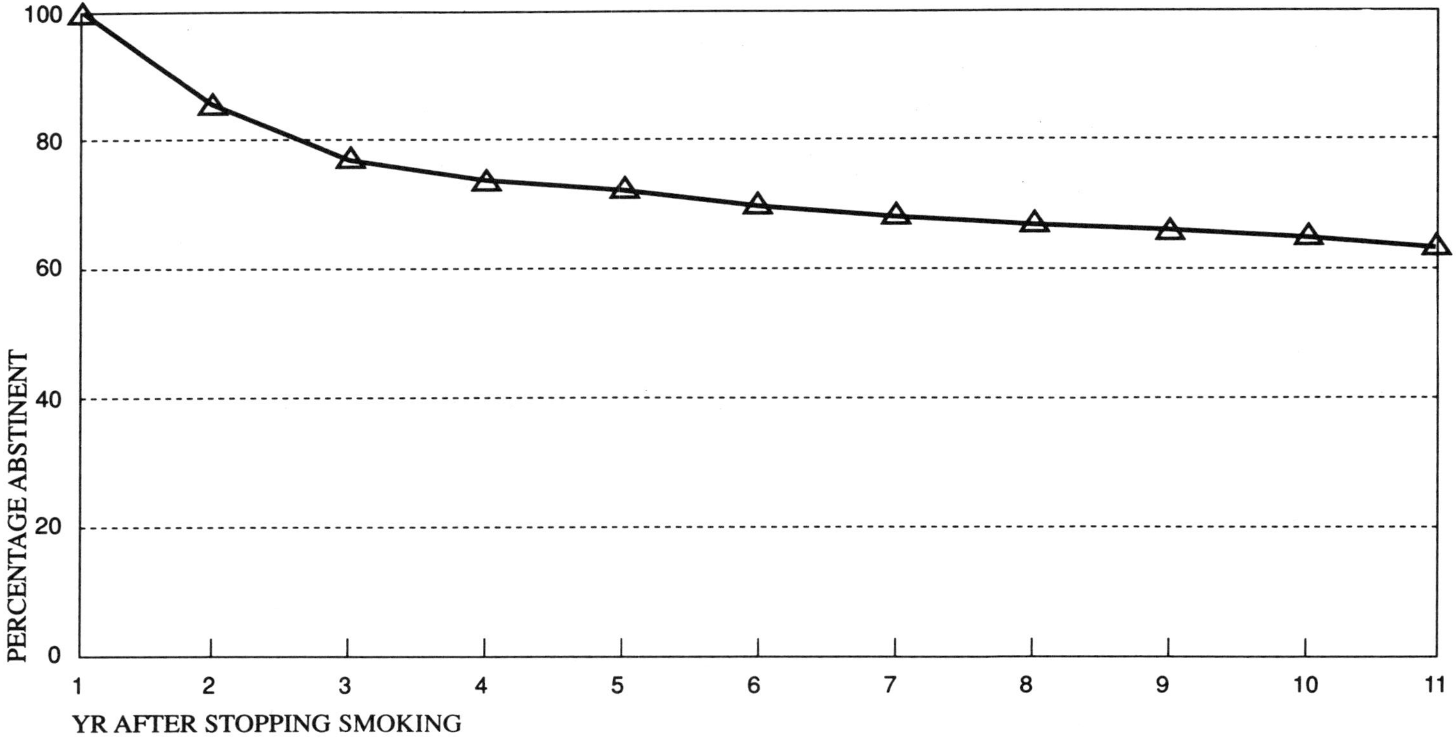

FIGURE 4.—Estimated duration of abstinence on first 1-year or longer quit attempt, product–limit method, N=3,363

SOURCE: NHANES-I Epidemiologic Followup Study 1982–84; OSH, unpublished data.

THE SMOKING CONTINUUM

A number of surveys have sought detailed information on respondents' quitting histories. An eight-point smoking continuum among ever smokers can be developed from the 1978, 1979, and 1980 NHIS tobacco supplements, the 1986 AUTS, and the 1987 NHIS. Smoking continuums for the four NHISs are presented in Table 2, and are similar over time.

The data in Table 2 can be used in various ways. For example, by focusing on those who were smoking during the year before the survey (categories 1 through 6), the proportion that tried to quit during that year (categories 3+4+5+6 divided by categories 1+2+3+4+5+6) and the proportion that quit during that year and were still abstinent at the time of the survey (categories 5+6 divided by categories 1+2+3+4+5+6) can be estimated. The proportion who tried to quit during the year before the survey was higher in 1987 (34 percent) than in 1978, 1979, and 1980 (27 to 29 percent). The proportion who quit during the year before the survey and were still abstinent at the time of the survey remained stable at 6 to 8 percent from 1978 to 1987.

Data are presented below on various components of the smoking continuum. Data from NHIS years not included in Table 2 are often presented in the following sections because, whereas these surveys did not provide all the questions necessary to construct a complete continuum, enough information to define one or more components of the continuum was collected. These data are broken down by education (Table 5 and Figures 5–9) because educational attainment is a strong sociodemographic predictor of smoking and quitting behavior (US DHHS 1989a; Pierce, Fiore et al. 1989). Data from other stratified analyses (i.e., gender, race, and age) are also presented in Table 5. The data on the continuum have been age-adjusted to the overall 1985 population.

Percentage of Ever Smokers Who Have Never Tried to Quit

There is no overall clear and significant trend from 1974 to 1987 in the percentage of ever smokers who have never tried to quit. Education has a consistent effect on quitting—lower levels of educational attainment are associated with a higher probability of never having tried to quit (Figure 5).

The difference between genders in the proportion of ever smokers who have never tried to quit has been decreasing with time (Table 5). While the proportion of females in this category has been decreasing over the years, it has remained fairly constant for males. The data also show that, on average, over time, females are more likely than males to have never tried to quit smoking.

Trend data broken down by race show that blacks have been consistently more likely than whites to have never tried to quit smoking; however, the difference between the races has been narrowing with time. The data also show that the likelihood of having ever tried to quit smoking increases with age. For all age categories, the percentage of ever smokers who have never tried to quit has been decreasing with time (especially for the oldest age group).

TABLE 5.—Selected measures of quitting activity (%), NHISs, United States, adults aged 20 and older[a]

		Gender		Race		Age (yr)				Education (yr)			
	Overall	Male	Female	Whites	Blacks	20–24	25–44	45–64	≥65	<12	12	13–15	≥16
Never tried to quit[b]													
1974	22.5	20.1	25.8	21.1	34.4	28.5	22.8	22.4	16.5	26.3	23.9	19.0	15.3
1987	18.7	18.5	19.5	17.7	26.5	26.6	20.3	16.9	11.0	25.5	18.5	16.7	13.9
Mean	23.4	22.0	25.6	22.6	30.1	31.7	24.7	22.2	15.3	28.0	24.2	20.0	16.9
Quit for at least 1 day[c]													
1978	27.8	25.8	30.2	26.9	36.5	41.6	27.8	22.5	26.4	26.7	27.4	30.2	29.2
1987	31.6	31.1	32.1	30.6	37.7	40.6	32.6	26.5	29.8	29.0	30.5	33.8	34.8
Mean	28.0	26.7	29.6	27.1	35.0	38.8	29.1	22.3	26.5	27.4	27.6	28.7	30.8
Off less than 1 yr[d]													
1965[e]	4.6	4.8	4.2	4.8	2.9	5.1	4.7	3.9	4.8	3.0	3.6	4.0	4.7
1987	4.6	4.5	4.7	4.5	4.9	6.2	5.5	3.6	2.5	4.1	4.5	4.8	4.8
Mean	4.3	4.3	4.4	4.3	3.7	6.9	5.0	2.9	2.6	3.0	4.5	4.8	5.3
Off 1–4 yr[f]													
1965[e]	8.0	8.7	6.7	8.2	6.1	6.5	7.8	7.6	10.0	7.4	9.1	9.0	14.1
1987	10.5	10.2	10.8	11.0	7.3	11.6	10.9	10.4	8.4	7.7	10.6	12.3	12.1
Mean	9.2	9.4	9.0	9.4	7.1	10.0	9.8	7.6	8.7	7.0	9.0	10.4	12.3
Off ≥5 yr[g]													
1965[e]	12.4	14.0	8.7	12.7	8.3	1.2	7.3	15.4	30.2	12.2	12.2	14.6	18.3
1987	29.8	32.8	25.5	30.9	20.7	4.7	22.1	36.7	58.3	22.4	27.4	32.6	42.0
Mean	21.7	24.3	17.5	20.8	14.3	2.9	15.2	27.0	46.4	18.1	21.9	25.2	33.1

NOTE: NHIS=National Health Interview Survey.
[a] Data were age-adjusted to the overall U.S. population in 1985.
[b] Never tried to quit = percentage of ever smokers who have never tried to quit.
[c] Quit for at least 1 day = percentage of those smoking at 12 mo prior to interview who quit for at least 1 day during those 12 mo.
[d] Off <1 yr = percentage of ever smokers who have been abstinent for <1 yr.
[e] 1966 (not 1965) is the first year for which data are available for the four education strata.
[f] Off 1–4 yr = percentage of ever smokers who have been abstinent for 1–4 yr.
[g] Off ≥5 yr= percentage of ever smokers who have been abstinent for at least 5 yr.

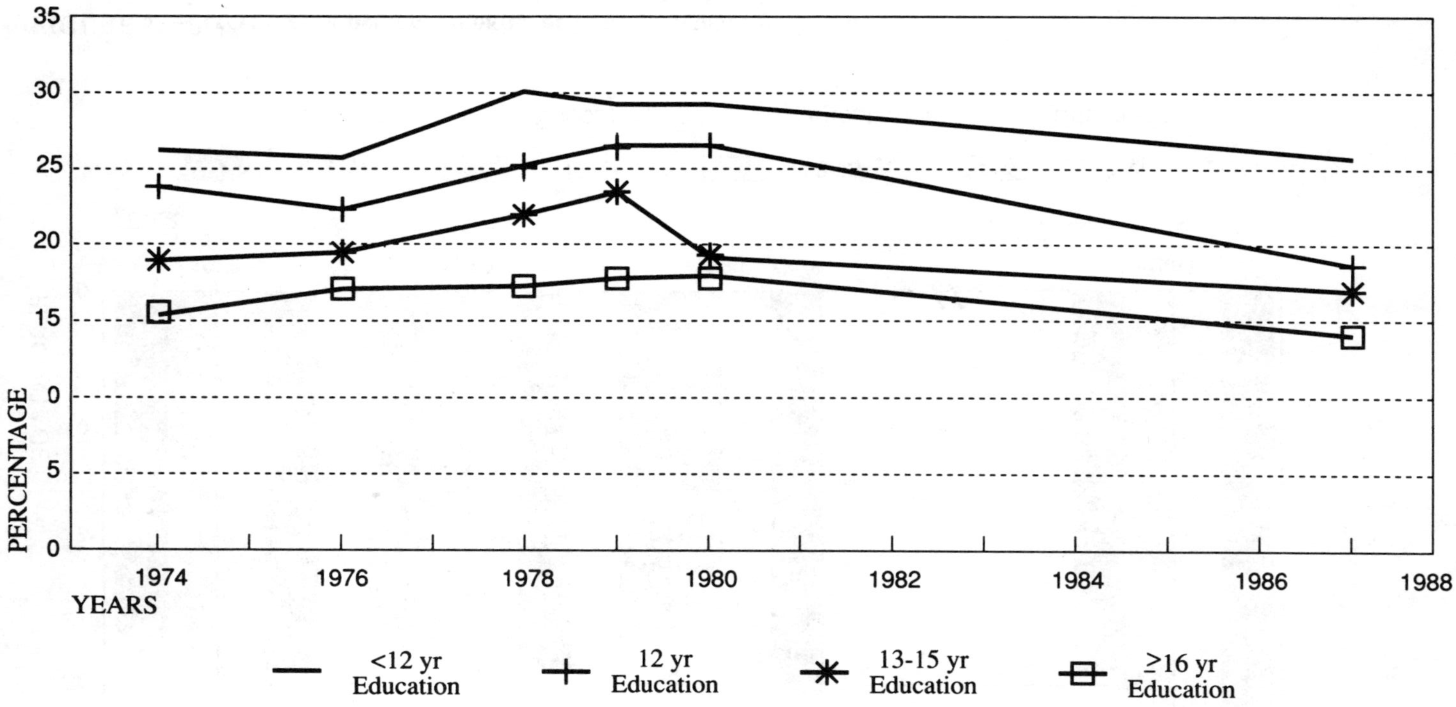

FIGURE 5.—Percentage of ever smokers who never tried to quit, by education, United States, 1974–87

SOURCE: NHISs 1974, 1976, 1978, 1979, 1980, 1987; OSH, unpublished data.

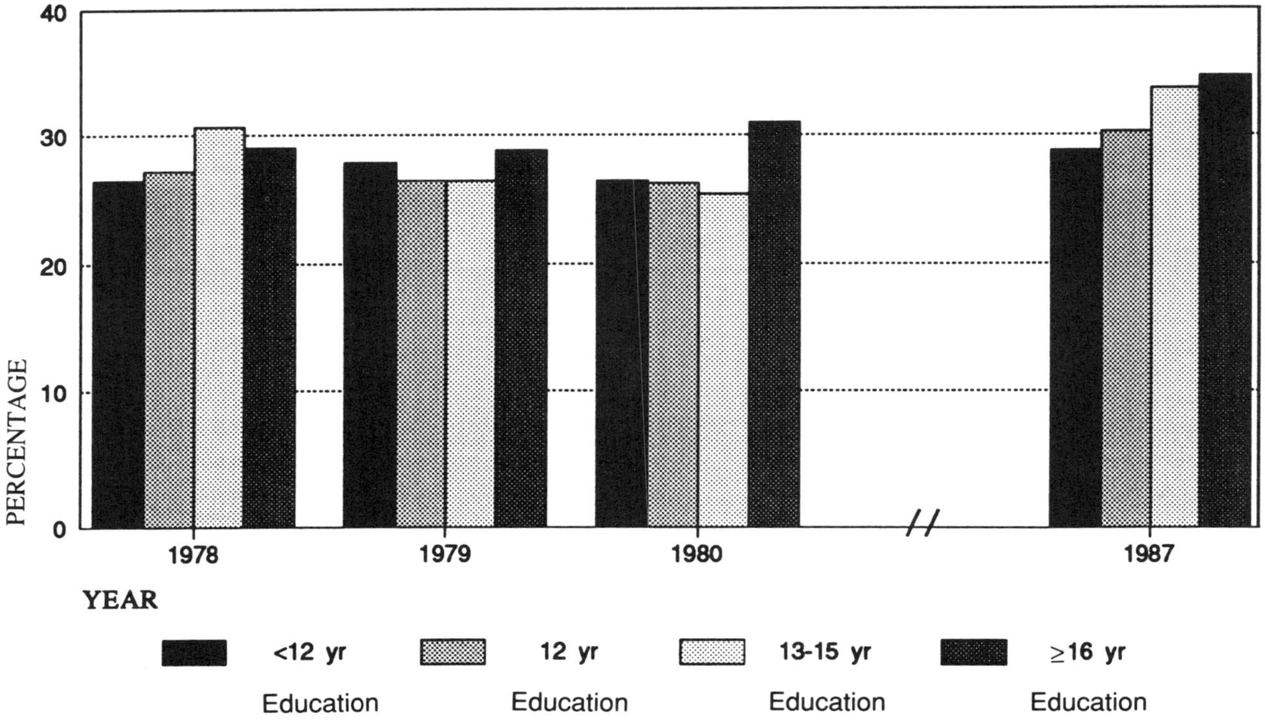

FIGURE 6.—Percentage of persons smoking at 12 months prior to the survey interview who quit for at least 1 day during those 12 months, United States, 1978–80, 1987, by education

SOURCE: NHISs 1978, 1979, 1980, 1987; OSH, unpublished data.

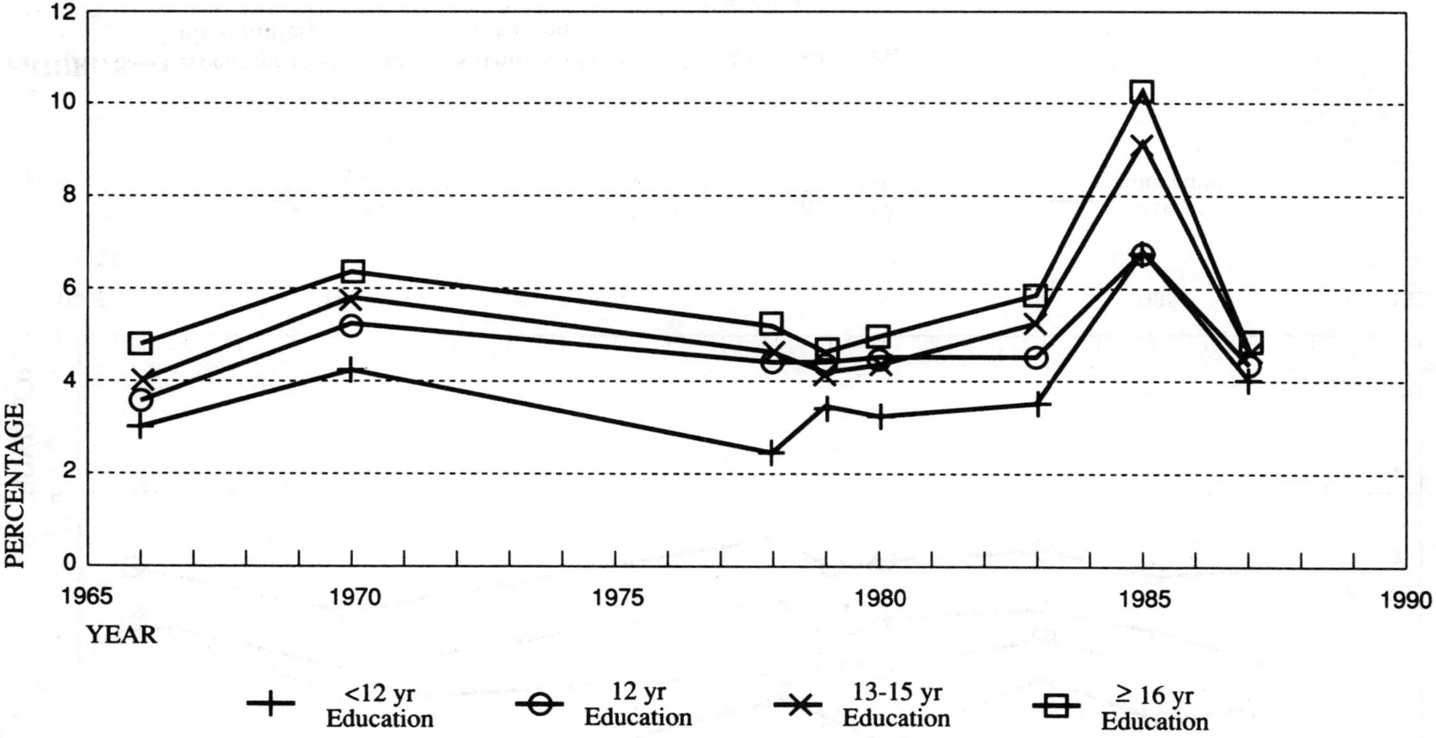

FIGURE 7.—Percentage of ever smokers who had been abstinent for less than 1 year, United States, 1966–87, by education
SOURCE: NHISs 1966, 1970, 1978, 1979, 1980, 1983, 1985, 1987; OSH, unpublished data.

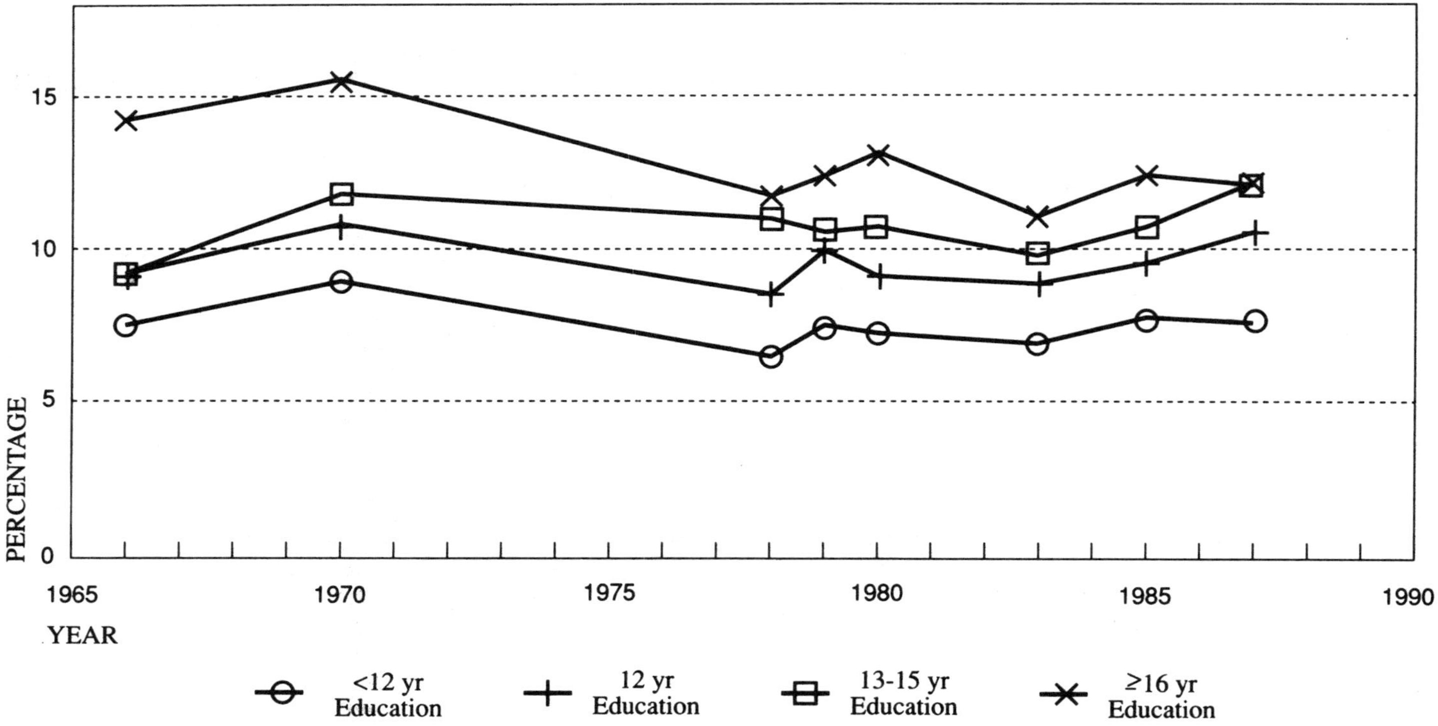

FIGURE 8.—Percentage of ever smokers who had been abstinent for 1–4 years, United States, 1966–87, by education

SOURCE: NHISs 1966, 1970, 1978, 1979, 1980, 1983, 1985, 1987; OSH, unpublished data.

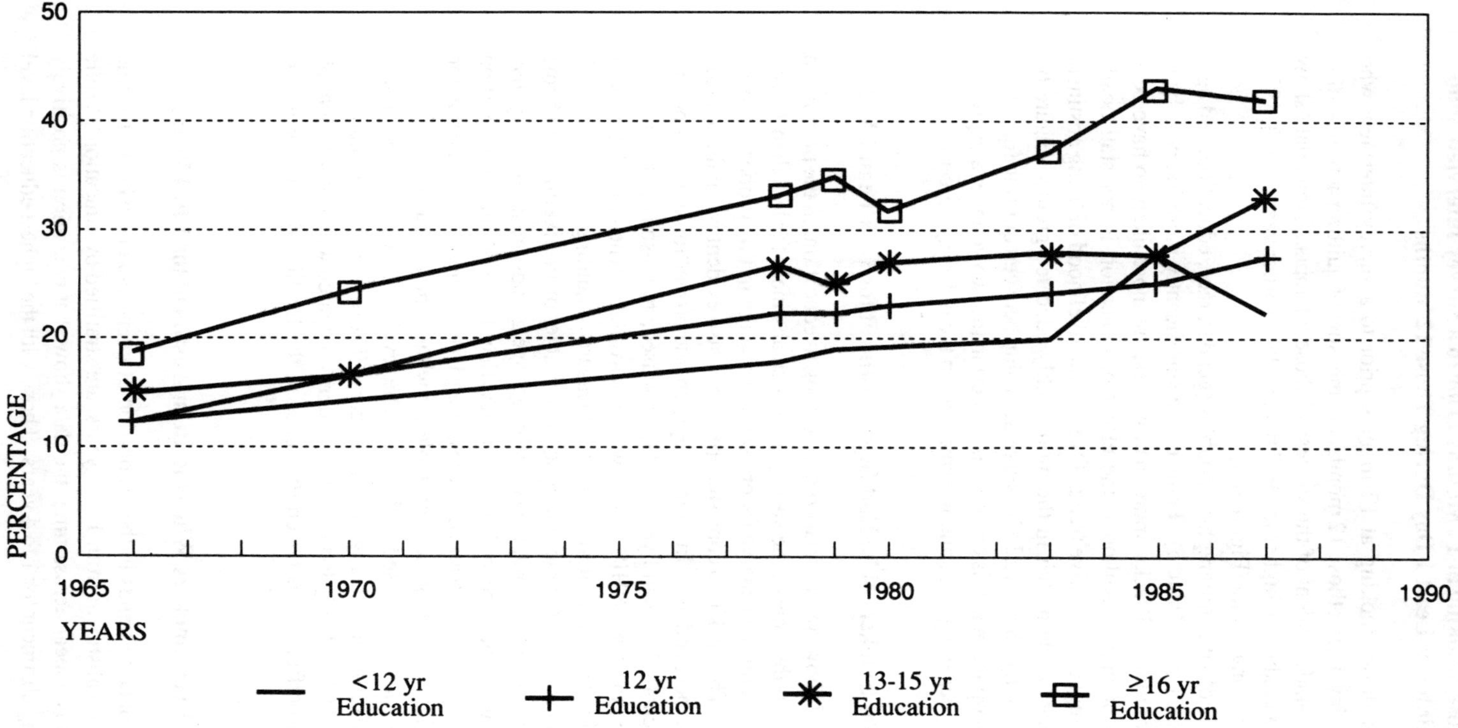

FIGURE 9.—Percentage of ever smokers who had been abstinent for 5 years or more, United States, 1966–87, by education

SOURCE: NHISs 1966, 1970, 1978, 1979, 1980, 1983, 1985, 1987; OSH, unpublished data.

Percentage of Those Smoking at 12 Months Prior to a Survey Interview Who Quit for at Least 1 Day During Those 12 Months

The percentage of those smoking at 12 months prior to a survey interview who stopped for at least 1 day during those 12 months is a measure of quitting activity—that is, quitting attempts—independent of the success of those attempts. Trend data show that this percentage was slightly higher in 1987 than in the 3 earlier years (1978, 1979, and 1980) in all educational strata (Figure 6).

Data show an effect of all demographic variables (gender, race, education, and age) on quitting for at least 1 day (Table 5). Females are significantly more likely to be in this category than are males. Blacks, more than whites, are more likely to have been abstinent for 1 day or more. Although the effect of education is not statistically significant, the data suggest a positive trend. Overall, the likelihood of being abstinent for at least 1 day tends to be higher in the more highly educated groups (Figure 6), especially in 1987. Finally, there is a J-shaped relationship between quitting for at least 1 day and age. The proportion in this category is highest in the two younger age groups, lowest in the 45–64-year-old group, and intermediate in the oldest age group.

Percentage of Ever Smokers Who Had Been Abstinent for Less Than 1 Year

The data in Figure 7 show trends, analyzed according to education, in the proportion of ever smokers who, at the time of the survey, had been abstinent for less than 1 year. In general, no stable trend over the years or absolute change in this proportion from 1965 to 1987 is seen. This lack of a consistent pattern is also evident when the data are classified by gender, race, and age. In every subgroup, the proportion of ever smokers who had been abstinent for less than 1 year in 1985 increased; the reason for this increase is unclear. Data from the 1988 NHIS, which were not available when this Report was prepared, should help clarify recent trends in this measure of quitting.

The data show effects of most of the demographic variables on the likelihood of being in this category (Table 5). In general, the two younger age groups are more likely than the two older age groups to have been abstinent for less than 1 year. A higher proportion of whites than blacks have been abstinent for less than 1 year. However, given that the trend in this proportion has been generally stable for whites and increasing for blacks, the gap between the races has closed with time. The level of education is positively associated with the likelihood of being in this category. Those with the least education (<12 years) are slightly less likely to be recent quitters compared with other education groups. There is no difference between the sexes in the likelihood of being in this category.

Percentage of Ever Smokers Who Had Been Abstinent for 1 to 4 Years

Figure 8 presents data on trends in the proportion of ever smokers, who at the time of the survey had been abstinent from 1 to 4 years, are stratified by education. While no consistent patterns appear across time, the data show that education is positively associated with being abstinent for 1 to 4 years. Those with the highest education level

(16+ years) are the most likely to have quit 1 to 4 years earlier, and those with the lowest educational level (<12 years) are the least likely.

The data also show that for 1965–1978, the proportion of males who had been abstinent for 1 to 4 years is slightly higher than that for females (although across the entire time period 1965–87, there is no difference in the proportions between the sexes). Given that the proportion off cigarettes for 1 to 4 years has been increasing significantly for females and remained stable for males with time, the gap between the genders has closed (Table 5). Whites are more likely than blacks to have been abstinent for 1 to 4 years. The data do not show any consistent patterns with respect to age. Across time, on average, the proportion of those in the 45–64-year age group in this category is slightly lower than in the other age groups.

Percentage of Ever Smokers Who Had Been Abstinent for at Least 5 Years

Data on the proportion of ever smokers who, at the time of the survey, had been abstinent for 5 years or more show positive trends with time for the overall population and for every population subgroup (trends across education shown in Figure 9). Overall, the proportion of ever smokers in this category has more than doubled from 12.4 percent in 1965 to 29.8 percent in 1987. Data from the 1955 Current Population Survey (the first large survey of tobacco use conducted among a probability sample of the U.S. population) indicate that 5.0 percent of those who ever smoked cigarettes were abstinent for at least 4.5 years in 1955 (Haenszel, Shimkin, Miller 1956).

The data also show strong effects of all four demographic variables on the likelihood of being abstinent for at least 5 years. Figure 9 shows that those with the most education (16+ years) are the most likely to have been abstinent for 5 years or more than those in the other categories. On average, over time, the data show that increasing education is associated with increasing likelihood of being in this category (Table 5). Also seen in the data are a gender effect (males are more likely than females to have been abstinent for 5+ years), a race effect (whites are more likely than blacks to be in this category), and a strong effect of age (increasing age is associated with increasing likelihood of being abstinent for at least 5 years). The age effect is due, at least in part, to the fact that older persons have had a longer opportunity to quit and maintain long-term abstinence compared with younger persons. The gaps between the races and across age groups (and to a lesser extent, across education) have been increasing with time.

Interpretation of Continuum Findings

In the period spanned by these data, a slightly increasing proportion of smokers are attempting to quit and are maintaining abstinence. Slightly less than a third of the people who were smoking at 12 months before the 1987 survey quit smoking for at least 1 day during those 12 months. Trends categorized by sociodemographic subgroups show that females, blacks, younger persons, and more highly educated persons are more likely than the appropriate comparison groups to have quit for at least 1 day during the last year.

One way to determine whether these quit attempts have been successful is to examine trends in the proportion of ever smokers who have been abstinent for 1 to 4 years. Although blacks are more likely than whites to have quit for 1 day or more, whites are more likely to have successfully maintained abstinence for 1 to 4 years. Younger smokers are more likely to have quit for 1 day or more than older smokers; however, there are only small absolute differences across age groups in the percentage who have been abstinent for 1 to 4 years. The positive trend across educational categories with respect to quitting for 1 day or more parallels important differences seen in the likelihood of being abstinent for 1 to 4 years. Those with the lowest level of education were the least likely to make an attempt to quit and the least likely to maintain long-term abstinence. Those with the highest level of education were the most likely to have made a quit attempt and the most likely to maintain long-term abstinence. Finally, although females were more likely than males to have quit for at least 1 day, there were no gender differences in abstinence for 1 to 4 years.

The data on the increasing proportion of ever smokers who have been off cigarettes for at least 5 years show that more ever smokers are entering this category by successfully quitting and abstaining than are exiting by death or relapse. Overall, this proportion has increased 242 percent between 1965 and 1987. Consistent with other data showing that males began quitting earlier than females (Fiore et al. 1989), proportionately more males than females are in this category. Similarly, whites began quitting earlier, and are therefore, more likely than blacks to have stopped smoking for 5 years or more. There is also evidence that those with the highest level of education have been abstinent for a longer period than those with less education. Finally, older people were more likely to have been abstinent for at least 5 years. This positive relationship reflects the accumulation of successful quitters with age and, probably to some extent, the benefits of cessation on survival.

OTHER MEASURES RELATED TO SMOKING CESSATION

Intention to Smoke in 5 Years

Intention to smoke or quit is a predictor of future smoking behavior (Collins, Emont, Zywiak, in press; Cummings et al. 1988; Pierce, Dwyer et al. 1987; Pederson, Baskerville, Wanklin 1982). Current and former smokers responding to the five OSH-sponsored surveys of tobacco use were asked to assess the likelihood that they would be smoking in 5 years. There is little change in the responses of former smokers since 1964. In each survey year, fewer than 3.2 percent of all former smokers responded that they would be smoking again in 5 years. Thus, former smokers overestimate the likelihood that they will remain abstinent. (See the previous Section, Long-Term Abstinence and Relapse.)

In Table 6, the predicted likelihood of future smoking behavior among current smokers is presented for each survey year by gender. The sharp dropoffs that occurred between 1966 and 1970 may have occurred as a result of the widespread television broadcast of antismoking public service announcements (PSAs) from 1968 to 1970

TABLE 6.—Percentage of those intending to smoke in 5 years, by gender, AUTSs, United States, 1964–86, current smokers aged 21 and older

Year	Definitely will be smoking Male	Definitely will be smoking Female	Probably will be smoking Male	Probably will be smoking Female	Total (definitely + probably) Male	Total (definitely + probably) Female
1964	25.2	20.1	50.6	54.4	75.8	74.5
1966	22.3	15.6	53.7	55.4	76.0	71.0
1970	10.9	10.2	39.1	41.1	50.0	51.3
1975	11.7	12.0	44.2	45.9	55.9	57.9
1986	7.3	6.4	35.2	38.8	42.6	45.3

NOTE: AUTS=Adult Use of Tobacco Survey.
SOURCE: AUTSs 1964, 1966, 1970, 1975, 1986.

under the Federal Communications Commission's Fairness Doctrine (US DHHS 1989a). Longitudinal data collected between 1964 and 1975 supported the hypothesis that the Fairness Doctrine PSAs influenced smokers' attitudes about quitting (Horn 1979). The percentage of smokers who "thought seriously about giving up smoking" increased from 56 percent before the PSAs to about 85 percent at the end of, and 5 years after, the PSAs. The proportion of smokers who tried to quit and the overall cessation rate also increased over the same timeframe.

The slight increases in intention to smoke from 1970 to 1975 might reflect a decay effect after the removal of the antismoking commercials. The reduction between 1975 and 1986 could reflect an increase in antismoking activity, such as the growth of the nonsmokers' rights movement (US DHHS 1989a).

Receipt of Advice to Quit from a Doctor

Advice to quit smoking by a doctor increases patient cessation rates (Glynn, Manley, Pechacek, 1990; Kottke et al. 1988; Schwartz 1987; US Preventive Services Task Force 1989). Data from Table 7 show that the percentage of current smokers who report having ever been advised by a doctor to stop smoking increased steadily for both genders between 1964 and 1987. Male current smokers were 3.1 times more likely to report having received advice from a doctor to stop smoking in 1987 than in 1964; female current smokers were 3.2 times more likely to have reported receipt of such advice in 1987 than in 1964.

The data for former smokers, while less consistent, also show increases with time. Male former smokers were 1.5 times more likely to report having received advice from a doctor to stop smoking in 1987 than in 1964. Female former smokers were 2.1 times more likely to report having received such advice in 1987 than in 1964.

In summary, large increases in the percentages of current and former smokers who reported having received advice to quit occurred between 1976 and 1987.

TABLE 7.—Percentage who report having ever received advice to quit from a doctor, by smoking status and gender, United States, 1964–87, adults aged 21 and older

	Current smokers		Former smokers	
Survey	Male	Female	Male	Female
AUTS 1964	15.0	16.6	22.3	15.9
AUTS 1966	16.9	18.8	27.8	21.8
AUTS 1970	21.8	25.0	20.0	20.1
NHIS 1974	25.2	27.8	22.6	18.9
AUTS 1975	26.2	28.2	24.2	23.7
NHIS 1976	26.8	30.2	24.4	19.3
AUTS 1986	40.0	53.1	26.4	27.8
NHIS 1987	46.6	53.8	33.6	32.8

NOTE: AUTS=Adult Use of Tobacco Survey; NHIS=National Health Interview Survey.

CONCLUSIONS

1. By 1987, more than 38 million Americans had quit smoking cigarettes, nearly half of all living adults who ever smoked.

2. The percentage of ever cigarette smokers who are former cigarette smokers (quit ratio) has increased from 29.6 percent in 1965 to 44.8 percent in 1987 at an average rate of 0.68 percentage points per year. The quit ratio has increased among men and women, among blacks and whites, and among all age and education subgroups. Between 1966 and 1987, the rate of increase in the quit ratio among college graduates was twice the rate among high school dropouts.

3. About one-third of all former cigarette smokers who have maintained abstinence for at least 1 year may eventually relapse. As the duration of abstinence increases, relapse becomes less likely.

4. Quitting activity, as measured by the proportion of people smoking at 12 months before a survey who quit for at least 1 day during those 12 months, has increased slightly over time. Between 1978 and 1987, this proportion increased from 27.8 to 31.6 percent.

5. Female smokers were more likely than male smokers to have quit smoking cigarettes for at least 1 day during the previous year; however, there were no gender differences in the proportion abstinent for 1 to 4 years. Men were more likely than women to have been abstinent for 5 years or more. These findings do not take into account the use of tobacco products other than cigarettes.

6. Black smokers were more likely than white smokers to have quit for at least 1 day during the previous year. Blacks, however, were less likely than whites to have been abstinent for 1 year or more.

7. Younger smokers (aged 20 to 44) were more likely than older smokers to have quit for at least 1 day during the previous year.

8. Smokers with less education tend to be less likely to have quit for at least 1 day during the previous year compared with those having more education. In addition, those with lower levels of education are less likely to have been abstinent for 1 year or more.

9. In 1964, about three-fourths of all current smokers predicted that they would "definitely" or "probably" be smoking in 5 years. In 1986, fewer than half of all current smokers felt the same way. Moreover, while more than 20 percent of current smokers in 1964 predicted that they would "definitely" be smoking in 5 years, only about 7 percent of current smokers in 1986 so predicted.

10. Current smokers in 1987 were more than three times as likely as current smokers in 1964 to report having received advice from a doctor to stop smoking.

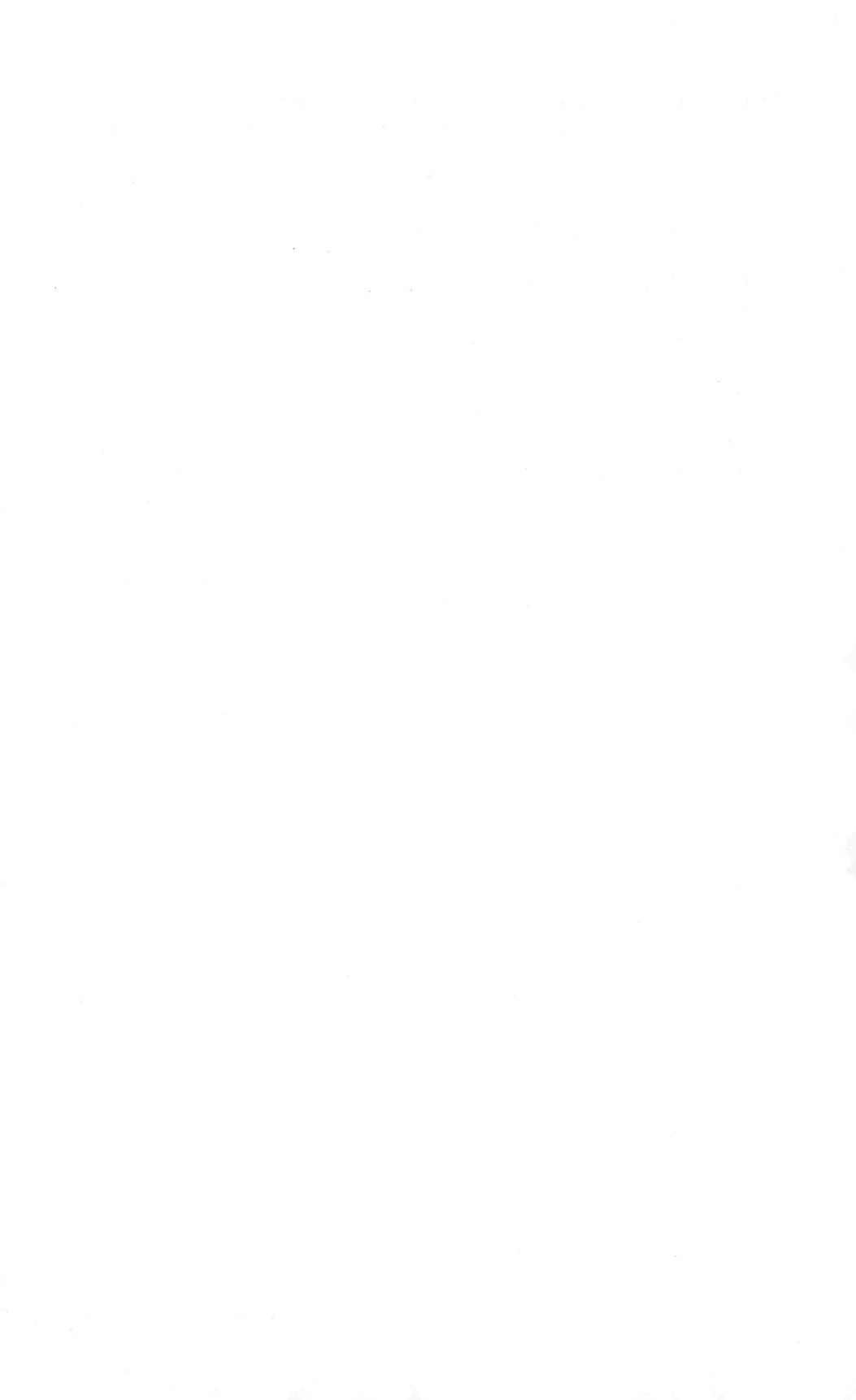

References

ANDA, R.F., WALLER, M.N., WOOTEN, K.G., MAST, E.E., ESCOBEDO, L.G., SANDERSON, L.M., STATE BRFSS COORDINATORS. Behavioral Risk Factor Surveillance, 1988. In: CDC Surveillance Summaries, June 1990. *Morbidity and Mortality Weekly Report* 1990; 39(SS-2):1–21.

CENTERS FOR DISEASE CONTROL. Smoking prevalence and cessation in selected States, 1981–1983 and 1985—The Behavioral Risk Factor Surveys. *Morbidity and Mortality Weekly Report* 47:740–743, 1986.

COHEN, S., LICHTENSTEIN, E., PROCHASKA, J., ROSSI, J., GRITZ, E., CARR, C., ORLEANS, C.T., SCHOENBACH, V.J., BIENER, L., ABRAMS, D., DICLEMENTE, C., CURRY, S., MARLATT, G.A., CUMMINGS, K.M., EMONT, S.L., GIOVINO, G.A., OSSIP-KLEIN, D. Debunking myths about self-quitting: Evidence from ten prospective studies of persons quitting smoking by themselves. *American Psychologist* 44(11):1355–1365, 1989.

COLLINS, R.L., EMONT, S.L., ZYWIAK, W.H. Social influence processes in smoking cessation: Postquitting predictors of longterm outcome. *Journal of Substance Abuse*, in press.

CUMMINGS, K.M., EMONT, S.L., JAEN, C., SCIANDRA, R. Format and quitting instructions as factors influencing the impact of a self-administered quit smoking program. *Health Education Quarterly* 15(2):199–216, 1988.

ELANDT-JOHNSON, R.C. Definition of rates: Some remarks on their use and misuse. *American Journal of Epidemiology* 102(4):267–271, October 1975.

FIORE, M.C., NOVOTNY, T.E., PIERCE, J.P., GIOVINO, G.A., HATZIANDREU, E.J., NEWCOMB, P.A., SURAWICZ, T.S., DAVIS, R.M. Methods used to quit smoking in the United States. Do cessation programs help? *Journal of the American Medical Association* 263(20):2760–2765, May 23/30, 1990.

FIORE, M.C., NOVOTNY, T.E., PIERCE, J.P., HATZIANDREU, E.J., PATEL, K.M., DAVIS, R.M. Trends in cigarette smoking in the United States. The changing influence of gender and race. *Journal of the American Medical Association* 261(1):49–55, January 6, 1989.

GLASGOW, R.E., LICHTENSTEIN, E. Long-term effects of behavioral smoking cessation interventions. *Behavior Therapy* 18:297–324, 1987.

GLYNN, T.J., MANLEY, M.W., PECHACEK, T.F. Physician-initiated smoking cessation program: The National Cancer Institute trials. In: Engstrom, P.F., Rimer, B., Mortenson, L.E. (eds.) *Advances in Cancer Control: Screening and Prevention Research.* New York: Wiley–Liss, Inc., 1990, pp. 11–25.

HAENSZEL, W., SHIMKIN, M.B., MILLER, H.P. Tobacco smoking patterns in the United States. Public Health Monograph 45, 111 pp., *Public Health Reports* 71(11): November 1956.

HAMMOND, E.C., GARFINKEL, L. The influence of health on smoking habits. *National Cancer Institute Monograph* 19:269–285, 1963.

HAMMOND, E.C., GARFINKEL, L. Changes in cigarette smoking. *Journal of the National Cancer Institute* 33(1):49–64, July 1964.

HORN, D. Who is quitting—and why. In: Schwartz, J.L. (ed.) *Progress in Smoking Cessation.* Proceedings of International Conference on Smoking Cessation, New York, June 21–23, 1978, American Cancer Society, pp. 27–31, 1979.

HUNT, W.A., BARNETT, L.W., BRANCH, L.G. Relapse rates in addiction programs. *Journal of Clinical Psychology* 27(4):455–456, October 1971.

JARVIS, M. Gender and Smoking: Do women really find it harder to give up? *British Journal of Addiction* 79(4):383–387, December 1984.

KABAT, G.C., WYNDER, E.L. Determinants of quitting smoking. *American Journal of Public Health* 77(10):1301–1305, October 1987.

KIRSCHT, J.P., BROCK, B.M., HAWTHORNE, V.M. Cigarette smoking and changes in smoking among a cohort of Michigan adults, 1980–1982. *American Journal of Public Health* 77(4):501–502, April 1987.

KOTTKE, T.E., BATTISTA, R.N., DEFRIESE, G.H., BREKKE, M.L. Attributes of successful smoking cessation interventions in medical practice. A meta-analysis of 39 controlled trials. *Journal of the American Medical Association* 259:2882–2889, May 20, 1988.

LANDO, H.A., MCGOVERN, P.G. Three-year data on a behavioral treatment for smoking: A follow-up note. *Addictive Behaviors* 7(2):177–181, 1982.

LEE, E.T. *Statistical Methods for Survival Data Analysis.* Belmont, California: Lifetime Learning Publications/Wadsworth, 1980.

LICHTENSTEIN, E., RODRIGUES, M.-R.P. Long-term effects of rapid smoking treatment for dependent cigarette smokers. *Addictive Behaviors* 2(2/3):109–112, 1977.

MACHLIN, S.R., KLEINMAN, J.C., MADANS, J.H. Validity of mortality analysis based on retrospective smoking information. *Statistics in Medicine* 8(8):997–1009, August 1989.

MADANS, J.H., KLEINMAN, J.C., COX, C.S., BARBANO, H.E., FELDMAN, J.J., COHEN, B., FINUCANE, F.F., CORNONI-HUNTLEY, J. 10 years after NHANES I: Report of initial followup, 1982–84. *Public Health Reports* 101(5):465–473, September–October 1986.

NATIONAL CENTER FOR HEALTH STATISTICS. *The Statistical Design of the Health Household-Interview Survey by Staff of the U.S. National Health Survey and the Bureau of the Census.* U.S. Department of Health, Education, and Welfare, Publication No. (PHS)583-4-A2, Hyattsville, Maryland, 1958.

NATIONAL CENTER FOR HEALTH STATISTICS. *The National Health Interview Survey Design, 1973–1984 and Procedures, 1975–1983.* Vital and Health Statistics, Series 1, No. 18. Public Health Service. DHHS Publication No. (HHS) 85-1320, 1985.

NATIONAL CENTER FOR HEALTH STATISTICS. In: Cohen, B.B., Barbano, H.E., Cox, C.S., Feldman, J.J., Finucane, F.F., Kleinman, J.C., Madans, J.H. *Plan and operation of the NHANES I Epidemiologic Followup Study 1982–84.* Vital Health and Statistics, Series 1, No. 22. Public Health Service. DHHS Publication No. (PHS) 87-1324, June 1987.

NATIONAL CENTER FOR HEALTH STATISTICS. Massey, J.T., Moore, T.F., Parsons, V.L., Tadros, W. *Design and Estimation for the National Health Interview Survey, 1985–94.* Series 2, No. 110, August 1989.

NOVOTNY, T.E., FIORE, M.C., HATZIANDREU, E.F., GIOVINO, G.A., MILLS, S.L., PIERCE, J.P. Trends in smoking by age and sex, United States, 1974–1987: The implications for disease impact. *Preventive Medicine*, in press.

OCKENE, J.K., HYMOWITZ, N., SEXTON, M., BROSTE, S.K. Comparison of patterns of smoking behavior change among smokers in the Multiple Risk Factor Intervention Trial (MRFIT). *Preventive Medicine* 11(6):621–638, November 1982.

OFFICE ON SMOKING AND HEALTH. Unpublished data.

OSSIP-KLEIN, D.J., BIGELOW, G., PARKER, S.R., CURRY, S., HALL, S., KIRKLAND, S. Task Force I: Classification and assessment of smoking behavior. In: Shumaker, S.A., Grunberg, N.E. (eds.). *Procedures of the National Working Conference on Smoking Relapse. Health Psychology* 5(Supplement):3–11, 1986.

PEDERSON, L.L., BASKERVILLE, J.C., WANKLIN, J.M. Multivariate statistical models for predicting change in smoking behavior following physician advice to quit smoking. *Preventive Medicine* 11(5):536–549, September 1982.

PIERCE, J.P., ALDRICH, R.N., HANRATTY, S., DWYER, T., HILL, D. Uptake and quitting smoking trends in Australia 1974–1984. *Preventive Medicine* 16(2):252–260, March 1987.

PIERCE, J.P., DWYER, T., CHAMBERLAIN, A., ALDRICH, R., SHELLEY, J., HANNAN, C.D. Targeting the smoker in an anti-smoking campaign. *Preventive Medicine* 16(6):816–824, November 1987.

PIERCE, J.P., FIORE, M.C., NOVOTNY, T.E., HATZIANDREU, E.J., DAVIS, R.M. Trends in cigarette smoking in the United States: Educational differences are increasing. *Journal of the American Medical Association* 261(1):56–60, January 6, 1989.

PIERCE, J.P., GIOVINO, G., HATZIANDREU, E., SHOPLAND, D. National age and sex differences in quitting smoking. *Journal of Psychoactive Drugs* 21(3):293–298, July–September 1989.

PROCHASKA, J.O., DICLEMENTE, C.C. Stages and processes of self-change of smoking: Toward an integrative model of change. *Journal of Consulting and Clinical Psychology* 51(3):390–395, 1983.

SCHOENBORN, C.A., BOYD, G.M. Smoking and other tobacco use: United States, 1987. National Center for Health Statistics (NCHS), *Vital and Health Statistics* 10(169), 1989.

SCHWARTZ, J.L. *Review and Evaluation of Smoking Cessation Methods: United States and Canada, 1978–1985.* U.S. Department of Health and Human Services, Public Health Service, National Institutes of Health. NIH Publication No. 87-2940, April 1987.

U.S. DEPARTMENT OF HEALTH AND HUMAN SERVICES. *The Health Consequences of Smoking for Women. A Report of the Surgeon General.* U.S. Department of Health and Human Services, Public Health Service, Office of the Assistant Secretary for Health, Office on Smoking and Health, 1980.

U.S. DEPARTMENT OF HEALTH AND HUMAN SERVICES. *The Health Consequences of Smoking: Cardiovascular Disease. A Report of the Surgeon General.* U.S. Department of Health and Human Services, Public Health Service, Office on Smoking and Health. DHHS Publication No.(PHS) 84-50204, 1983.

U.S. DEPARTMENT OF HEALTH AND HUMAN SERVICES. *The Health Consequences of Smoking: Nicotine Addiction. A Report of the Surgeon General, 1988.* U.S. Department of Health and Human Services, Public Health Service, Centers for Disease Control, Center for Health Promotion and Education, Office on Smoking and Health. DHHS Publication No. (CDC) 88-8406, 1988.

U.S. DEPARTMENT OF HEALTH AND HUMAN SERVICES. *Reducing the Health Consequences of Smoking: 25 Years of Progress. A Report of the Surgeon General.* U.S. Department of Health and Human Services, Public Health Service, Centers for Disease Control, Center for Chronic Disease Prevention and Health Promotion, Office on Smoking and Health. DHHS Publication No. (CDC) 89-8411, 1989a.

U.S. DEPARTMENT OF HEALTH AND HUMAN SERVICES. In: Pierce, J.P., Hatziandreu, E., Flyer, P., Hull, J., Maklan, D., Morganstein, D., Schreiber, G. *Tobacco Use in 1986—Methods and Basic Tabulations from Adult Use of Tobacco Survey.* Public Health Service, Centers for Disease Control, Office on Smoking and Health, U.S. Government Printing Office, 1989b.

U.S. DEPARTMENT OF HEALTH, EDUCATION, AND WELFARE. *Use of Tobacco. Practices, Attitudes, Knowledge, and Beliefs. United States—Fall 1964 and Spring 1966.* U.S. Department of Health, Education, and Welfare, Public Health Service, National Clearinghouse for Smoking and Health, July 1969.

U.S. DEPARTMENT OF HEALTH, EDUCATION, AND WELFARE. *Adult Use of Tobacco, 1970.* U.S. Department of Health, Education, and Welfare, Public Health Service, Center for Disease Control, National Clearinghouse for Smoking and Health, June 1973.

U.S. DEPARTMENT OF HEALTH, EDUCATION, AND WELFARE. *Adult Use of Tobacco—1975.* U.S. Department of Health, Education, and Welfare, Public Health Service, Center for Disease Control, National Clearinghouse for Smoking and Health, 1976.

U.S. DEPARTMENT OF HEALTH, EDUCATION, AND WELFARE. *Smoking and Health. A Report of the Surgeon General.* U.S. Department of Health, Education, and Welfare, Public Health Service, Office of the Assistant Secretary for Health, Office on Smoking and Health. DHEW Publication No. (PHS) 79-50066, 1979.

U.S. PREVENTIVE SERVICES TASK FORCE. *Guide to Clinical Preventive Services.* U.S. Department of Health and Human Services, Public Health Service, Office of the Assistant Secretary of Health, Office of Disease Prevention and Health Promotion, Baltimore: Williams and Wilkins, 1989, pp. 193–197.

WEST, D.W., GRAHAM, S., SWANSON, M., WILKINSON, G. Five year follow-up of a smoking withdrawal clinic population. *American Journal of Public Health* 67(6):536–544, 1977.

GLOSSARY

AARP	American Association of Retired Persons
ACS	American Cancer Society
AR	attributable risk
AUTS	Adult Use of Tobacco Survey
BM	bone mass
BMI	body mass index
BP	blood pressure
BPS	Baseline Prevalence Survey
BRFSS	Behavioral Risk Factor Surveillance System
BUPA	British United Providence Association
CASS	Coronary Artery Surgery Study
CC	closing capacity
CCDPHP	Center for Chronic Disease Prevention and Health Promotion
CDC	Centers for Disease Control
CHD	coronary heart disease
CI	confidence interval
cig	cigarettes
CNS	central nervous system
CO	carbon monoxide
COHb	carboxyhemoglobin
COPD	chronic obstructive pulmonary disease
CPS	Center for Preventive Services
CPS-I	Cancer Prevention Study I
CPS-II	Cancer Prevention Study II
CV	closing volume
CVD	cardiovascular disease
DBP	diastolic blood pressure
DHEW	Department of Health, Education, and Welfare
DHHS	Department of Health and Human Services
$D_{LCO}SB$	carbon monoxide diffusing capacity
DPA	dual photon absorptiometry
DSM-III-R	*Diagnostic and Statistical Manual of Mental Disorders*
FEV_1	1-sec forced expiratory volume
FVC_1	1-sec forced vital capacity
HANES	Health and Nutrition Examination Survey

HB$_s$Ag	hepatitis B surface antigen
HCN	hydrogen cyanide
HDL-C	high-density lipoprotein cholesterol
HMO	health maintenance organization
HR	heart rate
IARC	International Agency for Research on Cancer
LDL-C	low-density lipoprotein cholesterol
MI	myocardial infarction
MMEF	mid-maximum expiratory flow
MRC	Medical Research Council
MRFIT	Multiple Risk Factor Intervention Trial
NCHS	National Center for Health Statistics
NCI	National Cancer Institute
NHANES-I	National Health and Nutrition Examination Survey I
NHEFS	NHANES Epidemiologic Followup Study
NHIS	National Health Interview Survey
NHLBI	National Heart, Lung, and Blood Institute
NNS	National Natality Survey
OSH	Office on Smoking and Health
PBI	penile brachial index
PCA	percent cortical area
pDL	predicted diffusing capacity
PEF	peak expiratory flow
PHS	Public Health Service
POMS	Profile of Mood States
PPA	phenylpropanolamine
ppd	packs per day
PSA	public service announcement
REE	resting energy expenditure
RR	relative risk
SBP	systolic blood pressure
SCN$^-$	thiocyanate
SD	standard deviation
SES	socioeconomic status
SGA	small gestational age
SIDS	sudden infant death syndrome
SPA	single photon absorptiometry
ST	smokeless tobacco
STD	sexually transmitted disease
TLC	total lung capacity
TQ	Fagerstrom Tolerance Scale
VC	vital capacity
WHO	World Health Organization
WHR	ratio of waist to hip circumference

INDEX

A

Absenteeism, 89
Abstinence duration
    atherosclerosis severity, 199–200
    bladder cancer, 164
    cerebrovascular disease, 252–258
    COPD mortality, 345
    classifying smoking status, 26–27
    CHD mortality, 205–215, 223
    disease development, 129
    educational attainment, 606–608
    laryngeal cancer, 131–132
    locus of control, 542
    lung cancer diagnosis, 129–131
    lung cancer risk patterns, 110–122, 122–126
    multistage models, 126–128
    MI risk, 203–204
    overall mortality, 78–80
    relapse, 23–24, 595–598
    respiratory symptoms, 303
    self-efficacy, 541
    smoking continuum, 606–607
    withdrawal symptoms, 529–530
Abstinence
    long-term, 595–598
    performance, 525–526
Age at cessation, lung cancer, 125–126

Age factors
    abstinence duration, 606–608
    airway responsiveness, 338–340
    cerebrovascular disease, 251
    CHD mortality, 215–216, 223
    FEV_1 decline, 329–333
    menopause, 396–400
    overall mortality, 80
    quit ratio, 593–594
    respiratory symptoms, 286, 288–296
    smoking and cessation during pregnancy, 390–393
    smoking continuum, 599–608
Airway histopathology, former smokers, 108–109
Airway responsiveness
    age factors, 338–340
    clinical studies, 340–341
    cross-sectional studies, 338–339
    longitudinal studies, 339–340
    mechanisms, 338
    smoking and cessation, 337–341
Airways obstruction, see FEV_1
Alcohol consumption
    cessation, 524–525
    esophageal cancer, 152–155
    former smokers, 556–559
    hepatocellular cancer, 176
    laryngeal cancer, 132

619

oral cancer, 151–152
pancreatic cancer, 155–159
American Cancer Society Cancer Prevention Study-I, 26, 48–49, 75–78, 110, 124, 128, 250, 308, 432, 595–596
American Cancer Society Cancer Prevention Study-II, 48, 78–79, 110, 124, 129, 132, 159, 172, 215, 241, 245, 250, 252, 258, 308, 345
Anal cancer, 172–176
Analytic issues of consequence assessment, 55–57
Anxiety, 533–541
Aortic aneurysm, 241
Arrhythmias, 195
Arteriosclerosis obliterans, 244
Assessing smoking cessation, see Chapter 2
Asthma (see also Airway responsiveness)
  nosology, 279–280
  respiratory symptoms, 286
Atherosclerosis
  CHD development, 191–193
  severity, 199–200
Attributable risk, pregnancy outcome, 393–395

B

Behavioral consequences of cessation, see Chapter 11
Behavioral measures, 25–31
Bias, 46, 48, 52–55
Biochemical markers, 33–37
Birthweight
  cessation after conception, 383–387
  cessation before conception, 382–383
  continued smoking, 381–382
  low, attributable risk, 393–395
  smoking and cessation, 379–387
Bladder cancer, 159–165
Blood oxygen delivery, CHD development, 195–196
Body fat distribution, 495
Body weight, see Chapter 10
Bogus pipeline, 37
Bone loss, see Osteoporosis
Bone mineral content, 444–449
Breast cancer, 169
Breathlessness, see Respiratory symptoms
British Physicians Study, 79, 110, 128, 205, 308, 341
Bronchitis (see also Respiratory infections)
  mortality, 342–345
  nosology, 279

C

Caffeine use, cessation, 524–525
Cancers, nonrespiratory, see Chapter 5; see also specific sites
Cancers, respiratory, see Chapter 4; see also specific sites
Carbon monoxide, 34–35
Cardiovascular disease risk, estimated cessation effects, 197
Cardiovascular diseases, see Chapter 6
Carotid artery plaques, 246
Case–control study design, 49–50
Cerebral blood flow, 246, 251
Cerebrovascular disease
  abstinence duration, 252–258

age factors, 251
case–control studies, 246–249
cross-sectional studies, 246
development, 196
intervention studies, 251
oral contraceptives, 258–260
prospective cohort studies, 249–250
smoking and cessation, 245–260
smoking history, 251–252
summary of observational studies, 251
Cervical cancer, 165–169
Cessation
consequences assessment, 46–57
process and behavior assessment, 22–46
rate, see Quit ratio
stage model, 22–24
time trends, pregnancy, 393
timing, birthweight, 382–386
Chapter conclusions, 9–14
Chronic obstructive pulmonary disease
FEV_1 decline, 328–333
mortality, 341–348
nosology, 279–285
patients, 345–348
Cigar smoking
as cigarette replacement, 555–556
lung cancer, 124–125
trends, 593
Cigarette consumption
bladder cancer, 164
cerebrovascular disease, 251–252
FEV_1 decline, 329–333
laryngeal cancer, 132
lung cancer, 124
MI risk, 203
oral cancer, 151–152

overall mortality, 78–80, 86
pancreatic cancer, 155
pregnancy, 390–393
weight gain, 501–502
Cohort study design, 48–49
Conclusions
chapter, 9–14
volume, 8
Contextual issues, biochemical assessment, 37–46
Coping skills, 543–544
Coronary artery spasm, CHD development, 195
Coronary heart disease (CHD)
cross-sectional studies, 199–200
cessation, 197–240
development, 191–196
mortality, 205–224, 227–229
patients, 229–239
risk factors, 497–499
Cotinine, 36–37
Cough, see Respiratory symptoms
Craving, 523–524
Cross-sectional study design, 47–48

D

D-fenfluramine, weight control, 503–504
Demographic factors
pregnancy outcomes, attributable risk, 393–395
smoking and cessation during pregnancy, 390–393
Depression, 533–541
Diabetics, CHD mortality, 221–222
Diet, 500–502
Dietary changes, 484–486
Dietary practices, 554–555

Diffusing capacity, former smokers, 327–328
Disease development, abstinence duration, 129
DNA adduct levels, 109–110
Duodenal ulcers (see also Peptic ulcers)
  healing, 432–433
  recurrence, 433–439
Duration of abstinence, see Abstinence duration
Dyspnea, see Respiratory symptoms

E

Ecologic study design, 47
Ectopic pregnancy, 375–376
Educational attainment
  abstinence duration, 606–608
  quit ratio, 595
  smoking continuum, 599–608
Emphysema
  mortality, 342–345
  nosology, 279
Endometrial cancer, 169–172
Energy expenditure, 487–490
Enhancement models, performance, 525–526
Esophageal cancer, 152–155
Estrogen metabolism
  osteoporotic fractures, 443–444
  premature menopause, 398
Ethnic factors
  abstinence duration, 606–608
  quit ratio, 593
  smoking and cessation during pregnancy, 391–393
  smoking continuum, 599–608
Ex-smokers, see Former smokers

F

Fertility
  female, 372, 374–375
  male, 404–409
Fetal growth, 373, 379–387; see also Birthweight
Fetal mortality, 376–379
Forced expiratory volume in 1 second (FEV_1)
  cross-sectional population studies, 308–316
  decline, 328–337, 345–347
  longitudinal population studies, 328–337
Fibrinogens, former smokers, 194
Food intake, 484–486
Former smokers
  absenteeism, 89
  anal cancer, 172–176
  atherosclerosis severity, 199–200
  bladder cancer, 164
  breast cancer, 169
  cerebrovascular disease, 246–260
  cervical cancer, 166–169
  dietary practices, 554–555
  diffusing capacity, 327–328
  early menopause risk, 398–400
  endometrial cancer, 169–172
  esophageal cancer, 152–155
  established COPD, 345–348
  fibrinogen levels, 194
  health practices, 546–561
  health screening, 561–564
  health status, 87–91
  hepatocellular cancer, 176
  HDL-C levels, 192–193
  kidney cancer, 172

leukemia, 176
lung cancer risk patterns, 110–122
medical care utilization, 87
MI survival, 200–224
oral cancer, 147–152
ovarian cancer, 172
overall mortality, 78–80
penile cancer, 172–176
physical activity, 551–554
population percentage, 585
pulmonary function, 308–337
respiratory symptoms, 285–305
stomach cancer, 176
Fractures, see Osteoporosis
Framingham Heart Study, 80, 218–221, 230–235, 250, 258, 453, 497–498
Frequency issues, self-reports, 27–28

G

Gastric secretion, smoking, 429–430
Gastric ulcers (see also Peptic ulcers)
  healing, 440
  recurrence, 440–441
Gastrointestinal physiology, smoking, 429–430
Gender factors
  abstinence duration, 606–608
  alcohol consumption, 556–559
  bladder cancer, 164
  diet, 485–486
  dietary practices, 554–555
  esophageal cancer, 152–155
  MI survival, 237
  oral cancer, 147
  overall mortality, 80
  pancreatic cancer, 155
  physical activity, 551–554
  pipe or cigar smoking, 555–556
  postcessation weight gain, 473–483
  quit ratio, 588–593
  respiratory symptoms, 288–296, 303–304
  smoking continuum, 599–608
Gestational duration, 379–387; see also Birthweight

H

Health practices, former smokers, 546–561
Health risk changes, 497–500
Health screening, former smokers, 561–564
Health status, 87–91
Hemorrhagic stroke, see Cerebrovascular disease
Hepatocellular cancer, 176
High-density lipoprotein cholesterol (HDL-C) levels, former smokers, 192–193
Hormones, male reproduction, 401

I

Immune system, respiratory infections, 305–308
Impotence, male, 402–404
Infertility
  female, 372, 374–375
  male, 405–409
Influenza, see Respiratory infections
Inhalation practices, lung cancer, 124
Intention to smoke, 588, 608–609
Intermittent claudication, 243–244
Interpersonal interactions, 545–546
Intervention trials, study design, 50–51
Interviews, 25–29

623

Ischemic stroke, see Cerebrovascular disease

K

Kidney cancer, 172

L

Laryngeal cancer, 131–132
Leukemia, 176
Locus of control, 542–543
Long-term psychological and behavioral consequences and correlates, 532–546
Lung cancer
    abstinence duration, 110–122, 122–126, 126–128
    age at cessation, 125–126
    airway histopathology, 108–109
    smoking and cessation, 107–131
    cigar smokers, 125
    cigarette consumption, 124
    DNA adduct levels, 109–110
    diagnosis, 129–131
    inhalation practices, 124
    multistage models, 126–128
    nonfilter cigarettes, 124–125
    pathophysiologic mechanisms of smoking, 107–110
    pipe smokers, 125
    smoking duration, 122–123
    smoking history, 122–126

M

Major conclusions, 8
Measures of cessation, 22–46
Measures of quitting behavior, 584–588
Medical care utilization, 87

Menopause, premature, 396–400
Metabolic rate, 487–490
Methodologic issues of consequence assessment, 51–57
Methodologies, cessation assessment, see Chapter 2
Misclassification of smoking status, 49, 51, 52–55
Mood, 533–541
Morbidity (see also Chapter 3; specific causes)
    peptic ulcers, 431–432
    respiratory, 285–308
Mortality (see also Chapter 3; specific causes)
    bronchitis, 342–345
    COPD, 341–345, 347–348
    cohort studies, 75–83
    emphysema, 342–345
    fetal, neonatal, and perinatal, 374, 376–379
    overall, intervention studies, 84–86
    peptic ulcers, 432
    weight, 491–495
Mouth cancer, see Oral cancer
Multiple health habits, 559–561
Multiple primary cancers, 176–177
Multiple Risk Factor Intervention Trial, 24, 28, 50–51, 53, 86, 227–228, 333–335, 495, 498, 560–561, 595
Multistage models, lung cancer, 126–128
Myocardial infarct (MI) risk
    case–control studies, 200–204
    cigarette consumption, 203
    cohort studies, 205–224
    healthy persons, 200–229

intervention trials, 224–229
MI patients, 229–239
recurrent, 230–239

N

National Health and Nutrition Examination Survey, 24, 30, 431, 453, 583–584
National Health Interview Survey, 25, 390–391, 547–564, 583–584
National trends in smoking cessation, see Appendix
Neonatal mortality, 379–381
Neoplasms, see Cancers; see also specific sites
Nicotine polacrilex gum
  weight control, 502–504
  withdrawal symptoms, 528, 539
Nicotine withdrawal, 521–532
Nonbehavioral measures, 31–46
Nonfilter cigarettes, lung cancer, 124–125

O

Obesity, 490–497
Obstructive airways diseases, see Chapter 7
Occupational factors, respiratory symptoms, 296–299
Oral cancer
  alcohol consumption, 151–152
  cigarette consumption, 151–152
  former smokers, 147–152
  gender factors, 147
  smoking and cessation, 147–152
Oral contraceptives, cerebrovascular disease, 258–260
Osteoporosis, 443–453

Osteoporotic fractures, 449–453
Ovarian cancer, 172
Overweight, adverse medical and psychosocial outcomes, 490–497

P

Pancreatic cancer, 155–159
Pathophysiologic mechanisms of smoking
  cardiovascular diseases, 191–197
  laryngeal cancer, 131
  lung cancer, 107–110
  male reproduction, 400–401
  pregnancy, 371–374
  premature menopause, 396–398
  osteoporosis, 443–444
  respiratory diseases, 279–285
  skin wrinkling, 453–456
Penile cancer, 172–176
Peptic ulcer disease, 429–442
Peptic ulcers
  morbidity, 431–432
  mortality, 432
Performance, abstinence, 525–526, 530
Perinatal mortality
  attributable risk, 393–395
  smoking and cessation, 376–379
Peripheral arterial occlusive disease, 241–244
Peripheral artery disease
  development, 196, 243
  prognosis, 243–244
Phenylpropanolamine, weight control, 503–504
Phlegm production, see Respiratory symptoms
Physical activity, 486, 551–554
Physician advice, 588, 609

625

Physiologic measures, 32
Pipe smoking
  as cigarette replacement, 555–556
  lung cancer, 124–125
  trends, 593
Pneumonia, see Respiratory infections
Preeclampsia, 387
Pregnancy
  complications, 387
  outcome, 371–395
  prevalence of smoking and cessation, 390–393
  time trends in smoking and cessation, 393
  weight gain, 373
Prematurity, 386–387
Preterm delivery, 386–387, 395
Prevalence of smoking, pregnancy, 390–393
Process of smoking behavior change, 22–24
Psychological effects of cessation, see Chapter 11
Pulmonary function
  former smokers, 308–337
  smoking cessation, 316–328

Q

Questionnaires, 25–29
Quit attempts, 606
Quit ratio
  age trends, 593–594
  definition, 585,
  educational trends, 595
  gender trends, 588–593
  racial trends, 593
Quitting behavior, measures, 584–588

R

Racial factors, see Ethnic factors
Recidivism, 595–598; see also Relapse
Reduction of smoking, pregnancy, 387–389
Relapse, 23–24, 530–531, 595–598
Report
  conclusions, 8
  development, 8–9
  overview, 5–7
Reproduction
  female, 371–400
  male, 400–409
Reproduction, see Chapter 8
Respiratory cancers, see Chapter 4
Respiratory diseases, see Chapter 7
Respiratory function tests, see Spirometric parameters; Small airways function
Respiratory infections, 305–308
Respiratory morbidity, smoking cessation, 285–308
Respiratory symptoms
  abstinence duration, 303
  asthmatics, 286
  cessation clinics, 285–287
  cross-sectional population studies, 288–296
  longitudinal studies, 299–305
  occupational groups, 296–299
  reversal, possible mechanisms, 304
  smoking and cessation, 285–305
  smoking history, 299–303

S

Self-efficacy, 541–542
Self-management skills, 543–544